Autism: Importance of Neural Networks

Autism: Importance of Neural Networks

Edited by Jean Benet

AMERICAN
MEDICAL PUBLISHERS
www.americanmedicalpublishers.com

American Medical Publishers,
41 Flatbush Avenue,
1st Floor, New York,
NY 11217, USA

Visit us on the World Wide Web at:
www.americanmedicalpublishers.com

ISBN: 978-1-63927-284-6

Cataloging-in-Publication Data

Autism : importance of neural networks / edited by Jean Benet.
p. cm.
Includes bibliographical references and index.
ISBN 978-1-63927-284-6
1. Autism. 2. Neural networks (Neurobiology). 3. Autism spectrum disorders.
4. Hyperlexia. I. Benet, Jean.
RC553.A88 A98 2022
616.858 82--dc23

Table of Contents

Preface

The world is advancing at a fast pace like never before. Therefore, the need is to keep up with the latest developments. This book was an idea that came to fruition when the specialists in the area realized the need to coordinate together and document essential themes in the subject. That's when I was requested to be the editor. Editing this book has been an honour as it brings together diverse authors researching on different streams of the field. The book collates essential materials contributed by veterans in the area which can be utilized by students and researchers alike.

Autism spectrum disorders (ASD) are developmental disorders which originate in childhood. They are characterized by difficulties with social interaction and communication, and restricted and repetitive behavior. Autism is linked to a combination of genetic and environmental factors. A neural network is a circuit of neurons, interconnected by synapses to carry out a specific function when activated. It is presumed that there is a common cause at the neural level for the symptoms of autism, apart from genetic and cognitive reasons. Timely behavioral interventions or speech therapy can aid autistic children in gaining social and communication skills. This book unravels the recent studies on this subject. It includes contributions of experts and scientists which will provide innovative insights into this field. The topics covered in this book deal with the relationship between neural networks and autism.

Each chapter is a sole-standing publication that reflects each author´s interpretation. Thus, the book displays a multi-facetted picture of our current understanding of application, resources and aspects of the field. I would like to thank the contributors of this book and my family for their endless support.

Editor

1

Multisite functional connectivity MRI classification of autism: ABIDE results

Jared A. Nielsen[1,2], Brandon A. Zielinski[3], P. Thomas Fletcher[4], Andrew L. Alexander[5,6], Nicholas Lange[7,8], Erin D. Bigler[9,10], Janet E. Lainhart[5] and Jeffrey S. Anderson[1,10,11,12]*

[1] *Interdepartmental Program in Neuroscience, University of Utah, Salt Lake City, UT, USA*
[2] *Department of Psychiatry, University of Utah, Salt Lake City, UT, USA*
[3] *Departments of Pediatrics and Neurology, University of Utah and Primary Children's Medical Center, Salt Lake City, UT, USA*
[4] *School of Computing and Scientific Computing and Imaging Institute, University of Utah, Salt Lake City, UT, USA*
[5] *Waisman Laboratory for Brain Imaging and Behavior, Department of Psychiatry, University of Wisconsin, Madison, WI, USA*
[6] *Department of Medical Physics, University of Wisconsin, Madison, WI, USA*
[7] *Departments of Psychiatry and Biostatistics, Harvard University, Boston, MA, USA*
[8] *Neurostatistics Laboratory, McLean Hospital, Belmont, MA, USA*
[9] *Department of Psychology and Neuroscience Center, Brigham Young University, Provo, UT, USA*
[10] *The Brain Institute of Utah, University of Utah, Salt Lake City, UT, USA*
[11] *Department of Bioengineering, University of Utah, Salt Lake City, UT, USA*
[12] *Division of Neuroradiology, University of Utah, Salt Lake City, UT, USA*

Edited by:
Rajesh K. Kana, University of Alabama at Birmingham, USA

Reviewed by:
Ralph-Axel Müller, San Diego State University, USA
Gopikrishna Deshpande, Auburn University, USA

****Correspondence:***
Jeffrey S. Anderson, Interdepartmental Program in Neuroscience, University of Utah, 201 Presidents Cir, Salt Lake City, UT 84112, USA
e-mail: andersonjeffs@gmail.com

Background: Systematic differences in functional connectivity MRI metrics have been consistently observed in autism, with predominantly decreased cortico-cortical connectivity. Previous attempts at single subject classification in high-functioning autism using whole brain point-to-point functional connectivity have yielded about 80% accurate classification of autism vs. control subjects across a wide age range. We attempted to replicate the method and results using the Autism Brain Imaging Data Exchange (ABIDE) including resting state fMRI data obtained from 964 subjects and 16 separate international sites.

Methods: For each of 964 subjects, we obtained pairwise functional connectivity measurements from a lattice of 7266 regions of interest covering the gray matter (26.4 million "connections") after preprocessing that included motion and slice timing correction, coregistration to an anatomic image, normalization to standard space, and voxelwise removal by regression of motion parameters, soft tissue, CSF, and white matter signals. Connections were grouped into multiple bins, and a leave-one-out classifier was evaluated on connections comprising each set of bins. Age, age-squared, gender, handedness, and site were included as covariates for the classifier.

Results: Classification accuracy significantly outperformed chance but was much lower for multisite prediction than for previous single site results. As high as 60% accuracy was obtained for whole brain classification, with the best accuracy from connections involving regions of the default mode network, parahippocampaland fusiform gyri, insula, Wernicke Area, and intraparietal sulcus. The classifier score was related to symptom severity, social function, daily living skills, and verbal IQ. Classification accuracy was significantly higher for sites with longer BOLD imaging times.

Conclusions: Multisite functional connectivity classification of autism outperformed chance using a simple leave-one-out classifier, but exhibited poorer accuracy than for single site results. Attempts to use multisite classifiers will likely require improved classification algorithms, longer BOLD imaging times, and standardized acquisition parameters for possible future clinical utility.

Keywords: functional connectivity, fcMRI, classification, autism, ABIDE

INTRODUCTION

Brain imagingclassification strategies of autism have used information from structural MRI (Ecker et al., 2010a,b; Jiao et al., 2010; Uddin et al., 2011; Calderoni et al., 2012; Sato et al., 2013), functional MRI (Anderson et al., 2011d; Coutanche et al., 2011; Wang et al., 2012), diffusion tensor MRI (Lange et al., 2010; Ingalhalikar et al., 2011), positron emission tomography (Duchesnay et al., 2011), and magnetoencephalography (Roberts et al., 2010, 2011; Tsiaras et al., 2011; Khan et al., 2013). Such approaches have been undertaken for several clinical objectives. Sensitive and specific biomarkers for autism may contribute potentially useful biological information to diagnosis, prognosis, and treatment decision-making. It is hoped that imaging biomarkers may also help delineate subtypes of individuals with autism that may have common brain neuropathology and respond to similar treatment strategies, although different methodology will likely be required for subgrouping individuals than for classifying individuals by diagnosis. Such quantitative biomarkers may also serve as a metric for biological efficacy of potential behavioral or pharmacologic interventions. Finally, imaging biomarkers may help identify pathophysiologic mechanisms of autism in the brain that can guide investigations into the specific neural circuits, developmental windows, and genetic or environmental factors that may result in improved treatments.

Abnormal functional connectivity MRI (fcMRI) has been among the most replicated imaging metrics in autism. The proposed basis for fcMRI is that connected brain regions are likely to exhibit synchronized neural activity, which can be detected as covariance of slow fluctuations in Blood Oxygen Level Dependent (BOLD) signal between the regions. Initial reports of decreased functional connectivity in autism by three independent groups (Just et al., 2004; Villalobos et al., 2005; Welchew et al., 2005) have been followed by more than 50 primary reports of abnormal functional connectivity in autism in the literature, derived from fMRI data both in a resting state and acquired during cognitive tasks (Anderson, 2013).

Most reports show decreases in connectivity between distant brain regions, including nodes of the brain's default mode network (Cherkassky et al., 2006; Kennedy and Courchesne, 2008; Wiggins et al., 2011), social brain regions (Gotts et al., 2012; von dem Hagen et al., 2013), attentional regions (Koshino et al., 2005), language regions (Dinstein et al., 2011), interhemispheric homologues (Anderson et al., 2011a), and throughout the brain (Anderson et al., 2011d). Nevertheless, some reports have also shown abnormal increases in functional connectivity in autism (Muller et al., 2011) or unchanged connectivity (Tyszka et al., 2013). In particular, higher correlation between brain regions has been observed in negatively correlated connections (Anderson et al., 2011d), corticostriatal connections (Di Martino et al., 2011),visual search regions (Keehn et al., 2013), and brain network-level metrics (Anderson et al., 2013a; Lynch et al., 2013).

Despite the large and growing body of reports of abnormal functional connectivity in autism, uncertainty remains about the spatial distribution of decreased and increased connectivity and how this relates to the clinical heterogeneity of autism spectrum disorders (ASD). One of the challenges for answering these questions has been fractionation of the available data into individual site-specific studies with relatively small sample sizes. There is a need for analysis of multisite datasets that can improve statistical power, represent greater variance of disease and control samples, and allow replication across multiple sites with differential subject recruitment, imaging parameters, and analysis methods. Ultimately, clinically useful biomarkers will need to be replicated in diverse acquisition conditions that reflect community and academic imaging practices.

The advent of cooperative, publicly available datasets for resting state functional MRI is an important step forward. Multiple such datasets have now been released including the 1000 functional connectome project (Biswal et al., 2010), the ADHD 200 Consortium dataset (ADHD-200_Consortium, 2012), and most recently the Autism Brain Imaging Data Exchange (ABIDE) (Di Martino et al., 2013), consisting of images from 539 individuals with ASD and 573 typical control individuals, acquired at 16 international sites. In the present study, we evaluate classification accuracy of whole-brain functional connectivity across sites, and determine which abnormalities in connectivity across the brain are most informative for predicting autism from typical development, which imaging acquisition features lead to greatest accuracy, whether functional connectivity abnormalities covary with metrics of disease severity, and the extent to which abnormal functional connectivity is replicated across sites.

MATERIALS AND METHODS

SUBJECT SAMPLE

ABIDE consists of 1112 datasets comprised of 539 autism and 573 typically developing individuals (Di Martino et al., 2013). Each dataset consists of one or more resting fMRI acquisitions and a volumetric MPRAGE image. All data are fully anonymized in accordance with HIPAA guidelines, with analyses performed in accordance with pre-approved procedures by the University of Utah Institutional Review Board. All images were obtained with informed consent according to procedures established by human subjects research boards at each participating institution. Details of acquisition, informed consent, and site-specific protocols are available at http://fcon_1000.projects.nitrc.org/indi/abide/.

Inclusion criteria for subjects were successful preprocessing with manual visual inspection of normalization to MNI space of MPRAGE, coregistration of BOLD and MPRAGE images, segmentation of MPRAGE image, and full brain coverage from MNI $z > -35$ to $z < 70$ on all BOLD images. Inclusion criteria for sites were a total of at least 20 subjects meeting all other inclusion criteria. A total of 964 subjects met all inclusion criteria (517 typically developing subjects and 447 subjects with autism from 16 sites). Each site followed different criteria for diagnosing patients with autism or ascertaining typical development, however, the majority of the sites used the Autism Diagnostic Observation Schedule (Lord et al., 2000) and Autism Diagnostic Interview-Revised (Lord et al., 1994). Specific diagnostic criteria for each site can be found at fcon_1000.projects.nitrc.org/indi/abide/index.html.

Subject demographics for individuals satisfying inclusion criteria are shown in **Table 1**. Six different testing batteries were used to calculate verbal IQ and performance IQ, respectively. In addition to the IQ measures, the following measures were included in correlations with the classifier score (see **Table 1** for summary of behavioral measures):the Social Responsiveness Scale (Constantino et al., 2003) is a measure of social function and the Vineland Adaptive Behavior Scales (Sparrow et al., 1984) is a measure of daily functioning. See the ABIDE website for more information on the specific behavioral measures used. For handedness, categorical handedness (i.e., right-handed, left-handed, or ambidextrous) was used in the leave-one-out classifier (see details below). In the case that only a quantitative handedness measure was reported, positive values were converted to right-handed, negative values to left-handed, and a value of zero to ambidextrous. Fifteen subjects lacked a categorical

Table 1 | Subjects included from the ABIDE sample with demographic information.

	Age	ADI-R social	ADI-R verbal	ADOS total	Verbal IQ	Performance IQ	SRS total	Vineland
Number of subjects	964	348	349	348	781	796	335	201
Control	(426 M, 91 F)	0	0	32	413	425	160	80
Autism	(396 M, 51 F)	348	349	316	367	371	175	121
Control mean $\pm SD$	16.9 ± 7.56	NA	NA	1.25 ± 1.37	112 ± 13.3	108 ± 13.3	21.2 ± 16.2	105 ± 11.6
(Control range)	(6.47–56.2)	NA	NA	(0–4)	(67–147)	(67–155)	(0–103)	(77–131)
Autism mean $\pm SD$	16.6 ± 8.1	19.7 ± 5.65	15.9 ± 4.55	11.9 ± 3.81	105 ± 17.4	106 ± 17.2	91.6 ± 30.6	75 ± 13.2
(Autism range)	(7–64)	(2–30)	(2–26)	(2–22)	(50–149)	(59–157)	(6–164)	(41–106)

and quantitative measure of handedness. In those cases, a nearest neighbor classification function (ClassificationKNN.m in MATLAB) was used to assign categorical handedness. For the classifier, 862 subjects were right-handed, 95 were left-handed, and 7 were ambidextrous.

BOLD PREPROCESSING

Preprocessing was performed in MATLAB (Mathworks, Natick, MA) using SPM8 (Wellcome Trust, London) software. The following sequence of preprocessing steps was performed:

(1) Slice timing correction.
(2) Realign and reslice correction of motion for each volume relative to initial volume.
(3) Coregistration of BOLD images to MPRAGE anatomic sequence.
(4) Normalization of MPRAGE to MNI template brain, with normalization transformation also applied to coregistered BOLD images.
(5) Segmentation of gray matter, white matter, and CSF components of MPRAGE image (thorough clean).
(6) Voxelwisebandpass filter (0.001–0.1 Hz) and linear detrend
   (a) The lower limit of 0.001 Hz was chosen in order to be certain as much neural information was included as possible (Anderson et al., 2013b). The linear detrend removed much of the contribution of low frequencies given the relatively short time series available in the dataset.
(7) Extraction of mean time courses from the restriction masks applied to BOLD images from ROIs consisting of:
   (a) CSF segmented mask with bounding box $-35 < x < 35, -60 < y < 30, 0 < z < 30$.
   (b) White matter segmented mask overlapping with 10 mm radii spheres centered at $x = -27$, $y = -7$, $z = 30$, $x = 27, y = -7, z = 30$.
   (c) Mask of scalp and facial soft tissues (Anderson et al., 2011b).
(8) Voxelwise regression using glmfit.m (MATLAB Statistics Toolbox) software of CSF, WM, Soft tissue, and 6 motion parameters from realignment step from time series of each voxel of BOLD images.
(9) Motion scrubbing (Power et al., 2012) of framewise displacement and DVARS with removal of volumes before and after a root-mean-square displacement of >0.2 mm for either parameter and concatenation of remaining volumes. In 86.2% of the participants more than 50% of the volumes remained after motion scrubbing. Among the remaining participants with fewer than 50% retained volumes, the majority belonged to the autism group (8.8%, compared to 5.0% from the typically developing group; $p = 0.02$). The groups differed in the number of retained volumes when considering the entire sample of 964 subjects ($t = 4.11$, $p < 0.001$) and when considering only those with greater than 50% of the volumes remaining ($t = 2.04, p = 0.04$).
(10) No spatial smoothing was performed. The global mean signal and gray matter time courses were not regressed from voxelwise data (Saad et al., 2012, 2013; Jo et al., 2013).

ROI ANALYSIS

From preprocessed BOLD images for each subject, mean time course was extracted from 7266 gray matter ROIs. These ROIs from a lattice covering the gray.nii image (SPM8) from $z = -35$ to $z = 70$ at 5-mm resolution, with MNI coordinates of centroids previously reported (Anderson et al., 2011d). The ROIs averaged 4.9 ± 1.3 standard deviation voxels in size for 3 mm isotropic voxels. A 7266×7266 matrix of Fisher-transformed Pearson correlation coefficients was obtained for each subject from the ROI timecourses representing an association matrix of functional connectivity in each subject between all pairs of ROIs. Each pair of ROIs is termed a "connection" for the present analysis.

LEAVE-ONE-OUT CLASSIFIER

The classification approach is summarized in **Figure 1**. Overall, a leave-one-out classifier was used to generate a classification score for each of the 964 subjects, leaving out one subject at a time and calculating the classification score for the left out subject. The classification approach followed the approach reported previously, with slight modifications (Anderson et al., 2011d). First, the correlation measurements for the remaining 963 subjects were extracted for one of the 26.4 million connections from the 7266 × 7266 association matrix described above (**Figure 1**, Step 1). Second, a general linear model was fit to the measurements separately for autism (red fit line in **Figure 1**, Step 2) and control subjects (black fit line in **Figure 1**, Step 2) for the given connection with covariates of subject age, age-squared, gender, and handedness. From these data, estimated values for the left out subject for this connection were calculated based on the left out subject's age, gender, and handedness. A value was estimated separately from the remaining autism subjects (blue X in **Figure 1**, Step 2) and remaining control subjects (green X in **Figure 1**, Step 2).

Because each site used slightly different scanning hardware and parameters that may systematically bias results, the estimated values of the left out subject (blue and green X in **Figure 1**, Step 2) were adjusted by adding the difference of the site's mean value for that connection (minus the left out subject) from the mean value for that connection from all other sites. Finally, the actual value for the left out subject for the connection (green dot in **Figure 1**, Step 2) was subtracted from the estimated value obtained from autism subjects (blue vertical line on **Figure 1**, Step 2) and from the estimated value obtained from control subjects (green vertical line in **Figure 1**, Step 2). The difference of the absolute value of these two differences was then multiplied by the F-statistic for the difference between the remaining autism and control subjects. This process was iteratively carried out for all 26.4 million connections and then averaged across the 7265 connections in which each of 7266 ROIs participates. Then the averaged values for each of the 7266 ROIs were summed. The summed value was equal to the classification score for the subject. More negative values for the classification score predict the left out subject was a control subject, and more positive values for classification score predict the left-out subject was an autism subject.

BINS OF "CONNECTIONS"

Connections were grouped into bins in several different ways to aggregate groups of connections to test for accuracy in discriminating autism from control subjects. First, a measurement of correlation strength was obtained for each connection from 961 independent subjects from the 1000 Functional Connectome project using identical preprocessing steps (see y-axis of **Figure 6**). Subjects included in this sample have been previously described (Ferguson and Anderson, 2011). Second, Euclidean distance between each pair of ROIs was calculated from the centroid coordinates for the ROIs (see x-axis of **Figure 6**). Connections were grouped into 2-dimensional bins based on the strength of the correlation and the distance between the ROIs, with bin spacing of 0.05 units of Fisher-transformed correlation and 5-mm

Step 1: Create functional connectivity association matrices for 964 subjects and leave out a single subject.

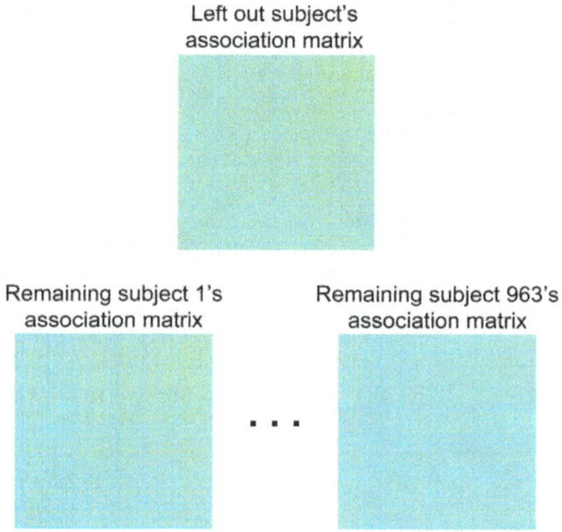

Step 2: General linear model was fit for autism and control groups separately. Differences between the left out subject's value and the autism and control group estimated values were calculated.

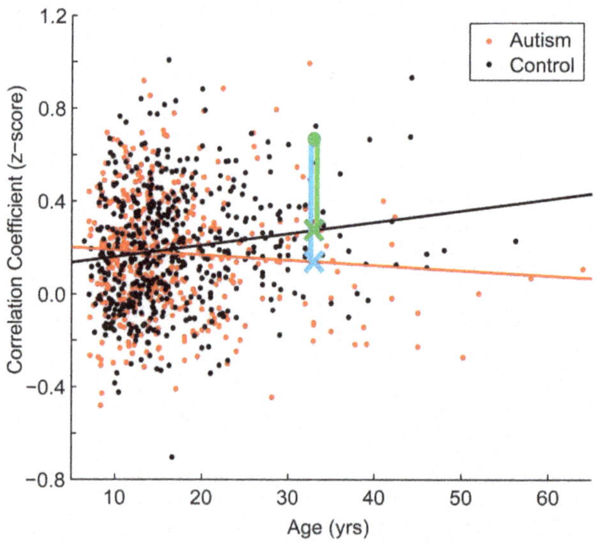

Step 3: The difference (i,.e., | Left Out - Autism | - | Left Out - Control |) was added to the running total for the subject for each binning scheme including the connection.

Step 4: Repeat steps 1-3 for all 26.4 million connections one at a time and for all 964 subjects, leaving one subject out at a time, until classifier score is totaled for each subject.

FIGURE 1 | Summary of classification approach. Step 1, Association matrices corresponding to the intrinsic connectivity between each pair of 7266 gray matter regions (about 26.4 million connections) are estimated

(Continued)

FIGURE 1 | Continued
for the left out subject and the 963 remaining subjects. Step 2, Plot depicting an example connection (i.e., single cell of the possible 26.4 million cells from the association matrices in Step 1) for the 964 subjects. The plot includes axes for correlation strength and age, however, the plot represents a multidimensional space that includes age-squared, gender, and handedness as covariates. *Black line*, fit line for the control group; *red line*, fit line for the autism group; *green data point*, left out subject (a control subject in this example); *green X*, estimated value for the control group; *blue X*, estimated value for autism group; *green vertical line*, difference between actual connection strength value for left out subject and estimated value for control group; *blue vertical line*, difference between actual connection strength value for left out subject and estimated value for autism group. Steps 3 and 4 are described in the text.

distance. The results for accurately classifying the subjects using this binning system are summarized in **Figure 6**.

A separate binning scheme was performed during the evaluation of a leave-one-out-classifier. For each left out subject, sets of connections were calculated that satisfied a two-tailed t-test between remaining autism and control subjects with p-values less than 0.01, 0.001, 0.0001, and 0.00001. These sets of connections varied slightly for each left out subject, since no data that can reflect the value of the left-out subject's connectivity measurement can be used in the classifier.

Classification accuracy, sensitivity, and specificity were calculated for the set of connections that differed between autism and control subjects at p-values of 0.01, 0.001, 0.0001, 0.00001 (**Figure 3A**). We used this last binning system because there is a tradeoff in using many connections in constructing the classifier scores and using fewer but more informative connections. We wanted to determine which thresholded bin yielded the highest accuracy.

STATISTICAL ANALYSES

For each bin of connections, a vector of 964 classification scores was obtained (one for each left out subject) and the classification score was thresholded at 0 (in the case of the strength/Euclidean distance bins, or at a threshold selected to optimize the area under a receiver operating characteristic curve for the case of the bins determined by p-values. Predicted diagnosis (autism vs. control) was compared to the actual diagnosis of each left out subject, and significant classification accuracy was determined by a binomial distribution. For 964 subjects, predicting 509 subjects (52.8%) correctly corresponded to an uncorrected p-value of less than 0.05, and predicting 531 subjects (55.1%) correctly corresponds to p-value of less than 0.001. Two-proportion z-tests were used to test the following: (1) whether there was a group difference in the proportion of subjects with less than 50% of the BOLD volumes remaining after motion scrubbing (results above in *BOLD preprocessing section*), (2) whether classification accuracy differed between the eyes open and eyes closed subjects, (3) whether classification accuracy differed between the male and female subjects, and (4) whether accuracy increased when considering only those subjects with greater than 50% of the BOLD volumes remaining after motion scrubbing, rather than all 964 subjects. Two-sample t-tests were used to determine if there was a group difference in the number of remaining volumes (results above in *BOLD preprocessing section*).

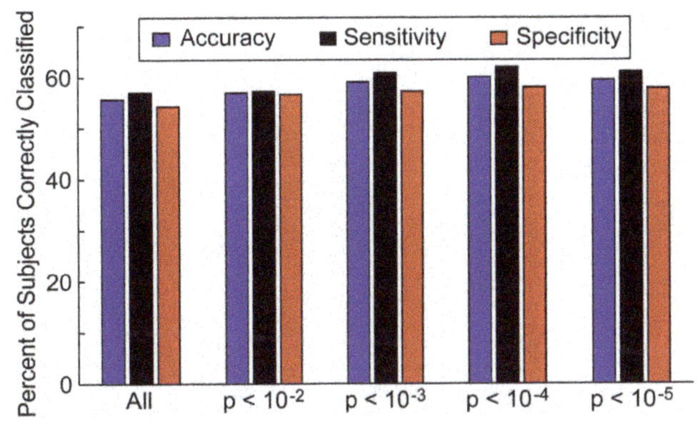

FIGURE 2 | Total accuracy, sensitivity, and specificity for leave-one-out classifier in 964 subjects. The total accuracy, sensitivity, and specificity are shown when all 26.4 million connections were included in the classifier and then for different p-value thresholds that determine which connections are included in the classifier.

RESULTS

First, we investigated the overall accuracy, sensitivity, and specificity of the leave-one-out classifier for all 964 subjects in the ABIDE consortium (**Figure 2**) and the 16 data collection sites individually (**Figure 3**). For the entire ABIDE consortium, we achieved the highest overall accuracy (60.0%), sensitivity (62.0%), and specificity (58.0%) when connections were included in the classification algorithm if group differences for the connection met a p-value threshold of less than 10^{-4}; whereas the lowest accuracy (55.7%), sensitivity (57.1%), and specificity (54.4%) were found when all 26.4 million connections were included in the leave-one out classifier. When considering only those subjects with greater than 50% of the BOLD volumes remaining after motion scrubbing, the accuracy for the five different p-value thresholds increased between 0.6% and 3.1%, although the difference was not significant compared to the accuracy for all 964 subjects ($p > 0.18$). No difference in classification accuracy was found between subjects who had their eyes open during the scan vs. those who had their eyes closed, after correcting for multiple comparisons using an FDR of $q < 0.05$. Also, no difference in classification accuracy was found between male and female subjects, after correcting for multiple comparisons using an FDR of $q < 0.05$.

We also compared the accuracy, sensitivity, and specificity across sites using different p-value thresholds for determining which connections to include in the leave-one-out classifier. The accuracy, sensitivity, and specificity varied at each site depending on the p-value threshold, however, we consistently achieved the highest accuracy at SBL (mean accuracy = 69.3%), USM (mean accuracy = 69.1%), Stanford (mean accuracy = 67.7%), and Pitt (mean accuracy = 65.4%); the highest sensitivity at SDSU (90.0%), Leuven (88.9%), SBL (84.0%), and Stanford (74.4%); and the highest specificity at USM (79.5%), Olin (75.0%), UCLA (71.5%), and KKI (70.6%).

Next, we determined whether the site's sample size or the number of imaging volumes from a single run related to the site's classification accuracy (**Figure 4**). The number of imaging volumes was positively correlated with accuracy ($r = 0.55$, $p = 0.03$).

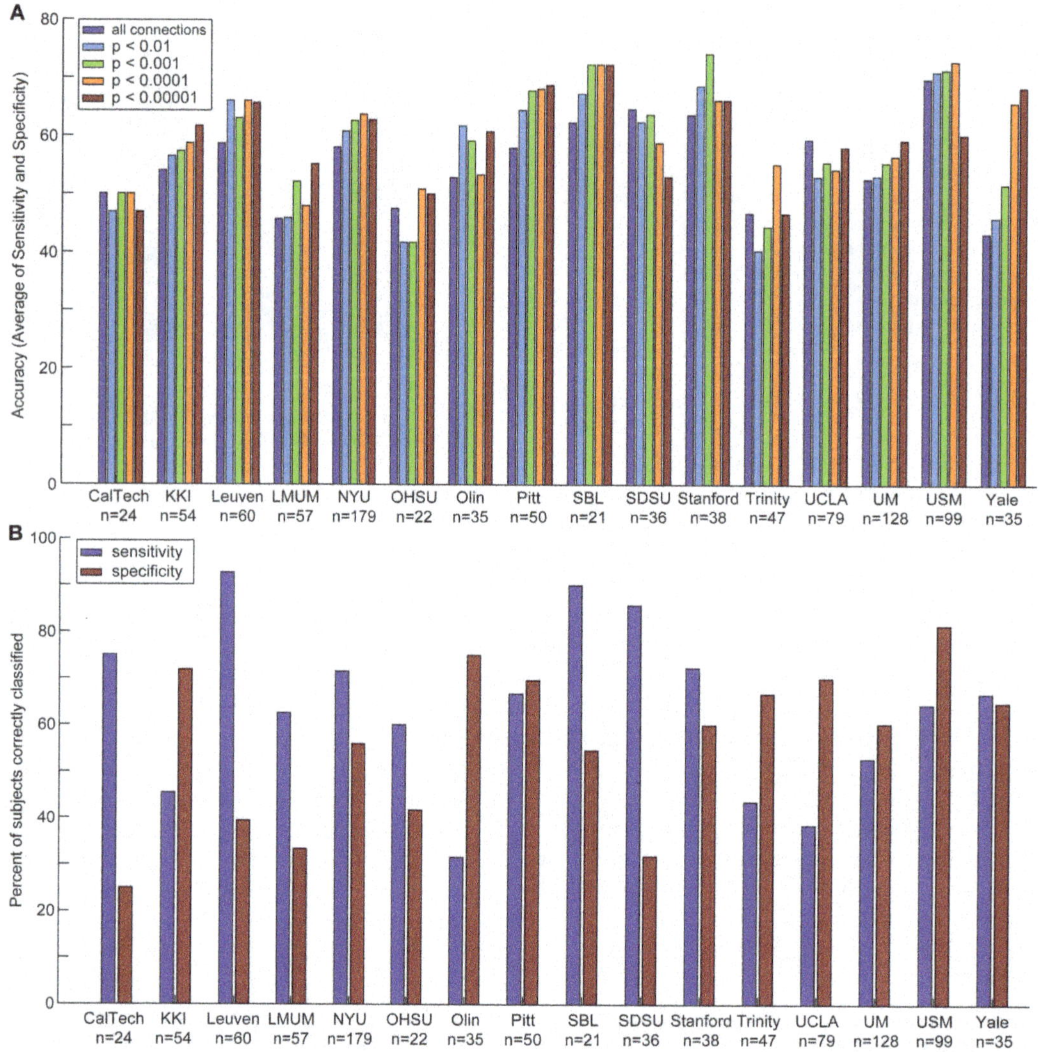

FIGURE 3 | Accuracy, sensitivity, and specificity for each data acquisition site. Accuracy **(A)** is shown for each data acquisition site at different *p*-value thresholds. The sensitivity and specificity **(B)** are shown for each data acquisition site at a threshold of $p < 0.0001$ (i.e., the threshold at which optimal total accuracy was obtained in **Figure 2**).

If the number of imaging volumes post-scrubbing was averaged across site, the relationship between number of imaging volumes and accuracy was no longer significant. Sample size did not correlate with site's classification accuracy ($r = 0.17$, $p = 0.53$).

We then determined which brain regions and connection characteristics accurately classified the ABIDE subjects. In **Figure 5**, the following brain regions (and the 7265 connections in which they were involved) resulted in the highest accuracy: parahippocampaland fusiform gyri, insula, medial prefrontal cortex, posterior cingulate cortex, Wernicke Area, and intraparietal sulcus. In **Figure 6**, two clusters of bins resulted in the highest accuracy. The first cluster included bins with short-range (10–25 mm) and medium-strength connections ($0.3 < z < 0.5$). The second cluster included bins with long-range (100–125 mm) and medium-strength connections ($0.15 < z < 0.4$).

Finally, we investigated the relationship between the subject's classifier score and behavioral measures (**Figure 7**). Estimates of symptom severity ($r = 0.13, p = 0.01$), as measured by the ADOS social + communication algorithm score, and SRS ($r = 0.17$, $p = 0.002$) positively correlated with the classifier score, however, symptom severity, as measured by the ADI-R verbal domain algorithm score ($r = -0.06$, $p = 0.30$) or social domain algorithm score ($r = -0.04$, $p = 0.51$), and performance IQ ($r = -0.03, p = 0.38$) did not correlate with the classifier score. Verbal IQ ($r = -0.07$, $p = 0.05$) and Vineland adaptive behavior composite score($r = 0.17$, $p = 0.002$) negatively correlate with the classifier score. In other words, as social function (lower SRS score is indicative of better social function), verbal IQ, and daily living skills increased and current level of symptom severity decreased, a subject was more likely to be classified as a control.

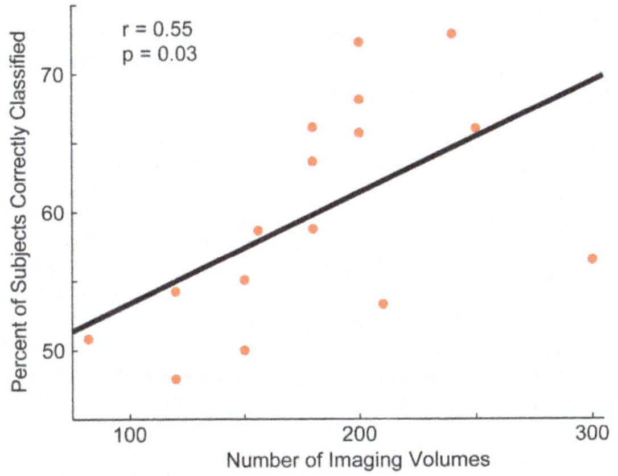

FIGURE 4 | Relationship between a site's total accuracy and the number of imaging volumes acquired by each site. Each site's total accuracy was calculated when using a $p < 0.0001$ threshold (i.e., the threshold at which optimal total accuracy was obtained in **Figure 2**) and correlated with the number of BOLD imaging volumes acquired during the resting-state sequence.

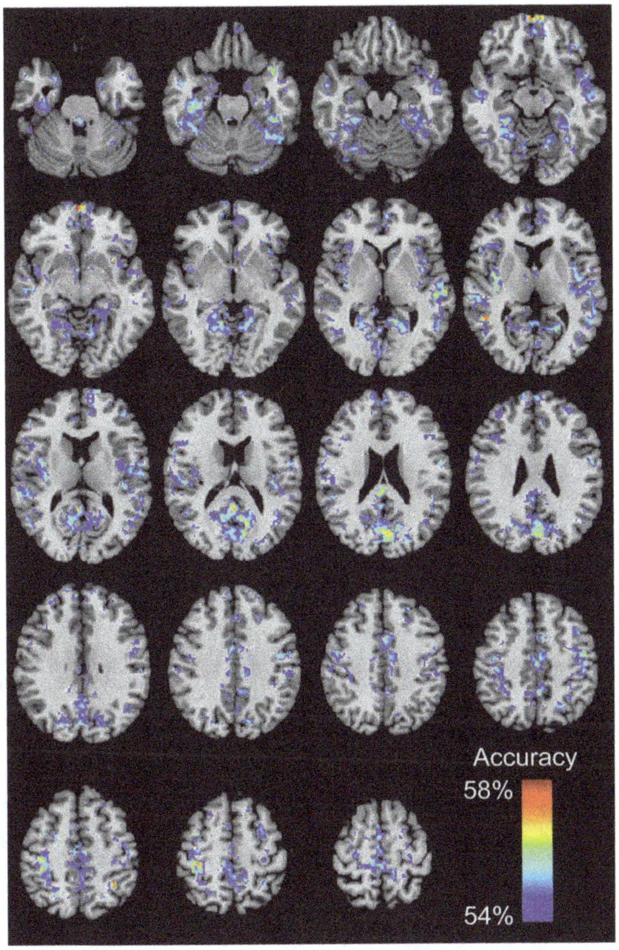

FIGURE 5 | Total accuracy for 7266 brain regions. Accuracy was determined for each of the 7266 brain regions independently by only taking into account the 7265 connections in which a given region was involved (no *p*-value threshold, all connections used). The minimum accuracy displayed for a single region is 53.95%, which was the false discovery rate corrected percentage for 7266 regions and a binomial cumulative distribution.

DISCUSSION

Functional connectivity MRI data from a set of 26.4 million "connections" per subject is able to successfully classify a subject as autistic or typically developing using a leave-one-out approach with an accuracy of 60.0% ($p < 2.2 \times 10^{-10}$), across a set of 964 subjects contributed from 16 different international sites. Overall specificity was 58.0% and overall sensitivity was 62.0%. Classification consisted of a weighted average of connections that used no information about the left out subject except for age, gender, site, and handedness. Using a weighted average of all 26.4 million connections resulted in a classification accuracy of 55.7% ($p = 0.00017$), with best accuracy (60.0%) achieved for a subset of connections that satisfied $p < 10^{-4}$ for a difference between autism and control among remaining subjects for each left-out subject. Classification scores significantly covaried with metrics of current disease severity including ADOS-G (as opposed to ADI-R, which incorporates disease severity at early ages), SRS, and verbal IQ metrics. Classification accuracy significantly improved in sites for which longer BOLD imaging times were used, but no relationship was found between number of subjects contributed by a site and classification accuracy.

Classification accuracy was lower in this multisite study despite its much larger sample size when compared with a prior study using similar methods from a single site (Anderson et al., 2011d). The prior study achieved ~80% accuracy, with 90% accuracy for subjects under 20 years of age in both a primary cohort and a replication sample of affected and unaffected individuals from multiplex families. Several reasons may explain this difference. Expanding a classifier to accommodate multisite data necessarily involves dealing with many additional sources of variance. The pulse sequence, magnetic field strength, scanner type, patient cohort and recruitment procedures, scan instructions (eyes open vs. closed vs. fixation), BOLD imaging length, age distribution, gender differences, and population ethnicity all varied across sites. Each of these variables has the potential to decrease sensitivity and specificity of functional connectivity measurements for autism. Nevertheless, a multisite cohort helps test generalizability of the results across different samples, making it more likely that connections identified as discriminatory between autism and control reflect disease properties rather than particulars of a single dataset.

Classification accuracy in the multisite cohort varied with the subset of connections used to construct the classifier. This finding reflected a tradeoff between improved accuracy when using more connections with decreased accuracy when including less specific connections in the classifier. This result argues against a homogenous regional distribution of connectivity abnormalities in autism in favor of a heterogeneous spatial distribution of connectivity disturbances that involves specific brain regions. Analysis of brain regions most affected in abnormal connections herein confirms the findings of previous reports:

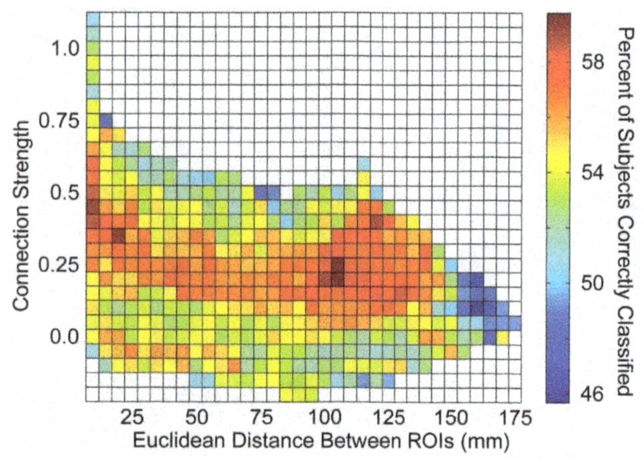

FIGURE 6 | Total accuracy across connection strength and distance between brain regions. The 26.4 million connections were divided up into bins based on the correlation strength of the connection (determined by an independent sample) and the distance between the connection's two endpoints. Accuracy is displayed for each bin with at least one connection.

areas of greatest abnormality included the insula, regions of the default mode network including posterior cingulate and medial prefrontal cortex, fusiform and parahippocampal gyri, Wernicke Area (posterior middle and superior temporal gyrus), and intraparietal sulcus (Anderson et al., 2011a,d; Gotts et al., 2012). All of these regions correspond to functional domains that are known to be impaired in autism, including attention, language, interoception, and memory. We note that some of these regions are in brain areas with relatively high susceptibility artifact and sensitivity to changes in brain shape (such as the medial prefrontal cortex). However, given the coherent distribution of the default mode network, we favor an interpretation of network-based differences attributable to autism rather than underlying structural or artifactual sources of these findings.

When interrogating subsets of connections from an independent dataset based on the Euclidean distance between ROIs and connection strength in a previous study, we found that the most informative connections consisted of typically strong connections between distant ROIs that were weaker in autism, and typically negatively correlated connections, that were less negative in autism (less anti-correlated) (Anderson et al., 2011d). In the current study, the connection bins based on strength and distance that showed greatest classification accuracy were not precisely the same connection bins found previously. Rather, they were adjacent to the bins in the previous study. This is the case because the classification algorithm in the current study takes advantage of larger numbers of connections. There was again a tradeoff between using more connections, given that individual connections exhibited relatively little information, and using sets of connections that differed more in autism. Thus, bins of medium strength connections ($0.3 < z < 0.5$) outperformed the more specific bins of stronger connections ($z > 0.5$) because the slightly weaker sets of connections included many more connections in the bin. This cautionary finding is relevant when attempting to identify the "optimal" set of connections for constructing candidate brain imaging biomarkers for ASD. Although specific affected regions appear to have autism connectivity abnormalities, classification schemes using only a small number of connections are likely to suffer from the high variance in metrics for individual connections.

This point is reinforced by a significant positive relationship between classification accuracy across sites and the length of BOLD imaging time per subject. Previous studies of test-retest reliability using functional connectivity MRI have shown that accuracy of results varies with one over the square root of BOLD imaging time (Van Dijk et al., 2010; Anderson et al., 2011c), with only moderate reproducibility when short BOLD imaging times such as 5 min are used (Shehzad et al., 2009; Van Dijk et al., 2010; Anderson et al., 2011c). This relationship would suggest that classifiers using information from many brain regions continue to show benefit from much longer imaging times, with continued improvements even after hours of imaging across multiple sessions per subject to the extent this is practical (Anderson et al., 2011c). Improvements in pulse sequence technology may also facilitate acquisition of greater numbers of volumes in shorter periods of time (Feinberg and Yacoub, 2012).The correlation between total imaging time and accuracy was more significant than the correlation between number of volumes used after scrubbing and accuracy. This might indicate that imaging time is more important than the number of volumes used. As multiband acquisition protocols become more prevalent (Setsompop et al., 2012), it will be important to determine the extent to which finer sampling vs. longer imaging time will contribute to specificity of BOLD fcMRI measurements.

In a prior study that examined the effect of BOLD imaging time on ability to identify functional connectivity values obtained from a single individual compared to a group mean, individual "connections" could only be reliably distinguished after 25 min of BOLD imaging time. The number of connections that could be reliably distinguished increased exponentially with imaging time for at least up to 10 h of total imaging time (Anderson et al., 2011c). Indeed, there is good theoretical basis that any desired accuracy can be obtained with sufficient imaging time, stretching into many hours. Although Van Dijk and colleagues report that the intrinsic connectivity measurements stabilize around 5 min of imaging time, they also state that noise continues to decrease at a rate of 1/sqrt(n), where n is the amount of imaging time (Van Dijk et al., 2010) (which is in accordance with our findings from (Anderson et al., 2011c). Moreover, they report that the stabilization is of composite network-level metrics rather than connections between small individual ROIs. In contrast, we have found that coarse network-level measurements are not particularly informative in classification compared to fine-grained metrics that take into account specific differences in the spatial distribution of connectivity. There may be no upper limit for continued improvements if more imaging time were obtained.

We found significant relationships between the classification score and some behavioral measures, such as social function and

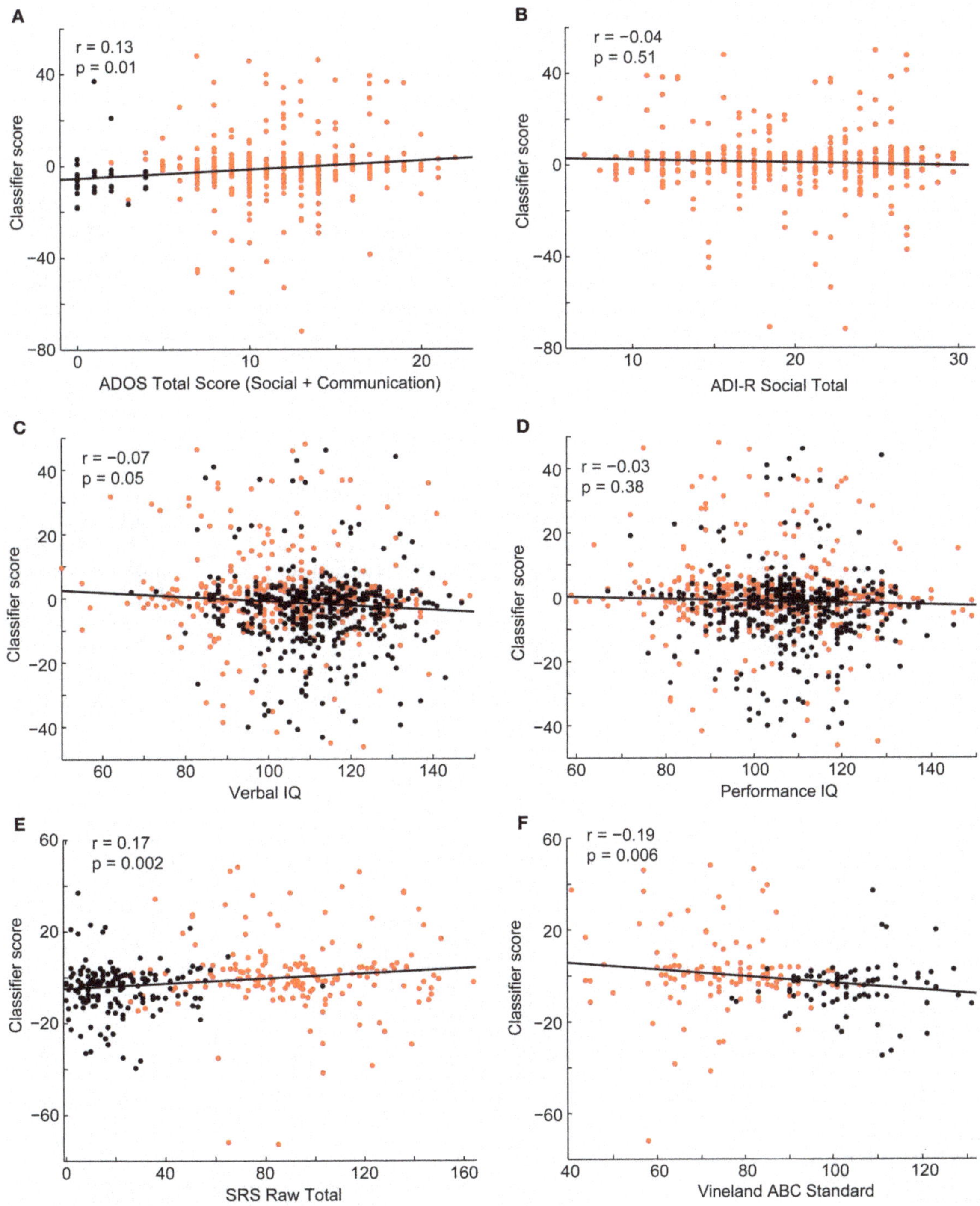

FIGURE 7 | Scatterplots depict the relationship between the classifier scores for control subjects (black) and subjects with autism (red) and the following behavioral measures: ADOS-G social + communication algorithm score (A), ADI-R social verbal algorithm score (B), verbal IQ (C), performance IQ (D), SRS total score (E), and Vineland Adaptive composite standard score (F). Correlation coefficients and corresponding *p*-values are included on the plots.

daily living skills, however, the proportion of variance in the behavioral measures that was explained by the linear relationship between the classification score and the behavioral measure was small (between 0.5 and 2.9%). This may be due to the overall poor accuracy of the classification approach. As accuracy and techniques for combining multisite data improves, we also expect an increase in the proportion of variance accounted for by the correlations.

Additional benefits may be achieved through improved classification algorithms that take advantage of machine learning techniques to allow more effective weighted combinations of connections. Similarly, multimodal classifiers remain a promising, relatively untapped method for characterizing diagnostic and prognostic information about autism. Given classification accuracies of single site datasets exceeding 80% for structural MRI (Ecker et al., 2010a,b; Jiao et al., 2010; Uddin et al., 2011; Calderoni et al., 2012; Sato et al., 2013), diffusion tensor MRI (Lange et al., 2010; Ingalhalikar et al., 2011), positron emission tomography (Duchesnay et al., 2011), and magnetoencephalography (Roberts et al., 2010, 2011; Tsiaras et al., 2011; Khan et al., 2013), it would be of great interest to determine whether different modalities identify similar cohorts of subjects correctly, and whether a combination neuroimaging approach that leverages these different features might be able to achieve even greater accuracy than any one alone.

Although multisite datasets such as those in ABIDE are invaluable for testing replicability of neuroimaging findings in autism, they contain inherent limitations that should be recognized. Large inhomogeneities in acquisition parameters, subject populations, and research protocols limit the sensitivity for detecting abnormalities. These inhomogeneities may overwhelm the ability of discriminating many findings, and may lead to overconfidence in a result as definitive because of the large sample of subjects used. There remains a need for replicating results in high-quality, carefully controlled individual datasets that may show increased sensitivity for some results compared to multisite data, as exhibited by classification accuracy in the present study. Preprocessing methods may also bias results in unpredictable ways, as has been suggested with head motion correction strategies (Power et al., 2012; Van Dijk et al., 2012) and regression procedures (Murphy et al., 2009; Anderson et al., 2011b; Saad et al., 2012). Datasets such as those in ABIDE will be of great value in testing multiple procedural manipulations in relatively large samples allowing determination of optimal processing methods for specific questions. Ultimately, it is unknown whether differences in resting state functional connectivity in autism arise from differential performance of the "resting" task or underlying differences in structural connectivity reflected in the measurements. Continuing comparison with structural metrics such as diffusion tensor imaging will help to clarify this point.

Nevertheless, it remains an attractive hypothesis that with longer imaging times, controlled acquisition strategies, integration of multimodal features, and improvement in classification methodology, neuroimaging may be able to contribute useful biological information to the clinical diagnosis and care of individuals with ASD and further elucidate pathophysiology and brain-based intermediate phenotypes.

ACKNOWLEDGMENTS

The analysis described was supported by NIH grant numbers K08MH092697 and R01MH084795, R01MH080826, the Flamm Family Foundation, the Morrell Family Foundation and by the Ben B. and Iris M. Margolis Foundation. The content is solely the responsibility of the authors and does not necessarily represent the official views of the National Institute of Mental Health or the National Institutes of Health. Funding sources for the datasets comprising the 1000 Functional Connectome Project are listed at fcon_1000.projects.nitrc.org/fcpClassic/FcpTable.html. Funding sources for the ABIDE dataset are listed at fcon_1000.projects.nitrcc.org/indi/abide.

REFERENCES

ADHD-200_Consortium. (2012). The ADHD-200 Consortium: a model to advance the translational potential of neuroimaging in clinical neuroscience. *Front. Syst. Neurosci.* 6:62. doi: 10.3389/fnsys.2012.00062

Anderson, J. S. (2013). "Cortical underconnectivity hypothesis in autism: evidence from functional connectivity MRI," in *Comprehensive Guide to Autism*, eds V. Patel, C. Martin, and V. Preedy (Berlin: Springer-Verlag) (in press). doi: 10.1007/SpringerReference_331190

Anderson, J. S., Druzgal, T. J., Froehlich, A., Dubray, M. B., Lange, N., Alexander, A. L., et al. (2011a). Decreased interhemispheric functional connectivity in autism. *Cereb. Cortex* 21, 1134–1146. doi: 10.1093/cercor/bhq190

Anderson, J. S., Druzgal, T. J., Lopez-Larson, M., Jeong, E. K., Desai, K., and Yurgelun-Todd, D. (2011b). Network anticorrelations, global regression, and phase-shifted soft tissue correction. *Hum. Brain Mapp.* 32, 919–934. doi: 10.1002/hbm.21079

Anderson, J. S., Ferguson, M. A., Lopez-Larson, M., and Yurgelun-Todd, D. (2011c). Reproducibility of functional connectivity measurements in single subjects. *AJNR Am. J. Neuroradiol.* 32, 548–555. doi: 10.3174/ajnr.A2330

Anderson, J. S., Nielsen, J. A., Froehlich, A. L., Dubray, M. B., Druzgal, T. J., Cariello, A. N., et al. (2011d). Functional connectivity magnetic resonance imaging classification of autism. *Brain* 134, 3742–3754. doi: 10.1093/brain/awr263

Anderson, J. S., Nielsen, J. A., Ferguson, M. A., Burback, M. C., Cox, E. T., Dai, L., et al. (2013a). Abnormal brain synchrony in Down Syndrome. *Neuroimage: Clinical* 2, 703–715. doi: 10.1016/j.nicl.2013.05.006

Anderson, J. S., Zielinski, B. A., Nielsen, J. A., and Ferguson, M. A. (2013b). Complexity of low-frequency blood oxygen level-dependent fluctuations covaries with local connectivity. *Hum. Brain Mapp.* doi: 10.1002/hbm.22251. [Epub ahead of print].

Biswal, B. B., Mennes, M., Zuo, X. N., Gohel, S., Kelly, C., Smith, S. M., et al. (2010). Toward discovery science of human brain function. *Proc. Natl. Acad. Sci. U.S.A.* 107, 4734–4739. doi: 10.1073/pnas.0911855107

Calderoni, S., Retico, A., Biagi, L., Tancredi, R., Muratori, F., and Tosetti, M. (2012). Female children with autism spectrum disorder: an insight from mass-univariate and pattern classification analyses. *Neuroimage* 59, 1013–1022. doi: 10.1016/j.neuroimage.2011.08.070

Cherkassky, V. L., Kana, R. K., Keller, T. A., and Just, M. A. (2006). Functional connectivity in a baseline resting-state network in autism. *Neuroreport* 17, 1687–1690. doi: 10.1097/01.wnr.0000239956.45448.4c

Constantino, J. N., Davis, S. A., Todd, R. D., Schindler, M. K., Gross, M. M., Brophy, S. L., et al. (2003). Validation of a brief quantitative measure of autistic traits: comparison of the social responsiveness scale with the autism diagnostic interview-revised. *J. Autism Dev. Disord.* 33, 427–433. doi: 10.1023/A:1025014929212

Coutanche, M. N., Thompson-Schill, S. L., and Schultz, R. T. (2011). Multi-voxel pattern analysis of fMRI data predicts clinical symptom severity. *Neuroimage* 57, 113–123. doi: 10.1016/j.neuroimage.2011.04.016

Di Martino, A., Kelly, C., Grzadzinski, R., Zuo, X. N., Mennes, M., Mairena, M. A., et al. (2011). Aberrant striatal functional connectivity in children with autism. *Biol. Psychiatry* 69, 847–856. doi: 10.1016/j.biopsych.2010.10.029

Di Martino, A., Yan, C. G., Li, Q., Denio, E., Castellanos, F. X., Alaerts, K., et al. (2013). The autism brain imaging data exchange: towards a large-scale evaluation of the intrinsic brain architecture in autism. *Mol. Psychiatry* doi: 10.1038/mp.2013.78. [Epub ahead of print].

Dinstein, I., Pierce, K., Eyler, L., Solso, S., Malach, R., Behrmann, M., et al. (2011). Disrupted neural synchronization in toddlers with autism. *Neuron* 70, 1218–1225. doi: 10.1016/j.neuron.2011.04.018

Duchesnay, E., Cachia, A., Boddaert, N., Chabane, N., Mangin, J. F., Martinot, J. L., et al. (2011).

Feature selection and classification of imbalanced datasets: application to PET images of children with autistic spectrum disorders. *Neuroimage* 57, 1003–1014. doi: 10.1016/j.neuroimage.2011.05.011

Ecker, C., Marquand, A., Mourao-Miranda, J., Johnston, P., Daly, E. M., Brammer, M. J., et al. (2010a). Describing the brain in autism in five dimensions—magnetic resonance imaging-assisted diagnosis of autism spectrum disorder using a multiparameter classification approach. *J. Neurosci.* 30, 10612–10623. doi: 10.1523/JNEUROSCI.5413-09.2010

Ecker, C., Rocha-Rego, V., Johnston, P., Mourao-Miranda, J., Marquand, A., Daly, E. M., et al. (2010b). Investigating the predictive value of whole-brain structural MR scans in autism: a pattern classification approach. *Neuroimage* 49, 44–56. doi: 10.1016/j.neuroimage.2009.08.024

Feinberg, D. A., and Yacoub, E. (2012). The rapid development of high speed, resolution and precision in fMRI. *Neuroimage* 62, 720–725. doi: 10.1016/j.neuroimage.2012.01.049

Ferguson, M. A., and Anderson, J. S. (2011). Dynamical stability of intrinsic connectivity networks. *Neuroimage* 59, 4022–4031. doi: 10.1016/j.neuroimage.2011.10.062

Gotts, S. J., Simmons, W. K., Milbury, L. A., Wallace, G. L., Cox, R. W., and Martin, A. (2012). Fractionation of social brain circuits in autism spectrum disorders. *Brain* 135, 2711–2725. doi: 10.1093/brain/aws160

Ingalhalikar, M., Parker, D., Bloy, L., Roberts, T. P., and Verma, R. (2011). Diffusion based abnormality markers of pathology: toward learned diagnostic prediction of ASD. *Neuroimage* 57, 918–927. doi: 10.1016/j.neuroimage.2011.05.023

Jiao, Y., Chen, R., Ke, X., Chu, K., Lu, Z., and Herskovits, E. H. (2010). Predictive models of autism spectrum disorder based on brain regional cortical thickness. *Neuroimage* 50, 589–599. doi: 10.1016/j.neuroimage.2009.12.047

Jo, H. J., Saad, Z. S., Gotts, S. J., Martin, A., and Cox, R. W. (2013). Correction: quantifying agreement between anatomical and functional interhemispheric correspondences in the resting brain. *PLoS ONE* 8:5. doi: 10.1371/annotation/cb15c6af-2153-49a9-8330- 45e40e6c296d

Just, M. A., Cherkassky, V. L., Keller, T. A., and Minshew, N. J. (2004). Cortical activation and synchronization during sentence comprehension in high-functioning autism: evidence of underconnectivity. *Brain* 127, 1811–1821. doi: 10.1093/brain/awh199

Keehn, B., Shih, P., Brenner, L. A., Townsend, J., and Muller, R. A. (2013). Functional connectivity for an "Island of sparing" in autism spectrum disorder: an fMRI study of visual search. *Hum. Brain Mapp.* 34, 2524–2537. doi: 10.1002/hbm.22084

Kennedy, D. P., and Courchesne, E. (2008). The intrinsic functional organization of the brain is altered in autism. *Neuroimage* 39, 1877–1885. doi: 10.1016/j.neuroimage.2007.10.052

Khan, S., Gramfort, A., Shetty, N. R., Kitzbichler, M. G., Ganesan, S., Moran, J. M., et al. (2013). Local and long-range functional connectivity is reduced in concert in autism spectrum disorders. *Proc. Natl. Acad. Sci. U.S.A.* 110, 3107–3112. doi: 10.1073/pnas.1214533110

Koshino, H., Carpenter, P. A., Minshew, N. J., Cherkassky, V. L., Keller, T. A., and Just, M. A. (2005). Functional connectivity in an fMRI working memory task in high-functioning autism. *Neuroimage* 24, 810–821. doi: 10.1016/j.neuroimage.2004.09.028

Lange, N., Dubray, M., Lee, J. E., Froimowitz, M., Froehlich, A., Adluru, N., et al. (2010). Atypical diffusion tensor hemispheric asymmetry: a potential DTI biomarker for autism. *Autism Res.* 3, 350–358. doi: 10.1002/aur.162

Lord, C., Risi, S., Lambrecht, L., Cook, E. H. Jr., Leventhal, B. L., Dilavore, P. C., et al. (2000). The autism diagnostic observation schedule-generic: a standard measure of social and communication deficits associated with the spectrum of autism. *J. Autism Dev. Disord.* 30, 205–223. doi: 10.1023/A:1005592401947

Lord, C., Rutter, M., and Le Couteur, A. (1994). Autism diagnostic interview-revised: a revised version of a diagnostic interview for caregivers of individuals with possible pervasive developmental disorders. *J. Autism Dev. Disord.* 24, 659–685. doi: 10.1007/BF02172145

Lynch, C. J., Uddin, L. Q., Supekar, K., Khouzam, A., Phillips, J., and Menon, V. (2013). Default mode network in childhood autism: posteromedial cortex heterogeneity and relationship with social deficits. *Biol. Psychiatry* 74, 212–219. doi: 10.1016/j.biopsych.2012.12.013

Muller, R. A., Shih, P., Keehn, B., Deyoe, J. R., Leyden, K. M., and Shukla, D. K. (2011). Underconnected, but how? A survey of functional connectivity MRI studies in autism spectrum disorders. *Cereb. Cortex* 21, 2233–2243. doi: 10.1093/cercor/bhq296

Murphy, K., Birn, R. M., Handwerker, D. A., Jones, T. B., and Bandettini, P. A. (2009). The impact of global signal regression on resting state correlations: are anti-correlated networks introduced? *Neuroimage* 44, 893–905. doi: 10.1016/j.neuroimage.2008.09.036

Power, J. D., Barnes, K. A., Snyder, A. Z., Schlaggar, B. L., and Petersen, S. E. (2012). Spurious but systematic correlations in functional connectivity MRI networks arise from subject motion. *Neuroimage* 59, 2142–2154. doi: 10.1016/j.neuroimage.2011.10.018

Roberts, T. P., Cannon, K. M., Tavabi, K., Blaskey, L., Khan, S. Y., Monroe, J. F., et al. (2011). Auditory magnetic mismatch field latency: a biomarker for language impairment in autism. *Biol. Psychiatry* 70, 263–269. doi: 10.1016/j.biopsych.2011.01.015

Roberts, T. P., Khan, S. Y., Rey, M., Monroe, J. F., Cannon, K., Blaskey, L., et al. (2010). MEG detection of delayed auditory evoked responses in autism spectrum disorders: towards an imaging biomarker for autism. *Autism Res.* 3, 8–18. doi: 10.1002/aur.111

Saad, Z., Reynolds, R. C., Jo, H. J., Gotts, S. J., Chen, G., Martin, A., et al. (2013). Correcting brain-wide correlation differences in resting-state FMRI. *Brain Connect.* 3, 339–352. doi: 10.1089/brain.2013.0156

Saad, Z. S., Gotts, S. J., Murphy, K., Chen, G., Jo, H. J., Martin, A., et al. (2012). Trouble at rest: how correlation patterns and group differences become distorted after global signal regression. *Brain Connect.* 2, 25–32. doi: 10.1089/brain.2012.0080

Sato, J. R., Hoexter, M. Q., Oliveira, P. P. Jr., Brammer, M. J., Murphy, D., and Ecker, C. (2013). Inter-regional cortical thickness correlations are associated with autistic symptoms: a machine-learning approach. *J. Psychiatr. Res.* 47, 453–459. doi: 10.1016/j.jpsychires.2012.11.017

Setsompop, K., Gagoski, B. A., Polimeni, J. R., Witzel, T., Wedeen, V. J., and Wald, L. L. (2012). Blipped-controlled aliasing in parallel imaging for simultaneous multislice echo planar imaging with reduced g-factor penalty. *Magn. Reson. Med.* 67, 1210–1224. doi: 10.1002/mrm.23097

Shehzad, Z., Kelly, A. M., Reiss, P. T., Gee, D. G., Gotimer, K., Uddin, L. Q., et al. (2009). The resting brain: unconstrained yet reliable. *Cereb. Cortex* 19, 2209–2229. doi: 10.1093/cercor/bhn256

Sparrow, S., Da, B., and Vc, D. (1984). *Vineland Adaptive Behavior Scales: Interview Edition, Survey form Manual.* Circle Pines, MN: A.G. Service.

Tsiaras, V., Simos, P. G., Rezaie, R., Sheth, B. R., Garyfallidis, E., Castillo, E. M., et al. (2011). Extracting biomarkers of autism from MEG resting-state functional connectivity networks. *Comput. Biol. Med.* 41, 1166–1177. doi: 10.1016/j.compbiomed.2011.04.004

Tyszka, J. M., Kennedy, D. P., Paul, L. K., and Adolphs, R. (2013). Largely typical patterns of resting-state functional connectivity in high-functioning adults with autism. *Cereb. Cortex* doi: 10.1093/cercor/bht040. [Epub ahead of print].

Uddin, L. Q., Menon, V., Young, C. B., Ryali, S., Chen, T., Khouzam, A., et al. (2011). Multivariate searchlight classification of structural magnetic resonance imaging in children and adolescents with autism. *Biol. Psychiatry* 70, 833–841. doi: 10.1016/j.biopsych.2011.07.014

Van Dijk, K. R., Hedden, T., Venkataraman, A., Evans, K. C., Lazar, S. W., and Buckner, R. L. (2010). Intrinsic functional connectivity as a tool for human connectomics: theory, properties, and optimization. *J. Neurophysiol.* 103, 297–321. doi: 10.1152/jn.00783.2009

Van Dijk, K. R., Sabuncu, M. R., and Buckner, R. L. (2012). The influence of head motion on intrinsic functional connectivity MRI. *Neuroimage* 59, 431–438. doi: 10.1016/j.neuroimage.2011.07.044

Villalobos, M. E., Mizuno, A., Dahl, B. C., Kemmotsu, N., and Muller, R. A. (2005). Reduced functional connectivity between V1 and inferior frontal cortex associated with visuomotor performance in autism. *Neuroimage* 25, 916–925. doi: 10.1016/j.neuroimage.2004.12.022

von dem Hagen, E. A., Stoyanova, R. S., Baron-Cohen, S., and Calder, A. J. (2013). Reduced functional connectivity within and between 'social' resting state networks in autism spectrum conditions. *Soc. Cogn. Affect. Neurosci.* 8, 694–701. doi: 10.1093/scan/nss053

Wang, H., Chen, C., and Fushing, H. (2012). Extracting multiscale pattern information of fMRI based functional brain connectivity with application on classification of autism spectrum disorders. *PLoS ONE* 7:e45502. doi: 10.1371/journal.pone.0045502

Welchew, D. E., Ashwin, C., Berkouk, K., Salvador, R., Suckling, J., Baron-Cohen, S., et al. (2005). Functional disconnectivity of the medial temporal lobe in Asperger's syndrome. *Biol. Psychiatry* 57, 991–998. doi: 10.1016/j.biopsych.2005.01.028

Wiggins, J. L., Peltier, S. J., Ashinoff, S., Weng, S. J., Carrasco, M., Welsh, R. C., et al. (2011). Using a self-organizing map algorithm to detect age-related changes in functional connectivity during rest in autism spectrum disorders. *Brain Res.* 1380, 187–197. doi: 10.1016/j.brainres.2010.10.102

2

Intrinsic functional network organization in high-functioning adolescents with autism spectrum disorder

Elizabeth Redcay[1]*, Joseph M. Moran[2,3], Penelope L. Mavros[4], Helen Tager-Flusberg[5], John D. E. Gabrieli[6,7] and Susan Whitfield-Gabrieli[6,7]

[1] Department of Psychology, University of Maryland, College Park, MD, USA
[2] Center for Brain Science, Harvard University, Cambridge, MA, USA
[3] United States Army Natick Soldier Research Development and Engineering Center, Natick, MA, USA
[4] Simons Center for the Social Brain at Massachusetts Institute of Technology, Cambridge, MA, USA
[5] Department of Psychology, Boston University, Boston, MA, USA
[6] McGovern Institute for Brain Research at Massachusetts Institute of Technology, Cambridge, MA, USA
[7] Department of Brain and Cognitive Sciences, Massachusetts Institute of Technology, Cambridge, MA, USA

Edited by:
Ralph-Axel Müller, San Diego State University, USA

Reviewed by:
Christian Sorg, Klinikum rechts der Isar Technische Universität München, Germany
Michal Assaf, Institute of Living, USA

****Correspondence:***
Elizabeth Redcay, Department of Psychology, University of Maryland, 1147 Biology-Psychology Building, College Park, MD 20742, USA
e-mail: redcay@umd.edu

Converging theories and data suggest that atypical patterns of functional and structural connectivity are a hallmark neurobiological feature of autism. However, empirical studies of functional connectivity, or, the correlation of MRI signal between brain regions, have largely been conducted during task performance and/or focused on group differences within one network [e.g., the default mode network (DMN)]. This narrow focus on task-based connectivity and single network analyses precludes investigation of whole-brain intrinsic network organization in autism. To assess whole-brain network properties in adolescents with autism, we collected resting-state functional connectivity MRI (rs-fcMRI) data from neurotypical (NT) adolescents and adolescents with autism spectrum disorder (ASD). We used graph theory metrics on rs-fcMRI data with 34 regions of interest (i.e., nodes) that encompass four different functionally defined networks: cingulo-opercular, cerebellar, fronto-parietal, and DMN (Fair et al., 2009). Contrary to our hypotheses, network analyses revealed minimal differences between groups with one exception. Betweenness centrality, which indicates the degree to which a seed (or node) functions as a hub within and between networks, was greater for participants with autism for the right lateral parietal (RLatP) region of the DMN. Follow-up seed-based analyses demonstrated *greater* functional connectivity in ASD than NT groups between the RLatP seed and another region of the DMN, the anterior medial prefrontal cortex. Greater connectivity between these regions was related to lower ADOS (Autism Diagnostic Observation Schedule) scores (i.e., lower impairment) in autism. These findings do not support current theories of underconnectivity in autism, but, rather, underscore the need for future studies to systematically examine factors that can influence patterns of intrinsic connectivity such as autism severity, age, and head motion.

Keywords: autism, resting-state functional connectivity, default mode network, intrinsic network organization, graph theory, functional MRI

INTRODUCTION

Atypical patterns of functional and structural connectivity are proposed to be a hallmark neurobiological feature of autism (Belmonte et al., 2004; Just et al., 2004; Courchesne and Pierce, 2005; Cherkassky et al., 2006). Most theories and data point to a pattern of underconnectivity, particularly for long-distance connections such as interhemispheric or anterior–posterior intra-hemispheric connections (Belmonte et al., 2004; Just et al., 2004; Anderson et al., 2011; Dinstein et al., 2011). Some also suggest an increase in local connections at the expense of long-distance connections (Courchesne and Pierce, 2005; Courchesne et al., 2007; Rippon et al., 2007). Recent findings, however, offer mixed support and suggest a more complex picture of connectivity differences in autism with evidence for both hypo- and hyper-connectivity for short- and long-distance connections, depending partly on the specific experimental and analytic methods used and age of the participants (e.g., Courchesne et al., 2007; Noonan et al., 2009; Khan et al., 2013; Lynch et al., 2013; review, Müller et al., 2011).

Structural connectivity findings, indexed by measures of white matter integrity from diffusion tensor imaging (DTI) (e.g., fractional anisotropy, or FA) or white matter volumes from structural MRI, reveal atypical connectivity patterns in autism but do not support general underconnectivity in autism. Rather, findings suggest developmentally *increased* white matter volume (Courchesne et al., 2001; Hazlett et al., 2006), particularly radiate white matter bundles supporting interhemispheric and cortico-cortical connections (Herbert et al., 2004) and increased FA in infants and young children with autism (e.g., Ben Bashat et al., 2007; Wolff et al., 2012), whereas later in development (e.g., adolescents and adults), FA is decreased (e.g., Barnea-Goraly et al., 2004; Lee et al., 2007; Nair et al., 2013).

Studies of *functional* connectivity, or the correlation in signal between brain regions, largely have supported the underconnectivity theory when functional connectivity has been assessed in the context of a task (review, Müller et al., 2011). This pattern of reduced long-distance connectivity (e.g., between regions of different hemispheres or lobes) is seen across domains of function including tasks involving language processing (e.g., Just et al., 2004; Kana et al., 2006), executive function (e.g., Just et al., 2007), and social processing (e.g., Mason et al., 2008; Kana et al., 2012; , but see Murphy et al., 2012), but notably these tasks also resulted in reduced activation in the autism spectrum disorder (ASD) group as compared to the neurotypical (NT) group. Thus, while informative, task-based functional connectivity analyses may reflect differences in performance during a task and may not reflect differences in intrinsic functional organization of the brain.

Task-independent studies of the "resting" brain provide a window with which to examine intrinsic functional network organization. As first noted by Biswal et al. (1995), even in the absence of a specific task, fluctuations in brain signal are temporally correlated within regions that are part of the same functional network. These large-scale functional networks can be identified using data-driven ICA (independent component analysis) analyses (e.g., Damoiseaux et al., 2006) or seed-based analyses (e.g., Fox et al., 2005) and are thought to reflect regions that have a history of co-activation. Indeed, differences in the organization or connection strength within these regions are related to developmental changes (e.g., Fair et al., 2009), training (Lewis et al., 2009), and individual differences, for example in memory (Wang et al., 2010), math abilities (Emerson and Cantlon, 2012), and face processing (Zhu et al., 2011), suggesting intrinsic network connectivity is behaviorally relevant.

There has been considerable divergence across studies in regards to the status of resting-brain functional connectivity in ASD. Like task-based studies, many studies of the resting brain in ASD (or those in which the task is used as a regressor of no interest) have revealed reduced functional connectivity in ASD, particularly for long-range connections (Cherkassky et al., 2006; Kennedy and Courchesne, 2008; Ebisch et al., 2011; Tsiaras et al., 2011; Murdaugh et al., 2012; Rudie et al., 2012; Washington et al., 2013). However, unlike task-based studies, a number of studies report findings that are inconsistent with a general theory of underconnectivity (e.g., Monk et al., 2009; Müller et al., 2011; Tyszka et al., 2013), and in some cases hyper-connectivity in ASD groups has been reported (Mizuno et al., 2006; Turner et al., 2006; Noonan et al., 2009; Di Martino et al., 2011; Shih et al., 2011; Lynch et al., 2013).

In sum, extant data suggest a general underconnectivity theory in autism is likely not the full story. Possibly, the age of the participant, the context in which connectivity is assessed (e.g., resting vs. task), and the specific networks examined may result in different findings between groups. Further, recent studies suggest that head motion may lead to systematic, spurious correlations which could mimic some of the same patterns of connectivity differences reported between autism and NT groups (Power et al., 2011). An incomplete picture of how each of these factors contributes to functional connectivity in autism still remains. One additional contributing factor is that most previous studies only focused on the strength of correlations within a single network rather than examining network organization with graph theoretical metrics. Recent advances in graph theory (or complex network) analyses for resting-state functional connectivity MRI (rs-fcMRI) data allow for characterization of whole-brain intrinsic network organization (e.g., review, Rubinov and Sporns, 2010; Bullmore and Bassett, 2011). Specifically, rather than focusing on the strength of region–region correlations, graph theory methods can examine the topological properties of each region within the context of all other regions of interest. For example, graph theory metrics can include measures of the integration (global efficiency, average path length), segregation (local efficiency, clustering coefficient), and centrality (betweenness centrality) of networks. Thus, these metrics can provide a more robust test of the theory of reduced long-distance and increased local connectivity by testing differences in measures of whole-brain network integration and segregation.

In the current study, we assessed whole-brain network properties in a group of adolescents with and without autism by using graph theory and seed-based analyses on rs-fcMRI data with functionally defined regions of interest. The functional regions of interest included 34 regions identified from previous meta-analyses (Dosenbach et al., 2006; Fair et al., 2009) that encompass four different functionally defined networks: cingulo-opercular (CO), cerebellar (C), fronto-parietal (FP), and default mode (DMN; Fair et al., 2009). These networks were chosen because previous research with these same networks has demonstrated a developmental pattern of progressive increases in long-distance connectivity between nodes of the same network and concurrent decreases in connectivity between anatomically proximal nodes of distinct networks (Fair et al., 2008, 2009). Furthermore, functions associated with these networks have all been implicated in autism (e.g., reviews, Di Martino et al., 2009; Minshew and Keller, 2010). Thus, examining these networks allows for a more rigorous test of the hypothesis of reduced long-distance and increased local connectivity in autism, across multiple networks that support varied functions.

MATERIALS AND METHODS

PARTICIPANTS

All participants gave written, informed consent and parental consent was obtained for participants under 18 years of age as approved by the Committee on the Use of Humans as Experimental Subjects (COUHES) at the Massachusetts Institute of Technology. Participants were compensated monetarily for their time. Participants were part of a multi-site study involving three visits for TD adolescents and four for the ASD group but only the resting-state functional MRI data are presented in the current study. Participant IQ was measured using the Kaufman Brief Intelligence Test (KBIT-2).

AUTISM SPECTRUM DISORDER PARTICIPANTS

We collected resting-state functional MRI data from 22 male adolescents and young adults (14–20 years; mean 17.3 ± 2.2 years; all male) with a clinical diagnosis of ASD or Asperger's disorder. Diagnosis was confirmed using a combination of the

Table 1 | Demographic and head motion information for NT and ASD groups and those ASD participants excluded due to excessive head motion.

	NT ($N = 14$)	ASD ($N = 14$)	ASD-excluded ($N = 7$)	NT vs. ASD (p-value)	ASD vs. ASD-excluded (p-value)
Age	17.7(1.8)	17.8(1.9)	15.8(2.5)	0.81	0.05
Full Scale IQ	119(9.6)	116.9(13.7)	98.3(24.4)	0.59	0.04
Verbal IQ	118(13.1)	116.3(15.1)	97(24.9)	0.75	0.04
Non-verbal IQ	115(10.3)	112.5(13.1)	99.7(27.3)	0.57	0.17
Motion outliers	2.2(3.8)	1.8(2.8)	45.9(17.3)	0.73	<0.0001°
ADOS Combined	N/A	9.5(1.3)	16.2(2.8)	N/A	0.02
ADOS Comm.	N/A	3(2)	4.2(2.3)	N/A	0.28
ADOS Social	N/A	6.5(2.8)	12(5.1)	N/A	0.007

Note: Data are mean (SD). Age is in years. IQ was measured using the Kaufman Brief Intelligence Test-2. ADOS Comm is the communication subscale. p-Value is based on a t-test comparing groups. °This difference is circular because these groups were created based on differences in motion outliers.

Autism Diagnostic Observation Schedule (ADOS) Module 3 or 4 (administered to the participant; Lord et al., 2000) and the Social Communication Questionnaire (SCQ; completed by the parent of the participant; Corsello et al., 2007). The SCQ is a questionnaire designed to screen for autism and all included ASD participants received an SCQ score greater than the suggested cut-off for ASD of 15 (mean 21.6; 16–28). All participants reached criteria for Autism or spectrum from the ADOS except 1 who was subsequently removed from the analyses. Seven participants were excluded from the analyses because of excessive movement artifact (see below for description) resulting in a final sample of 14 participants with ASD (**Table 1**). Information about co-morbid diagnoses and current medications were obtained through a phone screen with either the participant or parent if the participant was a minor. This information was not available for 2 of the 14 ASD participants. Six of the 12 participants reported use of medications associated with symptoms of neuropsychiatric disorders [ADHD (4), depression/anxiety (3), psychosis (2)]. Only two participants, however, reported any co-morbid neurological disorders and these were obsessive–compulsive disorder (1) and attention deficit hyperactivity disorder (2).

NEUROTYPICAL PARTICIPANTS

Twenty-three NT participants (14–20 years; all male) performed a resting-state scan. Participants were excluded if they reported any psychiatric or neurological disorders on a self-report screening questionnaire, which was filled out either by the participant or the parent. To screen for the presence of autism or autistic-like traits in the typical population, the participant's parents completed the SCQ screening described above. One participant who was no longer a minor completed the Autism Spectrum Quotient (AQ; Woodbury-Smith et al., 2005). No included participants received scores above the suggested threshold for autism screening. One was excluded due to excessive movement. Of the 22 remaining participants, 14 were matched as closely as possible to the ASD group on age. IQ scores did not differ significantly between groups (see **Table 1**).

MRI DATA ACQUISITION

Participants came to the Athinoula A. Martinos Imaging Center at the McGovern Institute for Brain Research at MIT for MRI data collection on a 3T Siemens Magnetom Tim Trio Scanner. We collected a structural MPRAGE image (128 sagittal slices, TE = 3.39 ms, TR = 25 ms, voxel size 1.3 mm × 1 mm × 1.3 mm) and a resting-state functional MRI scan (67 sagittal slices, TE = 30 ms, TR = 6000 ms, # of TRs = 64, voxel size = 2.0 mm isotropic) as part of a 90-min battery of tasks examining social processing that are not presented here. The last scan of the battery was the resting-state scan for which we asked participants to remain still with eyes open and fixated on a cross in the center of the screen. We chose a 6 s TR for the resting-state scan in order to achieve high spatial resolution with whole-brain coverage because previous work has demonstrated that array coils provide the biggest increases in temporal signal to noise ratio (tSNR) at high spatial resolutions (Triantafyllou et al., 2011). While this TR is unusually long, a study by Van Dijk et al. (2010), showed that there was no significant difference in the correlation strengths between the resting-state networks when compared between a TR of 2.5 and 5 s.

FUNCTIONAL MRI PREPROCESSING

All data were analyzed using SPM8[1], Nipype (Gorgolewski et al., 2011), the CONN functional connectivity toolbox ver 13e[2] (Whitfield-Gabrieli and Nieto-Castanon, 2012), and in-house Matlab (The Mathworks, Natick, MA, USA) scripts. All resting-state volumes were corrected for differences in the timing of slice acquisition. Functional data were realigned to the mean of all functional volumes in the timeseries using a 6° rigid spatial transformation, which provided the spatial deviation for each timepoint for translational (x, y, z) and rotational (roll, pitch, yaw) directions of movement. Functional data were then smoothed with a Gaussian smoothing kernel of 6 mm full-width half maximum, and normalized into standard Montreal Neurological Institute (MNI) space using non-linear transformations.

[1]www.fil.ion.ucl.ac.uk/spm

[2]http://www.nitrc.org/projects/conn/

ANALYSES OF HEAD MOTION

The artifact detection toolbox (ART)[3] was used to examine outliers in global signal and movement for each participant. Timepoints were marked as outliers if global signal exceeded three standard deviations of the mean or if movement exceeded 1 mm (across translational and rotational directions) of scan-to-scan deviation. Participants for whom greater than 20% of the run was marked as an outlier were removed from the analyses (seven ASD; one NT). Head motion has been shown to result in spurious patterns of correlations (both increased and decreased; e.g., Power et al., 2011). Thus to examine whether groups differed as a function of head motion we used between-group t-tests to test for differences in (1) the total number of outliers and (2) the sum across all volumes of the absolute value of the deviation (in mm) from the reference volume (i.e., the realignment parameters) for each of the six possible motion directions (i.e., x, y, z, roll, pitch, yaw). Using between group t-tests, we also examined whether those participants who were excluded from the analyses due to excessive head motion were systematically different from those included in terms of age, IQ, or autism severity (**Table 1**). No significant differences in head motion between groups were present for either the number of outliers (see **Table 1**) or realignment parameters in any of the six directions [x: $t(24) = -0.56$, $p < 0.58$; y: $t(24) = -0.58$, $p < 0.57$; z: $t(24) = 1.1$, $p < 0.28$; roll: $t(24) = 0.85$, $p < 0.41$; pitch: $t(24) = 0.18$, $p < 0.86$, yaw: $t(24) = 1.7$, $p < 0.11$). However, the ASD participants who were excluded due to excessive head motion had significantly lower Verbal Composite IQ scores, and higher (worse) social impairments as measured by the ADOS Reciprocal Social Interaction subscale and autism severity as measured by the Combined ADOS Communication and Reciprocal Social Interaction subscales. Excluded participants also showed a trend toward significantly younger ages (**Table 1**).

FUNCTIONAL CONNECTIVITY ANALYSES

To minimize the effects of head motion, whole-brain voxel-wise regression analyses were run for each seed region of interest with the six motion parameters from realignment and their temporal derivatives and each outlier timepoint entered separately as noise covariates. Additionally, using the aCompCor method (Behzadi et al., 2007) to account for physiological noise, covariates were included with a principal components analysis (PCA)-reduction (three dimensions) of the signal from white matter and CSF voxels based on each individual's unique segmented white matter and CSF masks. The residual datasets were then temporally filtered ($0.01 < f < 0.08$) to focus analyses to the low-frequency oscillations characteristic of resting-state networks.

Whole-brain regression analyses were computed for each of the 34 seed regions of interest (Fair et al., 2009; **Table 2**) on the preprocessed, "clean" datasets for each participant. These analyses resulted in a correlation value in each voxel for each of the 34 seed regions. Normalized correlation values were created by a Fishers r-to-z transform and used in subsequent analyses. Averaging the normalized correlation coefficients within each group for each region pair created correlation matrices for each of the 34 regions of interest (ROI). Two-way between group (ASD vs. NT) t-tests were run for each of the 561 ROI–ROI pairs to examine whether differences in connectivity strength between groups were present and specific to particular networks. False discovery rate (FDR; $q < 0.05$) was used to correct for multiple comparisons for the ROI–ROI comparisons.

Graph theory analyses were computed using the CONN functional connectivity toolbox. The unweighted ROI-to-ROI correlation matrices were first thresholded at a cost value of $k = 0.15$. Cost is a measure of the proportion of connections for each ROI in relation to all connections in the network. Rather than determining a fixed correlation value as a threshold (e.g., $r = 0.1$), using a cost threshold allows for roughly the same number of connections across participants by varying the correlation threshold for each participant to achieve the fixed cost threshold. When cost is equated across participants, direct comparisons across groups of network property differences can be made. Small world properties are observed in the range of costs $0.05 < k < 0.34$, where global efficiency is greater than that of a lattice graph and local efficiency is greater than that of a random graph (Achard and Bullmore, 2007). A cost threshold of .15 has also been demonstrated to provide a high degree of reliability when comparing session-specific estimates of graph theoretical measures across repeated runs or sessions (e.g., global efficiency $r = 0.95$, local efficiency $r = 0.9$; Whitfield-Gabrieli and Nieto-Castanon, 2012). We employed both one- and two-sided cost thresholds. In a one-sided cost threshold only positive correlations are considered, whereas two-sided includes both positive and negative correlations. To confirm that our findings generalize beyond these specific parameters, data were examined at a cost threshold of 0.05, 0.1, 0.2, and 0.25 and compared to the findings with our *a priori* cost threshold of 0.15.

The specific measures of interest were those of integration (global efficiency), segregation (local efficiency), and centrality (betweenness centrality). Between-group t-tests were used to compare network measures between groups with a FDR correction of $q < 0.05$. Global efficiency is calculated as the average of the inverse of the shortest path length between each ROI (or node) and all other ROIs. The shortest path length is defined as the fewest number of connections (or correlations) between two nodes. Thus, a network with high global efficiency would be one in which nodes are highly integrated so the path between nodes is consistently short. With cost kept constant, this measure can be thought of as reflecting global, long-distance connections within the brain. Local efficiency is calculated as the average inverse of the shortest path length between the neighbors of any given node (or ROI). In other words, local efficiency measures the extent to which nodes are part of a cluster of locally, interconnected nodes. Finally, we examined a measure of centrality, betweenness centrality, which measures the fraction of all shortest path lengths in a network that pass through a given node. Thus, if a node is directly connected to many other nodes in the network it will have a shorter overall path length and function as a hub within and between networks. For more details on graph theoretical measures see Bullmore and Bassett (2011) or Rubinov and Sporns (2010).

[3] http://www.nitrc.org/projects/artifact_detect/

Table 2 | Seed regions of interest.

Number	Network	Hemi	Region	X	V	Z
1	Cingulo-opercular	L	Anterior prefrontal cortex anterior insula/frontal	−28	51	15
2	Cingulo-opercular	L	Operculum	−35	14	5
3	Cingulo-opercular	L	Anterior thalamus dorsal anterior cingulate/medial superior	−12	−15	7
4	Cingulo-opercular	L	Frontal cortex	−1	10	46
5	Cingulo-opercular	R	Anterior prefrontal cortex anterior insula/frontal	27	50	23
6	Cingulo-opercular	R	Operculum	36	16	4
7	Cingulo-opercular	R	Anterior thalamus	10	−15	8
8	Cerebellar	L	Inferior cerebellum	−19	−78	−33
9	Cerebellar	L	Lateral cerebellum	−32	−66	−29
10	Cerebellar	R	Inferior cerebellum	18	−80	−33
11	Cerebellar	R	Lateral cerebellum	31	−61	−29
12	Default	L	Inferior temporal	−61	−33	−15
13	Default	L	Lateral parietal	−47	−67	36
14	Default	L	Parahippocampal gyrus	−22	−26	−16
IS	Default	L	Superior fronta	−14	38	52
16	Default	R	Inferior temporal	65	−17	−15
17	Default	R	Lateral parietal	53	−67	36
18	Default	R	Parahippocampal gyrus	25	−26	−14
19	Default	R	Superior frontaanterior medial prefrontal	17	37	52
20	Default	R	Cortex	1	54	21
21	Default	L	Posterior cingulate cortex	−2	−36	37
22	Default	R	Retrosplenial cortex ventromedial prefrontal	3	−51	8
23	Default	L	Cortex	−3	39	−2
24	Fronto-parietal	L	Inferior parietal lobe	−51	−51	36
25	Fronto-parietal	L	Intraparietal sulcus	−31	−59	42
26	Fronto-parietal	L	Dorsolateral prefrontal cortex	−43	22	34
27	Fronto-parietal	L	Frontal	−41	3	36
28	Fronto-parietal	L	Precuneus	−9	−72	37
29	Fronto-parietal	R	Inferior parietal lobe	51	−47	42
30	Fronto-parietal	R	Intraparietal sulcus	30	−61	39
31	Fronto-parietal	R	Dorsolateral prefrontal cortex	43	22	34
32	Fronto-parietal	R	Frontal	41	3	36
33	Fronto-parietal	R	Precuneus	10	−69	39
34	Fronto-parietal	LR	Mid cingulate cortex	0	−29	30

These regions of interest and coordinates are taken directly from Fair et al. (2009). Number corresponds to the number listed in ***Figure 1****.*

RESULTS

LARGELY TYPICAL NETWORK ORGANIZATION IN ASD

Comparison of normalized correlation matrices between groups revealed minimal differences, which do not survive correction for multiple comparisons. Similarly network analyses revealed largely typical patterns of connectivity in the ASD group as compared to the NT group. Contrary to our hypotheses we found no differences in measures of global or local efficiency. Only betweenness centrality, which indicates the degree to which a seed (or node) functions as a hub within and between networks, was significantly different between groups and it was *greater* for participants with autism for the right lateral parietal (RLatP) seed of the DMN ($t(26) = 3.52$; $p < 0.027$ FDR-corrected) only. This metric was only significantly different when both positive and negative correlations were used in the cost threshold. When only positive correlations were considered, greater betweenness centrality in RLatP remained larger in ASD than NT groups but not significantly ($t(26) = 1.57$, $p < 0.13$). This finding suggests both correlations and anti-correlations (i.e., negative correlations) drove differences between groups. This effect held when examining higher cost thresholds ($k = 0.2$ and 0.25) but not lower ($k = 0.1$ and 0.05).

EXPLORATION OF RIGHT LATERAL PARIETAL SEED CONNECTIVITY PATTERNS

Comparison of the 34 × 34 matrix of normalized correlation values between seed regions for each group suggests the higher betweenness centrality in ASD may be due to (1) greater long-distance connectivity within the default mode network [RLatP–anterior medial prefrontal cortex (aMPFC)] and (2) greater negative correlations with regions in cerebellar and control networks in participants with ASD (**Figure 1**). However, these ROI-to-ROI differences were not significant when controlling for multiple comparisons. To further investigate how differences in connectivity resulted in the difference in centrality between groups we conducted within- and between-group t-tests on correlation maps using the RLatP region as a seed region (**Figure 2, Table 3**). These maps demonstrate significantly *greater* functional connectivity in the ASD than NT group within medial prefrontal cortex using a FWE cluster correction of $p < 0.05$. The NT group showed higher connectivity between the RLatP seed and cerebellar tonsils [a region previously associated with the default mode network (Fox et al., 2005)]. Examination of correlation maps within each group suggests these regions of between-group differences are not driven only by negative correlations in one group.

Our findings of greater connectivity within long-distance regions of the default mode network and greater centrality in autism were surprising and thus we explored whether variance in RLatP connectivity was related to autism severity, as measured by the ADOS, IQ, or age. No significant relationships were seen for autism severity or IQ and betweenness centrality measures for the RLatP, although there was a trend toward *reduced* centrality with

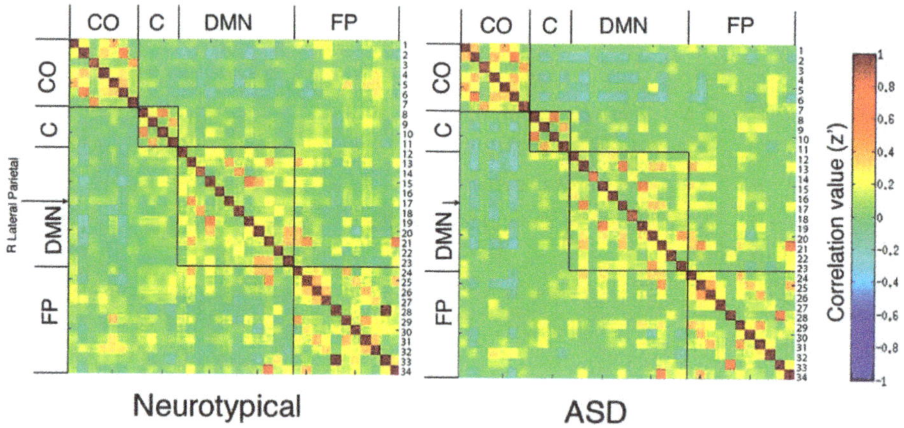

FIGURE 1 | Correlation matrices for neurotypical (A) and ASD (B) groups. Normalized correlation coefficients are reported for each of the 34 × 34 ROI correlations by group. These are organized by network based on Fair et al. (2009) (CO, cingulo-opercular; C, cerebellar; DMN, default mode network; FP, fronto-parietal). Each row is labeled with a number which corresponds to 1 of 34 seed regions (see **Table 2** for a list by number). Comparison of these matrices resulted in no significant differences between groups, when corrected for multiple comparisons. The right lateral parietal seed region (#17) of the DMN is identified with an arrow because that region showed a significant effect of group on centrality measures.

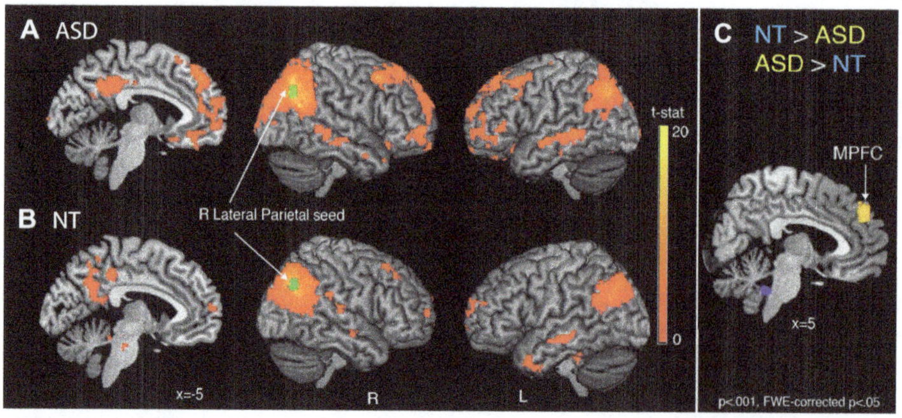

FIGURE 2 | Whole-brain functional connectivity maps with the right lateral parietal (RLatP) region (green) as a seed region are shown for the ASD group (A) and neurotypical group (B). Between-group comparisons **(C)** revealed one region of significantly greater connectivity from the RLatP seed in the ASD than NT group (yellow) which was the medial prefrontal cortex. The NT group showed greater connectivity between the RLatP seed and regions within the cerebellum (blue) than the ASD group. All maps are thresholded at $p < 0.001$, FWE cluster corrected at $p < 0.05$.

Table 3 | Functional connectivity from the right lateral parietal seed region.

Group region	Hemi	X	y	z	T	k
Neurotvpical						
Lateral parietal lobe	R	50	−70	36	21.28	2818
Posterior cingulate	L	−2	−34	46	7.76	2091
Lateral parietal lobe	L	−38	−74	40	8.74	1321
Parahippocampal gyms	L	−12	−36	−16	6.54	319
Superior temporal sulcus	R	−46	−32	−6	5.77	293
Superior frontal gyrus	L	−38	54	22	5.46	225
Middle frontal gyrus	R	26	32	40	6.87	210
Posterior insula	R	38	−28	16	6.06	196
anterior superior temporal sulcus	L	−50	10	−34	5.78	85
Superior frontal gyrus	R	28	66	10	6.06	81
Cerebellar tonsils	R	10	−40	−38	6.03	75
Parahippocampal gyrus	R	26	−30	−14	6.08	72
Brainstem/pons	R	2	−28	−26	8.06	65
Autism spectrum disorder						
Superior frontal gyrus	R	38	14	50	11.65	7006
Lateral parietal lobe	R	50	−62	22	18.56	3246
Lateral parietal lobe	L	−42	−74	38	11.95	1867
Posterior cingulate	R	12	−26	34	9.23	1710
Superior temporal sulcus	L	−54	−40	−4	10.29	552
Superior temporal sulcus	R	46	−36	−6	6.65	263
Superior frontal gyrus	L	40	58	0	8.41	211
Neurotvpical > autism spectrum disorder						
Cerebellum	L	−24	−40	−50	5.09	127
Cerebellar tonsils	R	8	−42	−38	5.65	123
Autism spectrum disorder > neurotypical						
Anterior medial prefrontal cortex	R	6	46	30	4.26	151

Regions were identified using $p < 0.001$, and FWE-cluster-correction of $p < 0.05$. Coordinates are given in MNI space. T-values from the peak voxel of the cluster and size (k) of the cluster are given. Clusters are organized by size.

age in the ASD group only [$r(13) = -0.48$, $p < 0.086$). Because the aMPFC was a region that showed significantly increased connectivity with RLatP in ASD in whole-brain analyses, we examined whether the strength of connectivity between the RLatP seed and the aMPFC seed was correlated with ADOS scores, IQ, or age. We found a negative correlation between the ADOS combined social-communication subscale and RLatP to aMPFC connectivity [$r(13) = -0.56$, $p < 0.046$), which was driven by the communication subscale [$r(13) = -0.67$, $p < 0.012$), suggesting lower connectivity within long-distance regions of the default mode network is related to more severe autism (**Figure 3**). No other correlations reached significance.

DISCUSSION

Overall, these data are consistent with recent studies suggesting largely typical patterns of functional connectivity in individuals with autism (Tyszka et al., 2013). Although network organization across four functional networks was examined, this relatively high-functioning group of adolescent males demonstrated only one significant difference in graph theoretical metrics of network organization: namely, betweenness centrality of the RLatP region of the DMN. Follow-up whole-brain voxel-wise analyses with the RLatP region as a seed region revealed *greater* connectivity in ASD to another region of the DMN, the aMPFC, as compared to NT controls.

Of the four functional networks examined in the current study, the DMN is the most consistently implicated in autism – though that may be largely due to a bias in the number of studies investigating this network alone. The DMN comprises a set of regions showing *deactivation* during goal-directed tasks, higher metabolic activity during rest, and relative activation during tasks requiring internally directed thought or social processing (e.g., Gusnard and Raichle, 2001). In autism, however, these regions do not show the typical pattern of deactivation during goal-directed tasks (Kennedy et al., 2006; Murdaugh et al., 2012) and show reduced activation during tasks of social-cognitive processing (e.g.,

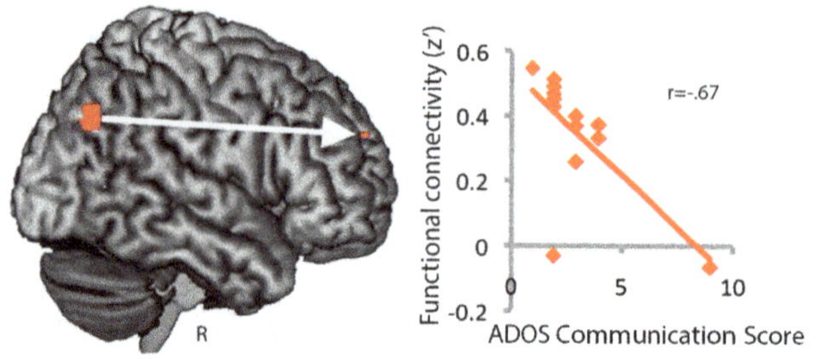

FIGURE 3 | Functional connectivity between the right lateral parietal and anterior medial prefrontal cortex regions in the default mode network is negatively correlated with ADOS communication scores in the ASD group. Higher scores indicate greater impairment.

Gilbert et al., 2009; Murdaugh et al., 2012, but see Dufour et al., in press). Furthermore, many previous studies have found a pattern of *reduced* DMN functional connectivity in ASD, particularly between long-distance frontal and parietal regions (Kennedy and Courchesne, 2008; Monk et al., 2009; Assaf et al., 2010; Weng et al., 2011; Murdaugh et al., 2012; Rudie et al., 2012; von dem Hagen et al., 2013, but see Lynch et al., 2013). Thus, while findings of atypical engagement of the DMN in autism is not new, the finding of *greater* functional connectivity between RLatP and medial prefrontal regions of the default mode network in ASD is inconsistent with many previous studies.

There are (at least) two factors that may account for differences between our study and previous studies finding reduced connectivity between groups. First, we matched groups on head motion parameters and used two measures to account for uncorrected head motion in subsequent analyses. While some previous studies demonstrated no significant differences in head motion between groups, four of the seven studies that showed reduced functional connectivity in the DMN did not compare head motion across groups. Differences in head motion between groups is a critical factor as previous studies have suggested that head motion may account for systematic and spurious correlations, particularly in reducing long-distance correlations while increasing short-distance correlations (Power et al., 2011). It remains unclear if "accounting" for head motion in the analysis is sufficient to eliminate group differences that may be due to motion.

Second, our final sample consisted of quite high-functioning individuals with autism. Many previous studies reporting reduced functional connectivity had, on average, slightly higher ADOS scores and lower IQs. Further, within the current study a significant relationship was found between functional connectivity between RLatP and MPFC and ADOS combined social-communication (and communication) scores, with greater impairment relating to lower functional connectivity. Taken together, these findings suggest lower-functioning autism may result in patterns of reduced connectivity. However, we offer caution in this interpretation because this relationship is counter-intuitive in the context of the current study. The ASD group had significantly greater connectivity than the NT group, which suggests that more severe autism should be related to greater connectivity, but instead the reverse is true. These data suggest a possible non-linear relationship between autism severity and functional connectivity in autism but this has yet to be systematically examined.

Systematically examining how level of functioning impacts connectivity patterns is especially challenging because lower-functioning individuals tend to have more motion artifact, and, as discussed above, head motion differences alone can lead to a pattern of reduced long-distance connectivity. In the current study, we used stringent criteria to exclude participants with excessive head motion and while this only resulted in loss of data from one NT participant, seven participants with ASD were removed from data analyses. These seven were significantly different from the rest of the ASD group not only because they moved more during the scan but also because they were younger, had higher ADOS scores (i.e., were more impaired), and had lower verbal and composite IQ scores. Thus, a significant, but necessary, challenge for further research is to characterize the functional significance of resting-state networks when head motion is equated across groups (Deen and Pelphrey, 2012), such as in the current study.

Although less common, this is not the first study to report hyper-connectivity within the default mode network in autism. Two previous studies also reported increased connectivity in ASD within default mode regions (Monk et al., 2009; Lynch et al., 2013), and for one (Lynch et al., 2013) this increased connectivity was found between frontal and parietal DMN regions similar to the current study. Specifically, Lynch et al. (2013) examined functional connectivity from regions within posteromedial cortex in 7–12-year-old children and reported greater connectivity in ASD from retrosplenial cortex, a region just inferior to the posterior cingulate and part of the default mode network, to several other regions including the aMPFC (though this particular connection was reduced in the ASD sample in Monk et al., 2009). Additionally, connectivity between posterior cingulate and several lateral and medial temporal regions showed greater connectivity in the ASD than NT groups – a finding similar to Monk et al. (2009).

The study of Lynch et al. (2013) was among the first to examine DMN connectivity during a resting baseline in young children with ASD. As such, they suggested the relatively novel finding of hyper-connectivity within the default mode network (and from posteromedial cortex to regions outside of the DMN) may be due to a developmental change in the pattern of connectivity differences between ASD and NT groups. This developmental story is consistent with other theories of connectivity in autism (e.g., Courchesne and Pierce, 2005; Pelphrey et al., 2011) as well as evidence of age-related changes in brain differences between autism and control groups (Redcay and Courchesne, 2005). In other words, whereas findings from older children and adults reveal reduced brain size, reduced measures of white matter integrity (e.g., FA) or reduced functional connectivity, findings from younger children reveal larger brain size (e.g., Courchesne et al., 2001; Hazlett et al., 2006), higher FA values (Wolff et al., 2012), and increased functional connectivity (Lynch et al., 2013). However, the current findings of DMN hyper-connectivity was in a sample of adolescents and the Monk et al. (2009) study was in adults. Thus, age-related differences may not completely account for patterns of increased functional connectivity within the default mode network.

While further research is needed to disentangle the factors contributing to relatively typical or *increased* connectivity in autism, we find the increased connectivity between the RLatP and aMPFC regions of the DMN in the current study intriguing. These regions play an important role in social processes that are atypical in individuals with autism, including mental state judgments of others (i.e., theory of mind) and of one's self (i.e., introspection) (e.g., Baron-Cohen et al., 1985; Frith and Happe, 1999; Saxe and Kanwisher, 2003; Saxe et al., 2006; Senju et al., 2009). While the medial prefrontal cortex plays a general role in mentalizing (Whitfield-Gabrieli et al., 2011), portions of RLatP cortex may play a more specific role in thinking about others thoughts and beliefs, or theory of mind (e.g., Saxe and Kanwisher, 2003; Saxe et al., 2006). Meta-analyses suggest the RLatP region of the default mode is at least partially overlapping with the right temporoparietal junction (RTPJ) often reported in studies of theory of mind processing (e.g., Schilbach et al., 2008; Spreng and Mar, 2012). Beyond social-cognitive processing, the RLatP lobe is also associated with shifts of spatial attention (Corbetta and Shulman, 2002), semantic processing (Binder et al., 1999), and narrative comprehension (e.g., Mar, 2011), all of which have been implicated as atypical in individuals with autism. Thus, greater connectivity within right parietal cortex could indicate less functional specialization of this region in ASD, similar to findings of right posterior temporal cortex (e.g., Shih et al., 2011). However, the current data do not directly address that hypothesis.

A notable limitation in this study, which claims minimal differences in functional connectivity between groups, is a small sample size. Nonetheless, the current findings of *greater* connectivity within the DMN in ASD adds to the small, growing body of literature suggesting inconsistent support for an underconnectivity theory of autism. A second limitation is the restricted range of high-functioning participants with autism who were able to complete the scan with minimal motion artifact. Even within this narrow range, a correlation was seen between a greater level of communicative impairment and lower functional connectivity between RLatP and medial prefrontal cortex and a trend toward increasing age and reduced betweenness centrality in ASD. Finally, a third limitation is the inclusion of data from participants currently on medication as some medications may affect the strength or patterns or brain activation; however, the sample is too small to determine whether medication had any systematic effects on functional connectivity. These data underscore the need for developmental studies of functional connectivity in high- and low-functioning individuals with autism in which head motion is tightly matched between groups.

ACKNOWLEDGMENTS

We gratefully acknowledge the Boston Autism Consortium for providing funding support for this project. We also wish to thank Dr. Charles A. Nelson, Dr. Tal Kenet, and Dr. Robert Joseph for their contributions to this multi-site project that made collection of these data possible, including recruitment and assessment of participants with ASD. We also thank Dr. Jasmin Cloutier and Daniel O'Young for assistance with data collection and the Athinoula A. Martinos Imaging Center at the McGovern Institute for Brain Research at MIT, particularly Dr. Christina Triantafyllou for development of the current resting-state imaging protocol. We also are grateful to the Eunice Kennedy Shriver National Institute of Child Health and Human Development for a postdoctoral fellowship to Elizabeth Redcay.

REFERENCES

Achard, S., and Bullmore, E. (2007). Efficiency and cost of economical brain functional networks. *PLoS Comput. Biol.* 3:e17. doi: 10.1371/journal.pcbi.0030017

Anderson, J. S., Druzgal, T. J., Froehlich, A., DuBray, M. B., Lange, N., Alexander, A. L., et al. (2011). Decreased interhemispheric functional connectivity in autism. *Cereb. Cortex* 21, 1134–1146. doi: 10.1093/cercor/bhq190

Assaf, M., Jagannathan, K., and Calhoun, V. (2010). Abnormal functional connectivity of default mode sub-networks in autism spectrum disorder patients. *Neuroimage* 53, 247–256. doi: 10.1016/j.neuroimage.2010.05.067.Assaf

Barnea-Goraly, N., Kwon, H., Menon, V., Eliez, S., Lotspeich, L., and Reiss, A. L. (2004). White matter structure in autism: preliminary evidence from diffusion tensor imaging. *Biol. Psychiatry* 55, 323–326. doi: 10.1016/j.biopsych.2003.10.022

Baron-Cohen, S., Leslie, A. M., and Frith, U. (1985). Does the autistic child have a "theory of mind"? *Cognition* 21, 37–46. doi: 10.1016/0010-0277(85)90022-8

Behzadi, Y., Restom, K., Liau, J., and Liu, T. T. (2007). A component based noise correction method (CompCor) for BOLD and perfusion based fMRI. *Neuroimage* 37, 90–101. doi: 10.1016/j.neuroimage.2007.04.042

Belmonte, M. K., Allen, G., Beckel-Mitchener, A., Boulanger, L. M., Carper, R. A., and Webb, S. J. (2004). Autism and abnormal development of brain connectivity. *J. Neurosci.* 24, 9228–9231. doi: 10.1523/JNEUROSCI.3340-04.2004

Ben Bashat, D., Kronfeld-Duenias, V., Zachor, D. A., Ekstein, P. M., Hendler, T., Tarrasch, R., et al. (2007). Accelerated maturation of white matter in young children with autism: a high b value DWI study. *Neuroimage* 37, 40–47. doi: 10.1016/j.neuroimage.2007.04.060

Binder, J. R., Frost, J. A., Hammeke, T. A., Bellgowan, P. S., Rao, S. M., and Cox, R. W. (1999). Conceptual processing during the conscious resting state. A functional MRI study. *J. Cogn. Neurosci.* 11, 80–95. doi: 10.1162/089892999563265

Biswal, B., Yetkin, F. Z., Haughton, V. M., and Hyde, J. S. (1995). Functional connectivity in the motor cortex of resting human brain using echo-planar MRI. *Magn. Reson. Med.* 34, 537–541. doi: 10.1002/mrm.1910340409

Bullmore, E. T., and Bassett, D. S. (2011). Brain graphs: graphical models of the human brain connectome. *Annu. Rev. Clin. Psychol.* 7, 113–140. doi: 10.1146/annurev-clinpsy-040510-143934

Cherkassky, V. L., Kana, R. K., Keller, T. A., and Just, M. A. (2006). Functional connectivity in a baseline resting-state network in autism. *Neuroreport* 17, 1687–1690. doi: 10.1097/01.wnr.0000239956.45448.4c

Corbetta, M., and Shulman, G. L. (2002). Control of goal-directed and stimulus-driven attention in the brain. *Nat. Rev. Neurosci.* 3, 201–215. doi: 10.1038/nrn755

Corsello, C., Hus, V., Pickles, A., Risi, S., Cook, E. H., Leventhal, B. L., et al. (2007). Between a ROC and a hard place: decision making and making decisions about using the SCQ. *J. Child Psychol. Psychiatry* 48, 932–940. doi: 10.1111/j.1469-7610.2007.01762.x

Courchesne, E., Karns, C. M., Davis, H. R., Ziccardi, R., Carper, R. A., Tigue, Z. D., et al. (2001). Unusual brain growth patterns in early life in patients with autistic disorder: an MRI study. *Neurology* 57, 245–254. doi: 10.1212/WNL.57.2.245

Courchesne, E., and Pierce, K. (2005). Why the frontal cortex in autism might be talking only to itself: local over-connectivity but long-distance disconnection. *Curr. Opin. Neurobiol.* 15, 225–230. doi: 10.1016/j.conb.2005.03.001

Courchesne, E., Pierce, K., Schumann, C. M., Redcay, E., Buckwalter, J. A., Kennedy, D. P., et al. (2007). Mapping early brain development in autism. *Neuron* 56, 399–413. doi: 10.1016/j.neuron.2007.10.016

Damoiseaux, J. S., Rombouts, S. A. R. B., Barkhof, F., Scheltens, P., Stam, C. J., Smith, S. M., et al. (2006). Consistent resting-state networks across healthy subjects. *Proc. Natl. Acad. Sci. U.S.A.* 103, 13848–13853. doi: 10.1073/pnas.0601417103

Deen, B., and Pelphrey, K. (2012). Perspective: brain scans need a rethink. *Nature* 491, S20. doi: 10.1038/491S20a

Di Martino, A., Kelly, C., Grzadzinski, R., Zuo, X.-N., Mennes, M., Mairena, M. A., et al. (2011). Aberrant striatal functional connectivity in children with autism. *Biol. Psychiatry* 69, 847–856. doi: 10.1016/j.biopsych.2010.10.029.Aberrant

Di Martino, A., Ross, K., Uddin, L. Q., Sklar, A. B., Castellanos, F. X., and Milham, M. P. (2009). Functional brain correlates of social and nonsocial processes in autism spectrum disorders: an activation likelihood estimation meta-analysis. *Biol. Psychiatry* 65, 63–74. doi: 10.1016/j.biopsych.2008.09.022

Dinstein, I., Pierce, K., Eyler, L., Solso, S., Malach, R., Behrmann, M., et al. (2011). Disrupted neural synchronization in toddlers with autism. *Neuron* 70, 1218–1225. doi: 10.1016/j.neuron.2011.04.018

Dosenbach, N. U. F., Visscher, K. M., Palmer, E. D., Miezin, F. M., Wenger, K. K., Kang, H. C., et al. (2006). A core system for the implementation of task sets. *Neuron* 50, 799–812. doi: 10.1016/j.neuron.2006.04.031

Dufour, N., Redcay, E., Young, L., Mavros, P. L., Moran, J. M., Triantafyllou, C., et al. (in press). Similar brain activation patterns during false belief tasks in a large sample of adults with and without autism. *PLoS ONE.*

Ebisch, S. J. H., Gallese, V., Willems, R. M., Mantini, D., Groen, W. B., Romani, G. L., et al. (2011). Altered intrinsic functional connectivity of anterior and posterior insula regions in high-functioning participants with autism spectrum disorder. *Hum. Brain Mapp.* 32, 1013–1028. doi: 10.1002/hbm.21085

Emerson, R. W., and Cantlon, J. F. (2012). Early math achievement and functional connectivity in the fronto-parietal network. *Dev. Cogn. Neurosci.* 2(Suppl. 1), S139–S151. doi: 10.1016/j.dcn.2011.11.003

Fair, D. A., Cohen, A. L., Dosenbach, N. U. F., Church, J. A., Miezin, F. M., Barch, D. M., et al. (2008). The maturing architecture of the brain's default network. *Proc. Natl. Acad. Sci. U.S.A.* 105, 4028–4032. doi: 10.1073/pnas.0800376105

Fair, D. A., Cohen, A. L., Power, J. D., Dosenbach, N. U. F., Church, J. A., Miezin, F. M., et al. (2009). Functional brain networks develop from a "local to distributed" organization. *PLoS Comput. Biol.* 5:e1000381. doi: 10.1371/journal.pcbi.1000381

Fox, M. D., Snyder, A. Z., Vincent, J. L., Corbetta, M., Van Essen, D. C., and Raichle, M. E. (2005). The human brain is intrinsically organized into dynamic, anticorrelated functional networks. *Proc. Natl. Acad. Sci. U.S.A.* 102, 9673–9678. doi: 10.1073/pnas.0504136102

Frith, U., and Happe, F. (1999). Theory of mind and self-consciousness: what is it like to be autistic? *Mind Lang.* 14, 82–89. doi: 10.1111/1468-0017.00100

Gilbert, S. J., Meuwese, J. D. I., Towgood, K. J., Frith, C. D., and Burgess, P. W. (2009). Abnormal functional specialization within medial prefrontal cortex in high-functioning autism: a multi-voxel similarity analysis. *Brain* 132, 869–878. doi: 10.1093/brain/awn365

Gorgolewski, K., Burns, C. D., Madison, C., Clark, D., Halchenko, Y. O., Waskom, M. L., et al. (2011). Nipype: a flexible, lightweight and extensible neuroimaging data processing framework in python. *Front. Neuroinform.* 5:13. doi: 10.3389/fninf.2011.00013

Gusnard, D. A., and Raichle, M. E. (2001). Searching for a baseline: functional imaging and the resting human brain. *Nat. Rev. Neurosci.* 2, 685–694. doi: 10.1038/35094500

Hazlett, H. C., Poe, M. D., Gerig, G., Smith, R. G., and Piven, J. (2006). Cortical gray and white brain tissue volume in adolescents and adults with autism. *Biol. Psychiatry* 59, 1–6. doi: 10.1016/j.biopsych.2005.06.015

Herbert, M. R., Ziegler, D. A., Makris, N., Filipek, P. A., Kemper, T. L., Normandin, J. J., et al. (2004). Localization of white matter volume increase in autism and developmental language disorder. *Ann. Neurol.* 55, 530–540. doi: 10.1002/ana.20032

Just, M. A., Cherkassky, V. L., Keller, T. A., Kana, R. K., and Minshew, N. J. (2007). Functional and anatomical cortical underconnectivity in autism: evidence from an FMRI study of an executive function task and corpus callosum morphometry. *Cereb. Cortex* 17, 951–961. doi: 10.1093/cercor/bhl006

Just, M. A., Cherkassky, V. L., Keller, T. A., and Minshew, N. J. (2004). Cortical activation and synchronization during sentence comprehension in high-functioning autism: evidence of underconnectivity. *Brain* 127(Pt 8), 1811–1821. doi: 10.1093/brain/awh199

Kana, R. K., Keller, T. A., Cherkassky, V. L., Minshew, N. J., and Just, M. A. (2006). Sentence comprehension in autism: thinking in pictures with decreased functional connectivity. *Brain* 129(Pt 9), 2484–2493. doi: 10.1093/brain/awl164

Kana, R., Libero, L., Hu, C., Deshpande, H., and Colburn, J. (2012). Functional brain networks and white matter underlying theory-of-mind in autism. *Soc. Cogn. Affect. Neurosci.* doi: 10.1093/scan/nss106 [Epub ahead of print].

Kennedy, D. P., and Courchesne, E. (2008). The intrinsic functional organization of the brain is altered in autism. *Neuroimage* 39, 1877–1885. doi: 10.1016/j.neuroimage.2007.10.052

Kennedy, D. P., Redcay, E., and Courchesne, E. (2006). Failing to deactivate: resting functional abnormalities in autism. *Proc. Natl. Acad. Sci. U.S.A.* 103, 8275–8280. doi: 10.1073/pnas.0600674103

Khan, S., Gramfort, A., Shetty, N. R., Kitzbichler, M. G., Ganesan, S., Moran, J. M., et al. (2013). Local and long-range functional connectivity is reduced in concert in autism spectrum disorders. *Proc. Natl. Acad. Sci. U.S.A.* 110, 3107–3112. doi: 10.1073/pnas.1214533110

Lee, J. E., Bigler, E. D., Alexander, A. L., Lazar, M., DuBray, M. B., Chung, M. K., et al. (2007). Diffusion tensor imaging of white matter in the superior temporal gyrus and temporal stem in autism. *Neurosci. Lett.* 424, 127–132. doi: 10.1016/j.neulet.2007.07.042

Lewis, C. M., Baldassarre, A., Committeri, G., Romani, G. L., and Corbetta, M. (2009). Learning sculpts the spontaneous activity of the resting human brain. *Proc. Natl. Acad. Sci. U.S.A.* 106, 17558–17563. doi: 10.1073/pnas.0902455106

Lord, C., Risi, S., Lambrecht, L., Cook, E. H., Leventhal, B. L., DiLavore, P. C., et al. (2000). The autism diagnostic observation schedule-generic: a standard measure of social and communication deficits associated with the spectrum of autism. *J. Autism Dev. Disord.* 30, 205–223. doi: 10.1023/A:1005592401947

Lynch, C. J., Uddin, L. Q., Supekar, K., Khouzam, A., Phillips, J., and Menon, V. (2013). Default mode network in childhood autism: posteromedial cortex heterogeneity and relationship with social deficits. *Biol. Psychiatry* 74, 212–219. doi: 10.1016/j.biopsych.2012.12.013

Mar, R. A. (2011). The neural bases of social cognition and story comprehension. *Annu. Rev. Psychol.* 62, 103–134. doi: 10.1146/annurev-psych-120709-145406

Mason, R., Williams, D., Kana, R., and Minshew, N. (2008). Theory of mind disruption and recruitment of the right hemisphere during narrative comprehension in autism. *Neuropsychologia* 46, 269–280. doi: 10.1016/j.neuropsychologia.2007.07.018

Minshew, N., and Keller, T. (2010). The nature of brain dysfunction in autism: functional brain imaging studies. *Curr. Opin. Neurol.* 23, 124–130. doi: 10.1097/WCO.0b013e32833782d4

Mizuno, A., Villalobos, M. E., Davies, M. M., Dahl, B. C., and Müller, R.-A. (2006). Partially enhanced thalamocortical functional connectivity in autism. *Brain Res.* 1104, 160–174. doi: 10.1016/j.brainres.2006.05.064

Monk, C., Peltier, S., and Wiggins, J. (2009). Abnormalities of intrinsic functional connectivity in autism spectrum disorders. *Neuroimage* 47, 764–772. doi: 10.1016/j.neuroimage.2009.04.069. Abnormalities

Müller, R.-A., Shih, P., Keehn, B., Deyoe, J. R., Leyden, K. M., and Shukla, D. K. (2011). Underconnected, but how? A survey of functional connectivity MRI studies in autism spectrum disorders. *Cereb. Cortex* 21, 2233–2243. doi: 10.1093/cercor/bhq296

Murdaugh, D. L., Shinkareva, S. V., Deshpande, H. R., Wang, J., Pennick, M. R., and Kana, R. K. (2012). Differential deactivation during mentalizing and classification of autism based on default mode network connectivity. *PloS ONE* 7:e50064. doi: 10.1371/journal.pone.0050064

Murphy, E. R., Foss-Feig, J., Kenworthy, L., Gaillard, W., and Vaidya, C. J. (2012). Atypical functional connectivity of the amygdala in childhood autism spectrum disorders during spontaneous attention to eye-gaze. *Autism Research and Treatment.* doi:10.1155/2012/652408

Nair, A., Treiber, J. M., Shukla, D. K., Shih, P., and Müller, R.-A. (2013). Impaired thalamocortical connectivity in autism spectrum disorder: a study of functional and anatomical connectivity. *Brain* 136(Pt 6), 1942–1955. doi: 10.1093/brain/awt079

Noonan, S., Haist, F., and Müller, R. (2009). Aberrant functional connectivity in autism: evidence from low-frequency bold fluctuations. *Brain Res.* 1262, 48–63. doi: 10.1016/j.brainres.2008.12.076.Aberrant

Pelphrey, K. A., Shultz, S., Hudac, C. M., and Vander Wyk, B. C. (2011). Research review: constraining heterogeneity: the social brain and its development in autism spectrum disorder. *J. Child Psychol. Psychiatry* 52, 631–644. doi: 10.1111/j.1469-7610.2010.02349.x

Power, J. D., Barnes, K. A., Snyder, A. Z., Schlaggar, B. L., and Petersen, S. E. (2011). Spurious but systematic correlations in functional connectivity MRI networks arise from subject motion. *Neuroimage* 59, 2142–2154. doi: 10.1016/j.neuroimage.2011.10.018

Power, J. D., Fair, D. A., Schlaggar, B. L., and Petersen, S. E. (2010). The development of human functional brain networks. *Neuron* 67, 735–748. doi: 10.1016/j.neuron.2010.08.017

Redcay, E., and Courchesne, E. (2005). When is the brain enlarged in autism? A meta-analysis of all brain size reports. *Biol. Psychiatry* 58, 1–9. doi: 10.1016/j.biopsych.2005.03.026

Rippon, G., Brock, J., Brown, C., and Boucher, J. (2007). Disordered connectivity in the autistic brain: challenges for the "new psychophysiology". *Int. J. Psychophysiol.* 63, 164–172. doi: 10.1016/j.ijpsycho.2006.03.012

Rubinov, M., and Sporns, O. (2010). Complex network measures of brain connectivity: uses and interpretations. *Neuroimage* 52, 1059–1069. doi: 10.1016/j.neuroimage.2009.10.003

Rudie, J. D., Hernandez, L. M., Brown, J. A., Beck-Pancer, D., Colich, N. L., Gorrindo, P., et al. (2012). Autism-associated promoter variant in MET impacts functional and structural brain networks. *Neuron* 75, 904–915. doi: 10.1016/j.neuron.2012.07.010

Saxe, R., and Kanwisher, N. (2003). People thinking about thinking people. The role of the temporoparietal junction in "theory of mind". *Neuroimage* 19, 1835–1842. doi: 10.1016/S1053-8119(03)00230-1

Saxe, R., Moran, J. M., Scholz, J., and Gabrieli, J. (2006). Overlapping and non-overlapping brain regions for theory of mind and self reflection in individual subjects. *Soc. Cogn. Affect. Neurosci.* 1, 229–234. doi: 10.1093/scan/nsl034

Schilbach, L., Eickhoff, S. B., Rotarska-Jagiela, A., Fink, G. R., and Vogeley, K. (2008). Minds at rest? Social cognition as the default mode of cognizing and its putative relationship to the "default system" of the brain. *Conscious. Cogn.* 17, 457–467. doi: 10.1016/j.concog.2008.03.013

Senju, A., Southgate, V., White, S., and Frith, U. (2009). Mindblind eyes: an absence of spontaneous theory of mind in Asperger syndrome. *Science* 325, 883–885. doi: 10.1126/science.1176170

Shih, P., Keehn, B., Oram, J. K., Leyden, K. M., Keown, C. L., and Müller, R.-A. (2011). Functional differentiation of posterior superior temporal sulcus in autism: a functional connectivity magnetic resonance imaging study. *Biol. Psychiatry.* 70, 270–277. doi: 10.1016/j.biopsych.2011.03.040

Spreng, R. N., and Mar, R. A. (2012). I remember you: a role for memory in social cognition and the functional neuroanatomy of their interaction. *Brain Res.* 1428, 43–50. doi: 10.1016/j.brainres.2010.12.024

Triantafyllou, C., Polimeni, J., and Wald, L. (2011). Physiological noise and signal-to-noise ratio in fmri with multi-channel array coils. *Neuroimage* 55, 597–606. doi: 10.1016/j.neuroimage.2010.11.084. Physiological

Tsiaras, V., Simos, P. G., Rezaie, R., Sheth, B. R., Garyfallidis, E., Castillo, E. M., et al. (2011). Extracting biomarkers of autism from MEG resting-state functional connectivity networks. *Comput. Biol. Med.* 41, 1166–1177. doi: 10.1016/j.compbiomed.2011.04.004

Turner, K. C., Frost, L., Linsenbardt, D., McIlroy, J. R., and Müller, R.-A. (2006). Atypically diffuse functional connectivity between caudate nuclei and cerebral cortex in autism. *Behav. Brain Funct.* 2, 34. doi: 10.1186/1744-9081-2-34

Tyszka, J. M., Kennedy, D. P., Paul, L. K., and Adolphs, R. (2013). Largely typical patterns of resting-state functional connectivity in high-functioning adults with autism. *Cereb. Cortex* doi: 10.1093/cercor/bht040

Van Dijk, K. R. A., Hedden, T., Venkataraman, A., Evans, K. C., Lazar, S. W., and Buckner, R. L. (2010). Intrinsic functional connectivity as a tool for human connectomics: theory, properties, and optimization. *J. Neurophysiol.* 103, 297–321. doi: 10.1152/jn.00783.2009

von dem Hagen, E. A. H., Stoyanova, R. S., Baron-Cohen, S., and Calder, A. J. (2013). Reduced functional connectivity within and between "social" resting state networks in autism spectrum conditions. *Soc. Cogn. Affect. Neurosci.* 8, 694–701. doi: 10.1093/scan/nss053

Wang, L., Laviolette, P., O'Keefe, K., Putcha, D., Bakkour, A., Van Dijk, K. R. A., et al. (2010). Intrinsic connectivity between the hippocampus and posteromedial cortex predicts memory performance in cognitively intact older individuals. *Neuroimage* 51, 910–917. doi: 10.1016/j.neuroimage.2010.02.046

Washington, S. D., Gordon, E. M., Brar, J., Warburton, S., Sawyer, A. T., Wolfe, A., et al. (2013). Dysmaturation of the default mode network in autism. *Hum. Brain Mapp.* doi:10.1002/hbm.22252 [Epub ahead of print].

Weng, S., Wiggins, J. L., Peltier, S. J., Carrasco, M., Risi, S., Lord, C., et al. (2011). Alterations of resting state functional connectivity in the default network in adolescents with autism spectrum disorders. *Brain Res.* 131, 202–214. doi: 10.1016/j.brainres.2009.11.057

Whitfield-Gabrieli, S., Moran, J. M., Nieto-Castañón, A., Triantafyllou, C., Saxe, R., and Gabrieli, J. D. E. (2011). Associations and dissociations between default and self-reference networks in the human brain. *Neuroimage* 55, 225–232. doi: 10.1016/j.neuroimage.2010.11.048

Whitfield-Gabrieli, S., and Nieto-Castanon, A. (2012). Conn: a functional connectivity toolbox for correlated and anticorrelated brain networks. *Brain Connect.* 2, 125–141. doi: 10.1089/brain.2012.0073

Wolff, J., Gu, H., and Gerig, G. (2012). Differences in white matter fiber tract development present from 6 to 24 months in infants with autism. *Am. J. Psychiatry* 169, 589–600. doi: 10.1176/appi.ajp.2011.11091447

Woodbury-Smith, M. R., Robinson, J., Wheelwright, S., and Baron-Cohen, S. (2005). Screening adults for Asperger Syndrome using the AQ: a preliminary study of its diagnostic validity in clinical practice. *J. Autism Dev. Disord.* 35, 331–335. doi: 10.1007/s10803-005-3300-7

Zhu, Q., Zhang, J., Luo, Y. L. L., Dilks, D. D., and Liu, J. (2011). Resting-state neural activity across face-selective cortical regions is behaviorally relevant. *J. Neurosci.* 31, 10323–10330. doi: 10.1523/JNEUROSCI.0873-11.2011

3

In vivo detection of reduced Purkinje cell fibers with diffusion MRI tractography in children with autistic spectrum disorders

***Jeong-Won Jeong*[1,2]*, *Vijay N. Tiwari*[1,2], *Michael E. Behen*[1,2], *Harry T. Chugani*[1,2] and *Diane C. Chugani*[1,2]**

[1] *Department of Pediatrics and Neurology, Wayne State University, Detroit, MI, USA*
[2] *Translational Imaging Laboratory, PET center, Children's Hospital of Michigan, Detroit, MI, USA*

Edited by:
Ralph-Axel Müller, San Diego State University, USA

Reviewed by:
Jeffrey Jon Hutsler, University of Nevada, Reno, USA
Naama Barnea-Goraly, Stanford University, USA

****Correspondence:***
Jeong-Won Jeong, Department of Pediatrics and Neurology, Wayne State University, 3901 Beaubien Boulevard, Detroit, MI 48201, USA
e-mail: jeongwon@pet.wayne.edu

Postmortem neuropathology studies report reduced number and size of Purkinje cells (PC) in a majority of cerebellar specimens from persons diagnosed with autism spectrum disorders (ASD). We used diffusion weighted MRI tractography to investigate whether structural changes associated with reduced number and size of PC, could be detected *in vivo* by measuring streamlines connecting the posterior-lateral region of the cerebellar cortex to the dentate nucleus using an independent component analysis with a ball and stick model. Seed regions were identified in the cerebellar cortex, and streamlines were identified to two sorting regions, the dorsal dentate nucleus (DDN) and the ventral dentate nucleus (VDN), and probability of connection and measures of directional coherence for these streamlines were calculated. Tractography was performed in 14 typically developing children (TD) and 15 children with diagnoses of ASD. Decreased numbers of streamlines were found in the children with ASD in the pathway connecting cerebellar cortex to the right VDN (p-value = 0.015). Reduced fractional anisotropy (FA) values were observed in pathways connecting the cerebellar cortex to the right DDN (p-value = 0.008), the right VDN (p-value = 0.010) and left VDN (p-value = 0.020) in children with ASD compared to the TD group. In an analysis of single subjects, reduced FA in the pathway connecting cerebellar cortex to the right VDN was found in 73% of the children in the ASD group using a threshold of 3 standard errors of the TD group. The detection of diffusion changes in cerebellum may provide an *in vivo* biomarker of Purkinje cell pathology in children with ASD.

Keywords: Purkinje cell, dentate nucleus, autism spectrum disorders, diffusion weighted MRI, independent component analysis tractography with a ball and stick model

INTRODUCTION

Autism spectrum disorders (ASD) are prevalent neurodevelopmental disorders characterized by impaired language development, repetitive or stereotyped behaviors, and difficulties in socio-emotional interactions (Kanner and Eisenberg, 1957; Fonbonne, 2003). Many neuroimaging studies demonstrate that the development of the cerebellum is abnormal in children with ASD, both neuroanatomically and functionally. For instance, abnormalities in cerebellar size, morphology, and function have been reported and correlated with behavioral deficits in functional domains (Abell et al., 1999; Courchesne et al., 2001; McAlonan et al., 2002; Akshoomoff et al., 2004; McAlonan et al., 2005; Fatemi et al., 2012). Neuropathology studies have shown significant reductions in Purkinje cells (PC) in the posterior-lateral cerebellar hemisphere in brain specimens from patients with ASD (Bauman and Kemper, 1985, 2005; Ritvo et al., 1986; Bailey et al., 1998; Whitney et al., 2009). In addition, decreased size of PC in autism brain specimens has been reported (Fatemi et al., 2002).

The PC are the primary efferent neurons of the cerebellar cortex. Loss of PC may result in altered cerebellar cortical efferent signals (Tsai et al., 2012) and may be associated with some of the symptoms that have been identified in children with ASDs including problems with motor control and learning (Hoxha et al., 2013). The dentate nuclei lie in a key position within the cerebellum, serving to integrate inputs from the PC efferents (Batini et al., 1992). Previous studies have reported no changes in cell number or size of the dentate nuclei in samples of children with ASDs (Bauman and Kemper, 1985; Yip et al., 2009). However, a recent diffusion weighted MRI (DW-MRI) study demonstrated alterations in white matter in the dentatorubrothalamic pathway in high and low functioning children with ASD (Jeong et al., 2012). This study divided the dentate nucleus into four subdivisions, dorso-rostal, dorso-caudal, ventro-rostal, and ventro-caudal, in order to investigate four different dentatorubrothalamic pathways associated with motor and non-motor domains (Küper et al., 2011). It was found that children with ASD had significant differences in fractional anisotropy (FA), axial diffusivity (AD), and radial diffusivity (RD) in the dentatorubrothalamic tracts originating in both the dorso-rostal and ventro-caudal portions of the dentate nucleus compared to a typically developing (TD) control group. These diffusion changes were highly correlated with deficits in daily living skills and communication, respectively (Jeong et al., 2012).

To date, no neuroimaging studies have investigated white matter connecting the cerebellar cortex to the dentate nucleus in children with ASD. This is due to several technical challenges involved in accurately defining these pathways, and in particular, the problem of crossing fibers. In order to address this problem, the present study applied a newly developed tractography method for DW-MRI termed the "independent component analysis with a ball and stick model" (ICA+BSM) (Jeong et al., 2013). This method was developed to resolve the orientation of multiple fiber bundles in clinical DW-MRI data and thereby increase the feasibility of detecting changes in efferent white matter in young children with autism, potentially related to decreases in number and size of PC neurons in cerebellar cortex shown postmortem. In addition to the crossing fiber problem, clinical MRI scans performed on children with ASD are performed under sedation, while MRI studies of TD children performed for research purposes are conducted without sedation due to ethical issues. Comparing data in which one group is sedated and the other is not may be result in between-group differences in movement and physiological artifacts (Walker et al., 2011, 2012) related to the effects of sedation, potentially confounding the identification of hypothesized differences in diffusion metrics between diagnostic groups (i.e., ASD vs. TD). In order to address the problems of motion and physiological artifacts, we assessed the magnitude of these artifacts in the cerebellum and corrected for them using iRESTORE (Chang et al., 2012).

We hypothesized that decreased number and size of the PC may result in reduced directional coherence and detection of streamlines connecting cerebellar cortex with dentate nuclei. Decreased PC cell number and size might also cause significant changes in other conventional DW-MRI metrics such as FA, AD, RD, streamline volume (SV), and streamline count (SC) (Song et al., 2002, 2005; Budde et al., 2009; Jones et al., 2013). Such changes in DW-MRI metrics may provide *in vivo* measures related to the previous pathology findings (Bauman and Kemper, 1985; Ritvo et al., 1986; Bailey et al., 1998; Bauman and Kemper, 2005; Whitney et al., 2009). This study assessed diffusion differences between children with ASD and TD children, while assessing potential artifacts associated with these measurements.

METHODS AND MATERIALS

SUBJECTS

This study included 15 children with ASD (age: 6.2 ± 3.1 years, range: 3.6–13.3 years, 11 boys) and 14 TD children (TD, age: 6.8 ± 3.1, range = 4.0–14.0 years, 11 boys). These subjects are a subset of subjects included in a previous study of the dentatorubrothalamic pathway (Jeong et al., 2012). The children with ASD were referred from the Children's Hospital of Michigan Pediatric Neurology Clinic based upon a clinical diagnosis of autistic disorder, Asperger disorder, or pervasive developmental disorder not otherwise specified made by pediatric neurologists using the *Diagnostic and Statistical Manual of Mental Disorders, 4th edition*, criteria.

Inclusion and exclusion criterion for ASD were detailed in our previous study (Jeong et al., 2012). In brief, inclusion criteria for the study required that children with clinical diagnoses of ASD meet criteria for an autism spectrum disorder according to the ADI-R. In the present study 12 of the children met or exceeded the clinical cutoff on all three sections of the ADI-R [(a) Qualitative Abnormalities in Reciprocal Social Behavior, (b) Qualitative Abnormalities in Communication, and (c) Restricted, Repetitive, and Stereotyped Patterns of Behavior] and received diagnoses of Autistic Disorder. The remaining three children met or exceeded the cutoffs for criteria (a) and (c) and were diagnosed with Asperger's Disorder. Adaptive behavior was measured using the Vineland Adaptive Behavior Scales. The Vineland Adaptive Behavior Scales-2nd Edition (VABS) is a caregiver-reported semi-structured interview that yields measures of the child's adaptive behavior functioning in four domains (communication, daily living, socialization, and motor skills), as well as an overall adaptive behavior composite. The measure is used extensively in research studies on children with developmental disabilities and has excellent reliability and validity (Sparrow et al., 1984). Neurological disorders were excluded in the ASD group, including seizure disorders (patients with abnormal EEG without seizures were not excluded), PKU, tuberous sclerosis complex, Rett Syndrome, Fragile X, Down Syndrome and traumatic brain injury. The Human Investigation Committee at Wayne State University granted permission for the retrieval and analysis of the clinical data and MRI scans of children with ASD. Written informed consent was obtained for the children in the TD group.

MRI DATA ACQUISITION AND PROCESSING

A 3T Signa EXCITE scanner (GE Healthcare, Waukesha, WI) equipped with an eight channel phased-array head coil was utilized to acquire the whole brain DW-MRI data at $TR/TE = 12{,}500/88.7$ ms, voxel size = $1.88 \times 1.88 \times 3$ mm. A multislice single-shot echo-planer spin-echo sequence was employed to obtain the measurements at a diffusion weighting of $b = 1000\,\text{s/mm}^2$ and 55 diffusion gradient directions. An additional acquisition at $b = 0\,\text{s/mm}^2$ was also obtained to normalize the diffusion weighted signals at individual gradient directions. Parallel imaging of DW data acquired with the eight-channel EXCITE head coil was accomplished using the array spatial sensitivity encoding technique with an acceleration factor of 2. A three-dimensional fast spoiled gradient echo sequence (FSPGR) was acquired for each subject at TR/TE/TI of 9.12/3.66/400 ms, slice thickness of 1.2 mm, and planar resolution of $0.94 \times 0.94\,\text{mm}^2$. Since the participants in the ASD group underwent clinical scans, they were sedated during their scans. TD children were not sedated, but their movements were carefully monitored during the scans. In order to quantify head motion, an estimated head motion index (sum of displacements) was obtained from individual children in the TD and the ASD groups. For each child, a, $b = 0$ image was selected as a target image for co-registering the 55 $b = 1000$ images. Six motion parameters including three translation and three rotation parameters in *x,y,z* were estimated for each $b = 1000$ image using SPM 8 (http://www.fil.ion.ucl.ac.uk/spm/). For each parameter, the absolute displacement between adjacent images was averaged to assess the degree of head motion (Ling et al., 2012). The summation of the six motion assessments was used to denote the overall degree of head motion for each child.

We utilized a software package called the Tolerably Obsessive Registration and Tensor Optimization Indolent Software Ensemble (TORTOISE version 1.4.0. available from https://science.nichd.nih.gov/confluence/display/nihpd/TORTOISE) in order to (1) preprocess the DW-MRI data for correction of motion and eddy current distortion using DIFF_PREP, (2) estimate diffusion tensor data using informed Robust Estimation of Tensors by Outlier Rejection (iRESTORE) using DIFF_CALC, and (3) calculate the maps of FA, AD, and RD from the tensors of iRESTORE. The iRESTORE method utilizes an iterative non-linear least square fitting with equal weight to identify optimal outlier data on a voxel-by-voxel basis (Chang et al., 2012). It removes the identified data from consideration in the final tensor fitting, and performs conventional fitting on the remaining data points. It was designed to remove physiological noise artifacts and head motion in DW-MRI data acquired at low angular resolution.

ICA+BSM TRACTOGRAPHY

The ICA+BSM tractography was performed using the TORTOISE-corrected DW-MRI data to identify the crossing fiber components in voxels of small clusters where dimensionality reduction and BSM fitting are sequentially applied to isolate the multiple diffusion components that are independently attenuated in each direction of the diffusion sensitizing gradients (Jeong et al., 2013). An eleven-neighborhood window was defined at each voxel of the white matter to create a diffusion data matrix with row vectors indicating the diffusion-weighted signals at every voxel of the window. Multiple diffusion tensors (up to 3) were estimated by iterating two complementary steps, hidden source decomposition using fast ICA and the multi-compartment ball-stick model.The resulting tensors were utilized to resolve the major fiber directions existing at the voxel and were finally applied for subsequent tractography. At each seeding point, tracking was started in the direction of the most prominent stick compartment. The step size was 0.2 voxels width, and the turning angle threshold was 60°. The propagation direction was calculated by applying trilinear interpolation on the directions of the stick compartments having a fraction >0.15, provided from 8 nearby voxels of the current point. For each nearby voxel, only the direction that had the smallest turning angle was considered for interpolation. In order to smooth the streamlines, each subsequent direction was determined by the previous direction with 0.5 weighting and the incoming direction with 0.5 weighting.

VISUALIZATION OF TRACTS CONNECTING THE CEREBELLAR CORTEX WITH THE DENTATE NUCLEI

To generate tracts containing the PC efferent fibers from the ICA+BSM tractography of individual subjects, the current study defined seeding points at the posterior-lateral region of the cerebellar cortex (e.g., cerebellum crus 1 and 2). The conventional FreeSurfer process (http://surfer.nmr.mgh.harvard.edu) was applied to the high resolution FSPGR images in order to segment the cerebellar cortex in each hemisphere. The resulting cerebellar cortex was then masked by the standard templates of cerebellum crus 1 and 2 (available at http://www.cyceron.fr/index.php/fr/plateforme/freeware). To seed the streamlines containing the PC efferent fibers, the masked region was finally registered to the b0 image via rigid body transformation using SPM 8 (http://www.fil.ion.ucl.ac.uk/spm/). A total of 2000 seeding points were uniformly distributed over all the voxels of the registered seed region.

An ROI approach was utilized to sort the tracts connecting from the seed region to each of two dentate ROIs, the dorsal dentate nucleus (DDN) and the ventral dentate nucleus (VDN), which are considered to be the motor and non-motor domains of the dentate nucleus (Küper et al., 2011). The two subdivisions of the dentate nucleus in template space [using "Spatially Unbiased Infratentorial Template (SUIT)"] were separately transformed into the FSPGR space of the individual subjects by applying the inverse of the deformation field that fits the cerebellar cortex of the individual FSPGR image to that of the SUIT space (Diedrichsen, 2006, available at http://www.icn.ucl.ac.uk/motorcontrol/imaging/suit.htm). The SUIT normalized ROIs in the FSPGR space were registered to the b0 space by applying the rigid body transformation obtained between the FSPGR and b0 image using SPM 8 (http://www.fil.ion.ucl.ac.uk/spm/). **Figure 1** illustrates an example of the cerebellar cortex seeding ROIs and the two dentate subregion sorting ROIs (DDN, VDN) that were objectively located in the b0 image. For each of the pathways projecting to the DDN and VDN, a streamline visitation map was created by the number of streamlines passing each voxel. Voxels having more than 5 visits were assumed to belong to each pathway, and the values of FA, AD, and RD for the voxels in each pathway was averaged for comparison. SV was measured by summing the volume of all voxels belonging to the pathway. SC was calculated by counting the total number streamlines per pathway. FA, AD, RD, SC, and SV were separately measured for each pathway bilaterally and compared to quantify diffusion metrics potentially associated with decreased PC size and number in children with ASD.

STATISTICAL ANALYSIS

Separate multi-variate general linear model analyses using four different dependent variables (left DDN, left VDN, right DDN,

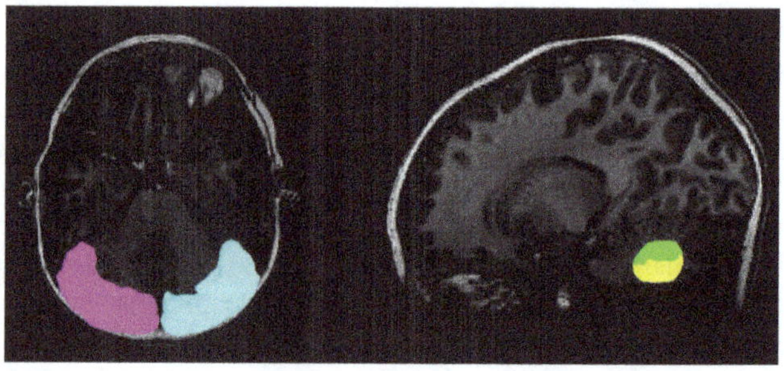

FIGURE 1 | Regions of interest to track streamlines containing PC efferent axons. The posterior-lateral cortex of the cerebellum (seed region, magenta for left, cyan for right) and two subdivisions of the dentate nucleus (target region, green for DDN, yellow for VDN) were objectively placed for the tractography using the SUIT normalization procedure.

right VDN) were applied for each diffusion parameter to investigate differences between the TD and ASD groups. For these analyses, age and head-motion were used as covariates where head-motion was assessed for the individual subjects by summing the absolute differences of displacement estimates between adjacent $b = 1000$ images in six motion parameters, including three translations and three rotations (Ling et al., 2012). Finally, all diffusion parameters were correlated with developmental and behavioral variables (VABS assessments of motor, communication, daily living skills, and socialization) within the ASD group. For these analyses, age and head-motion were used as covariates, and partial Pearson correlation coefficients were obtained. SPSS 21.0 was used for the statistical analyses.

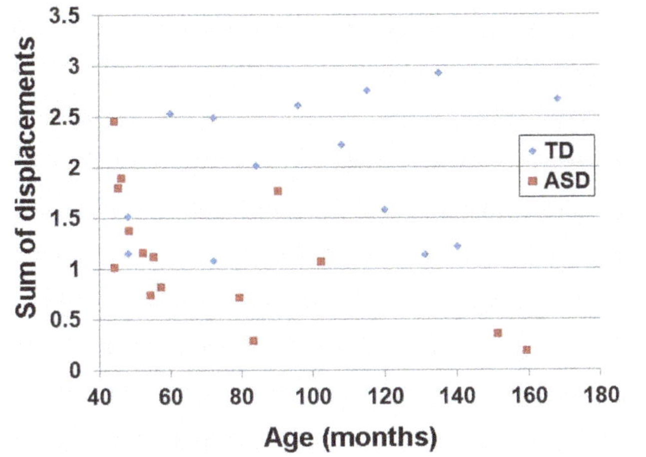

FIGURE 2 | Estimated head motion index (sum of displacements) obtained from individual children in the TD and the ASD groups. For each child, *a*, $b = 0$ image was selected as a target image for co-registering the 55 $b = 1000$ images. Six motion parameters including three translation and three rotation parameters in *x,y,z* were estimated for each $b = 1000$ image. For each parameter, the absolute displacement between adjacent images was averaged to assess the degree of head motion (Ling et al., 2012). The summation of the six motion assessments was used to denote overall degree of head motion for each child. Note that this index has no unit since two physical metrics (mm and radian) are summed.

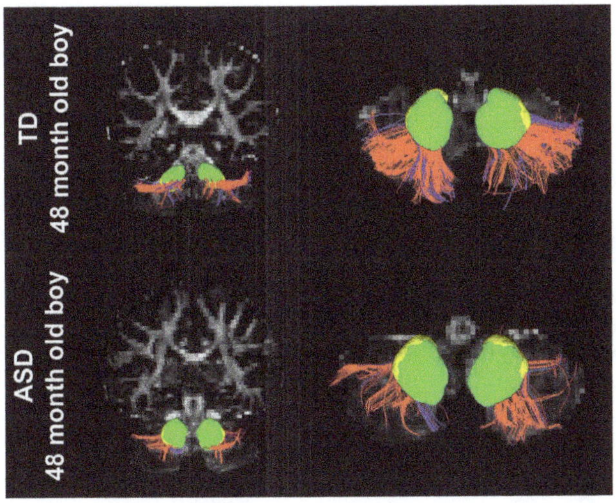

FIGURE 3 | Streamlines connecting the posterior-lateral cerebellar cortex with the DDN (red) and the VDN (blue) in two age-matched boys, (top) TD and (bottom) ASD. It is visually apparent that the boy with ASD shows significantly reduced streamline number and volume compared to the TD child; total streamline volume of both sides = 13985 and 8933 mm^3 for the TD child and the child with ASD, respectively.

RESULTS

ASSESSMENT OF MOTION AND PHYSIOLOGICAL ARTIFACTS

The estimated head motion index (sum of displacements) obtained from individual children in the TD and the ASD groups is shown in **Figure 2**. Head motion is higher in the TD group than in the ASD group, as expected due to sedation of the ASD group (group average ± standard deviation of the sum of motion displacements: 2.00 ± 0.67 for the TD group and 1.12 ± 0.63 for the ASD group). Analyses with iRESTORE identified more outlier

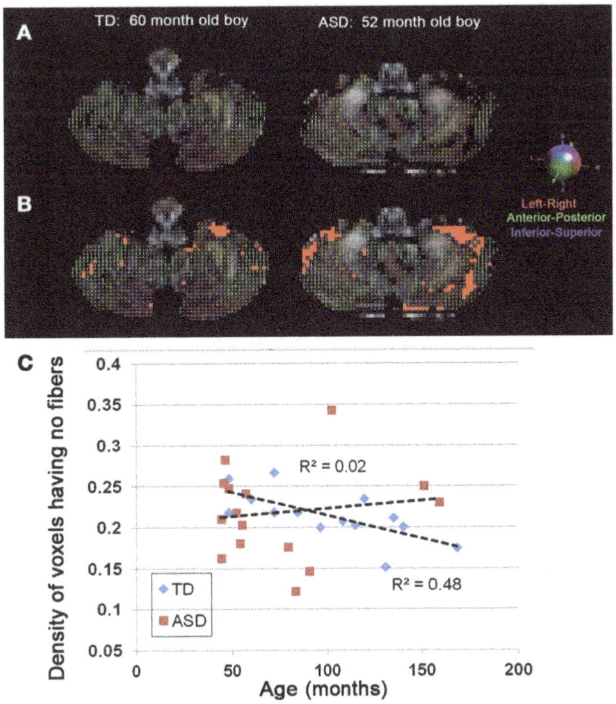

FIGURE 4 | (A) Directions of stick compartments obtained by the ICA+BSM in two boys, (left) TD and (right) ASD. Each colored bar represents primary orientation of individual axonal bundle within the voxel of cerebellar white matter. **(B)** Voxels having no stick compartments were denoted by red boxes. **(C)** The density of cerebellar voxels having no stick compartments was evaluated in individual children in both the TD and ASD groups. To avoid a confound of size of the cerebellum, the total number of voxels having no stick compartments was normalized by total number of voxels in entire cerebellum which yields the density of voxels having no stick compartments. The TD group shows a significant age-related decrease in the density of voxels having no stick compartments ($R^2 = 0.48$, $p = 0.0044$), while the ASD group shows no age related decrease ($R^2 = 0.02$, $p = 0.619$).

data points in the TD group (9.1 ± 1.3%) than in the ASD group (7.2 ± 0.6%).

VISUALIZATION OF TRACTS CONNECTING THE CEREBELLAR CORTEX WITH THE DENTATE NUCLEI

Figure 3 shows representative examples of streamlines connecting the cerebellar cortex and the dentate nuclei in age-matched boys with TD and ASD. It is visually apparent in this figure that the SV in the posterio-lateral cerebellar cortex is reduced in the child with ASD, compared with the TD child. Although the decrease in streamlines was striking in some children with ASD as shown here, there was great variability among the children in the group. Both SC and SV were significantly lower only in the pathway projecting to the right VDN ($p = 0.015$ and 0.048 for SC and SV, respectively) in ASD group, compared to the TD group. Representative examples of directional compartments of streamlines identified by the ICA+BSM tractography (i.e., primary eigenvectors of the stick compartments) are shown in **Figure 4A**. The directional stick compartments are reduced near the voxels of the cerebellar cortex in the child with ASD (marked by red in **Figure 4B**), which may result in fewer streamlines in the child with ASD, compared with the TD child. Interestingly, age-related reduction of no stick voxels normalized by total cerebellum volume (i.e., density of voxels having no fibers) was notable in the TD group ($R^2 = 0.48$, $p = 0.0044$) but not in the ASD group ($R^2 = 0.02$, $p = 0.619$, **Figure 4C**).

COMPARISON OF DIFFUSION PARAMETERS

Tables 1, 2 summarize changes in four different diffusion parameters measured along pathways connecting the posterior-lateral cerebellar cortex with the dentate nuclei obtained from the TD and ASD groups. The mean values of the diffusion parameters showing significant group differences are given in **Figure 5A**. The multi-variate analyses revealed that FA was significantly lower in three pathways in the ASD group, compared to the TD group: pathways projecting to the right DDN ($p = 0.008$) and pathways projecting to the VDN bilaterally (left: $p = 0.020$, right: $p = 0.010$). In the left VDN and the right DDN, the reduced FA was apparent at all ages in children with ASD (**Figure 5B**). AD was significantly lower in the pathway projecting to the left DDN ($p =$

Table 1 | Fractional anisotropy (FA), axial diffusivity (AD), and radial diffusivity (RD) of the pathways connecting the posterior-lateral cerebellar cortex with the dentate nuclei.

Pathway	Group	*FA*		*AD* [10^4 mm/s^2]		*RD* [10^4 mm/s^2]	
		Mean ± *SD*	*p*-value	Mean ± *SD*	*p*-value	Mean ± *SD*	*p*-value
Left DDN	TD	0.27 ± 0.03	0.083	8.97 ± 0.37	0.002**	5.76 ± 0.44	0.956
	ASD	0.24 ± 0.03		8.46 ± 0.38		5.85 ± 0.38	
	$TD_{\le 5y.o}$	0.26 ± 0.03	0.161	9.14 ± 0.23	0.000**	5.93 ± 0.57	0.640
	$ASD_{\le 5y.o}$	0.23 ± 0.03		8.53 ± 0.25		6.04 ± 0.33	
	$TD_{>5y.o}$	0.28 ± 0.03	0.224	8.53 ± 0.25	0.054	5.66 ± 0.34	0.552
	$ASD_{>5y.o}$	0.26 ± 0.02		8.36 ± 0.54		5.56 ± 0.28	
Left VDN	TD	0.27 ± 0.03	0.020*	9.13 ± 1.12	0.040*	6.03 ± 0.80	0.273
	ASD	0.24 ± 0.02		8.51 ± 0.78		5.90 ± 0.32	
	$TD_{\le 5y.o}$	0.25 ± 0.03	0.071	9.06 ± 0.47	0.094	6.02 ± 0.49	0.9556
	$ASD_{\le 5y.o}$	0.23 ± 0.03		8.60 ± 0.44		6.03 ± 0.29	
	$TD_{>5y.o}$	0.27 ± 0.03	0.121	9.17 ± 1.40	0.219	6.04 ± 0.96	0.421
	$ASD_{>5y.o}$	0.25 ± 0.02		8.39 ± 0.54		5.70 ± 0.26	
Right DDN	TD	0.28 ± 0.03	0.008*	9.06 ± 0.97	0.514	5.76 ± 1.00	0.396
	ASD	0.24 ± 0.04		8.84 ± 0.51		5.93 ± 0.44	
	$TD_{\le 5y.o}$	0.28 ± 0.02	0.092	9.15 ± 0.40	0.181	5.74 ± 0.43	0.505
	$ASD_{\le 5y.o}$	0.24 ± 0.04		8.87 ± 0.31		5.91 ± 0.44	
	$TD_{>5y.o}$	0.29 ± 0.04	0.0161*	9.03 ± 1.20	0.673	5.78 ± 1.23	0.727
	$ASD_{>5y.o}$	0.24 ± 0.02		9.03 ± 1.20		5.97 ± 0.48	
Right VDN	TD	0.27 ± 0.03	0.010*	9.03 ± 1.24	0.630	5.84 ± 1.29	0.316
	ASD	0.23 ± 0.03		8.80 ± 0.52		6.05 ± 0.59	
	$TD_{\le 5y.o}$	0.26 ± 0.02	0.083	9.10 ± 0.45	0.221	5.59 ± 0.25	0.1222
	$ASD_{\le 5y.o}$	0.23 ± 0.03		9.10 ± 0.45		5.94 ± 0.43	
	$TD_{>5y.o}$	0.27 ± 0.03	0.030*	8.98 ± 1.55	0.780	5.99 ± 1.61	0.7667
	$ASD_{>5y.o}$	0.23 ± 0.01		8.79 ± 0.72		6.20 ± 0.78	

DDN, dorsal dentate nucleus; VDN, ventral dentate nucleus; SD, standard deviation; Group mean and SD were reported for TD (n = 14), ASD (n = 15).
**, **p-value < 0.05 and 0.005, respectively (α = 0.05).*

Table 2 | Streamline count (SC) and streamline volume (SV) of the pathways connecting cerebellar cortex to the dentate nuclei.

Pathway	Group	*SC*		*SV* [mm³]	
		Mean ± *SD*	***p*-value**	**Mean ± *SD***	***p*-value**
Left DDN	TD	328.86 ± 245.73	0.511	4822.93 ± 2483.78	0.776
	ASD	221.23 ± 143.57		3668.28 ± 1676.55	
	$TD_{\leq 5y.o}$	226.40 ± 146.10	0.400	3896.02 ± 1735.3	0.593
	$ASD_{\leq 5y.o}$	314.33 ± 195.65		4485.94 ± 2012.32	
	$TD_{>5y.o}$	385.78 ± 277.92	0.189	5337.88 ± 2771.98	0.579
	$ASD_{>5y.o}$	222.00 ± 85.46		4665.23 ± 870.83	
Left VDN	TD	401.64 ± 291.83	0.230	5258.36 ± 2660.71	0.333
	ASD	198.27 ± 134.62		3304.01 ± 1558.77	
	$TD_{\leq 5y.o}$	307.40 ± 73.39	0.544	4665.23 ± 870.83	0.354
	$ASD_{\leq 5y.o}$	253.00 ± 183.93		3932.81 ± 1777.67	
	$TD_{>5y.o}$	454.00 ± 356.47	0.172	5517.18 ± 3259.20	0.431
	$ASD_{>5y.o}$	234.17 ± 114.64		4389.26 ± 1033.49	
Right DDN	TD	430.93 ± 219.79	0.196	5604.90 ± 1962.33	0.416
	ASD	271.19 ± 153.14		4048.79 ± 1557.02	
	$TD_{\leq 5y.o}$	360.40 ± 178.18	0.305	5174.30 ± 1688.04	0.446
	$ASD_{\leq 5y.o}$	286.11 ± 85.31		4599.61 ± 1068.87	
	$TD_{>5y.o}$	470.11 ± 240.39	0.389	5844.13 ± 2156.96	0.462
	$ASD_{>5y.o}$	470.11 ± 240.39		4981.64 ± 2160.28	
Right VDN	TD	533.34 ± 247.84	0.015*	5990.62 ± 1967.36	0.048*
	ASD	279.38 ± 124.69		3769.70 ± 1376.23	
	$TD_{\leq 5y.o}$	487.80 ± 212.29	0.064	6039.14 ± 752.26	0.017*
	$ASD_{\leq 5y.o}$	305.33 ± 126.87		4348.83 ± 1223.67	
	$TD_{>5y.o}$	558.78 ± 274.33	0.050	5963.66 ± 2450.37	0.215
	$ASD_{>5y.o}$	296.17 ± 131.23		4510.55 ± 1424.99	

*DDN, dorsal part of dentate nucleus; VDN, ventral part of dentate nucleus; SD, standard deviation; Group mean and SD were reported for TD (n = 14), ASD (n = 15). *p-value < 0.005, respectively (α = 0.05).*

0.002) and to the left VDN ($p = 0.040$) in ASD group, compared to the TD group. However, RD was not significantly different in any of the pathways in ASD group compared to the TD group. Both SC and SV were significantly lower in the pathway projecting to right VDN in ASD group, compared to the TD group ($p = 0.015$, 0.048 for SC and SV, respectively). The FA difference between the ASD and TD groups for the right DDN pathway was more significant in older children (>5 y.o, **Table 1**), while the reduced AD in left DDN and VDN, and SV in the right VDN were more prominent in younger children (≤5 y.o, **Tables 1, 2**).

Figure 6 presents the cumulative density functions of FA, AD, SC, and SV measured from separate pathways showing significant changes between the TD and ASD groups. The ASD group shows significantly higher probability to have lower FA (left VDN, right DDN, right VDN), lower AD (left DDN, left VDN), lower SC (right VDN), and lower SV (right VDN) than the TD group, probably due to the reduced directional coherence of streamlines in ASD group. Furthermore, as reported in **Table 3**, FA was 3 standard errors below the mean of the TD group in 10 of 15 ASD cases (67%) for the right DDN pathway. For the right VDN pathway, a total 11 of the 15 ASD cases (73%) showed the reduced FA being 3 standard errors below the mean of the TD group.

There was a trend for a positive correlation between FA of right DDN and daily living skills ($R = 0.39$, $p = 0.084$). There were no other correlations between diffusion parameters (AD, RD, SC, SV) and VABS variables (communication, socialization, and motor skills).

DISCUSSION

The present study demonstrates that the ICA+BSM tractography method can be used to detect differences in the cerebellar white matter that contain PC efferent pathways. Although the pathological origin of reduced directional coherence remains unclear in DW-MRI, the decreases in FA, AD, SC, and SV in the ASD group were hypothesized based upon previous pathology studies showing reduced numbers and size of PC in postmortem brain from subjects with autism (Bauman and Kemper, 1985, 2005; Ritvo et al., 1986; Bailey et al., 1998; Fatemi et al., 2002; Whitney et al., 2009). In addition to decreased numbers and size of PC in ASDs, there is also evidence for neuroinflammation throughout the brain in ASD; such inflammation is reported to be more prominent in cerebellum (Vargas et al., 2005; Suzuki et al., 2013). Changes associated with glial proliferation and inflammatory processes might be one source of the decreased directional

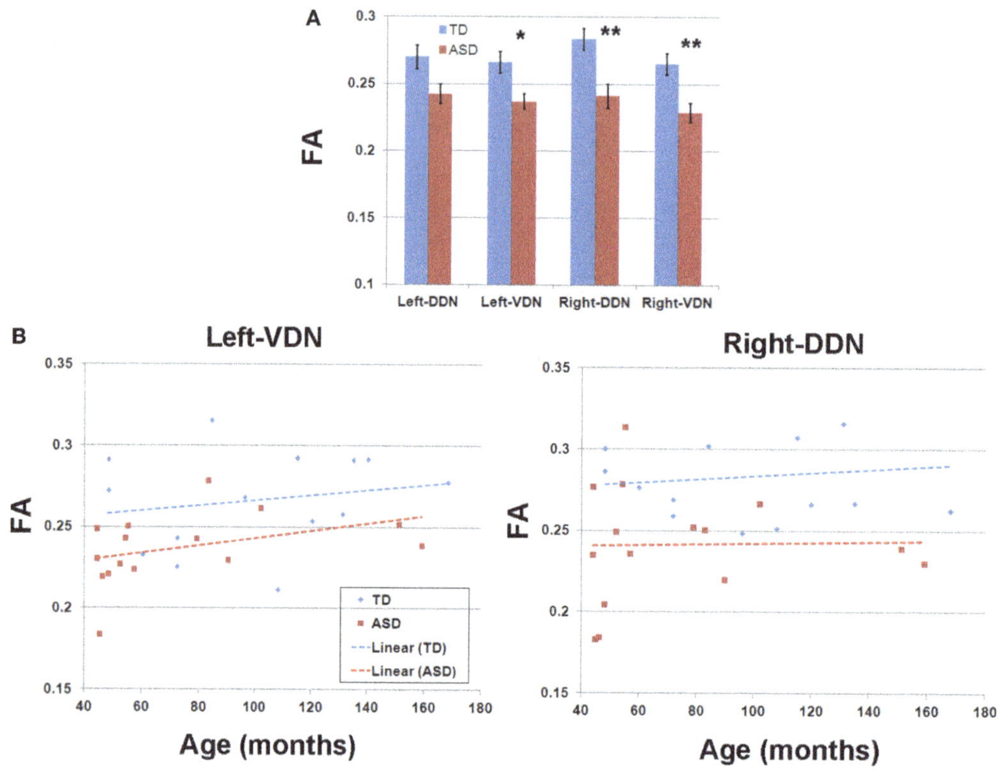

FIGURE 5 | (A) Group mean values and standard errors of fractional anisotropy (FA) obtained from four pathways of the PC efferent streamlines. *, ***p*-value < 0.05 and 0.005, respectively ($\alpha = 0.05$). **(B)** FA values and ages of individual subjects obtained from left VDN pathway (left) and right DDN pathway (right) showing the most significant group differences.

coherence in children with ASD observed in the present study. We found that 73.3% of children with ASD (11 of 15 studied ASD cases, **Table 3**) showed reduced FA in fibers connecting cerebellar cortex to right VDN using a threshold 3 standard errors below the mean of the TD group. Similarly, Palmen et al. reported that 72.4% of subjects with ASD (21 of 29 studied cases) had a decreased number of PC (Palmen et al., 2004). Thus, the diffusion methods in the current study detected white matter pathology in pathways connecting the lateral cerebellar cortex to the dentate nuclei in a similar portion of cases as in postmortem pathology showing decreased PC in lateral posterio-lateral cerebellar cortex.

The mechanisms for the observed decreases in numbers of PC and other cerebellar pathology may reflect different etiologies. There is evidence for ASD genetic risk factors involving mutations in genes involved in cerebellar development such as Engrailed2 (Gharani et al., 2004) and the tuberous sclerosis genes TSC1 and TSC2 (Reith et al., 2011, 2013; Tsai et al., 2012), maternal infection and preterm birth (Pinto-Martin et al., 2011; Limperopoulos et al., 2014). Each mechanism might involve different aspects of PC development and maintenance. For example, PC might not be sufficiently generated, may fail to migrate to the proper layer or may degenerate later in development. There is evidence from human pathology studies that cells are formed, but are then lost. Bauman and Kemper (1994) hypothesized that that the PC loss occurred early in development at or before 30 weeks of gestation, associated with absence of glial cell hyperplasia and the preservation of neurons in the inferior olive. Whitney et al. (2009) suggested that PC are lost during the last trimester or early postnatal period potentially due to the preservation of basket and stellate cells in neuropathology samples from autistic subjects where there is PC loss. More recently, Wegiel et al. (2013) compared autism and control postmortem tissue and focused on the floccular region of cerebellar cortex. They reported focal areas of dysplasia in the flocculus with not only decreased PC, but also misaligned PC and loss of basket and stellate cells.

Mouse models in which the tuberous sclerosis genes TSC1 (Tsai et al., 2012) or TSC2 (Reith et al., 2013) are knocked down specifically in PC produced an increase in PC size followed by a progressive loss of PC. PC loss has been reported in two of four patients with TSC (Reith et al., 2011). Cerebellar abnormalities have also been shown following hypoxic or hypoxic-ischemic forebrain injury at postnatal day 2 in the neonatal rat (Biran et al., 2011). In this model, there were decreased numbers of PC and a decrease in the thickness of the molecular cell layer in multiple cerebellar lobules at postnatal day 21. The timing of the injury in this model would be similar to a very preterm infant born at 28 weeks gestation. An increased risk of ASD has been reported in preterm infants (Pinto-Martin et al., 2011) and infants with very low birthweight (Moss and Chugani, 2014). Furthermore, injury to the premature cerebellum in humans was significantly linked to

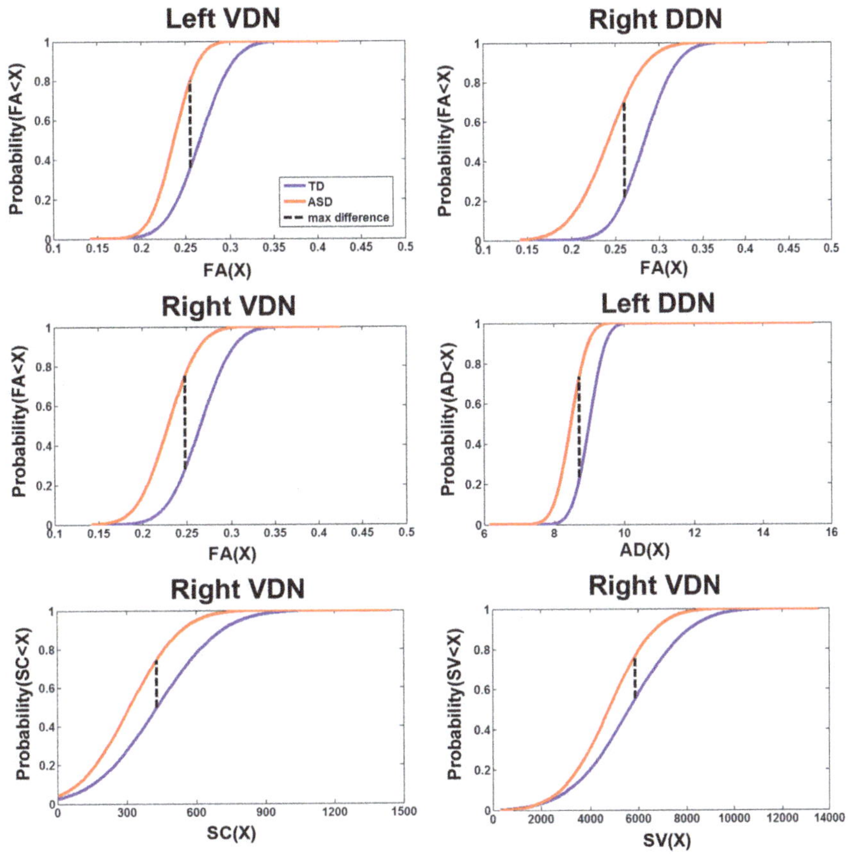

FIGURE 6 | Cumulative density functions of the diffusion parameters showing the significant group differences reported in Figure 5A. Probabilities (parameter ≤X) were measured from the TD ($n = 14$) and ASD ($n = 15$) groups in the corresponding pathways showing significant group differences. The ASD group shows significantly higher probability to have a reduction in each parameter than the TD group in all pathways.

Table 3 | Percentage of children with ASD showing significant changes in diffusivity parameters in the pathways connecting the cerebellar cortex with the dentate nuclei compared to the values of the TD group.

Pathway	Criterion	*FA*	*AD*	*RD*	*SC*	*SV*
Left DDN	<lower 10% (TD)	27	53	0	0	0
	<Mean(TD)—3*SE(TD)	60	73	13	27	20
Left VDN	<lower 10% (TD)	33	0	0	0	7
	<Mean(TD)—3*SE(TD)	53	27	13	33	20
Right DDN	<lower 10% (TD)	53	0	0	0	7
	<Mean(TD)—3*SE(TD)	73	13	7	27	20
Right VDN	<lower 10% (TD)	47	0	0	7	0
	<Mean(TD)—3*SE(TD)	67	7	0	40	33

DDN, dorsal dentate nucleus; VDN, ventral dentate nucleus; SE, standard error; Group mean and SE were evaluated from TD (n = 14) and ASD (n = 15).

autism (Limperopoulos et al., 2014). Preterm birth has also been associated with prenatal infection. Utilizing two mouse models, one involving maternal infection with the influenza virus, a second of maternal inflammation using poly I:C, Shi et al. (2009) found decreased numbers of PC and heterotopic PC in lobule VII, as well as delayed migration of granule cells in lobules VI and VII. Thus, there is evidence for multiple genetic and environmental risks for ASD that may lead to decreased PC number with or without changes in other cerebellar cell types and affecting different cerebellar cortical regions.

LIMITATIONS OF THE STUDY

Two common problems encountered in DW-MRI are (1) head motion and physiological artifacts (i.e., cardiac pulsation) and (2) the existence of multiple fiber orientations within an imaging voxel (referred to as the "intra-voxel crossing fiber problem"). A recent study reported that head motion resulted in a positive bias for the calculation of FA even though a standard correction method was applied to DW-MRI data (Ling et al., 2012). Indeed, it was also found that cardiac pulsation might influence the diffusion signals leading to over-estimation of the FA in cerebellum and underestimation of the FA in the genu and splenium of the corpus callosum in healthy adults (Walker et al., 2011). Since the ASD group was sedated and the TD group was not, there likely was more motion in the TD group. In addition, sedation of the ASD group may have systemically affected the heart rate and the breathing cycle resulting in altered patterns of physiological noise in the ASD group compared to the TD group. These types of artifacts were reported to be dominant in cerebellum (Walker et al., 2011, 2012).

To minimize the effects of these artifacts on the quality of the DW-MRI data, the present study utilized the iRESTORE tensor fitting to reduce variance and normalize the mean value of the metrics (Walker et al., 2011; Chang et al., 2012). iRESTORE fitting minimizes the variability of the metrics in the cerebellum by removing artifacts produced by both uncorrected head motion and the physiological noise including cardiac pulsation and respiration drop-out. Even though the iRESTORE tensor fitting was utilized to minimize the effect of physiological artifacts in both groups, the fitting algorithm might not correct the artifacts at all cerebellar voxels since the present study acquired the data without cardiac gating. In order to further correct for head motion, amount of head movement was included as a covariate in the statistical analyses. The group differences (i.e., $\sim$10% reduction in FA) remained statistically significant even after covarying for age and head motion.

To address the intra-voxel crossing fiber problem, we utilized a novel tractography model called "ICA+BSM" which can provide the most accurate recovery of multiple streamlines in clinical DWI data, compared with other tractography methods (Jeong et al., 2013). Although the ICA+BSM was utilized to solve the problem of crossing fibers in the present study, it may not guarantee a complete solution for every voxel. In addition, the present study utilized SC as a measure of probable connection between the seeding region and the sorting ROI. Thus, the false estimates of PC efferent related streamlines may reflect uncertain change in geometry such as curvature, density, and length, suggesting that SC may be suboptimal to measure the degree of probable connection in PC efferent fibers (Jones et al., 2013). Further, the present study defined seeding points only in posterior-lateral cortex of cerebellum (see **Figure 1**) and therefore the methodology in the present this study would not detect PC pathology in other cerebellar cortical regions.

Additional limitations of the present study include the large age range of participants, the small sample size, the use of clinical diagnosis with ADI-R without a measure of direct observation (i.e., Autism Diagnostic Observation Schedule, ADOS) which is the current gold standard diagnostic instrument, and limited spatial-angular resolution of DWI data including the relatively small number of diffusion sensitizing gradients at a single b value. In addition, although the main connection between the cerebellar cortex and the dentate nuclei consists of PC efferent fibers, there is evidence of reciprocal afferents from the dentate to the cerebellum in several species (Brown and Graybiel, 1976; Tolbert et al., 1978). Finally, the apparent hemispheric asymmetry (more differences detected in pathways on the right side) in our study might be related to incomplete spatial normalization to identify cerebellar cortex and dentate nucleus in children with ASD. Although the present study successfully imaged changes in tracts containing PC efferent streamlines by combining conventional SUIT approach with FreeSurfer analysis, the current SUIT normalization scheme was reported to achieve about 94% of maximal overlap across participants and $\pm$1.5 mm of registration error to locate the dentate nucleus in x-y-z axis (Diedrichsen et al., 2011). The error probably increases in younger children with ASD due to greater mismatch to the template. On the other hand, the right lateralized findings are consistent with other studies reporting differences in function in right and left cerebellum. For example, strongly right lateralized cerebellar intrinsic functional connectivity in the posterior lobe of cerebellum (crus I and II) with contralateral cerebral association cortex was reported in a study using resting state fMRI (Wang et al., 2013). Finally, functional asymmetries of tryptophan metabolism in cerebellum in children with ASD were also detected on α-^{11}C-methyl-L-tryptophan positron emission tomography (Chugani et al., 1997; Eluvathingal et al., 2006).

CONCLUSION

In summary, we used diffusion weighted MRI tractography to investigate whether structural abnormalities in cerebellar white matter (i.e., decreased PC numbers and size) that have been identified in postmortem specimens of individuals with ASD diagnoses could be detected *in vivo* in children with ASDs. Using this method we found reduced number and volume of streamlines from cerebellar cortex to dentate nuclei and reduced directional coherence in children with ASD diagnoses compared to TD children. Importantly, this method detected the white matter abnormalities at a similar proportion as has been reported in postmortem studies of ASD samples. Still, given the some of the limitations discussed above, these results are preliminary and further validation of this approach and replication of the above findings are warranted.

REFERENCES

Abell, F., Krams, M., Ashburner, J., Passingham, R., Friston, K., Frackowiak, R., et al. (1999). The neuroanatomy of autism: a voxel-based whole brain analysis of structural scans. Neuroreport 10, 1647–1651. doi: 10.1097/00001756-199906030-00005

Akshoomoff, N., Lord, C., Lincoln, A. J., Courchesne, R. Y., Carper, R. A., Townsend, J., et al. (2004). Outcome classification of preschool children with autism spectrum disorders using MRI brain measures. J. Am. Acad. Child Adolesc. Psychiatry 43, 349–357. doi: 10.1097/00004583-200403000-00018

Bailey, A., Luthert, P., Dean, A., Harding, B., Janota, I., Montgomery, M., et al. (1998). A clinicopathological study of autism. Brain 121, 889–905. doi: 10.1093/brain/121.5.889

Batini, C., Compoint, C., Buisseret-Delmas, H., Danile, M., and Guegan, M. (1992). Cerebellar nuclei and the nucleocortical projections in the rat: retrograde tracking coupled to GABA and glutamate immunohistochemistry. J. Comp. Neurol. 315, 74–84. doi: 10.1002/cne.903150106

Bauman, M. L., and Kemper, T. L. (1985). Histoanatomic observations of the brain in early infantile autism. Neurology 35, 866–874. doi: 10.1212/WNL.35.6.866 Bauman, M. L., and Kemper, T. L. (1994). "Neuroanatomic observations of the brain in autism," in The Neurobiology of Autism, eds M. L. Bauman and T. L. Kemper (Baltimore: The Johns Hopkins University Press), 119–145.

Bauman, M. L., and Kemper, T. L. (2005). Neuroanatomic observations of the brain in autism: a review and future directions. Int. J. Dev. Neurosci. 23, 183–187. doi: 10.1016/j.ijdevneu.2004.09.006

Biran, V., Heine, V. M., Verney, C., Sheldon, R. A., Vexler, Z. S., Rowitch, D. H., et al.(2011). Cerebellar abnormalities following hypoxia alone compared to hypoxic-ischemic forebrain injury in the developing rat brain. Neurobiol. Dis. 41, 138–146. doi: 10.1016/j.nbd.2010.09.001

Brown, G. B., and Graybiel, A. M. (1976). Afferents to the cerebellar cortex in the cat: evidence for an intrinsic pathway leading from the deep nuclei to the cortex. Brain Res. 110, 601–611. doi: 10.1016/0006-8993(76)90869-6

Budde, M. D., Xie, M., Cross, A. H., and Song, S. K. (2009). Axial diffusivity is the primary correlate of axonal injury in the experimental autoimmune encephalomyelitis spinal cord: a quantitative pixelwise analysis. J. Neurosci. 29, 2805–2815. doi: 10.1523/JNEUROSCI.4605-08.2009

Chang, L. C., Walker, L., and Pierpaoli, C. (2012). Informed RESTORE: a method for robust estimation of diffusion tensor from low redundancy datasets in the presence of physiological noise artifacts. Magn. Reson. Med. 68, 1654–1663. doi: 10.1002/mrm.24173

Chugani, D. C., Muzik, O., Rothermel, R., Behen, M., Chakraborty, P., Mangner, T., et al. (1997). Altered serotonin synthesis in the dentatothalamocortical pathway in autistic boys. Ann. Neurol. 42, 666–669. doi: 10.1002/ana.410420420

Courchesne, E., Karns, C. M., Davis, H. R., Ziccardi, R., Carper, R. A., Tigue, Z. D., et al. (2001). Unusual brain growth patterns in early life in patients with autistic disorder: an MRI study. Neurology 57, 245–254. doi: 10.1212/WNL. 57.2.245

Diedrichsen, J. (2006). A spatially unbiased atlas template of the human cerebellum. Neuroimage 33, 127–138. doi: 10.1016/j.neuroimage.2006.05.056

Diedrichsen, J., Maderwald, S., Küper, M., Thürling, M., Rabe, K., Gizweski, E. R., et al. (2011). Imaging the deep cerebellar nuclei: a probabilistic atlas and normalization procedure. Neuroimage 54, 1786–1794. doi: 10.1016/j.neuroimage.2010.10.035

Eluvathingal, T. J., Behen, M. E., Chugani, H. T., Janisse, J., Bernardi, B., Chakraborty, P., et al. (2006). Cerebellar lesions in tuberous sclerosis complex: neurobehavioral and neuroimaging correlates. J. Child Neurol. 21, 846–851. doi: 10.1177/08830738060210100301

Fatemi, S. H., Aldinger, K. A., Ashwood, P., Bauman, M. L., Blaha, C. D., Blatt, G. J., et al. (2012). Consensus paper: pathological role of the cerebellum in autism. Cerebellum, 11, 777–807. doi: 10.1007/s12311-012-0355-9

Fatemi, S. H., Halt, A. R., Realmuto, G., Earle, J., Kist, D. A., Thuras, P., et al. (2002). Purkinje cell size is reduced in cerebellum of patients with autism. Cell. Mol. Neurobiol. 22, 171–175. doi: 10.1023/A:1019861721160

Fonbonne, E. (2003). Epidemiological surveys of autism and other pervasive developmental disorders: an update. J. Autism Dev. Disord 33, 365–382. doi: 10.1023/A:1025054610557

Gharani, N., Benayed, R., Mancuso, V., and Brzustowicz, L. M., Millonig, J.

H. (2004). Association of the homeobox transcription factor, ENGRAILED 2, 3, with autism spectrum disorder. Mol. Psychiatry. 9, 474–484. doi: 10.1038/sj.mp.4001498

Hoxha, E., Tonini, R., Montarolo, F., Croci, L., Consalez, G. G., and Temapia, F. (2013). Motor dysfunction and cerebellar Purkinje cell firing impart- ment in Ebf2 null mice. Mol. Cell. Neurosci. 52, 51–61. doi: 10.1016/j.mcn.2012.09.002

Jeong, J. W., Asano, E., Yeh, F. C., Chugani, D. C., and Chugani, H. T. (2013). Independent component analysis tractography combined with a ball-stick model to isolate intravoxel crossing fibers of the corticospinal tracts in clinical diffusion MRI. Magn. Reson. Med. 70, 441–53. doi: 10.1002/mrm. 24487

Jeong, J. W., Chugani, D. C., Behen, M. E., Tiwari, V. N., and Chugani, H. T. (2012). Altered white matter structure of the dentatorubrothalamic pathway in children with autistic spectrum disorders. Cerebellum 114, 957–971. doi: 10.1007/s12311-012-0369-3

Jones, D. K., Knösche, T. R., and Turner, R. (2013). White matter intergrity, fiber count, and other fallacies: The do's and don'ts of diffusion MRI. Neuroimage 73, 239–254. doi: 10.1016/j.neuroimage.2012.06.081

Kanner, L., and Eisenberg, L. (1957). Early infantile autism. Psychiatr. Res. Rep. Am. Psychiatr. Assoc. 7, 55–65.

Küper, M., Dimitrova, A., Thürling, M., Maderwald, S., Roths, J., Elles, H. G., et al. (2011). Evidence for a motor and a non-motor domain in the human dentate nucleus-an fMRI study. Neuroimage 54, 2612–2622. doi: 10.1016/j.neuroimage.2010.11.028

Limperopoulos, C., Chilingaryan, G., Sullivan, N., Guizard, N., Robertson, R. L., and du Plessis, A. J. (2014). Injury to the premature cerebellum: outcome is related to remote cortical development. Cereb. Cortex 24, 728–736. doi: 10.1093/cercor/bhs354

Ling, J., Merideth, F., Caprihan, A., Pena, A., Teshiba, T., and Mayer, A. R. (2012). Head injury or head motion? assessment and quantification of motion artifacts in diffusion tensor imaging studies. Hum. Brain Mapp. 33, 50–62. doi: 10.1002/hbm.21192

McAlonan, G. M., Cheung, V., Cheung, C., Suckling, J., Lam, G. Y., Tai, K. S., et al. (2005). Mapping the brain in autism. A voxel-based MRI study of vol- umetric difference and intercorrelations in autism. Brain 128, 268–276. doi: 10.1093/brain/awh332

McAlonan, G. M., Daly, E., Kumari, V., Critchley, H. D., van Amlsvoort, T., Suckling, J., et al. (2002). Brain anatomy and sensorimotor gating in Asperger's syndrome. Brain 125, 1584–1606. doi: 10.1093/brain/awf150

Moss, B. G., and Chugani, D. C. (2014). Increased risk of very low birth weight, rapid postnatal growth, and autism in underweight and obese mothers. Am. J. Health Promot. 28, 181–188. doi: 10.4278/ajhp.120705-QUAN-325

Palmen, S., van Engeland, H., Hof, P. R., and Schmitz, C. (2004). Neuropathological findings in autism. Brain 127, 2572–2583. doi: 10.1093/brain/awh287

Pinto-Martin, J. A., Levy, S. E., Feldman, J. F., Lorenz, J. M., Paneth, N., and Whitaker, A. H. (2011). Prevalence of autism spectrum disorder in adolescents born weighing <2000 grams. Pediatrics 128, 883–891. doi: 10.1542/peds.2010-2846

Reith, R. M., McKenna, J., Wu, H., Hashmi, S. S., Cho, S. H., Dash, P. K., et al. (2013). Loss of Tsc2 in Purkinje cells is associated with autistic-like behavior in a mouse model of tuberous sclerosis complex. Neurobiol. Dis. 51, 93–103. doi: 10.1016/j.nbd.2012.10.014

Reith, R. M., Way, S., McKenna, J. 3rd., Haines, K., and Gambello, M. J. (2011). Loss of the tuberous sclerosis complex protein tuberin causes Purkinje cell degeneration. Neurobiol. Dis. 43, 113–122. doi: 10.1016/j.nbd. 2011.02.014

Ritvo, E. R., Freeman, B. J., Scheibel, A. B., Duong, T., Robinson, H., Guthrie, D., et al. (1986). Lower Purkinje cell counts in the cerebella of four autistic subjects: initial findings of the UCLA-NSAC autopsy research report. Am. J. Psychiatry 143, 862–866.

Shi, L., Smith, S. E., Malkova, N., Tse, D., Su, Y., and Patterson, P. H. (2009). Activation of the maternal immune system alters cerebellar development in the offspring. Brain Behav. Immun. 23, 116–123. doi: 10.1016/j.bbi.2008.07.012

Song, S. K., Sun, S. W., Ju, W. K., Lin, S. J., Cross, A. H., and Neufeld, A. H. (2002). Dysmyelination revealed through MRI as increased radial (but unchanged axial) diffusion of water. Neuroimage 17, 1429–1436. doi: 10.1006/nimg.2002.1267

Song, S. K., Yoshino, J., Le, T. Q., Lin, S. J., Sun, S. W., Cross, A. H., et al. (2005). Demylination increases radial diffusivity in corpus callosum of mouse brain. Neuroimage 26, 132–140. doi: 10.1016/j.neuroimage.2005.01.028

Sparrow, S. S., Balla, D. A., Cicchetti, D. V., and Doll, E. A. (1984). Vineland Adaptive Behavior Scales. Circle Pines, MN: American Guidance Service.

Suzuki, K., Sugihara, G., Ouchi, Y., Nakamura, K., Futatsubashi, M., Takebayashi, K., et al. (2013). Microglial activation in young adults with autism spectrum disorder. JAMA Psychiatry 70, 49–58. doi: 10.1001/jamapsychiatry. 2013.272

Tolbert, D. L., Bantli, H., and Bloedel, J. R. (1978). Organizational features of the cat and monkey cerebellar nucleocortical projection. J. Comp. Neurol. 182, 39–56. doi: 10.1002/cne.901820104

Tsai, P. T., Hull, C., Chu, Y., Greene-Colozzi, E., Sadowski, A. R., Leech, J. M., et al. (2012). Autistic-like behavior and cerebellar dysfunction in Purkinje cell Tsc1 mutant mice. Nature 488, 647–651. doi: 10.1038/nature11310

Vargas, D. L., Nascimbene, C., Krishnan, C., Zimmerman, A. W., and Pardo, C. A. (2005). Neuroglial activation and neuroinflammation in the brain of patients with autism. Ann. Neurol. 57, 67–81. doi: 10.1002/ana.20315

Walker, L., Chang, L. C., Koay, C. G., Sharma, N., Cohen, L., Verma, R., et al. (2011). Effects of physiological noise in population analysis of diffu- sion tensor MRI data. Neuroimage 54, 1168–1177. doi: 10.1016/j.neuroimage.2010.08.048

Walker, L., Gozzi, M., Lenroot, R., Thurm, A., Behseta, B., Swedo, S., et al.

(2012). Diffusion tensor imaging in young children with autism: biolog ical effects and potential confounds. Biol. Psychiatry 71, 1043–1051. doi: 10.1016/j.biopsych.2012.08.001

Wang, D., Buckner, R. L., and Liu, H. (2013). Cerebellar asymmetry and its rela- tion to cerebral asymmetry estimated by intrinsic functional connectivity. J. Neurophysiol. 109, 46–57. doi: 10.1152/jn.00598.2012

Wegiel, J., Kuchna, I., Nowicki, K., Imaki, H., Wegiel, J., Ma, S. Y., et al. (2013). Contribution of olivofloccular circuitry developmental defects to atypical gaze in autism. Brain Res. 1512, 106–1122. doi: 10.1016/j.brainres. 2013.03.037

Whitney, E. R., Kemper, T. L., Rosens, D. L., Bauman, M. L., and Blatt, G. J. (2009). Density of cerebellar basket and stellate cells in autism: evidence for a late developmental loss of Purkinje cells. J. Neurosci. Res. 87, 2245–2254. doi: 10.1002/ jnr.22056

Yip, J., Soghomonian, J. J., and Blatt, G. J. (2009). Decreased GAD65 mRNA levels in select subpopulations in the cerebellar dentate nuclei in autism: an in situ hybridization study. Autism Res. 2, 50–59. doi: 10.1002/ aur.62

4

Identification of neural connectivity signatures of autism using machine learning

Gopikrishna Deshpande[1,2], Lauren E. Libero[3], Karthik R. Sreenivasan[1], Hrishikesh D. Deshpande[3] and Rajesh K. Kana[3]*

[1] *AU MRI Research Center, Department of Electrical and Computer Engineering, Auburn University, Auburn, AL, USA*
[2] *Department of Psychology, Auburn University, Auburn, AL, USA*
[3] *Department of Psychology, University of Alabama at Birmingham, Birmingham, AL, USA*

Edited by:
Lucina Q. Uddin, Stanford University, USA

Reviewed by:
Baxter P. Rogers, Vanderbilt University, USA
Joao Sato, Universidade Federal do ABC, Brazil

***Correspondence:**
Rajesh K. Kana, Department of Psychology, University of Alabama, Birmingham, CIRC 235G, 1719 6th Ave South, Birmingham, AL 35294-0021, USA
e-mail: rkana@uab.edu

Alterations in interregional neural connectivity have been suggested as a signature of the pathobiology of autism. There have been many reports of functional and anatomical connectivity being altered while individuals with autism are engaged in complex cognitive and social tasks. Although disrupted instantaneous correlation between cortical regions observed from functional MRI is considered to be an explanatory model for autism, the causal influence of a brain area on another (effective connectivity) is a vital link missing in these studies. The current study focuses on addressing this in an fMRI study of Theory-of-Mind (ToM) in 15 high-functioning adolescents and adults with autism and 15 typically developing control participants. Participants viewed a series of comic strip vignettes in the MRI scanner and were asked to choose the most logical end to the story from three alternatives, separately for trials involving physical and intentional causality. The mean time series, extracted from 18 activated regions of interest, were processed using a multivariate autoregressive model (MVAR) to obtain the causality matrices for each of the 30 participants. These causal connectivity weights, along with assessment scores, functional connectivity values, and fractional anisotropy obtained from DTI data for each participant, were submitted to a recursive cluster elimination based support vector machine classifier to determine the accuracy with which the classifier can predict a novel participant's group membership (autism or control). We found a maximum classification accuracy of 95.9% with 19 features which had the highest discriminative ability between the groups. All of the 19 features were effective connectivity paths, indicating that causal information may be critical in discriminating between autism and control groups. These effective connectivity paths were also found to be significantly greater in controls as compared to ASD participants and consisted predominantly of outputs from the fusiform face area and middle temporal gyrus indicating impaired connectivity in ASD participants, particularly in the social brain areas. These findings collectively point toward the fact that alterations in causal connectivity in the brain in ASD could serve as a potential non-invasive neuroimaging signature for autism.

Keywords: autism, effective connectivity, fMRI, classification, machine learning, theory-of-mind

INTRODUCTION

A biological origin for autism spectrum disorders (ASD) had been proposed even in the earliest published accounts of the disorder (Kanner, 1943; Asperger, 1944). Despite several decades of research since then, a focal neurobiological marker for autism has been rather elusive. Brain imaging techniques in the last decade, particularly functional and structural MRI, have pointed to disrupted cortical connectivity as a defining neural feature of ASD (Kana et al., 2011; Just et al., 2012). Neuroimaging studies have reported functional under connectivity (weaker synchronization of activated brain areas) between frontal and posterior brain areas (Just et al., 2004, 2007; Villalobos et al., 2005; Kana et al., 2006, 2007, 2009; Koshino et al., 2008; Mason et al., 2008; Solomon et al., 2009; Damarla et al., 2010; Jones et al., 2010; Mizuno et al., 2011; Schipul et al., 2011), and intact or increased functional connectivity within relatively posterior brain areas (Villalobos et al., 2005; Kana et al., 2006; Damarla et al., 2010; Kana et al., under review). Similar findings have also been reported during task-free resting state in autism (Cherkassky et al., 2006; Assaf et al., 2010; Murdaugh et al., 2012). Furthermore, diffusion tensor imaging (DTI) studies have reported disruptions in anatomical connectivity in ASD (Barnea-Goraly et al., 2004, 2010; Alexander et al., 2007; Keller et al., 2007; Jou et al., 2011; see Travers et al., 2012 for a review). Although there is converging evidence for connection abnormalities, the neural connectivity model of ASD is based primarily on functional connectivity, with some contributing evidence from white matter integrity. While the insights gained from these models are valuable, functional connectivity is a method for assessing zero-lag correlations, and does not provide insight into the time-lagged relationships and direction of such causal influence.

Effective connectivity, on the other hand, refers to the influence one neural system exerts over another with respect to a given experimental context (Buchel and Friston, 2000), thus helping uncover more information about how brain areas communicate. Effective connectivity can provide information about the transfer of information from one node to another, and differentiate between top-down vs. bottom-up effects. Thus, effective connectivity findings have enriched models of cognitive function by emphasizing the dynamic and interactive nature of neural instantiations (McIntosh et al., 2010). Studying such interactions is important not only for understanding typical brain functioning, but also is critical in learning more about diseases. Considering relatively consistent reports of disruptions in functional connectivity in ASD, it is perhaps a logical and valuable next step to study how information transfer is accomplished in ASD brains. Of particular interest is to explore the information transfer among brain areas that are part of a team to perform higher-order cognitive and social functions, which people with ASD particularly struggle with.

Understanding the information transfer, or the lack of it, between specific nodes in the brain may help uncover the neural bases of behavioral and social problems in ASD. It should be noted that only four previous studies have examined effective connectivity between brain regions in ASD (Bird et al., 2006; Wicker et al., 2008; Shih et al., 2010; Shen et al., 2012). These studies only permit limited inferences as they used a small number of regions and made prior assumptions about the underlying connectional architecture. This is because they used confirmatory methods such as dynamic causal modeling (Friston et al., 2003) and structural equation modeling (McIntosh and Gozales-Lima, 1994) in their studies. In contrast, the present study applies multivariate autoregressive (MVAR) modeling for obtaining Granger causality between a large number of brain regions. This is an exploratory technique which does not make any prior assumptions about the underlying connectional architecture. In addition, it is capable of obtaining condition-specific causal influences between a large number of brain regions using relatively shorter time series. According to the principle of Granger causality, the directional causal influence from time series X to time series Y can be inferred if past values of time series X help predict the present and future values of the time series Y (Granger, 1969). MVAR models have been used to characterize the predictive relationship between the time series from different brain regions in many previous studies (Roebroeck et al., 2005; Abler et al., 2006; Deshpande et al., 2008, 2009b; Sathian et al., 2011). But according to many recent studies, the spatial variability of the hemodynamic response is considered to be of vascular origin, and hence confounding the Granger causal estimates obtained from raw fMRI time series (David et al., 2008; Deshpande et al., 2010b). Removing the smoothing effect of the hemodynamic response function (HRF) will increase the effective temporal resolution of the signal in addition to accounting for the inter-subject and inter-regional variability of the HRF (Handwerker et al., 2004). This can be accomplished using blind hemodynamic deconvolution methods where in the underlying hidden neuronal variable for the fMRI time series can be estimated. We employed this approach in this study by deconvolving the hemodynamic response from fMRI time series using a Cubature Kalman filter (CKF) (Havlicek et al., 2011). Subsequently, these hidden neuronal variables were input into the MVAR model to obtain directional connectivity measures.

Investigating the directional interactions among brain areas in ASD could supplement functional connectivity findings, and potentially may serve as a neural signature for the disorder. Thus, connection abnormalities at anatomical, functional, and causal levels may be considered for potential diagnosis of ASD and/or to supplement the behavior-based diagnosis. However, such attempts will need to test and validate the diagnostic utility of connection abnormalities in ASD. Questions pertaining to diagnostic utility may be best answered through pattern classification analyses using sophisticated machine learning algorithms (Deshpande et al., 2010a; Weygandt et al., 2011; Shinkareva et al., 2013). In this regard, earlier studies have used pattern recognition and machine learning algorithms reliably in classification. Craddock et al. (2009) showed that by using resting state functional connectivity metrics as features in SVM based machine learning classifier, Major Depressive Disorder (MDD) patients were successfully distinguished from healthy controls. In another study, the treatment type provided to patients with MDD was accurately identified using SVM classifier based on the effective connectivity measures (Deshpande et al., 2009a). A pattern recognition approach using structural networks as biomarkers was proposed (Marquand et al., 2013) for classification of Parkinson's Disorder. This method of analysis accurately predicted the diagnosis in patients with Parkinson disorders. A study by Mirowski and colleagues (2009) showed that machine learning classifiers can be successfully used in prediction of seizures in patients with epilepsy. Given the success of pattern recognition and classification methods based on machine learning techniques in other fields and contexts, they could potentially prove to be useful to correctly identify participants with ASD after replication and fine tuning. In these lines, diagnostic information (although preliminary) has been obtained from even short fMRI BOLD sequences, such as characterization of subject age (Dosenbach et al., 2010), classification of dementia (Chen et al., 2011), and autism (Anderson et al., 2011; Murdaugh et al., 2012; Wang et al., 2012). For a neurodevelopmental disorder such as ASD, which is currently diagnosed solely by behavioral observation and in-person interviews by clinicians, classification by brain imaging signatures could be applied to gain more accurate (and perhaps earlier) diagnosis of the disorder. Classification studies have utilized a wide range of data sources to differentiate participants into ASD and TD groups, including functional connectivity (Anderson et al., 2011; Murdaugh et al., 2012; Wang et al., 2012), voxel based morphometry (Uddin et al., 2011; Calderoni et al., 2012), fMRI activation patterns (Coutanche et al., 2011), EEG (Duffy and Als, 2012), and DTI (Ingalhalikar et al., 2011). Yet, none of these methods are currently employed to diagnose the disorder. Issues remain regarding generalizability, such as whether the classification techniques can still be accurately applied to younger children. When other disorders also show functional connectivity and resting state abnormalities, such as schizophrenia (Lawrie et al., 2002; Meyer-Lindenberg et al., 2005; Garrity et al., 2007) and ADHD (Tian et al., 2006; Cubillo et al., 2010), it begs the question about the specificity of these metrics to ASD. However, notably, effective connectivity markers have not been used in classification of ASD individuals. In this regard, effective connectivity could be an additional data source utilized to add to classification of ASD participants, potentially providing sufficient information to serve as a biomarker for the disorder. In other words, effective connectivity could contribute significantly to the global connectivity-based neural characterization of ASD. Also, whereas traditional statistical analyses can uncover significant group differences in brain activation and connectivity, classification analyses can serve to identify brain imaging signatures which are not only able to separate or distinguish the groups, but also predict the group membership of a new subject.

In the current study we explored the causal influences between brain regions that may underlie the processing of theory-of-mind (ToM) in young adults with ASD and typically developing (TD) control participants. The original fMRI study on ToM was published earlier (Kana et al., 2012), reporting findings of brain activity, functional connectivity and white matter integrity. In the current study, we obtained causal connectivity between 18 brain regions activated in the ToM task in our previous publication (Kana et al., 2012). We used these causal connectivity weights along with the following metrics from our previous study—assessment scores, functional connectivity values and fractional anisotropy (FA) obtained from DTI data—as features for classification. We employed recursive cluster elimination to select important features and a support vector machine (SVM) classifier to classify participants into ASD and TD based on the entire feature set. This paper is novel in that it takes into consideration different aspects of brain connectivity, instead of a single index, to characterize the nature of brain functioning in individuals with ASD for classification purposes.

METHOD

PARTICIPANTS

Fifteen adolescents and young adults with high-functioning ASD (mean age: 21.14 years) and 15 age-and-IQ-matched individuals with typical development (TD) (mean age: 22.18 years) participated in this fMRI study. Functional connectivity, structural connectivity, behavioral data, and brain activation measures from the same participants were reported elsewhere (Kana et al., 2012). All participants were required to have an IQ of 80 or above measured by the Wechsler Abbreviated Scale of Intelligence (WASI). The participants with ASD were recruited from the University of Alabama ASD Clinic and surrounding service providers. The study was approved by the Institutional Review Board of the University of Alabama at Birmingham, and all participants provided informed consent for their participation in the study. Participants with ASD had received a previous diagnosis of an ASD based on Autism Diagnostic Interview (ADI-R) symptoms, and Autism Diagnostic Observation Schedule (ADOS). Eight of the 15 ASD participants in this study had received a diagnosis of Asperger's Disorder. The TD participants were recruited through newspaper advertisements and through the University of Alabama at Birmingham's Psychology 101 course subject pool. They were screened through a parent-report (for participants younger than 18 years) or self-report history questionnaire to rule out neurological disorders, such as ASD, ADHD, or Tourette's Disorder, that could potentially confound the results. All participants completed the Autism Spectrum Quotient (AQ) questionnaire (Baron-Cohen et al., 2001b), and the Reading the Mind in the Eyes (RME) test (Baron-Cohen et al., 2001a). Demographic information about the participants is shown in **Table 1.**

EXPERIMENTAL PARADIGM AND IMAGING PARAMETERS

The stimuli consisted of a series of black and white comic strip vignettes (adapted from Brunet et al., 2000) depicting scenarios that demand either a physical causal attribution or an intentional causal attribution to arrive at a logical ending. The first part of the vignette was presented for 5 s and the participants' task was to choose a logical ending to the story from the three choices in the second panel presented for 6 s. The entire vignette remained on the screen for a total of 11 s. The experiment was designed in an event-related format. All data were collected using a Siemens 3.0 Tesla Allegra head-only scanner (*Siemens* Medical Inc., Erlangen, Germany). For functional imaging, a single-shot gradient-recalled echo-planar pulse sequence was used for rapid image acquisition ($TR = 1000$ ms, $TE = 30$ ms, flip angle = 60 degrees). Seventeen adjacent oblique-axial slices were acquired in an interleaved sequence with 5 mm slice thickness, 1 mm slice gap, a $24 \times 24\,cm^2$ field of view (FOV), and a 64×64 matrix, resulting in an in-plane resolution of $3.75 \times 3.75 \times 5\,mm^3$. More information on the experimental paradigm and imaging parameters for the 3D MPRAGE structural MRI data and diffusion weighted echo-planar imaging data can be found in Appendix A (for further details, please refer to Kana et al., 2012).

Table 1 | Demographic information of the ASD and TD control participants.

	Autism N = 15					Control N = 15					Group difference	
	Mean	Range	*SD*	Median	IQR	Mean	Range	*SD*	Median	IQR	*t*-value	*p*-value
Age	21.14	16–29	0.99	20.08	5	22.28	16–34	1.08	21.83	3.3	0.77	0.44
VIQ	104.8	74–139	5.02	102	31	113.93	98–127	2.2	116	14	1.66	0.11
PIQ	107.7	73–129	4.33	106	25	107.2	89–124	2.48	108	6	0.11	0.92
FSIQ	106.93	80–140	4.84	105	35	112	96–128	2.24	113	13	0.94	0.35
MIE	19.07	15–24	0.7	20	4	21.6	18–24	0.55	22	4	2.84	0.01
AQ	26.5	9–38	2.04	29	12	14.06	4–22	1.45	14	9	5.47	<0.001

DATA ANALYSES

Head motion correction and regions of interest (ROI) definition

Within-group brain activation was examined for the whole group (ASD + TD) of participants (see Kana et al., 2012). Functional ROIs were defined on the group activation map for the whole group (ASD + TD) for the contrast (Intentional Causality + Physical Causality) vs. Fixation, so that it best represented the study. Because head motion can impact connectivity analyses (Satterthwaite et al., 2012; Van Dijk et al., 2012), a conservative threshold of 0.5 mm was set for head motion in any direction. In addition, the root mean square (RMS) values of head motion were measured in three translational directions (x, y, and z) and three rotations (pitch, roll, and yaw) for each individual participant in the study (see Appendix B **Table B1**). We examined group differences in head motion on this data using a Mann-Whitney U Test, which is a non-parametric test and may be more appropriate in case assumptions about normality of sample distributions are not met.

Eighteen ROIs were identified: supplementary motor area (SMA), left and right inferior frontal gyrus (LIFG, RIFG), left and right precentral cortex (LPRCN, RPRCN), left and right middle temporal gyrus (LMTG, RMTG), right superior temporal gyrus (RSTG), left and right inferior parietal lobule (LIPL, RIPL), left and right fusiform gyrus (LFFG, RFFG), left and right superior parietal lobule (LSPL, RSPL), left and right middle occipital gyrus (LMOG, RMOG), and left and right temporal parietal junction (LTPJ, RTPJ). A sphere was defined for each cluster (with a radius ranging from 8 to 12 mm) that best captured the cluster of activation in the contrast map for each group. The radius was selected to specifically encompass as much of the activation cluster as possible, without including surrounding (not significantly activated) areas. Selecting ROIs of the same radius or utilizing anatomically defined ROIs may entail those ROIs not encompassing the entire cluster of activation, or may include tissue that is not significantly active for the task. As a result, extracting time courses from ROIs defined in these ways may result in time series variability that does not reflect the cognitive task being processed.

The effective connectivity model

Let l fMRI time series be represented as $X(t) = [x_1(t)x_2(t)\ldots x_l(t)]$. Below, we present a model linking observed fMRI time series to underlying latent neuronal variables. A dynamic state-space model can be described as follows.

$$\tilde{h}^l_T = \begin{bmatrix} h^l_T \\ u^l_T \\ \theta^l_T \end{bmatrix} = \begin{bmatrix} f(h^l_{T-1}, u^l_{T-1}, \theta^l_{T-1}) \\ u^l_{T-1} \\ \theta^l_{T-1} \end{bmatrix} + \begin{bmatrix} P^l_{T-1} \\ Q^l_{T-1} \\ R^l_{T-1} \end{bmatrix} \quad (1)$$

Where h is the hidden neuronal state variable, u is the exogenous input and θ represents the HRF parameter variables. f is the function which links the current neuronal state to the previous neuronal states, exogenous inputs and parameters. The subscript T indicates continuous time and the superscript l indicates the number of time series in the model. P, Q, and R are the zero mean Gaussian state noise vectors. The observation equation links the state to observation variables as given below.

$$x_l(t) = \boldsymbol{m}(\tilde{h}^l_t) + \varepsilon_{t-1} \quad (2)$$

where ε is the measurement noise, t is discrete time and $\boldsymbol{m}$ is the measurement function which links the state variables to measurement variables. The exogenous inputs u, which is the experimental boxcar function, and $x_l(t)$ are the inputs to the model. As demonstrated before, using the CKF (Havlicek et al., 2011), the hidden neuronal variables can be estimated successfully. The CKF performs very efficient joint estimation of the hidden neuronal state variables and parameters. In addition, since Eq. 1 represents a continuous time model, the neuronal variables can be estimated with a highly improved temporal resolution up to 10 times smaller than the TR. When the hidden neuronal state variables $h_l(t)$ are input into the MVAR model, we get the following equation.

$$\begin{bmatrix} h_1(t) \\ h_2(t) \\ \cdot \\ \cdot \\ h_l(t) \end{bmatrix} = \begin{bmatrix} 0 & a_{12}(0) & \cdots & a_{1l}(0) \\ a_{21}(0) & 0 & & a_{2l}(0) \\ \cdot & \cdot & 0 & \cdot \\ \cdot & \cdot & & \cdot \\ a_{l1}(0) & a_{l2}(0) & \cdots & 0 \end{bmatrix} \times \begin{bmatrix} h_1(t) \\ h_2(t) \\ \cdot \\ \cdot \\ h_l(t) \end{bmatrix} + \sum_{j=1}^{p} \begin{bmatrix} a_{11}(j) & a_{12}(j) & \ldots & a_{1l}(j) \\ a_{21}(j) & a_{22}(j) & & a_{2l}(j) \\ \cdot & \cdot & & \cdot \\ \cdot & \cdot & & \cdot \\ a_{l1}(j) & a_{l2}(j) & \ldots & a_{ll}(j) \end{bmatrix} \times \begin{bmatrix} h_1(t-j) \\ h_2(t-j) \\ \cdot \\ \cdot \\ h_l(t-j) \end{bmatrix} + \begin{bmatrix} e_1(t) \\ e_2(t) \\ \cdot \\ \cdot \\ e_l(t) \end{bmatrix} \quad (3)$$

where p is the model order estimated by the Akaike/Bayesian information criterion (Deshpande et al., 2009b), a represent the model coefficients and e represents the error of the MVAR model. From the above equation it can be observed that $a(0)$ represents the instantaneous influences between the time series, and the Granger causal influences between them is indicated by $a(j)$, $j = 1 \ldots . p$. Both terms are used in the model because including both instantaneous and causal terms in the model minimizes the "leakage" of instantaneous correlation into causality (Deshpande et al., 2010c). The multivariate model we have used is less sensitive to the effects of missing variables than the traditionally used pairwise bivariate models (Kuś et al., 2004). Also, since we included all 18 regions which were activated in the effect of interest, it guaranteed to a certain level that all regions involved in the task were indeed included in the model.

Effective connectivity analysis

Mean time series from 18 activated regions were obtained for each of the 15 participants with ASD and the 15 typical control participants. Using the boxcar function corresponding to "intentional causality" as the exogenous input, hidden neuronal variables corresponding to normalized mean fMRI time series were obtained and input into the MVAR model. The Granger causal relationships between the 18 regions for each participant (ASD and TD) were obtained. The number of coefficients in the MVAR model is equal to k^2p (k is the number of time series and p is the model order) (Kuś et al., 2004). This must be smaller than the number of time points in each time series. We had 18 ROI time series, each of length 460. Since we used a first order model, $k^2p = 324$ which is less than 460. Therefore, we were able to estimate the model.

Classification using support vector machine

The statistical separation of neural signatures (e.g., t-test) does not guarantee generalizability or predictive power of those signatures for diagnosis. Therefore, in this study, we also used machine learning approaches for identification of metrics which can accurately classify individuals with ASD from individuals with typical development. A Recursive Cluster Elimination based Support Vector Machine (RCE-SVM) (Deshpande et al., 2010a) was used in this study to classify the participants based on granger causal path weights between the 18 ROIs, functional connectivity z-scores for all pairs of the 18 ROIs, assessment scores (AQ and RME scores) and FA values for the white matter tract extending into the temporal lobe as the input features. The functional connectivity, assessment and DTI FA values were obtained from our prior study (Kana et al., 2012).

Our choice of SVM for classification was motivated by its wide applicability as a machine learning approach (Vapnik, 1995) for classification in many different fields (Wang, 2005). Previous studies have demonstrated that using discriminatory features enhances SVM classification (Craddock et al., 2009). Therefore, to enhance the performance of the SVM classifier, filtering and wrapper methods for feature selection have been used. Filtering methods are based on extraction of features that are statistically different between classes. They can be extracted using statistical tests such as a t-test. The wrapper approach is based on iteratively eliminating features to minimize the prediction error. RCE is one of the wrapper methods that is an iterative process were the feature selection and classification steps are embedded with each other. The main steps of the RCE-SVM algorithm, shown in the flowchart in **Figure 1**, are the cluster step, the SVM scoring step and the RCE step. Initially, the features that were input into the classifier were divided into training and testing data sets. Fifty such splits were carried out in order to ensure the generalizability of the results. In the clustering step, k-means algorithm (Yang et al., 2003) was used to cluster the training data into n clusters. The number of clusters was first set to the number of features, and was progressively decreased by one until there were no empty clusters. The n obtained by this iteration served as the initial n for the RCE-SVM loop.

In the SVM scoring step, each cluster was scored based on its ability to differentiate the two categories by applying linear SVM. In order to rate the clusters, the training data was randomly partitioned into 10 non-overlapping subsets of equal sizes (10 folds). Using 9 subsets, the linear SVM was trained and performance was calculated using the remaining subset. Different

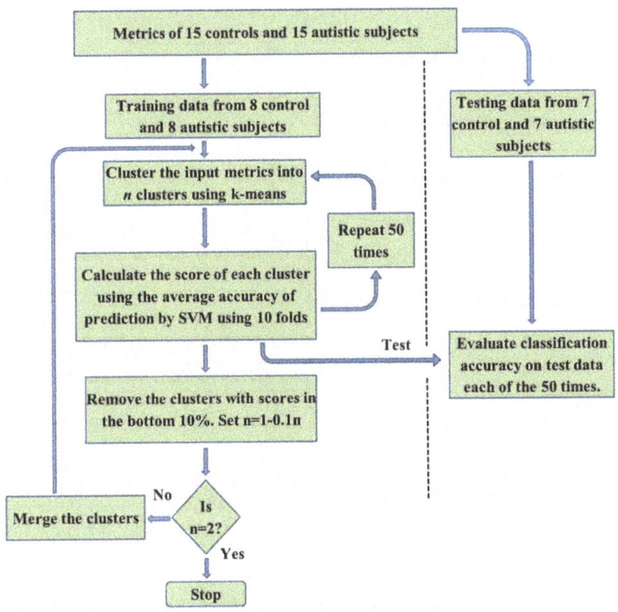

FIGURE 1 | A flow-chart depicting the Recursive Cluster Elimination based Support Vector Machine (RCE-SVM) procedure.

possible partitions were taken into account by repeating the clustering and cross validation procedure 50 times. For each of these 50 repetitions, the classification accuracy of SVM was ascertained using the test data. The average value of this accuracy, taking into account the repetitions and all the folds was assigned as the score of the cluster. The bottom 10% of low score clusters were eliminated in the RCE step. The remaining features were merged and the value of n was decreased by 10% and the cluster step, the SVM scoring step and the RCE step were repeated again in an iterative manner. After each iteration, the performance of the classifier was assessed using the testing data and lesser number of features compared to the earlier iteration. When the number of clusters was equal to two, the procedure was stopped. Complete separation of testing and training data in this algorithm eliminates bias in performance accuracy (Kriegeskorte et al., 2009). The accuracy at every RCE-SVM loop was calculated as a mean value of accuracy obtained over 50 repetitions of each loop and each train-test split, using the feature clusters of test data available at the corresponding loop and split. The statistical significance of mean accuracies was calculated by estimating the p-values of a binomial null distribution $B(\eta,\rho)$, η being the number of participants and ρ is the probability of accurate classification as in previous studies (Pereira et al., 2009). Only accuracies whose p-values were less than 0.05 after correcting for multiple comparisons using Bonferroni method were considered as statistically significant.

The causal connectivity weights obtained from the MVAR model, the behavioral assessment scores, the functional connectivity z-scores for each ROI pair, and DTI FA metrics for each of the 30 subjects (15 ASD and 15 TD) were input into the RCE-SVM classifier to determine the accuracy with which the classifier can predict a novel subject's group membership (autism or control).

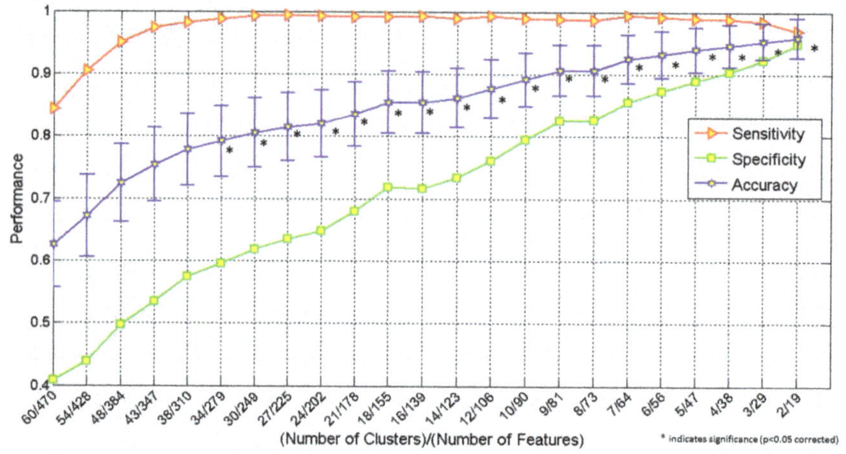

FIGURE 2 | Graph showing classification accuracy, sensitivity and specificity obtained by simultaneously using the following features: behavioral scores, functional connectivity, effective connectivity and fractional anisotropy obtained from DTI. The X-axis shows number of clusters/number of features and the Y-axis, the performance (classification accuracy, sensitivity and specificity). *indicates significance ($p < 0.05$ corrected).

RESULTS

The main results of this study are summarized as follows: (1) The effective connectivity path weights were able to successfully classify participants by diagnosis with 95.9% accuracy. These path weights were the most discriminative features among all the different metrics used in classification; (2) Effective connectivity paths most important for classification were significantly reduced ($p < 0.05$) in ASD participants compared to typical control participants; and (3) The paths that were among the top ranked features in the classification analysis were found to be negatively correlated with the AQ and positively correlated with the RME test scores.

The first set of results pertains to a pattern classification analysis involving several indices of connectivity (functional connectivity, effective connectivity, white matter integrity) and performance accuracy in this ToM task. In this analysis, utilizing 2 feature clusters comprised of 19 metrics, the classification accuracy reached a maximum accuracy of 95.9% (specificity 94.8%, and sensitivity 96.9%). It should be noted that all of the 19 features were effective connectivity paths. **Figure 2** demonstrates the increase in performance of classification with decreasing number of features (and removal of uninformative features). The p-values for all the accuracy values shown in **Figure 2** can be seen in **Table 2.**

Second, the causal connectivity weights of the 19 paths which led to maximum accuracy of 95.9% showed clear separation between participants with autism (blue) and typical control participants (green) as shown in **Figure 3**, with these paths showing significantly ($p < 0.05$ corrected using Bonferroni method for 18 paths; for one of the paths $p < 0.05$ uncorrected) weaker connectivity in participants with ASD compared to TD controls. Many of these connections are between regions that are part of the social brain network (LTPJ, RTPJ, LFFG, RFFG, LMTG, RMTG, RIFG) which may prove critical in accomplishing the ToM task used in this study. It is noteworthy that there may be other paths which are significantly different between the groups. Here, we restrict ourselves to finding the statistical separation of features which have the highest ability for predicting the diagnosis of a given subject. We do so primarily because we are interested in features with predictive ability rather than those which just "differ" between the groups. Please refer to Appendix B **Figures B1, B2** in order to gain a qualitative understanding of the functional and effective

Table 2 | Classification accuracy values and the corresponding *p*-values obtained at each step of the RCE algorithm.

Accuracy	*p*-Value
0.625	0.100244
0.672	0.049369
0.724	0.008062
0.754	0.002611
0.778	0.002611
0.792	0.000715
0.805	0.000715
0.815	0.000715
0.82	0.000162
0.835	0.000162
0.855	2.97×10^{-05}
0.854	2.97×10^{-05}
0.862	2.97×10^{-05}
0.876	2.97×10^{-05}
0.892	4.22×10^{-06}
0.906	4.22×10^{-06}
0.906	4.22×10^{-06}
0.925	4.34×10^{-07}
0.932	4.34×10^{-07}
0.939	4.34×10^{-07}
0.945	4.34×10^{-07}
0.953	2.89×10^{-08}
0.959	2.89×10^{-08}

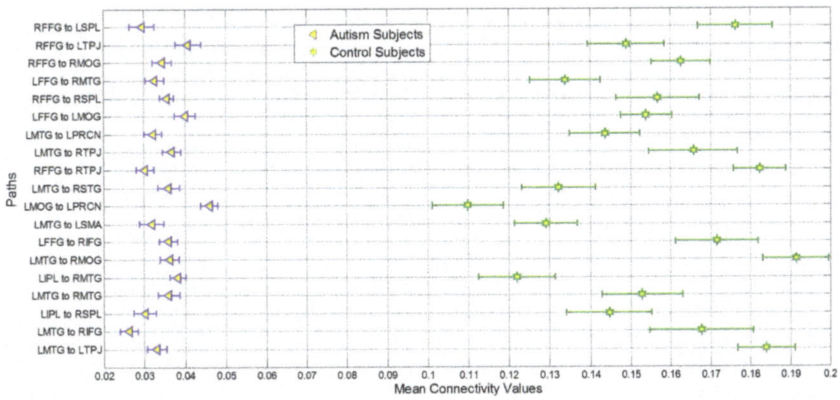

FIGURE 3 | Mean of nineteen paths which was most important for giving maximum classification accuracy for autism and control groups. All paths had significantly decreased connectivity ($p < 0.05$ corrected using Bonferroni method for 18 paths; for one of the paths $p < 0.05$ uncorrected) in the Autism group as compared to controls. The bars represent standard errors.

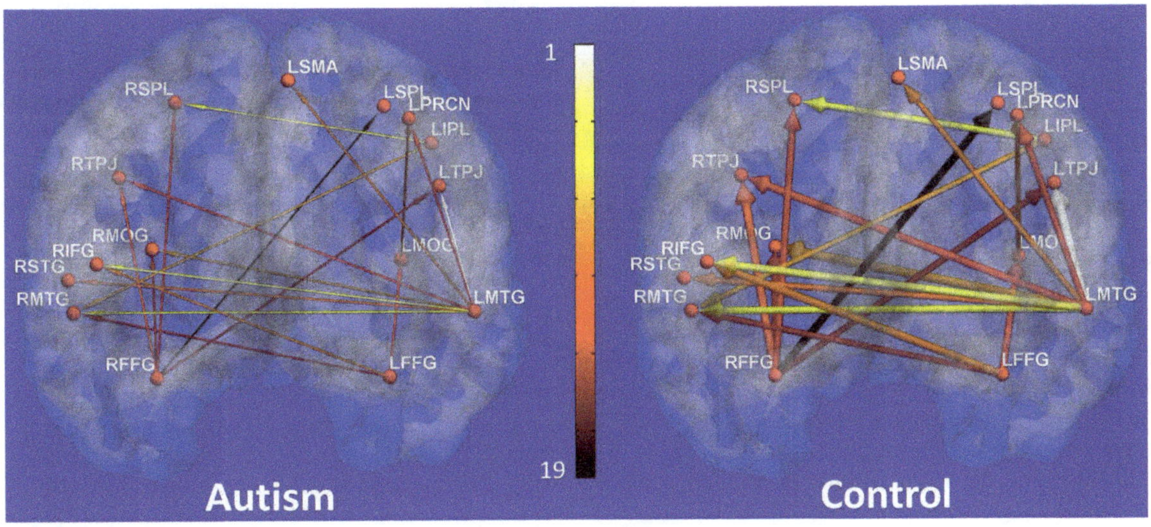

FIGURE 4 | The nineteen paths whose effective connectivity values were top-ranked features for classification of the two groups (Autism and Controls) with the maximum accuracy (Left panel: participants with autism; and right panel: control participants). The width of the arrows represents the path strength and the color of the path indicates its rank obtained during classification with 1 being the most significant and 19 being the least significant.

connectivity paths, respectively, between all 18 ROIs in both ASD and TD groups.

The 19 effective connectivity paths which were most important in classification are shown in **Figure 4**. The left panel shows these paths in ASD participants and the right panel in control participants. The width of the arrows illustrates the path weight in the corresponding group and the color represents the rank of the path obtained during classification.

Third, a correlation analysis was also performed between the features that were ranked highest in classification and gave rise to maximum accuracy, and assessment scores (AQ and RME). Given that the top-ranked features are not guaranteed to have normal distribution, we used Spearman's non-parametric correlation method to determine whether the top-ranked features were correlated with behavior. This analysis (including all participants in the study) revealed a significant negative correlation between several effective connectivity paths and the AQ scores as well as a significant positive correlation between effective connectivity paths and RME scores (see **Table 3** for specific paths, correlation and p-values). These results suggest that as autism symptom severity increased, the effective connectivity of the top-ranked paths decreased; and as the theory-of-mind ability increased, effective connectivity of the top-ranked paths also increased. This provides a second-level test of the behavioral relevance of the top-ranked paths, which is to be expected given the fact that diagnosis was based on behavioral symptoms. As a cautionary note, these results should not be construed as a general discovery regarding brain connectivity features in autism which correlate with behavioral symptoms.

Neuroimaging data, especially brain connectivity analyses are prone to be influenced by head motion and signal quality. We conducted several different measures to make sure that our data

Table 3 | Paths correlated with Autism Quotient (AQ) scores and Reading Mind in Eye (RME) scores.

Paths correlated with Autism Quotient (AQ) scores					Paths correlated with Reading Mind in Eye (RME) scores				
Source region	**→**	**Sink region**	***p*-Value**	**Correlation coefficient**	**Source region**	**→**	**Sink region**	***p*-Value**	**Correlation coefficient**
LMTG	→	*LTPJ*	0.0003	−0.6137	*LMTG*	→	*LTPJ*	0.0311	0.3941
LMTG	→	*RIFG*	0.0007	−0.5837	*LMTG*	→	*RIFG*	0.0183	0.4279
LMTG	→	*RMTG*	0.0001	−0.6466	*LMTG*	→	*RMTG*	0.0455	0.3679
LMTG	→	*RMOG*	0.0006	−0.5901	*LMTG*	→	*RMOG*	0.0325	0.3912
LFFG	→	*RIFG*	0.0061	−0.4889	*LFFG*	→	*RIFG*	0.0428	0.3723
LMTG	→	*LSMA*	0.0006	−0.5930	*LMTG*	→	*LSMA*	0.0421	0.3734
RFFG	→	*RTPJ*	0.0028	−0.5274	*RFFG*	→	*RTPJ*	0.0373	0.3819
LFFG	→	*RMTG*	0.0119	−0.4531	*LFFG*	→	*RMTG*	0.0151	0.4395
RFFG	→	*RMOG*	0.0098	−0.4642	*RFFG*	→	*RMOG*	0.0035	0.5169
RFFG	→	*LSPL*	0.0187	−0.4266	*RFFG*	→	*LSPL*	0.0417	0.3741
LMTG	→	RSTG	0.0391	−0.3785	LIPL	→	RSPL	0.0082	0.4735
LMTG	→	RTPJ	0.0319	−0.3926	LFFG	→	LMOG	0.0213	0.4186
					RFFG	→	RSPL	0.0425	0.3727

The paths in red were correlated with both AQ and RME.

and the reported results were not influenced by quality related issues. First, the root mean square (RMS) values for each subject and each head motion parameter were obtained (see Appendix B **Table B1**). The RMS values were then submitted to a non-parametric Mann-Whitney *U* test, which also revealed no significant difference in motion in x [$U_{(28)} = 66$, $Z = -1.929$, $p = 0.06$], y [$U_{(28)} = 93$, $Z = -0.809$, $p = 0.42$], and z [$U_{(28)} = 96$, $Z = -0.684$, $p = 0.49$] translational directions. Nor was there a significant group difference in rotation in pitch [$U_{(28)} = 68$, $Z = -1.846$, $p = 0.06$], roll [$U_{(28)} = 107$, $Z = -0.228$, $p = 0.82$], and yaw [$U_{(28)} = 93$, $Z = -0.809$, $p = 0.42$]. These results indicate that there were no statistical differences in head motion between the two groups, assuming a *p*-value threshold of 0.05. However, there was a non-significant trend ($p = 0.06$) for translation in x direction and the degree of rotation in pitch to differ between the groups.

Further, we obtained the mean value of frame wise displacement (FD) for each subject as a quality control (QC) metric and investigated whether they correlated with any of the 19 top-ranked paths obtained from classification across the entire sample. The instantaneous motion of the head was expressed as a scalar quantity using the formula, $FD_i = |\Delta d_{ix}| + |\Delta d_{iy}| + |\Delta d_{iz}| + |\Delta\alpha_i| + |\Delta\beta_i| + |\Delta\gamma_i|$, where $\Delta d_{ik} = d_{(j-1)k} - d_{ik}$ and k is any of the 3 translational parameters (*x*, *y*, *z*) or rotational parameters (α, β, γ). We converted the rotational displacements from degrees to millimeters by calculating displacement on the surface of a sphere of radius 50 mm, assuming that the approximate mean distance from the center of the head to the cerebral cortex is 50 mm. The above procedure of calculating FD and correlating its mean with connectivity metrics obtained from individual subjects has been recommended recently for either confirming or ruling out the influence of head motion on connectivity measures (Power et al., 2012; Satterthwaite et al., 2012; Van Dijk et al., 2012; Satterthwaite et al., 2013; Yan et al., 2013). The QC-connectivity Spearman's correlations and corresponding *p*-values indicating their statistical significance are shown in **Table 4**. It is evident that none of the QC-connectivity correlations were statistically significant ($p > 0.05$). Given these evidence, any significant group differences for imaging metrics was probably not due to head motion. We did not use the scrubbing method described in Power et al. (2012), where removal of certain parts of the time series (scrubbing) creates an artificial discontinuity in the data. This may not be a problem while using Pearson's correlation coefficient as zero-lag synchronization in the data does not depend on the temporal ordering in the data as long as the correspondence between the variables being examined is preserved. However, other methods which are sensitive to temporal ordering in the data cannot use scrubbing.

Table 4 | The Spearman's correlation between mean frame wise displacement (our quality control metric) and the Granger causality weights for the top ranked 19 paths.

Source region	→	Sink region	*p*-Value	Correlation coefficient
LMTG	→	LTPJ	0.869	−0.031
LMTG	→	RIFG	0.958	0.010
LIPL	→	RSPL	0.984	−0.003
LMTG	→	RMTG	0.701	−0.073
LIPL	→	RMTG	0.547	0.115
LMTG	→	RMOG	0.856	−0.035
LFFG	→	RIFG	0.309	0.192
LMTG	→	LSMA	0.741	−0.063
LMOG	→	LPRCN	0.827	0.042
LMTG	→	RSTG	0.725	−0.067
RFFG	→	RTPJ	0.599	0.099
LMTG	→	RTPJ	0.827	−0.042
LMTG	→	LPRCN	0.665	−0.083
LFFG	→	LMOG	0.702	−0.073
RFFG	→	RSPL	0.322	−0.187
LFFG	→	RMTG	0.623	0.094
RFFG	→	RMOG	0.404	−0.158
RFFG	→	LTPJ	0.703	−0.073
RFFG	→	LSPL	0.866	0.032

The paths shown in the table are ordered according to the rank obtained during classification with 1 being the most significant and 19 being the least significant (first path is Rank − 1 and the last path is Rank − 19).

Granger causality is one such method which is indeed sensitive to temporal ordering in the data and hence we did not use scrubbing.

Differences in signal to noise ratio (SNR) can also impact Granger causality estimates (Nalatore et al., 2007) when the SNR is low. On the other hand, when SNR = 2, which is typically the case for task-based fMRI, we have previously showed using simulations that Granger causality estimates are accurate in the absence of hemodynamic variability (which is the case here since we deconvolved the hemodynamic response) (Deshpande et al., 2010b). We calculated effective SNR of the deconvolved fMRI time series by estimating the variance of the entire deconvolved signal, i.e., the hidden neuronal variable, and divided it by the variance of the deconvolved signal during non-stimulation phases. We then populated the SNRs of each ROI in autism and control groups to two different samples and performed a nonparametric Wilcoxon ranksum to find statistical differences. The SNR was significantly higher ($p < 0.05$, z-value = 20.1) in the ASD group (SNR = 4.13 ± 0.01) as compared to the control group (SNR = 3.2 ± 0.03). The SNRs for both groups were high enough so that SNR differences between the groups will not impact Granger causality. SNR has an impact on Granger causality only when the SNR is low.

DISCUSSION

The goals of this study were: (1) to investigate effective connectivity among brain areas during intentional causal attribution in ASD and (2) to utilize machine learning techniques to classify participants based on effective connectivity weights from this study, and behavior assessment scores, functional connectivity, and fractional anisotropy obtained from DTI data from our previous study (Kana et al., 2012). Using SVM based classification, we found that the causal connectivity path weights had the highest discriminative power to separate groups by diagnosis with high accuracy. It was uncovered that the top-ranked causal connectivity paths were also significantly weaker between social brain regions in young adults with ASD as compared to their TD peers and correlated with the ASD symptom severity (AQ) scores and theory-of-mind ability as measured by the RME test.

An application of characterizing brain connectivity patterns is to test whether such patterns can differentiate individuals with ASD from typically developing control participants such that the diagnostic label of a new participant can be determined based on imaging data. Thus, in this study we conducted a classification analysis using the effective connectivity measures, functional connectivity values, fractional anisotropy obtained from DTI data and the causal attribution task performance scores to get a fair assessment of which metric possesses the highest discriminative power. A maximum classification accuracy of 95.9% was obtained with 2 clusters and 19 features, all of these being effective connectivity paths. These results suggest that significantly weaker causal influence between brain regions during ToM processing in ASD is sufficient to separate adults with ASD from typical control participants. The discriminative patterns found in this study using SVM may have clinical applications in the long-run. Accurate separation of ASD adults from TD peers may provide potential value for clinicians, particularly in cases when behavioral observation and clinical interviews are not sufficient enough to determine a diagnosis. The key finding of differences in the causal influence of brain regions for ToM in ASD in this study adds to the relatively limited literature on effective connectivity in ASD. In addition, while previous studies explored effective connectivity in ASD during language processing, facial and emotional processing, and imitation, the current study examined effective connectivity in the context of a ToM task, which has not been studied in ASD to date. The current study expands what we know about inferring mental states in ASD, and provides insight into the causal relationships of brain regions during ToM processing. In addition, this study, to our knowledge, is the first to use effective connectivity measures for classification purposes in ASD. While this method will require some fine tuning, validation in a larger sample, and replication through multiple studies to be applied within clinical settings, the causal relationships between brain areas related to ToM holds promise for separating individuals with ASD from typical controls or from other disorders. Nevertheless, the current study marks the first attempt at using effective connectivity measures as inputs for a classification analysis of ASD subjects, therefore marking the first step in the direction of more accurate classification of the disorder.

Weaker effective connectivity of the 19 top-ranked paths found in participants with ASD in this study involved paths and regions that are found to be part of the social brain network. Several nodes, such as the TPJ, MTG, RIFG, IPL, FFG, and SMA have been associated with processing theory-of-mind, face processing, and the mirror neuron system. These findings are in line with previous studies of effective connectivity in ASD (Wicker et al., 2008; Shih et al., 2010). Our results also include significant functional alterations in social brain and visuospatial brain regions (e.g., TPJ, IFG, IPL, FFG, etc.) seen previously in functional connectivity findings (Kana et al., 2006, 2009, 2012; Just et al., 2007; Koshino et al., 2008; Mason et al., 2008), suggesting some consistency in disrupted connectivity across different modalities of connectivity and providing further support for disrupted connectivity accounts of ASD (Just et al., 2004; Kana and Just, 2011; Schipul et al., 2011; Kana et al., 2012). The findings here supplement the functional connectivity results in our previous study utilizing the same ToM stimuli, where ASD participants displayed significantly reduced functional connectivity between temporal and frontal regions, and weaker connectivity between networks made up of ventral premotor regions and TPJ (Kana et al., 2012). Our results in the current study further these previous findings by illustrating the directionality of connectivity. We found that, for ToM processing in TD participants, significantly stronger (compared to ASD group) causal connections existed among the 19 top-ranked paths which included the nodes that are associated with social cognition. So, here we find that the critical regions of the social brain are not as well coordinated with others, that they should be sharing information with, in participants with ASD. This lack of synchrony and reduced flow of information may represent a critical problem of bandwidth (maximal rate of data transfer supported by a communication channel) in ASD, where some information is getting by, but at a much lower rate than what would be needed for complex ToM connections (Just et al., 2012).

In a correlation analysis using assessment measures and effective connectivity paths for the entire sample of participants, we found the paths that were among the top ranked features in the classification analysis were correlated with AQ and RME scores. While the AQ showed significant negative correlation, the RME showed significant positive correlation with connectivity paths. Similarly, participants with better ToM skills had stronger effective connectivity during this causal attribution task. It should be noted that most of these connection paths involved information transfer to different regions mainly from the temporal lobe (LMTG, and bilateral FFG). While FFG has been associated with face processing and processing socially salient stimuli (Schultz, 2005), middle and superior temporal areas have been found to be involved in social cognition, especially in taking intentional stance, as seen in the current study, on social scenarios (Mosconi et al., 2005). The correlations found in our study reveal how social abilities such as ToM skill can influence information transfer in the brain. In addition, it also points out that severe autism symptoms may have a neural basis in reduced causal brain connectivity from the temporal lobe. As noted earlier, the correlation analysis was performed across the entire sample and we restricted it to the top-ranked 19 paths because we feel that the covariance of a brain imaging based metric with a behavioral assessment score is clinically meaningful only if the imaging metric under consideration has the power to predict the diagnostic label of a new subject. Therefore, there may very well be other connectivity paths in the brain which may be correlated with behavior (but which lack the discriminative ability) which we have not discussed here.

In conclusion, this study provides preliminary evidence to support a hypothesis that metrics based on directional brain connectivity obtained from a task engaging social brain areas may provide highly discriminative features for predicting whether a given subject has ASD or not. Studies involving larger sample size, and replication of these findings across multiple studies would be required to fully test the extent of this hypothesis and investigate its clinical implications.

ACKNOWLEDGMENTS

The authors would like to thank the UAB department of Psychology and the Civitan-McNulty Scientist Award to Rajesh K. Kana as well as support from Auburn University MRI Research Center to Gopikrishna Deshpande as sources of funding support for this study.

REFERENCES

Abler, B., Roebroeck, A., Goebel, R., Hose, A., Schfnfeldt-Lecuona, C., Hole, G., et al. (2006). Investigating directed influences between activated brain areas in a motor-response task using fMRI. *Magn. Reson. Imaging* 24, 181–185. doi: 10.1016/j.mri.2005.10.022

Alexander, A. L., Lee, J. E., Lazar, M., Boudos, R., DuBray, M. B., Oakes, T. R., et al. (2007). Diffusion tensor imaging of the corpus callosum in autism. *Neuroimage* 34, 61–73. doi: 10.1016/j.neuroimage.2006.08.032

Anderson, J. S., Nielsen, J. A., Froehlich, A. L., DuBray, M. B., Druzgal, T. J., Cariello, A. N., et al. (2011). Functional connectivity magnetic resonance imaging classification of autism. *Brain* 134(Pt. 12), 3742–3754. doi: 10.1093/brain/awr263

Asperger, H. (1944). "Die 'autistichen Psychopathen' im Kindersalter," in *Archive fur psychiatrie und Nervenkrankheiten*, Vol. 117, Reprinted in Autism and Asperger syndrome, ed U. Frith (Cambridge: Cambridge University Press), 76–136.

Assaf, M., Jagannathan, K., Calhoun, V., Miller, L., Stevens, M. C., Sahl, R., et al. (2010). Abnormal functional connectivity of default mode sub-networks in autism spectrum disorder patients. *Neuroimage* 53, 247–256. doi: 10.1016/j.neuroimage.2010.05.067

Barnea-Goraly, N., Kwon, G., Menon, B., Eliez, S., Lotspeich, L., and Reiss, A. L. (2004). White matter structure in autism: preliminary evidence from diffusion tensor imaging. *Biol. Psychiatry* 55, 323–326. doi: 10.1016/j.biopsych.2003.10.022

Barnea-Goraly, N., Lotspeich, L. J., and Reiss, A. L. (2010). Similar white matter aberrations in children with autism and their unaffected siblings: a diffusion tensor imaging study using tract based spatial statistics. *Arch. Gen. Psychiatry* 67, 1052–1060. doi: 10.1001/archgenpsychiatry.2010.123

Baron-Cohen, S., Wheelwright, S., Hill, J., Raste, Y., and Plumb, I. (2001a). The "reading the mind in the eyes" test revised version: a study with normal adults, and adults with Asperger syndrome or high-functioning autism. *J. Child Psychol. Psychiatry* 42, 241–251. doi: 10.1111/1469-7610.00715

Baron-Cohen, S., Wheelwright, S., Skinner, R., Martin, J., and Clubley, E. (2001b). The autism spectrum quotient (AQ): evidence from Asperger syndrome/high functioning autism, males and females, scientists and mathematicians. *J. Autism Dev. Disord.* 31, 5–17. doi: 10.1023/A:1005653411471

Bird, G., Catmur, C., Silani, G., Frith, C., and Frith, U. (2006). Attention does not modulate neural responses to social stimuli in autism spectrum disorders. *Neuroimage* 31, 1614–1624. doi: 10.1016/j.neuroimage.2006.02.037

Brunet, E., Sarfati, Y., Hardy-Baylé, M. C., and Decety, J. (2000). A PET investigation of the attribution of intentions with a nonverbal task. *Neuroimage* 11, 157–166. doi: 10.1006/nimg.1999.0525

Buchel, C., and Friston, K. J. (2000). Assessing interactions among neuronal systems using functional neuroimaging. *Neural Netw.* 13, 871–882. doi: 10.1016/S0893-6080(00)00066-6

Calderoni, S., Reticom, A., Biagi, L., Tancredi, R., Muratori, F., and Tosetti, M. (2012). Female children with autism spectrum disorder: an insight from mass-univariate and pattern classification analyses. *Neuroimage* 59, 1013–1022. doi: 10.1016/j.neuroimage.2011.08.070

Chen, G., Ward, D., Xie, C., Li, W., Wu, Z., Jones, J., et al. (2011). Classification of Alzheimer disease, mild cognitive impairment, and normal cognitive status with large-scale network analysis based on resting-state functional MR imaging. *Radiology* 259, 213–221. doi: 10.1148/radiol.10100734

Cherkassky, V., Kana, R., Keller, T., and Just, M. (2006). Functional connectivity in a baseline resting-state network in autism. *Neuroreport* 17, 1687–1690. doi: 10.1097/01.wnr.0000239956.45448.4c

Coutanche, M. N., Thompson-Schill, S. L., and Schultz, R. T. (2011). Multi-voxel pattern analysis of fMRI data predicts clinical symptom severity. *Neuroimage* 57, 113–123. doi:10.1016/j.neuroimage.2011.04.016

Craddock, R., Holtzheimer, I. P., Hu, X., and Mayberg, H. (2009). Disease state prediction from resting state functional connectivity. *Magn. Reson. Med.* 62, 1619–1628. doi: 10.1002/mrm.22159

Cubillo, A., Rozmin, H., Ecker, C., Giampietro, V., Taylor, E., and Rubia, K. (2010). Reduced activation and inter-regional functional connectivity of fronto-striatal networks in adults with childhood Attention-Deficit Hyperactivity Disorder (ADHS) and persisting symptoms during tasks of motor inhibition and cognitive switching. *J. Psychiatry Res.* 44, 629–639. doi: 10.1016/j.jpsychires.2009.11.016

Damarla, S. R., Keller, T. A., Kana, R. K., Cherkassky, V. L., Williams, D. L., Minshew, N. J., et al. (2010). Cortical underconnectivity coupled with preserved visuospatial cognition in autism: evidence from an fMRI study of an embedded figures task. *Autism Res.* 3, 273–279. doi: 10.1002/aur.153

David, O., Guillemain, I., Saillet, S., Reyt, S., Deransart, C., Segebarth, C., et al. (2008). Identifying neural drivers with functional MRI: an electrophysiological validation. *PLoS Biol.* 6:2683–2697. doi: 10.1371/journal.pbio.0060315

Deshpande, G., Hu, X., Stilla, R., and Sathian, K. (2008). Effective connectivity during haptic perception: a study using granger causality analysis of functional magnetic resonance imaging data. *Neuroimage* 40, 1807–1814. doi: 10.1016/j.neuroimage.2008.01.044

Deshpande, G., James, G., Craddock, R., Mayberg, H., and Hu, X. (2009a). "Predicting treatment in patients with major depression using granger-based connectivity and support vector machines," in *Proceedings of ISMRM 17th Scientific Meeting 2009* (Honolulu, HI), 3362.

Deshpande, G., LaConte, S., James, G., Peltier, S., and Hu, X. (2009b). Multivariate Granger causality analysis of brain networks. *Hum. Brain Mapp.* 30, 1361–1373. doi: 10.1002/hbm.20606

Deshpande, G., Li, Z., Santhanam, P., Coles, C. D., Lynch, M. E., Hamann, S., et al. (2010a). Recursive cluster elimination based support vector machine for disease state prediction using resting state functional and effective brain connectivity. *PLoS ONE* 5:e14277. doi: 10.1371/journal.pone.0014277

Deshpande, G., Sathian, K., and Hu, X. (2010b). Effect of hemodynamic variability on Granger causality analysis of fMRI. *Neuroimage* 52, 884–896. doi: 10.1016/j.neuroimage.2009.11.060

Deshpande, G., Sathian, K., and Hu, X. (2010c). Assessing and compensating for zero-lag correlation effects in time-lagged granger causality analysis of fMRI. *IEEE Trans. Biomed. Eng.* 57, 1446–1456. doi: 10.1109/TBME.2009.2037808

Dosenbach, N. U., Nardos, B., Cohen, A. L., Fair, D. A., Power, J. D., Church, J. A., et al. (2010). Prediction of individual brain maturity using fMRI. *Science* 329, 1358–1361. doi: 10.1126/science.1194144

Duffy, F. H., and Als, H. (2012). A stable pattern of EEG spectral coherence distinguishes children with autism from neuro-typical controls – a large case control study. *BMC Med.* 10, 64. doi: 10.1186/1741-7015-10-64

Friston, J. K., Holmes, A. P., Worsley, K. J., Poline, J. B., Frith, C. D., and Frackowiak, R. S. J. (1995). Statistical parametric maps in functional imaging: a general linear approach. *Hum. Brain Mapp.* 2, 189–210. doi: 10.1002/hbm.460020402

Friston, K., Harrison, L., and Penny, W. (2003). Dynamic causal modeling. *Neuroimage* 19, 1273–1302. doi: 10.1016/S1053-8119(03)00202-7

Garrity, A. G., Pearlson, G. D., McKiernan, K., Lloyd, D., Kiehl, K. A., and Calhoun, V. D. (2007). Aberrant "deafult mode" functional connectivity in schizophrenia. *Am. J. Psychiatry* 164, 450–457. doi: 10.1176/appi.ajp.164.3.450

Granger, C. (1969). Investigating causal relations by econometric models and cross-spectral methods. *Econometrica* 37, 424–438. doi: 10.2307/1912791

Handwerker, D., Ollinger, J., and D'Esposito, M. (2004). Variation of BOLD hemodynamic responses across subjects and brain regions and their effects on statistical analyses. *Neuroimage* 21, 1639–1651. doi: 10.1016/j.neuroimage.2003.11.029

Havlicek, M., Friston, K., Jan, J., Brazdil, M., and Calhoun, V. (2011). Dynamic modeling of neuronal responses in fMRI using cubature Kalman filtering. *Neuroimage* 56, 2109–2128. doi: 10.1016/j.neuroimage.2011.03.005

Ingalhalikar, M., Parker, D., Bloy, L., Roberts, T. P. L., and Verma, R. (2011). Diffusion based abnormality markers of pathology: toward learned diagnostic prediction of ASD. *Neuroimage* 57, 918–927. doi: 10.1016/j.neuroimage.2011.05.023

Jones, T. B., Bandettini, P. A., Kenworthy, L., Case, L. K., Milleville, S. C., Martin, A., et al. (2010). Sources of group differences in functional connectivity: an investigation applied to autism spectrum disorder. *Neuroimage* 49, 401–414. doi: 10.1016/j.neuroimage.2009.07.051

Jou, R., Jackowski, A., Papademetris, X., Rajeevan, N., Staib, L., and Volkmar, F. (2011). Diffusion tensor imaging in autism spectrum disorders: preliminary evidence of abnormal neural connectivity. *Aust. N.Z. J. Psychiatry* 45, 153–162. doi: 10.3109/00048674.2010.534069

Just, M., Cherkassky, V., Keller, T., and Minshew, N. (2004). Cortical activation and synchronization during sentence comprehension in high-functioning autism: evidence of underconnectivity. *Brain* 127, 1811–1821. doi: 10.1093/brain/awh199

Just, M. A., Cherkassky, V. L., Keller, T. A., Kana, R. K., and Minshew, N. J. (2007). Functional and anatomical cortical underconnectivity in autism: evidence from an fMRI study of an executive function task and corpus callosum morphometry. *Cereb. Cortex* 17, 951–961. doi: 10.1093/cercor/bhl006

Just, M. A., Keller, T. A., Malave, V. L., Kana, R. K., and Varma, S. (2012). Autism as a neural systems disorder: a theory of frontal-posterior underconnectivity. *Neurosci. Biobehav. Rev.* 36, 1292–1313. doi: 10.1016/j.neubiorev.2012.02.007

Kana, R., Keller, T., Cherkassky, V., Minshew, N., and Just, M. (2006). Sentence comprehension in autism: thinking in pictures with decreased functional connectivity. *Brain* 129, 2484–2493. doi: 10.1093/brain/awl164

Kana, R. K., and Just, M. A. (2011). "Autism as a disorder of functional brain connectivity," in *Handbook of Autism Spectrum Disorders*, eds D. G. Amaral, D. Geschwind, and G. Dawson (New York, NY: Oxford University Press), 981–989. doi: 10.1093/med/9780195371826.003.0061

Kana, R. K., Keller, T. A., Minshew, N. J., and Just, M. A. (2007). Inhibitory control in high-functioning autism: decreased activation and underconnectivity in inhibition networks. *Biol. Psychiatry* 62, 198–206. doi: 10.1016/j.biopsych.2006.08.004

Kana, R. K., Keller, T. A., Cherkassky, V. L., Minshew, N. J., and Just, M. A. (2009). Atypical frontal-posterior synchronization of Theory-of-Mind regions in autism during mental state attribution. *Soc. Neurosci.* 4, 135–152. doi: 10.1080/17470910802198510

Kana, R. K., Libero, L. E., and Moore, M. S. (2011). Disrupted cortical connectivity theory as an explanatory model for autism spectrum disorders. *Phys. Life Rev.* 8, 410–437. doi: 10.1016/j.plrev.2011.10.001

Kana, R. K., Libero, L. E., Hu, C. P., Deshpande, H. D., and Colburn, J. S. (2012). Functional brain networks and white matter underlying theory-of-mind in autism. *Soc. Cogn. Affect. Neurosci.* 7, 1–8. doi: 10.1093/scan/nss106

Kanner, L. (1943). Autistic disturbances of affective contact. *Nervous Child* 2, 217–250.

Keller, T. A., Kana, R. K., and Just, M. A. (2007). A developmental study of the structural integrity of white matter in autism. *Neuroreport* 18, 23–27. doi: 10.1097/01.wnr.0000239965.21685.99

Koshino, H., Kana, R. K., Keller, T. A., Cherkassky, V. L., Minshew, N. J., and Just, M. A. (2008). fMRI investigation of working memory for faces in autism: visual coding and underconnectivity with frontal areas. *Cereb. Cortex* 18, 289–300. doi: 10.1093/cercor/bhm054

Kriegeskorte, N., Simmons, W., Bellgowan, P., and Baker, C. (2009). Circular analysis in systems neuroscience: the dangers of double dipping. *Nat. Neurosci.* 12, 535–540.doi: 10.1038/nn.2303

Kuś, R., Kamiñski, M., and Blinowska, K. (2004). Determination of EEG activity propagation: pair-wise versus multichannel estimate. *IEEE Trans. Biomed. Eng.* 51, 1501–1510. doi: 10.1109/TBME.2004.827929

Lawrie, S. M., Buechel, C., Whalley, H. C., Frith, C. D., Friston, K. J., and Johnstone, E. C. (2002). Reduced frontotemporal functional connectivity in schizophrenia associated with auditory hallucinations. *Biol. Psychiatry* 51, 1008–1011. doi: 10.1016/S0006-3223(01)01316-1

Lieberman, M., and Cunningham, W. (2009). Type I and Type II error concerns in fMRI research: rebalancing the scale. *Soc. Cogn. Affect. Neurosci.* 4, 423–428. doi: 10.1093/scan/nsp052

Marquand, A.F., Filippone, M., Ashburner, J., Girolami, M., Mourao-Miranda, J., Barker, G. L., et al. (2013). Automated, high accuracy classification of parkinsonian disorders: a pattern recognition approach. *PLoS ONE* 8:e69237. doi:10.1371/journal.pone.0069237

Mason, R. A., Williams, D. L., Kana, R. K., Minshew, N., and Just, M. A. (2008). Theory-of-Mind disruption and recruitment of the right hemisphere during narrative comprehension in autism. *Neuropsychologia* 46, 269–280. doi: 10.1016/j.neuropsychologia.2007.07.018

McIntosh, A., and Gozales-Lima, F. (1994). Structural equation modelling and its application to network analysis in functional brain imaging. *Hum. Brain Mapp.* 2, 2–22. doi: 10.1002/hbm.460020104

McIntosh, A. R., Kovacevic, N., Lippe, S., Garrett, D., Grady, C., and Jirsa, V. (2010). The development of a noisy brain. *Arch. Ital. Biol.* 148, 323–337.

Meyer-Lindenberg, A. S., Olsen, R. K., Kohn, P. D., Brown, T., Egan, M. D., Weinberger, D. R., et al. (2005). Regionally specific disturbance of dorsolateral prefrontal-hippocampal functional connectivity in schizophrenia. *Arch. Gen. Psychiatry* 62, 379–386. doi: 10.1001/archpsych.62.4.379.

Mirowski, P., Madhavan, D., LeCun, Y., and Kuzniecky, R. (2009). Classification of patterns of EEG synchronization for seizure prediction. *Clin. Neurophysiol.* 120, 1927–1940. doi: 10.1016/j.clinph.2009.09.002

Mizuno, A., Liu, Y., Williams, D. L., Keller, T. A., Minshew, N. J., and Just, M. A. (2011). The neural basis of deictic shifting in linguistic perspective-taking in high-functioning autism. *Brain* 134(Pt. 8), 2422–2435. doi: 10.1093/brain/awr151

Mosconi, M. W., Mack, P. B., McCarthy, G., and Pelphrey, K. A. (2005). Taking an "intentional

stance" on eye-gaze shifts: a functional neuroimaging study of social perception in children. *Neuroimage* 27, 247–252. doi: 10.1016/j.neuroimage.2005.03.027
Murdaugh, D. L., Shinkareva, S. V., Deshpande, H. R., Wang, J., Pennick, M. R., and Kana, R. K. (2012). Differential deactivation during mentalizing and classification of autism based on default mode connectivity. *PLoS ONE* 7:e50064. doi: 10.1371/journal.pone.0050064
Nalatore, H., Ding, M., and Rangarajan, G. (2007). Mitigating the effects of measurement noise on Granger causality. *Phys. Rev. E Stat. Nonlin. Soft Matter Phys.* 75(3 Pt 1), 031123. doi: 10.1103/PhysRevE.75.031123
Pereira, F., Mitchell, T., and Botvinick, M. (2009). Machine learning classifiers and fMRI: a tutorial overview. *Neuroimage* 45, S199–S209. doi: 10.1016/j.neuroimage.2008.11.007
Power, J., Barnes, K., Snyder, A., Schlaggar, B., and Petersen, S. (2012). Spurious but systematic correlations in functional connectivity MRI networks arise from subject motion. *Neuroimage* 59, 2142–2154. doi: 10.1016/j.neuroimage.2011.10.018
Roebroeck, A., Formisano, E., and Goebel, R. (2005). Mapping directed influence over the brain using Granger causality and fMRI. *Neuroimage* 25, 230– 242. doi: 10.1016/j.neuroimage.2004.11.017
Sathian, K., Lacey, S., Stilla, R., Gibson, G., Deshpande, G., Hu, X., et al. (2011). Dual pathways for haptic and visual perception of spatial and texture information. *Neuroimage* 57, 462–475. doi: 10.1016/j.neuroimage.2011.05.001
Satterthwaite, T. D., Elliott, M. A., Gerraty, R. T., Ruparel, K., Loughead, J., Calkins, M. E., et al. (2013). An improved framework for confound regression and filtering for control of motion artifact in the preprocessing of resting-state functional connectivity data. *Neuroimage* 64, 240–256. doi: 10.1016/j.neuroimage.2012.08.052
Satterthwaite, T. D., Wolf, D. H., Loughead, J., Ruparel, K., Elliott, M. A., Hakonarson, H., et al. (2012). Impact of in-scanner head motion on multiple measures of functional connectivity: relevance for studies of neurodevelopment in youth. *Neuroimage* 60, 623–632. doi: 10.1016/j.neuroimage.2011.12.063
Schipul, S., Keller, T., and Just, M. (2011). Inter-regional brain communication and its disturbance in autism. *Front. Syst. Neurosci.* 5:10. doi: 10.3389/fnsys.2011.00010
Schultz, R. T. (2005). Developmental deficits in social perception in autism: the role of the amygdala and fusiform face area. *Int. J. Dev. Neurosci.* 23, 125–141. doi: 10.1016/j.ijdevneu.2004.12.012
Shen, M. D., Shih, P., Ottl, B., Keehn, B., Leyden, K. M., Gaffrey, M. S., et al. (2012). Atypical lexicosematntic function of extrastriate cortex in autism spectrum disorder: evidence from functional and effective connectivity. *Neuroimage* 62, 1780–1791. doi: 10.1016/j.neuroimage.2012.06.008
Shih, P., Shen, M., Ottl, B., Keehn, B., Gaffrey, M., and Muller, R-A. (2010). Atypical network connectivity for imitation in autism spectrum disorder. *Neuropsychologia* 48, 2931–2939. doi: 10.1016/j.neuropsychologia.2010.05.035
Shinkareva, S. V., Wang, J., and Wedell, D. H. (2013). Examining similarity structure: multidimensional scaling and related approaches in neuroimaging. *Comput. Math. Methods Med.* 2013, 796183. doi: 10.1155/2013/796183
Solomon, M., Ozonoff, S. J., Ursu, S., Ravizza, S., Cumings, N., Ly, S., et al. (2009). The neural substrates of cognitive control deficits in autism spectrum disorders. *Neuropsychologia* 47, 2515–2526. doi: 10.1016/j.neuropsychologia.2009.04.019
Tian, L., Jiang, T., Wang, Y., Zang, Y., He, Y., Liang, M., et al. (2006). Altered resting-state functional connectivity patterns of anterior cingulate cortex in adolescents with attention deficit hyperactivity disorder. *Neurosci. Lett.* 400, 39–43. doi: 10.1016/j.neulet.2006.02.022
Travers, B. G., Adluru, N., Ennis, C., Tromp do, P. M., Destiche, D., Doran, S., et al. (2012). Diffustion tensor imaging in autism spectrum disorder: a review. *Autism Res.* 5, 289–313. doi: 10.1002/aur.1243
Uddin, L., Vinod, M., Young, C. B., Ryali, S., Chen, T., Khouzam, A., et al. (2011). Multivariate searchlight classification of structural magnetic resonance imaging in children and adolescents with autism. *Biol. Psychiatry* 70, 833–841. doi: 10.1016/j.biopsych.2011.07.014
Van Dijk, K. R. A., Sabuncu, M. R., and Buckner, R. L. (2012). The influence of head motion on intrinsic functional connectivity MRI. *Neuroimage* 59, 431–438. doi: 10.1016/j.neuroimage.2011.07.044
Vapnik, V. (1995). *The Nature of Statistical Learning Theory.* New York, NY: Springer. doi: 10.1007/978-1-4757-2440-0
Villalobos, M. E., Mizuno, A., Dahl, B. C., Kemmotsu, N., and Muller, R.-A. (2005). Reduced functional connectivity between V1 and inferior frontal cortex associated with visuomotor performance in autism. *Neuroimage* 25, 916–925. doi: 10.1016/j.neuroimage.2004.12.022
Wang, L. (2005). *Support Vector Machines: Theory and Applications.* New York, NY: Springer.
Wang, G., Chen, C., and Fushing, H. (2012). Extracting multiscale pattern information of fMRI based functional brain connectivity with application on classification of autism spectrum disorders. *PLoS ONE* 7:e45502. doi: 10.1371/journal.pone.0045502
Weygandt, M., Hackmack, K., Pfüller, C., Bellmann-Strobl, J., Paul, F., Zipp, F., et al. (2011). MRI pattern recognition in multiple sclerosis normal-appearing brain areas. *PLoS ONE* 6:e21138. doi: 10.1371/journal.pone.0021138
Wicker, B., Fonlupt, P., Hubert, B., Tardif, C., Gepner, B., and Deruelle, C. (2008). Abnormal cerebral effective connectivity during explicit emotional processing in adults with autism spectrum disorder. *Soc. Cogn. Affect. Neurosci.* 3, 135–143. doi: 10.1093/scan/nsn007
Yan, C. G., Cheung, B., Kelly, C., Colcombe, S., Craddock, R. C., Di Martino, A., et al. (2013). A comprehensive assessment of regional variation in the impact of head micromovements on functional connectomics. *Neuroimage* 76, 183–201. doi: 10.1016/j.neuroimage.2013.03.004
Yang, X., Lin, D., Hao, Z., Liang, Y., Liu, G., and Han, X. (2003). A fast SVM training algorithm based on the set segmentation and k-means clustering. *Prog. Nat. Sci.* 13, 750–755. doi: 10.1080/10020070312331344360

5

Reconceptualizing functional brain connectivity in autism from a developmental perspective

Lucina Q. Uddin[1]*, Kaustubh Supekar[1] and Vinod Menon[1,2,3]

[1] Department of Psychiatry and Behavioral Sciences, Stanford University School of Medicine, Stanford, CA, USA
[2] Program in Neuroscience, Stanford University School of Medicine, Stanford, CA, USA
[3] Department of Neurology and Neurological Sciences, Stanford University School of Medicine, Stanford, CA, USA

Edited by:
Rajesh K. Kana, University of Alabama at Birmingham, USA

Reviewed by:
Qingbao Yu, The Mind Research Network, USA
R. Matthew Hutchison, Western University, Canada
Timothy A. Keller, Carnegie Mellon University, USA
Diane L. Williams, Duquesne University, USA

***Correspondence:**
Lucina Q. Uddin, Department of Psychiatry and Behavioral Sciences, Stanford University School of Medicine, 401 Quarry Rd., Stanford, CA 94305-5719, USA
e-mail: lucina@stanford.edu

While there is almost universal agreement amongst researchers that autism is associated with alterations in brain connectivity, the precise nature of these alterations continues to be debated. Theoretical and empirical work is beginning to reveal that autism is associated with a complex functional phenotype characterized by both hypo- and hyper-connectivity of large-scale brain systems. It is not yet understood why such conflicting patterns of brain connectivity are observed across different studies, and the factors contributing to these heterogeneous findings have not been identified. Developmental changes in functional connectivity have received inadequate attention to date. We propose that discrepancies between findings of autism related hypo-connectivity and hyper-connectivity might be reconciled by taking developmental changes into account. We review neuroimaging studies of autism, with an emphasis on functional magnetic resonance imaging studies of intrinsic functional connectivity in children, adolescents and adults. The consistent pattern emerging across several studies is that while intrinsic functional connectivity in adolescents and adults with autism is generally reduced compared with age-matched controls, functional connectivity in younger children with the disorder appears to be increased. We suggest that by placing recent empirical findings within a developmental framework, and explicitly characterizing age and pubertal stage in future work, it may be possible to resolve conflicting findings of hypo- and hyper-connectivity in the extant literature and arrive at a more comprehensive understanding of the neurobiology of autism.

Keywords: autism spectrum disorders, brain development, functional connectivity, puberty, fMRI

INTRODUCTION

Autism spectrum disorder (ASD) is a neurodevelopmental disorder characterized by impaired social interaction and communication, repetitive behaviors, and restricted interests. According to the latest reports, ASD affects nearly 1 in 88 children, and the prevalence continues to grow (Investigators, 2012). The recognition of the increasing prevalence of ASD has placed a mandate on understanding its neurobiological foundations. As highlighted in several articles appearing in this special topic, one of the most well-documented observations in the autism literature is that the brains of individuals with the disorder exhibit aberrant functional connectivity or inter-regional communication (Belmonte et al., 2004). Functional connectivity as measured from functional magnetic resonance imaging (fMRI) data is defined as "temporal correlations between remote neurophysiological events" (Friston, 1994). Functional connectivity is typically measured using one of three approaches: (1) regression analysis using a seed region of interest (Greicius et al., 2003; Fox et al., 2005), (2) full or partial correlation analysis of multiple regions of interest (Ryali et al., 2012), or (3) independent component analysis (ICA) of the entire imaging dataset to identify spatial maps with common temporal profiles (Beckmann and Smith, 2004; Cole et al., 2010). These measures have been used to characterize large-scale networks in the human brain (Bressler and Menon, 2010; Sporns, 2011), and have paved the way for increasingly sophisticated investigations of brain connectivity in ASD (Kennedy and Adolphs, 2012).

Temporal correlations in blood oxygen level dependent (BOLD) fMRI signals are thought to arise from signal propagation and dynamical slowing down of fluctuations in anatomically constrained neural networks (Deco et al., 2013). Consistent with this, empirical studies using human ECoG have shown that slow (<0.1 Hz) spontaneous fluctuations of firing rate and gamma local field potentials are correlated with spontaneous fMRI fluctuations (Nir et al., 2008). Intrinsic functional connectivity measured during resting state fMRI may reflect a history of task-dependent coactivation, and likely serves to organize and coordinate neuronal activity, or might represent dynamic predictions about expected patterns of use (Fox and Raichle, 2007).

Several investigations have reported that functional connectivity between brain regions is weaker in high-functioning ASD, leading to long-distance cortical "under-connectivity" theories of autism (Courchesne and Pierce, 2005; Geschwind and Levitt,

Abbreviations: ASD, Autism spectrum disorder; fMRI, Functional magnetic resonance imaging; DMN, Default mode network; ICA, Independent component analysis.

2007; Schipul et al., 2011; Just et al., 2012). However, there is emerging evidence that challenges these models and suggests that functional connectivity between brain regions can be stronger in ASD (Uddin et al., 2013). It is not yet understood why such conflicting patterns of brain connectivity results are observed across different studies, and factors contributing to these heterogeneous findings have not been identified. A more nuanced account capturing patterns of both task-related and intrinsic hypo- and hyper-connectivity observed in autism is essential for characterizing aberrant brain organization in the disorder (Kana et al., 2011; Muller et al., 2011; Vissers et al., 2011). Recent attempts to provide explanations for the discrepant findings in the literature have delineated both methodological issues (Muller et al., 2011) and conceptual issues (Vissers et al., 2011). Here we propose that yet another source of inconsistency exists, namely that developmental changes in functional connectivity have received inadequate attention to date. We posit that discrepancies between findings of autism-related hypo-connectivity and hyper-connectivity might be reconciled by taking developmental stage into account.

The idea that critical periods of plasticity during brain development represent particularly vulnerable stages during which aberrant maturational process can occur is not a new one. In 2003 Rubenstein and Merzenich first introduced the theory that autism may arise from an increased ratio of excitation/inhibition in developing neural systems subserving sensory, mnemonic, social, and emotional processes. Hyperexcitability as a result of this imbalance has been hypothesized to contribute to poorly functionally differentiated and inherently unstable cortex in autism (Rubenstein and Merzenich, 2003). As summarized in a recent review characterizing autism as a critical period disorder, excessive plasticity at the wrong times could result in noisy and unstable processing, yet a brain that lacks appropriate levels of plasticity early in life might remain hyper- or hypo-connected and unresponsive to environmental changes early in life (LeBlanc and Fagiolini, 2011).

One of the earliest signs of autism is enlarged head circumference or macrocephaly (Lainhart et al., 1997). Infants and young children with ASD show signs of early brain overgrowth (Courchesne et al., 2003). Postmortem studies of children with ASD show that they have an overabundance or excess numbers of neurons in the prefrontal cortex (Courchesne et al., 2011). Animal models likewise provide evidence for hyper-connectivity at very early time points in development (Testa-Silva et al., 2011). There is a profound inconsistency between these observations and "under-connectivity" or hypo-connectivity theories that by and large do not account for the possibility of an early phase of neural hyper-connectivity in ASD.

The EEG literature has long reflected an understanding that stabilization and pruning of connections during development plays a central role in the development of cognitive and perceptual functions during critical periods early in life. Uhlhaas and colleagues summarize decades of work to hypothesize that "in ASDs abnormal brain maturation during early prenatal and postnatal periods results in cortical circuits that are unable to support the expression of high-frequency oscillations during infancy. These impaired oscillations might in turn reduce the temporal precision of coordinated firing patterns and thereby disturb activity-dependent circuit selection during further development" (Uhlhaas et al., 2010). These developmental perspectives from animal models and electrophysiological studies should be integrated into the fMRI community, which has struggled to reconcile inconsistent findings with regards to functional brain connectivity in ASD over the past several years.

There has been rapid progress in understanding changes in functional connectivity accompanying typical development with the advent of resting-state fMRI (Uddin et al., 2010). For example, it is now known that subcortical areas are more strongly functionally coupled with primary sensory, association, and paralimbic areas in children, whereas adults show stronger cortico-cortical functional connectivity between paralimbic, limbic, and association areas (Supekar et al., 2009). More generally, several studies have demonstrated that over development, functional brain networks shift from a local anatomical emphasis to a more distributed architecture (Fair et al., 2009; Kelly et al., 2009). It has recently been suggested that motion-related artifacts can have a significant impact on functional connectivity estimates (Power et al., 2012; Van Dijk et al., 2012) in such a way that makes it difficult to study developmental differences. While the appropriate treatment of motion-related artifacts is as yet an unresolved issue in the field (see Satterthwaite et al., 2012, 2013), findings from other imaging modalities including diffusion tensor imaging corroborate functional connectivity findings of increased integrity of long-distance connections with development (Supekar et al., 2010; Uddin et al., 2011). These and other insights from developmental cognitive neuroscience can and should inform theories of atypical development of functional connectivity in autism.

The majority of functional neuroimaging studies of autism have been conducted in adolescents or adults, in part due to practical limitations related to scanning very young children (Yerys et al., 2009). Evidence from these studies of older individuals generally supports the hypo-connectivity theory of autism. However, the lack of available empirical data from younger children with the disorder has made it difficult to test the extent to which the hypo-connectivity theory generalizes to younger age groups. Although calls for data sharing in autism research have been put forth in the past (Belmonte et al., 2008), only recently have large neuroimaging datasets been released. One recent grassroots data sharing initiative (http://fcon_1000.projects.nitrc.org/indi/abide/) has made pre-publication datasets of neuroimaging data collected from individuals between the ages of 6 and 60 available to researchers to facilitate and accelerate the discovery of the functional architecture of the autistic brain (Di Martino et al., 2013a). Still, at this time relatively little has been published addressing the issue of functional brain connectivity in young children with ASD.

The purpose of this review is to (1) summarize the current status of the field by highlighting key findings from studies using fMRI to examine task-related and intrinsic functional connectivity in individuals with ASD across various age groups, (2) reveal critical gaps in the literature which have led to an inconsistent characterization of functional connectivity in ASD, and (3) argue that a developmental perspective can help reconcile some extant contradictory findings, and is necessary for future progress in the field.

FUNCTIONAL BRAIN CONNECTIVITY IN AUTISM: REVIEW

Autism is a disorder with early life onset and variable developmental trajectory (Stefanatos, 2008). Functional neuroimaging studies of young children are thus especially critical for developing accurate models of the underlying neurobiology of the disorder. Thus, it is perhaps surprising that very few fMRI studies have addressed the question of how the brain is functionally organized in childhood ASD, at developmental stages more proximal to the onset of the disorder (Akshoomoff et al., 2002; Amaral, 2010). Below we survey fMRI studies of ASD examining task-based functional connectivity and resting-state functional connectivity with the goal of providing an overview of the existing literature and highlighting the dearth of developmental studies of functional connectivity in ASD.

TASK-BASED FUNCTIONAL CONNECTIVITY

Task-based functional connectivity measures the synchronization of activation levels between brain regions during the performance of a given cognitive task. Since the initial fMRI reports of hypo-connectivity in autism (Just et al., 2004), task-related reductions in inter-regional brain connectivity during language (Just et al., 2004; Mason et al., 2008; Jones et al., 2010), working memory (Koshino et al., 2005, 2008), mental imagery (Kana et al., 2006), executive functions (Just et al., 2007), cognitive control (Kana et al., 2007; Solomon et al., 2009; Agam et al., 2010), visuomotor coordination (Villalobos et al., 2005) and social cognition (Kleinhans et al., 2008; Kana et al., 2009) have been documented. However, reports of brain hyper-connectivity in ASD also exist in the domains of visuomotor processing (Mizuno et al., 2006; Turner et al., 2006), visual search (Shih et al., 2011), emotion processing (Welchew et al., 2005), memory (Noonan et al., 2009), and language (Shih et al., 2010). These findings are comprehensively reviewed elsewhere (Thai et al., 2009; Schipul et al., 2011; Vissers et al., 2011). A recent review of studies conducted mainly in adults highlights several methodological variables including concatenation of specific task blocks, the use of low-pass filtering, regression of main effects of task, and methods for selecting regions-of-interest that result in considerable heterogeneity between studies with respect to how functional connectivity is conceptualized and analyzed. The authors suggest that such variables may partially account for discrepancies in connectivity results, and that hypo-connectivity findings may be contingent upon these methodological choices (Muller et al., 2011). For example, Muller and colleagues surveyed 32 studies and found that the use of low-pass filtering of fMRI data more often produced results inconsistent with the general under-connectivity theory (Muller et al., 2011).

Recognizing and documenting methodological issues is a critical first step toward synthesizing findings in the "functional connectivity in autism" literature and identifying robust and replicable results. Overall, task-based functional connectivity studies largely support the hypo-connectivity theory, however, the majority of these report results from older adolescents and adults. Additionally, task-based approaches produce results that cannot be easily generalized to other cognitive states, and differences between groups in task performance can make interpretation of hypo- and hyper-connectivity results difficult. The emergence of resting-state fMRI as a means for characterizing the intrinsic functional architecture of the brain, unconfounded by task and behavioral effects, has facilitated data collection from younger typically developing (TD) children and children with ASD (Uddin et al., 2010).

RESTING-STATE FUNCTIONAL CONNECTIVITY

Since the initial demonstration by Biswal and colleagues that coherent spontaneous low-frequency fluctuations in BOLD signal can be detected within functional systems in the absence of task performance (Biswal et al., 1995), the use of resting-state fMRI in neuroscience has grown exponentially. Applications in clinical neuroscience have been particularly useful, and have provided insights into systems-level cortical and subcortical anomalies of functional connectivity in neurodevelopmental disorders such as attention-deficit/hyperactivity disorder (ADHD, Castellanos and Proal, 2012) and schizophrenia (Yu et al., 2012). Surprisingly, however, there are relatively few published resting-state functional connectivity studies examining individuals with ASD. Extant studies have by and large focused on adolescents or adults with the disorder, with a few notable exceptions.

The earliest published intrinsic functional connectivity study of autism was conducted by Cherkassky and colleagues, who used a seed region-of-interest (ROI) approach to demonstrate functional hypo-connectivity in anterior–posterior connections in adolescents and adults with ASD (Cherkassky et al., 2006). Using an ROI-based approach in another study, Kennedy and colleagues demonstrated disrupted intrinsic connectivity of the default mode network (DMN), but not the dorsal attention network, in a group of adolescents and adults with autism (Kennedy and Courchesne, 2008). Others have replicated this finding of reduced DMN connectivity in adults (Monk et al., 2009), as well as adolescents (Weng et al., 2010) with ASD. Similar findings of decreased functional connectivity of the DMN in adults with ASD have been obtained using data-driven ICA approaches (Assaf et al., 2010), as well as studies combining both seed correlation and ICA (von dem Hagen et al., 2013). Whole-brain connectivity approaches have also provided evidence of hypo-connectivity of social processing-related brain circuits in adolescents with ASD (Gotts et al., 2012), though a recent systematic investigation using both ROI-based and ICA-based analytic approaches found very few examples of functional hypo-connectivity in adults with ASD compared with age-matched control participants (Tyszka et al., 2013). A study of adolescents and adults revealed decreased intrinsic functional connectivity of the insular cortex in high-functioning ASD (Ebisch et al., 2010). As summarized in **Table 1**, the studies that have reported group differences in the direction of autism-related intrinsic hypo-connectivity were all conducted in either adolescent or adult high-functioning (average or above average IQ) samples. The nascent literature on childhood ASD, in contrast, paints a very different picture.

In a group of children between 7 and 14 years of age, Di Martino and colleagues found that children with ASD exhibit functional hyper-connectivity compared with TD peers. They found increased functional connectivity between striatal subregions and heteromodal association and limbic cortices including insula and superior temporal gyrus (Di Martino et al., 2011).

Table 1 | Resting-state functional connectivity MRI studies in ASD.

Publication	Ages examined	Gender and sample size	Intrinsic functional connectivity method and results
Dinstein et al., 2011	ASD: 2.42 Range: 1–3.83 TD: 2.33 Range: 1.08–3.83	29 ASD; 30 TD; gender not reported	Interhemispheric hypo-connectivity between left and right superior temporal gyri and left and right inferior frontal gyri (seed-based during auditory stimulation)
Di Martino et al., 2011	ASD: 10.4 ± 1.7 TD: 10.9 ± 1.6 Range: 7.6–13.5	20 ASD (17 male); 20 TD (14 male)	Hyper-connectivity of striatum with insula and superior temporal gyrus (seed-based)
Uddin et al., 2013	ASD: 9.96 ± 1.59 Range: 7.52–11.88 TD: 9.95 ± 1.60 Range: 7.75–12.43	20 ASD (16 male); 20 TD (16 male)	Hyper-connectivity within salience, default mode, frontotemporal, motor, and visual networks (ICA)
Lynch et al., 2013	ASD: 9.96 ± 1.59 TD: 9.88 ± 1.61 Range: 7–12	20 ASD (16 male); 19 TD (15 male)	Hyper-connectivity within default mode network (seed-based)
Washington et al., 2013	ASD: 10.88 ± 2.27 TD: 10.08 ± 3.17 Range: 6–17	24 ASD (21 male); 24 TD (21 male)	Hyper-connectivity within default mode, visual, and motor networks (ICA), internodal default mode hypo-connectivity (seed-based)
Rudie et al., 2012	ASD: 13.57 TD: 12.79	38 ASD (32 male); 33 TD (28 male)	Hypo-connectivity within default mode network (seed-based)
Weng et al., 2010	ASD: 15 ± 1.45 years Range: 13–17 TD: 16 ± 1.44 years Range: 13–18	16 ASD (15 male); 15 TD (14 male)	Hypo-connectivity within default mode network (seed-based)
Assaf et al., 2010	ASD: 15.7 ± 3.0 Range: 11–20 TD: 17.1 ± 3.6 Range: 10–23	15 ASD (14 male); 15 TD (13 male)	Hypo-connectivity within default mode sub-network (ICA)
Ebisch et al., 2010	ASD: 15.79 ± 1.93 TD: 15.95 ± 1.65 Range: 12–20	14 ASD (10 male); 15 TD (13 male)	Hypo-connectivity of insular cortex with amygdala (seed-based)
Gotts et al., 2012	ASD: 16.92 ± 2.66 TD: 17.86 ± 3.00 Range: 12–23	31 ASD (29 male); 29 TD (28 male)	Whole-brain hypo-connectivity
Cherkassky et al., 2006	ASD: 24 ± 10.6 years TD: 24 ± 9.0 years	57 ASD (53 male); 57 TD (52 male)	Hypo-connectivity between anterior cingulate and posterior cingulate (seed-based)
Kennedy and Courchesne, 2008	ASD: 26.5 ± 12.8 years Range: 15.7–52.1 TD: 27.5 ± 10.9 years Range: 15.9–45.4	12 ASD (12 male); 12 TD (12 male)	Hypo-connectivity within default mode network (seed-based)
Monk et al., 2009	ASD: 26 ± 5.93 years TD: 27 ± 6.1 years	12 ASD (11 male); 12 TD (10 male)	Hypo-connectivity within default mode network (seed-based)
Anderson et al., 2011	ASD: 22.4 ± 7.2 Range: 12–42 TD: 21.1 ± 6.5 Range: 8–34	53 ASD (53 male); 39 TD (39 male)	Interhemispheric hypo-connectivity between left and right insula and left and right parieto-occipital regions

(Continued)

Table 1 | Continued

Publication	Ages examined	Gender and sample size	Intrinsic functional connectivity method and results
Tyszka et al., 2013	ASD: 27.4 ± 2.4 TD: 28.5 ± 2.5	19 ASD (15 male); 20 TD (17 male)	No group differences in whole-brain connectivity (ICA)
von dem Hagen et al., 2013	ASD: 30 ± 8: Range: 19–40 TD: 25 ± 6 Range: 19–36	15 ASD (15 male); 24 TD (24 male)	Hypo-connectivity within default mode network (ICA and seed-based)
Mueller et al., 2013	ASD: 35.5 ± 11.4 TD: 33.3 ± 9.0	12 ASD (9 male); 12 TD (8 male)	Hypo-connectivity within dorsal attention, default mode, and left fronto-parietal network (ICA)

ASD, autism spectrum disorder; TD, typically developing; only studies using resting state fMRI methods are included.

Recently, we demonstrated that children aged 7–12 with autism exhibit hyper-connectivity of several major large-scale brain networks important for cognitive functions. A widely-used method for comparing brain networks between groups is dual regression ICA. Dual regression employs a set of spatial maps derived from the initial group ICA in a linear model fit against each individual fMRI dataset, resulting in matrices describing the temporal dynamics of the corresponding networks for each subject (Beckmann et al., 2005; Filippini et al., 2009). Using this approach, we found that children with ASD exhibited greater functional connectivity than TD children within the DMN, salience, fronto-temporal, motor, and visual networks (Uddin et al., 2013). This somewhat surprising hyper-connectivity result also emerged using complementary analytic approaches and was replicated in several independent datasets (Supekar et al., 2012), and by other groups examining wider age ranges (6–17-year-olds) (Washington et al., 2013). Further, we have found that even within the DMN, hypo- vs. hyper-connectivity results can be observed in children with ASD depending on the precise anatomical location of ROIs within the posterior medial cortex (Lynch et al., 2013). Another recent study of children aged 9–18 found mixed patterns of hypo- and hyper-connectivity between ROIs across the entire brain (Rudie et al., 2013). Rudie and colleagues also report data from graph theoretical analyses demonstrating that while "small worldness" was similar between groups, network level reductions in modularity and clustering as well as shorter characteristic path lengths were observed in children and adolescents with ASD. Some reports of hypo-connectivity between specific ROIs in children with ASD have been published recently (Dinstein et al., 2011; Abrams et al., 2013).

These recent findings raise an important question: If childhood autism is characterized by functional hyper-connectivity, and adults with autism exhibit functional hypo-connectivity, why has the field been slow to examine this important developmental discontinuity? One possible explanation is that the hypo-connectivity theory of ASD has been so dominant that investigators finding contradictory findings have been reluctant to publish their results. This idea has been discussed in a recent Simons Foundation blog (http://sfari.org/news-and-opinion/specials/2013/connectivity/guest-blog-negative-results). A survey of presentations at recent meetings of the International Meeting for Autism Research (IMFAR) and the Organization for Human Brain Mapping (OHBM) suggests that this may in fact be the case. Deen and colleagues conducted ROI-based analyses on data collected from children aged ~13 with ASD and TD control participants. In a poster presented at IMFAR in 2011, they report: "A number of group differences were found in both directions, with no trend toward more differences in the direction of TD>ASD ...in the ROI analysis, 19 correlations were stronger in the TD group, while 38 were stronger in the ASD group" (Deen and Pelphrey, 2011). In an HBM poster from the 2012 meeting, You and colleagues reported using a "connectivity degree"—computed by counting, for each voxel, the number of voxels meeting a correlation threshold of $r > 0.25$ inside (local) and outside (distant) its neighborhood defined as a sphere of 14 mm radius (Sepulcre et al., 2010)—to find that degree of functional connectivity was higher in 7–13-year-old children with ASD than TD children (You et al., 2012). These initial findings of functional hyper-connectivity in children with ASD are only now beginning to surface, and may have been initially received with skepticism due to their inconsistency with the hypo-connectivity theory.

DEVELOPMENTAL MODEL OF FUNCTIONAL BRAIN CONNECTIVITY IN ASD

We propose that the discrepancies between the adult ASD and childhood ASD findings with respect to whole-brain functional connectivity may be reconciled by considering critical developmental factors such as the onset of puberty, which signals the beginning of adolescence and has a major impact on brain structure and function. Puberty typically begins between 9 and 12 years of age, and creates a surge of hormones that trigger rapid physical growth, sexually dimorphic alterations in facial structure, metabolic changes, and several social, behavioral, and emotional changes (Crone and Dahl, 2012). Studies of brain development in animals suggest that the hormonal events surrounding puberty exert significant effects on brain maturation (Cahill, 2006). Relatively few neuroimaging studies have explored the role of puberty in human brain development (Blakemore et al., 2010; Crone and Dahl, 2012; Galvan et al., 2012), though it was noted long ago that measurements of peak gray matter volume coincide with the onset of puberty (Giedd et al., 1999; Blakemore, 2012).

The age-related discontinuity in the autism neuroimaging literature between findings from children and adults coincides with this developmental period. As summarized in **Table 1**, studies of children under the age of 12 (presumably predominantly pre-pubertal) find considerable evidence for functional hyper-connectivity in ASD, whereas the studies reporting data collected from adolescents and adults (presumably predominantly post-pubertal) reveal functional hypo-connectivity in ASD. A schematic model of this proposed developmental shift is depicted in **Figure 1**.

A growing body of literature documents age-related increases in white matter volume (Lenroot and Giedd, 2006), which may be related to increases in long-range functional connectivity from childhood through adolescence and into adulthood (Fair et al., 2008; Kelly et al., 2009). Recent reports of strengthening of structural and functional connectivity with age have shed light on typical developmental processes (Hagmann et al., 2010; Supekar et al., 2010; Uddin et al., 2011). Similar developmental studies of brain connectivity in ASD do not yet exist. In concert with studies of the effects of puberty on typical brain development, this work will help to explain the developmental shift that is suggested by the existing literature of functional connectivity in autism.

CHALLENGES AND GAPS IN THE LITERATURE

LACK OF LONGITUDINAL DATA AND DATA FROM YOUNGER PARTICIPANTS

The most critical gap in the literature on functional brain connectivity in ASD is the lack of longitudinal studies tracking the same individuals as they progress from pre- to post-pubertal stages of development (Wass, 2011). There are a few longitudinal findings from structural neuroimaging studies spanning the developmental period discussed in this review. One report found significantly greater decreases in gray matter volume in children with autism scanned at two time points (age ~11 and at 30-month follow-up) compared with TD children (Hardan et al., 2009).

While very few studies have examined functional connectivity in young children and toddlers with autism (Dinstein et al., 2011), some have started to use structural measures to examine high-risk infants, including siblings of children with autism. Wolff and colleagues report that infants with ASD showed higher fractional anisotropy (FA) of most fiber tracts at 6 months followed by a slower change over time relative to infants without ASD such that

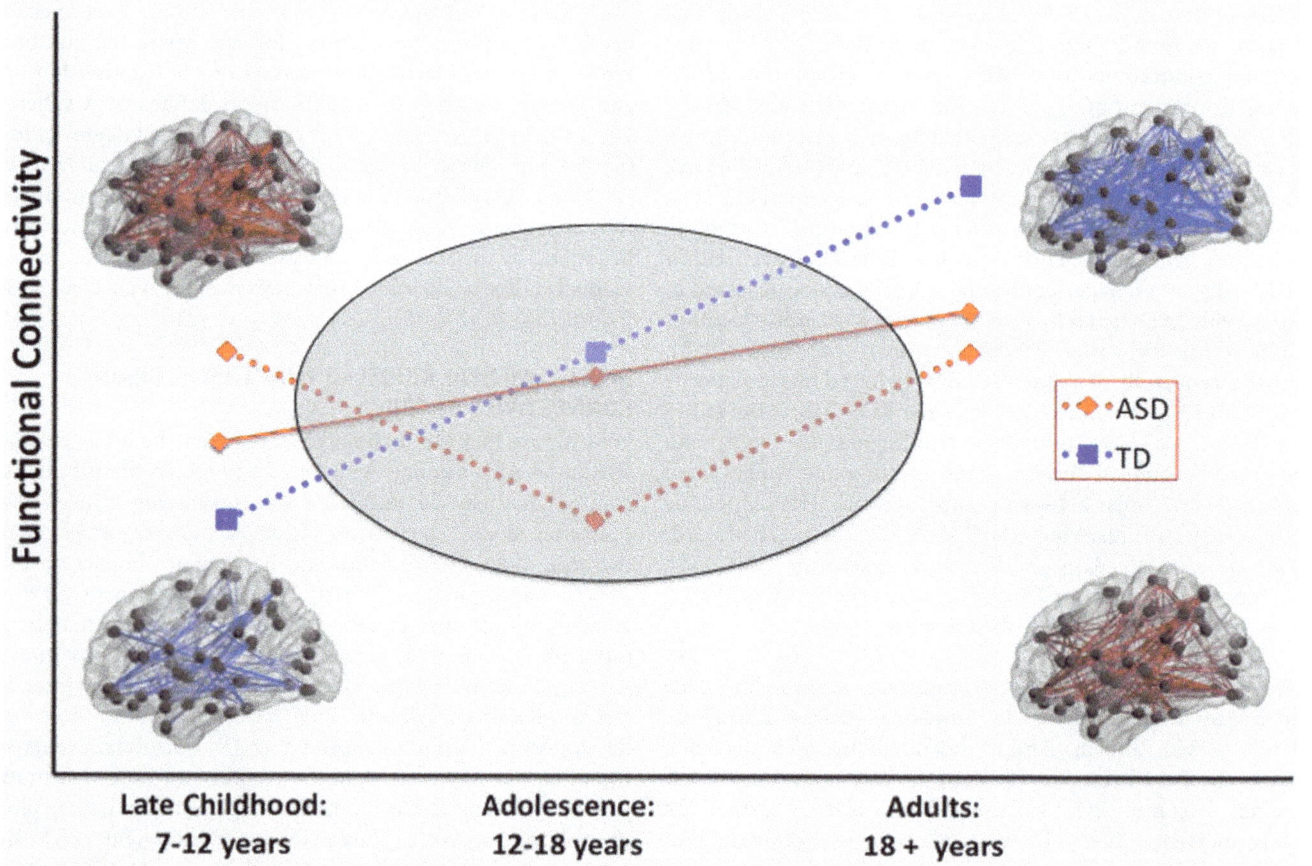

FIGURE 1 | Schematic model of two scenarios that could explain a developmental shift from intrinsic hyper-to hypo-connectivity in ASD. In scenario 1 (solid red line), the ASD group shows a less steep developmental increase in functional connectivity over the age span compared with the TD group. In scenario 2 (dashed red line), the ASD group shows anomalous patterns of connectivity across the pubertal period. Resting-state functional connectivity MRI studies provide evidence for widespread hyper-connectivity in children with ASD in contrast to hypo-connectivity observed in adolescents and adults with ASD. To reconcile these findings, it will be necessary to conduct longitudinal studies that span the developmental period surrounding puberty (gray oval). ASD, autism spectrum disorders; TD, typical development.

by 24 months of age, the infants with ASD had lower FA values (Wolff et al., 2012). This study suggests that aberrant development of white matter may precede the manifestation of autistic symptoms in the first year of life, and highlights the importance of longitudinal data and data from young children and infants with the disorder.

LACK OF PUBERTAL STAGE ASSESSMENT

As highlighted throughout, a potentially informative way of stratifying a sample would be to group individuals by pubertal stage to examine brain maturation as a function of sexual maturity in ASD. Explicit characterization of pubertal stage in research participants can be accomplished in one of several ways. The most widely used tool is the Tanner scale for assessing pubertal development. Tanner staging characterizes individuals along a puberty scale from 1 to 5 on the basis of pubic hair and breast development in females, and pubic hair and genital development in males (Tanner and Whitehouse, 1976). A physical exam carried out by a trained clinician is the typical mode of administration. While there are several limitations to Tanner staging (including ethnic homogeneity of the scale), the test is the current gold standard for puberty assessment. Self-report versions of the scale have also been developed [e.g., the Petersen Developmental Scale (PDS) (Petersen et al., 1988)]. Hormonal assays can also in principle be used to assess pubertal stage, but practical considerations limit their utility Blakemore et al. (2010). Adopting one of these approaches to pubertal assessment when studying adolescents will likely contribute to clarity and interpretability of neuroimaging findings in this population.

INSUFFICIENT CHARACTERIZATION OF HETEROGENEITY

One significant obstacle to understanding the brain basis of ASD is the fact that the disorder (indeed, disorders) encompasses a wide range of abilities and levels of functioning. Almost no functional brain imaging data is available from individuals who are considered "low-functioning." Additionally, because of the 4:1 male:female ratio in diagnosis (Werling and Geschwind, 2013), males with the disorder are much more prevalent and therefore receive the majority of attention from researchers. As a consequence, very little is known about gender-specific functional connectivity differences associated with the disorder. It has recently been shown that individuals with variants of the MET gene show differential patterns of resting-state functional connectivity, such that differences between ASD and controls were moderated by genotype (Rudie et al., 2012). This study highlights the important point that studies of disorders characterized by considerable heterogeneity, such as ASD, may need to be particularly mindful of potential genetic differences within their samples.

Reports of relationships between efficiency of functional brain networks and IQ (van den Heuvel et al., 2009) as well as between regional node properties and IQ (Wu et al., 2013) are beginning to emerge. Important directions for future work include assessing interactions between diagnostic category, IQ, and functional connectivity measures. One can speculate that a unique developmental trajectory might exist for children with ASD on the low-functioning end of the spectrum, compared with high-functioning ASD and typical development.

DIRECT COMPARISONS BETWEEN TASK-BASED AND RESTING-STATE FUNCTIONAL CONNECTIVITY

Both task-based and resting-state fMRI have been applied to the study of functional connectivity in ASD. However, to date no empirical work has investigated both types of measures in the same individual. It is clear that methodological choices in both task- and resting-state approaches can affect outcomes in autism neuroimaging studies (Muller et al., 2011). Further, it is increasingly recognized that intrinsic and evoked brain states interact in complex and unpredictable ways (He, 2013). As the field moves closer toward understanding the ways in which task-based and resting-state measures can meaningfully capture brain dynamics, it will continue to inform functional connectivity theories of autism and allow investigators to more confidently predict the conditions under which aberrant brain connectivity in ASD will manifest.

RELATIONSHIPS BETWEEN FUNCTIONAL AND STRUCTURAL CONNECTIVITY

As the focus of the current review is to summarize findings from the fMRI functional connectivity literature, and structural findings have recently been reviewed elsewhere (Schipul et al., 2011; Vissers et al., 2011), we have included only a limited discussion of the links between structural and functional connectivity here. Relationships between functional and structural connectivity are complex, even in the neurotypical adult brain (Damoiseaux and Greicius, 2009), and these relationships undergo significant changes with development (Supekar et al., 2010; Uddin et al., 2011). In a previously published review of structural connectivity changes in ASD (Vissers et al., 2011), it is noted by the authors that few studies exist simultaneously examining functional and structural changes in ASD. To our knowledge, there are only three reports that do so. In a study by Rudie and colleagues, the authors report that structural connectivity (measured by FA) between the medial prefrontal cortex and posterior cingulate cortex did not show significant differences between ASD and TD children (Rudie et al., 2012). This group has also recently shown that there are no significant differences between groups with respect to structure-function correlations assessed at the whole brain level (Rudie et al., 2013). Finally, it was recently shown that in adults with ASD, reduced functional and structural connectivity can be observed in the right temporo-parietal junction and left frontal lobe (Mueller et al., 2013). The dearth of studies examining structure-function relationships and their development in ASD leaves several open questions that will need to be addressed by future multimodal imaging approaches.

ASSESSING WHOLE BRAIN vs. REGION-SPECIFIC PATTERNS OF FUNCTIONAL CONNECTIVITY

An important area for future work will be to understand functional connectivity abnormalities in ASD at the global level, across the whole brain, as well as in specific functional networks or sets of nodes. There is already evidence to suggest that in children with the disorder, widespread hyper-connectivity can be observed (Supekar et al., 2012; Uddin et al., 2013) alongside both hypo-connectivity (Abrams et al., 2013; Lynch et al., 2013) and hyper-connectivity (Di Martino et al., 2011) between subsets of specific regions. The immediate challenge will be to develop metrics to more systematically assess region-specific and large-scale patterns of connectivity and apply them uniformly to different age groups of individuals with ASD and TD controls.

CLINICAL IMPLICATIONS: BRAIN-BASED BIOMARKERS

One of the goals of functional imaging of neurodevelopmental disorders is to quantify brain connectivity in ways that may eventually be used to develop brain-based biomarkers for objectively identifying children with disorders. Anderson and colleagues demonstrate that functional connectivity based classifiers perform more accurately on datasets from younger individuals (<20 years of age) with ASD (Anderson et al., 2011). These findings underscore the importance of understanding age-related changes in functional connectivity in ASD, as they have clear implications for the development of increasingly sophisticated approaches to diagnosis and evaluation of response to treatment. Functional connectivity measures can also aid in understanding unique and shared neural markers in ASD and comorbid conditions such as ADHD (Di Martino et al., 2013b). Our recent demonstration of high levels of classification accuracy based on examination of specific intrinsic large-scale networks in 7–12 year-old children highlights the utility of using data from narrower developmental windows to identify potential biomarkers for the disorder (Uddin et al., 2013).

SUMMARY AND FUTURE DIRECTIONS

Inadequate attention to critical age-related developmental stages has impeded our understanding of functional brain connectivity in ASD. Here we have (1) reviewed the emerging literature on intrinsic functional brain connectivity in ASD, (2) identified results of hypo- and hyper-connectivity as being partially attributable to the age of participants examined, and (3) proposed that longitudinal studies examining pre- and post-pubertal individuals with ASD are sorely needed to resolve current controversies regarding the nature of brain connectivity abnormalities in the disorder. A developmental perspective will contribute greatly to future research efforts in autism neuroimaging.

ACKNOWLEDGMENTS

The authors gratefully acknowledge Carl Feinstein for insightful discussions. This work was supported by a National Institute of Mental Health Career Development Award [K01MH092288] to Lucina Q. Uddin, as well as grants from the Singer Foundation, the Stanford Institute for Neuro-Innovation and Translational Neurosciences, and the National Institutes of Health [DC011095 and MH084164] to Vinod Menon. The content is solely the responsibility of the authors and does not necessarily represent the official views of the NIMH or the NIH.

REFERENCES

Abrams, D. A., Lynch, C. J., Cheng, K. M., Phillips, J., Supekar, K., Ryali, S., et al. (2013). Underconnectivity between voice-selective cortex and reward circuitry in children with autism. *Proc. Natl. Acad. Sci. U.S.A.* 110, 12060–12065. doi: 10.1073/pnas.1302982110

Agam, Y., Joseph, R. M., Barton, J. J., and Manoach, D. S. (2010). Reduced cognitive control of response inhibition by the anterior cingulate cortex in autism spectrum disorders. *Neuroimage* 52, 336–347. doi: 10.1016/j.neuroimage.2010.04.010

Akshoomoff, N., Pierce, K., and Courchesne, E. (2002). The neurobiological basis of autism from a developmental perspective. *Dev. Psychopathol.* 14, 613–634. doi: 10.1017/S0954579402003115

Amaral, D. G. (2010). The promise and the pitfalls of autism research: an introductory note for new autism researchers. *Brain Res.* 1380, 3–9. doi: 10.1016/j.brainres.2010.11.077

Anderson, J. S., Druzgal, T. J., Froehlich, A., DuBray, M. B., Lange, N., Alexander, A. L., et al. (2011). Decreased interhemispheric functional connectivity in autism. *Cereb. Cortex* 21, 1134–1146. doi: 10.1093/cercor/bhq190

Assaf, M., Jagannathan, K., Calhoun, V. D., Miller, L., Stevens, M. C., Sahl, R., et al. (2010). Abnormal functional connectivity of default mode sub-networks in autism spectrum disorder patients. *Neuroimage* 53, 247–256. doi: 10.1016/j.neuroimage.2010.05.067

Beckmann, C. F., DeLuca, M., Devlin, J. T., and Smith, S. M. (2005). Investigations into resting-state connectivity using independent component analysis. *Philos. Trans. R. Soc. Lond., B, Biol. Sci.* 360, 1001–1013. doi: 10.1098/rstb.2005.1634

Beckmann, C. F., and Smith, S. M. (2004). Probabilistic independent component analysis for functional magnetic resonance imaging. *IEEE Trans. Med. Imaging* 23, 137–152. doi: 10.1109/TMI.2003.822821

Belmonte, M. K., Allen, G., Beckel-Mitchener, A., Boulanger, L. M., Carper, R. A., and Webb, S. J. (2004). Autism and abnormal development of brain connectivity. *J. Neurosci.* 24, 9228–9231. doi: 10.1523/JNEUROSCI.3340-04.2004

Belmonte, M. K., Mazziotta, J. C., Minshew, N. J., Evans, A. C., Courchesne, E., Dager, S. R., et al. (2008). Offering to share: how to put heads together in autism neuroimaging. *J. Autism Dev. Disord.* 38, 2–13. doi: 10.1007/s10803-006-0352-2

Biswal, B., Yetkin, F. Z., Haughton, V. M., and Hyde, J. S. (1995). Functional connectivity in the motor cortex of resting human brain using echo-planar MRI. *Magn. Reson. Med.* 34, 537–541. doi: 10.1002/mrm.1910340409

Blakemore, S. J. (2012). Imaging brain development: the adolescent brain. *Neuroimage* 61, 397–406. doi: 10.1016/j.neuroimage.2011.11.080

Blakemore, S. J., Burnett, S., and Dahl, R. E. (2010). The role of puberty in the developing adolescent brain. *Hum. Brain Mapp.* 31, 926–933. doi: 10.1002/hbm.21052

Bressler, S. L., and Menon, V. (2010). Large-scale brain networks in cognition: emerging methods and principles. *Trends Cogn. Sci.* 14, 277–290. doi: 10.1016/j.tics.2010.04.004

Cahill, L. (2006). Why sex matters for neuroscience. *Nat. Rev. Neurosci.* 7, 477–484. doi: 10.1038/nrn1909

Castellanos, F. X., and Proal, E. (2012). Large-scale brain systems in ADHD: beyond the prefrontal-striatal model. *Trends Cogn. Sci.* 16, 17–26. doi: 10.1016/j.tics.2011.11.007

Cherkassky, V. L., Kana, R. K., Keller, T. A., and Just, M. A. (2006). Functional connectivity in a baseline resting-state network in autism. *Neuroreport* 17, 1687–1690. doi: 10.1097/01.wnr.0000239956.45448.4c

Cole, D. M., Smith, S. M., and Beckmann, C. F. (2010). Advances and pitfalls in the analysis and interpretation of resting-state FMRI data. *Front. Syst. Neurosci.* 4:8. doi: 10.3389/fnsys.2010.00008

Courchesne, E., Carper, R., and Akshoomoff, N. (2003). Evidence of brain overgrowth in the first year of life in autism. *JAMA* 290, 337–344. doi: 10.1001/jama.290.3.337

Courchesne, E., Mouton, P. R., Calhoun, M. E., Semendeferi, K., Ahrens-Barbeau, C., Hallet, M. J., et al. (2011). Neuron number and size in prefrontal cortex of children with autism. *JAMA* 306, 2001–2010. doi: 10.1001/jama.2011.1638

Courchesne, E., and Pierce, K. (2005). Why the frontal cortex in autism might be talking only to itself: local over-connectivity but long-distance disconnection. *Curr. Opin. Neurobiol.* 15, 225–230. doi: 10.1016/j.conb.2005.03.001

Crone, E. A., and Dahl, R. E. (2012). Understanding adolescence as a period of social-affective engagement and goal flexibility. *Nat. Rev. Neurosci.* 13, 636–650. doi: 10.1038/nrn3313

Damoiseaux, J. S., and Greicius, M. D. (2009). Greater than the sum of its parts: a review of studies combining structural connectivity and resting-state functional connectivity. *Brain Struct. Funct.* 213, 525–533. doi: 10.1007/s00429-009-0208-6

Deco, G., Ponce-Alvarez, A., Mantini, D., Romani, G. L., Hagmann, P., Corbetta, M. (2013). Resting-state functional connectivity emerges from structurally and dynamically shaped slow linear fluctuations. *J. Neurosci.* 33, 11239–11252.

Deen, B., and Pelphrey, K. A. (2011). "Large-Scale Cortical Functional Connectivity in Children with Autism Spectrum Disorders," in *Paper presented at the International Meeting for Autism Research*, San Diego, CA.

Di Martino, A., Kelly, C., Grzadzinski, R., Zuo, X. N., Mennes, M., Mairena, M. A., et al. (2011). Aberrant striatal functional connectivity in children with autism. *Biol. Psychiatry* 69, 847–856. doi: 10.1016/j.biopsych.2010.10.029

Di Martino, A., Yan, C. G., Li, Q., Denio, E., Castellanos, F. X., Alaerts, K., et al. (2013a). The autism brain imaging data exchange: towards a large-scale evaluation of the intrinsic brain architecture in autism. *Mol. Psychiatry*. doi: 10.1038/mp.2013.78. [Epub ahead of print].

Di Martino, A., Zuo, X. N., Kelly, C., Grzadzinski, R., Mennes, M., Schvarcz, A., et al. (2013b). Shared and distinct intrinsic functional network centrality in autism and attention-deficit/hyperactivity disorder. *Biol. Psychiatry*. doi: 10.1016/j.biopsych.2013.02.011. [Epub ahead of print].

Dinstein, I., Pierce, K., Eyler, L., Solso, S., Malach, R., Behrmann, M., et al. (2011). Disrupted neural synchronization in toddlers with autism. *Neuron* 70, 1218–1225. doi: 10.1016/j.neuron.2011.04.018

Ebisch, S. J., Gallese, V., Willems, R. M., Mantini, D., Groen, W. B., Romani, G. L., et al. (2010). Altered intrinsic functional connectivity of anterior and posterior insula regions in high-functioning participants with autism spectrum disorder. *Hum. Brain Mapp.* 32, 1013–1028. doi: 10.1002/hbm.21085

Fair, D. A., Cohen, A. L., Dosenbach, N. U., Church, J. A., Miezin, F. M., Barch, D. M., et al. (2008). The maturing architecture of the brain's default network. *Proc. Natl. Acad. Sci. U.S.A.* 105, 4028–4032. doi: 10.1073/pnas.0800376105

Fair, D. A., Cohen, A. L., Power, J. D., Dosenbach, N. U., Church, J. A., Miezin, F. M., et al. (2009). Functional brain networks develop from a "local to distributed" organization. *PLoS Comput. Biol.* 5:e1000381. doi: 10.1371/journal.pcbi.1000381

Filippini, N., MacIntosh, B. J., Hough, M. G., Goodwin, G. M., Frisoni, G. B., Smith, S. M., et al. (2009). Distinct patterns of brain activity in young carriers of the APOE-epsilon4 allele. *Proc. Natl. Acad. Sci. U.S.A.* 106, 7209–7214. doi: 10.1073/pnas.0811879106

Fox, M. D., and Raichle, M. E. (2007). Spontaneous fluctuations in brain activity observed with functional magnetic resonance imaging. *Nat. Rev. Neurosci.* 8, 700–711. doi: 10.1038/nrn2201

Fox, M. D., Snyder, A. Z., Vincent, J. L., Corbetta, M., Van Essen, D. C., and Raichle, M. E. (2005). The human brain is intrinsically organized into dynamic, anticorrelated functional networks. *Proc. Natl. Acad. Sci. U.S.A.* 102, 9673–9678. doi: 10.1073/pnas.0504136102

Friston, K. (1994). Functional and effective connectivity in neuroimaging: a synthesis. *Hum. Brain Mapp.* 2, 56–78. doi: 10.1002/hbm.460020107

Galvan, A., Van Leijenhorst, L., and McGlennen, K. M. (2012). Considerations for imaging the adolescent brain. *Dev. Cogn. Neurosci.* 2, 293–302. doi: 10.1016/j.dcn.2012.02.002

Geschwind, D. H., and Levitt, P. (2007). Autism spectrum disorders: developmental disconnection syndromes. *Curr. Opin. Neurobiol.* 17, 103–111. doi: 10.1016/j.conb.2007.01.009

Giedd, J. N., Blumenthal, J., Jeffries, N. O., Castellanos, F. X., Liu, H., Zijdenbos, A., et al. (1999). Brain development during childhood and adolescence: a longitudinal MRI study. *Nat. Neurosci.* 2, 861–863. doi: 10.1038/13158

Gotts, S. J., Simmons, W. K., Milbury, L. A., Wallace, G. L., Cox, R. W., and Martin, A. (2012). Fractionation of social brain circuits in autism spectrum disorders. *Brain* 135, 2711–2725. doi: 10.1093/brain/aws160

Greicius, M. D., Krasnow, B., Reiss, A. L., and Menon, V. (2003). Functional connectivity in the resting brain: a network analysis of the default mode hypothesis. *Proc. Natl. Acad. Sci. U.S.A.* 100, 253–258. doi: 10.1073/pnas.0135058100

Hagmann, P., Sporns, O., Madan, N., Cammoun, L., Pienaar, R., Wedeen, V. J., et al. (2010). White matter maturation reshapes structural connectivity in the late developing human brain. *Proc. Natl. Acad. Sci. U.S.A.* 107, 19067–19072. doi: 10.1073/pnas.1009073107

Hardan, A. Y., Libove, R. A., Keshavan, M. S., Melhem, N. M., and Minshew, N. J. (2009). A preliminary longitudinal magnetic resonance imaging study of brain volume and cortical thickness in autism. *Biol. Psychiatry* 66, 320–326. doi: 10.1016/j.biopsych.2009.04.024

He, B. J. (2013). Spontaneous and task-evoked brain activity negatively interact. *J. Neurosci.* 33, 4672–4682. doi: 10.1523/JNEUROSCI.2922-12.2013.

Investigators. (2012). Prevalence of autism spectrum disorders–autism and developmental disabilities monitoring network, 14 sites, United States, 2008. *MMWR. Surveill. Summ.* 61, 1–19.

Jones, T. B., Bandettini, P. A., Kenworthy, L., Case, L. K., Milleville, S. C., Martin, A., et al. (2010). Sources of group differences in functional connectivity: an investigation applied to autism spectrum disorder. *Neuroimage* 49, 401–414. doi: 10.1016/j.neuroimage.2009.07.051

Just, M. A., Cherkassky, V. L., Keller, T. A., Kana, R. K., and Minshew, N. J. (2007). Functional and anatomical cortical underconnectivity in autism: evidence from an FMRI study of an executive function task and corpus callosum morphometry. *Cereb. Cortex* 17, 951–961. doi: 10.1093/cercor/bhl006

Just, M. A., Cherkassky, V. L., Keller, T. A., and Minshew, N. J. (2004). Cortical activation and synchronization during sentence comprehension in high-functioning autism: evidence of underconnectivity. *Brain* 127(Pt 8), 1811–1821. doi: 10.1093/brain/awh199

Just, M. A., Keller, T. A., Malave, V. L., Kana, R. K., and Varma, S. (2012). Autism as a neural systems disorder: a theory of frontal-posterior underconnectivity. *Neurosci. Biobehav. Rev.*36, 1292–1313. doi: 10.1016/j.neubiorev.2012.02.007

Kana, R. K., Keller, T. A., Cherkassky, V. L., Minshew, N. J., and Just, M. A. (2006). Sentence comprehension in autism: thinking in pictures with decreased functional connectivity. *Brain* 129(Pt 9), 2484–2493. doi: 10.1093/brain/awl164

Kana, R. K., Keller, T. A., Cherkassky, V. L., Minshew, N. J., and Just, M. A. (2009). Atypical frontal-posterior synchronization of Theory of Mind regions in autism during mental state attribution. *Soc. Neurosci.* 4, 135–152. doi: 10.1080/17470910802198510

Kana, R. K., Keller, T. A., Minshew, N. J., and Just, M. A. (2007). Inhibitory control in high-functioning autism: decreased activation and underconnectivity in inhibition networks. *Biol. Psychiatry* 62, 198–206. doi: 10.1016/j.biopsych.2006.08.004

Kana, R. K., Libero, L. E., and Moore, M. S. (2011). Disrupted cortical connectivity theory as an explanatory model for autism spectrum disorders. *Phys. Life Rev.* 8, 410–437. doi: 10.1016/j.plrev.2011.10.001

Kelly, A. M., Di Martino, A., Uddin, L. Q., Shehzad, Z., Gee, D. G., Reiss, P. T., et al. (2009). Development of anterior cingulate functional connectivity from late childhood to early adulthood. *Cereb. Cortex* 19, 640–657. doi: 10.1093/cercor/bhn117

Kennedy, D. P., and Adolphs, R. (2012). The social brain in psychiatric and neurological disorders. *Trends Cogn. Sci.* 16, 559–572. doi: 10.1016/j.tics.2012.09.006

Kennedy, D. P., and Courchesne, E. (2008). The intrinsic functional organization of the brain is altered in autism. *Neuroimage* 39, 1877–1885. doi: 10.1016/j.neuroimage.2007.10.052

Kleinhans, N. M., Richards, T., Sterling, L., Stegbauer, K. C., Mahurin, R., Johnson, L. C., et al. (2008). Abnormal functional connectivity in autism spectrum disorders during face processing. *Brain* 131, 1000–1012. doi: 10.1093/brain/awm334

Koshino, H., Carpenter, P. A., Minshew, N. J., Cherkassky, V. L., Keller, T. A., and Just, M. A. (2005). Functional connectivity in an fMRI working memory task in high-functioning autism. *Neuroimage* 24, 810–821. doi: 10.1016/j.neuroimage.2004.09.028

Koshino, H., Kana, R. K., Keller, T. A., Cherkassky, V. L., Minshew, N. J., and Just, M. A. (2008). fMRI investigation of working memory for faces in autism: visual coding and underconnectivity with frontal areas. *Cereb. Cortex* 18, 289–300. doi: 10.1093/cercor/bhm054

Lainhart, J. E., Piven, J., Wzorek, M., Landa, R., Santangelo, S. L., Coon, H., et al. (1997). Macrocephaly in children and adults with autism. *J. Am. Acad. Child Adolesc. Psychiatry* 36, 282–290. doi: 10.1097/00004583-199702000-00019

LeBlanc, J. J., and Fagiolini, M. (2011). Autism: a "critical period" disorder?

Neural Plast. 2011, 921680. doi: 10.1155/2011/921680

Lenroot, R. K., and Giedd, J. N. (2006). Brain development in children and adolescents: insights from anatomical magnetic resonance imaging. *Neurosci. Biobehav. Rev.* 30, 718–729. doi: 10.1016/j.neubiorev.2006.06.001

Lynch, C. J., Uddin, L. Q., Supekar, K., Khouzam, A., Phillips, J., and Menon, V. (2013). Default mode network in childhood autism: posteromedial cortex heterogeneity and relationship with social deficits. *Biol. Psychiatry* 74, 212–219. doi: 10.1016/j.biopsych.2012.12.013

Mason, R. A., Williams, D. L., Kana, R. K., Minshew, N., and Just, M. A. (2008). Theory of Mind disruption and recruitment of the right hemisphere during narrative comprehension in autism. *Neuropsychologia* 46, 269–280. doi: 10.1016/j.neuropsychologia.2007.07.018

Mizuno, A., Villalobos, M. E., Davies, M. M., Dahl, B. C., and Muller, R. A. (2006). Partially enhanced thalamocortical functional connectivity in autism. *Brain Res.* 1104, 160–174. doi: 10.1016/j.brainres.2006.05.064

Monk, C. S., Peltier, S. J., Wiggins, J. L., Weng, S. J., Carrasco, M., Risi, S., et al. (2009). Abnormalities of intrinsic functional connectivity in autism spectrum disorders. *Neuroimage* 47, 764–772. doi: 10.1016/j.neuroimage.2009.04.069

Mueller, S., Keeser, D., Samson, A. C., Kirsch, V., Blautzik, J., Grothe, M., et al. (2013). Convergent findings of altered functional and structural brain connectivity in individuals with high functioning autism: a multimodal MRI Study. *PLoS ONE* 8:e67329. doi: 10.1371/journal.pone.0067329

Muller, R. A., Shih, P., Keehn, B., Deyoe, J. R., Leyden, K. M., and Shukla, D. K. (2011). Underconnected, but how? A survey of functional connectivity MRI studies in autism spectrum disorders. *Cereb. Cortex* 21, 2233–2243. doi: 10.1093/cercor/bhq296

Nir, Y., Mukamel, R., Dinstein, I., Privman, E., Harel, M., Fisch, L., et al. (2008). Interhemispheric correlations of slow spontaneous neuronal fluctuations revealed in human sensory cortex. *Nat. Neurosci.* 11, 1100–1108. doi: 10.1038/nn.2177

Noonan, S. K., Haist, F., and Muller, R. A. (2009). Aberrant functional connectivity in autism: evidence from low-frequency BOLD signal fluctuations. *Brain Res.* 1262, 48–63. doi: 10.1016/j.brainres.2008.12.076

Petersen, A. C., Crockett, L., Richards, M., and Boxer, A. (1988). Self-report measure of pubertal status: reliability, validity, and initial norms. *J. Youth Adolesc.* 17, 117–133. doi: 10.1007/BF01537962

Power, J. D., Barnes, K. A., Snyder, A. Z., Schlaggar, B. L., and Petersen, S. E. (2012). Spurious but systematic correlations in functional connectivity MRI networks arise from subject motion. *Neuroimage* 59, 2142–2154. doi: 10.1016/j.neuroimage.2011.10.018

Rubenstein, J. L., and Merzenich, M. M. (2003). Model of autism: increased ratio of excitation/inhibition in key neural systems. *Genes Brain Behav.* 2, 255–267. doi: 10.1034/j.1601-183X.2003.00037.x

Rudie, J. D., Brown, J. A., Beck-Pancer, D., Hernandez, L. M., Dennis, E. L., Thompson, P. M., et al. (2013). Altered functional and structural brain network organization in autism. *Neuroimage Clin.* 2, 79–94. doi: 10.1016/j.nicl.2012.11.006

Rudie, J. D., Hernandez, L. M., Brown, J. A., Beck-Pancer, D., Colich, N. L., Gorrindo, P., et al. (2012). Autism-associated promoter variant in MET impacts functional and structural brain networks. *Neuron* 75, 904–915. doi: 10.1016/j.neuron.2012.07.010

Ryali, S., Chen, T., Supekar, K., and Menon, V. (2012). Estimation of functional connectivity in fMRI data using stability selection-based sparse partial correlation with elastic net penalty. *Neuroimage* 59, 3852–3861. doi: 10.1016/j.neuroimage.2011.11.054

Satterthwaite, T. D., Elliott, M. A., Gerraty, R. T., Ruparel, K., Loughead, J., Calkins, M. E., et al. (2013). An improved framework for confound regression and filtering for control of motion artifact in the preprocessing of resting-state functional connectivity data. *Neuroimage* 64, 240–256. doi: 10.1016/j.neuroimage.2012.08.052

Satterthwaite, T. D., Wolf, D. H., Loughead, J., Ruparel, K., Elliott, M. A., Hakonarson, H., et al. (2012). Impact of in-scanner head motion on multiple measures of functional connectivity: relevance for studies of neurodevelopment in youth. *Neuroimage* 60, 623–632. doi: 10.1016/j.neuroimage.2011.12.063

Schipul, S. E., Keller, T. A., and Just, M. A. (2011). Inter-regional brain communication and its disturbance in autism. *Front. Syst. Neurosci.* 5:10. doi: 10.3389/fnsys.2011.00010

Sepulcre, J., Liu, H., Talukdar, T., Martincorena, I., Yeo, B. T., and Buckner, R. L. (2010). The organization of local and distant functional connectivity in the human brain. *PLoS Comput. Biol.* 6:e1000808. doi: 10.1371/journal.pcbi.1000808

Shih, P., Keehn, B., Oram, J. K., Leyden, K. M., Keown, C. L., and Muller, R. A. (2011). Functional differentiation of posterior superior temporal sulcus in autism: a functional connectivity magnetic resonance imaging study. *Biol. Psychiatry* 70, 270–277. doi: 10.1016/j.biopsych.2011.03.040

Shih, P., Shen, M., Ottl, B., Keehn, B., Gaffrey, M. S., and Muller, R. A. (2010). Atypical network connectivity for imitation in autism spectrum disorder. *Neuropsychologia* 48, 2931–2939. doi: 10.1016/j.neuropsychologia.2010.05.035

Solomon, M., Ozonoff, S. J., Ursu, S., Ravizza, S., Cummings, N., Ly, S., et al. (2009). The neural substrates of cognitive control deficits in autism spectrum disorders. *Neuropsychologia* 47, 2515–2526. doi: 10.1016/j.neuropsychologia.2009.04.019

Sporns, O. (2011). From simple graphs to the connectome: networks in neuroimaging. *Neuroimage* 62, 881–886. doi: 10.1016/j.neuroimage.2011.08.085

Stefanatos, G. A. (2008). Regression in autistic spectrum disorders. *Neuropsychol. Rev.* 18, 305–319. doi: 10.1007/s11065-008-9073-y

Supekar, K., Musen, M., and Menon, V. (2009). Development of large-scale functional brain networks in children. *PLoS Biol.*7:e1000157. doi: 10.1371/journal.pbio.1000157

Supekar, K., Uddin, L. Q., Khouzam, A., Phillips, J., Gaillard, W., Kenworthy, L., et al. (2012). "Widespread brain hyperconnectivity in children with autism," in *Paper Presented at the Organization for Human Brain Mapping*, (Beijing).

Supekar, K., Uddin, L. Q., Prater, K., Amin, H., Greicius, M. D., and Menon, V. (2010). Development of functional and structural connectivity within the default mode network in young children. *Neuroimage* 52, 290–301. doi: 10.1016/j.neuroimage.2010.04.009

Tanner, J. M., and Whitehouse, R. H. (1976). Clinical longitudinal standards for height, weight, height velocity, weight velocity, and stages of puberty. *Arch. Dis. Child.* 51, 170–179. doi: 10.1136/adc.51.3.170

Testa-Silva, G., Loebel, A., Giugliano, M., de Kock, C. P., Mansvelder, H. D., and Meredith, R. M. (2011). Hyperconnectivity and slow synapses during early development of medial prefrontal cortex in a mouse model for mental retardation and autism. *Cereb. Cortex* 22, 1333–1342. doi: 10.1093/cercor/bhr224

Thai, N. J., Longe, O., and Rippon, G. (2009). Disconnected brains: what is the role of fMRI in connectivity research? *Int. J. Psychophysiol.* 73, 27–32.

Turner, K. C., Frost, L., Linsenbardt, D., McIlroy, J. R., and Muller, R. A. (2006). Atypically diffuse functional connectivity between caudate nuclei and cerebral cortex in autism. *Behav. Brain Funct.* 2, 34. doi: 10.1186/1744-9081-2-34

Tyszka, J. M., Kennedy, D. P., Paul, L. K., and Adolphs, R. (2013). Largely typical patterns of resting-state functional connectivity in high-functioning adults with autism. *Cereb. Cortex.* doi: 10.1093/cercor/bht040. [Epub ahead of print].

Uddin, L. Q., Supekar, K., Lynch, C. J., Khouzam, A., Phillips, J., Feinstein, C., et al. (2013). Salience network-based classification and prediction of symptom severity in children with autism. *JAMA Psychiatry.* doi: 10.1001/jamapsychiatry.2013.104. [Epub ahead of print].

Uddin, L. Q., Supekar, K., and Menon, V. (2010). Typical and atypical development of functional human brain networks: insights from resting-state FMRI. *Front. Syst. Neurosci.* 4:21. doi: 10.3389/fnsys.2010.00021

Uddin, L. Q., Supekar, K. S., Ryali, S., and Menon, V. (2011). Dynamic reconfiguration of structural and functional connectivity across core neurocognitive brain networks with development. *J. Neurosci.* 31, 18578–18589. doi: 10.1523/JNEUROSCI.4465-11.2011

Uhlhaas, P. J., Roux, F., Rodriguez, E., Rotarska-Jagiela, A., and Singer, W. (2010). Neural synchrony and the development of cortical networks. *Trends Cogn. Sci.* 14, 72–80. doi: 10.1016/j.tics.2009.12.002

van den Heuvel, M. P., Stam, C. J., Kahn, R. S., and Hulshoff Pol, H. E. (2009). Efficiency of functional brain networks and intellectual performance. *J. Neurosci.* 29, 7619–7624. doi: 10.1523/JNEUROSCI.1443-09.2009

Van Dijk, K. R., Sabuncu, M. R., and Buckner, R. L. (2012). The influence of head motion on intrinsic functional connectivity MRI. *Neuroimage* 59, 431–438. doi: 10.1016/j.neuroimage.2011.07.044

Villalobos, M. E., Mizuno, A., Dahl, B. C., Kemmotsu, N., and Muller, R. A. (2005). Reduced functional connectivity between V1 and inferior frontal cortex associated with visuomotor performance in autism. *Neuroimage* 25, 916–925. doi: 10.1016/j.neuroimage.2004.12.022

Vissers, M. E., Cohen, M. X., and Geurts, H. M. (2011). Brain connectivity and high functioning autism: a promising path of research that needs refined models, methodological convergence, and stronger behavioral links. *Neurosci. Biobehav. Rev.* 36, 604–625. doi: 10.1016/j.neubiorev.2011.09.003

von dem Hagen, E. A. H., Stoyanova, R. S., Baron-Cohen, S., and Calder, A. J. (2013). Reduced functional connectivity within and between 'social' resting state networks in autism spectrum conditions. *Soc. Cogn. Affect. Neurosci.* doi: 10.1093/scan/nss053. [Epub ahead of print].

Washington, S. D., Gordon, E. M., Brar, J., Warburton, S., Sawyer, A. T., Wolfe, A., et al. (2013). Dysmaturation of the default mode network in autism. *Hum. Brain Mapp.* doi: 10.1002/hbm.22252. [Epub ahead of print].

Wass, S. (2011). Distortions and disconnections: disrupted brain connectivity in autism. *Brain Cogn.* 75, 18–28. doi: 10.1016/j.bandc.2010.10.005

Welchew, D. E., Ashwin, C., Berkouk, K., Salvador, R., Suckling, J., Baron-Cohen, S., et al. (2005). Functional disconnectivity of the medial temporal lobe in Asperger's syndrome. *Biol. Psychiatry* 57, 991–998. doi: 10.1016/j.biopsych.2005.01.028

Weng, S. J., Wiggins, J. L., Peltier, S. J., Carrasco, M., Risi, S., Lord, C., et al. (2010). Alterations of resting state functional connectivity in the default network in adolescents with autism spectrum disorders. *Brain Res.* 1313, 202–214. doi: 10.1016/j.brainres.2009.11.057

Werling, D. M., and Geschwind, D. H. (2013). Sex differences in autism spectrum disorders. *Curr. Opin. Neurol.* 26, 146–153. doi: 10.1097/WCO.0b013e32835ee548

Wolff, J. J., Gu, H., Gerig, G., Elison, J. T., Styner, M., Gouttard, S., et al. (2012). Differences in white matter fiber tract development present from 6 to 24 months in infants with autism. *Am. J. Psychiatry* 169, 589–600. doi: 10.1176/appi.ajp.2011.11091447

Wu, K., Taki, Y., Sato, K., Hashizume, H., Sassa, Y., Takeuchi, H., et al. (2013). Topological organization of functional brain networks in healthy children: differences in relation to age, sex, and intelligence. *PLoS ONE* 8:e55347. doi: 10.1371/journal.pone.0055347

Yerys, B. E., Jankowski, K. F., Shook, D., Rosenberger, L. R., Barnes, K. A., Berl, M. M., et al. (2009). The fMRI success rate of children and adolescents: typical development, epilepsy, attention deficit/hyperactivity disorder, and autism spectrum disorders. *Hum. Brain Mapp.* 30, 3426–3435. doi: 10.1002/hbm.20767.

You, X., Norr, M., Murphy, E., Sokoloff, J., Yerys, B., Gaillard, W., et al. (2012). "Atypical development of local and distant intrinsic functional connectivity in ASD," in *Paper Presented at the Organization for Human Brain Mapping*, (Beijing).

Yu, Q., Allen, E. A., Sui, J., Arbabshirani, M. R., Pearlson, G., and Calhoun, V. D. (2012). Brain connectivity network in schizophrenia underlying resting state functional magnetic resonance imaging. *Curr. Top. Med. Chem.* 12, 2415–2425. doi: 10.2174/156802612805289890

6

Decreased frontal gyrification correlates with altered connectivity in children with autism

Marie Schaer[1,2]*, Marie-Christine Ottet[2], Elisa Scariati[2], Daniel Dukes[3,4], Martina Franchini[2], Stephan Eliez[2,5] and Bronwyn Glaser[2]

[1] Stanford Cognitive and Systems Neuroscience Laboratory, Stanford University School of Medicine, Palo Alto, CA, USA
[2] Office Médico-Pédagogique, Department of Psychiatry, University of Geneva School of Medicine, Geneva, Switzerland
[3] Cognitive Science Centre, University of Neuchâtel, Neuchâtel, Switzerland
[4] Swiss Center for Affective Sciences, University of Geneva, Geneva, Switzerland
[5] Department of Genetic Medicine and Development, University of Geneva School of Medicine, Geneva, Switzerland

Edited by:
Diane Chugani,
Wayne State University, USA

Reviewed by:
Christine Ecker, Institute of Psychiatry, King's College, UK
Jeong-Won Jeong, Wayne State University, USA

***Correspondence:**
Marie Schaer, Stanford Cognitive and Systems Neuroscience Laboratory, Stanford University School of Medicine, 1070 Arastradero Road, Suite 220, Palo Alto, CA 94304, USA
e-mail: marie.schaer@unige.ch

The structural correlates of functional dysconnectivity in autism spectrum disorders (ASD) have been seldom explored, despite the fact that altered functional connectivity is one of the most frequent neuropathological observations in the disorder. We analyzed cerebral morphometry and structural connectivity using multi-modal imaging for 11 children/adolescents with ASD and 11 matched controls. We estimated regional cortical and white matter volumes, as well as vertex-wise measures of cortical thickness and local Gyrification Index (*l*GI). Diffusion Tensor Images (DTI) were used to measure Fractional Anisotropy (FA) and tractography estimates of short- and long-range connectivity. We observed four clusters of *l*GI reduction in patients with ASD, three were located in the right inferior frontal region extending to the inferior parietal lobe, and one was in the right medial parieto-occipital region. Reduced volume was found in the anterior corpus callosum, along with fewer inter-hemispheric frontal streamlines. Despite the spatial correspondence of decreased gyrification and reduced long connectivity, we did not observe any significant relationship between the two. However, a positive correlation between *l*GI and local connectivity was present in all four clusters in patients with ASD. Reduced gyrification in the inferior fronto-parietal and posterior medial cortical regions lends support for early-disrupted cortical growth in both the mirror neuron system and midline structures responsible for social cognition. Early impaired neurodevelopment in these regions may represent an initial substrate for altered maturation in the cerebral networks that support complex social skills. We also demonstrate that gyrification changes are related to connectivity. This supports the idea that an imbalance between short- and long-range white matter tracts not only impairs the integration of information from multiple neural systems, but also alters the shape of the brain early on in autism.

Keywords: cortical folding, cerebral morphometry, tractography, neuroimaging, autism spectrum disorder

INTRODUCTION

Autism is a heterogeneous disorder characterized by a triad of symptoms including impairments in social interactions, delayed development of spoken language, and repetitive patterns of behavior. To satisfactorily account for the observed clinical heterogeneity in autism, the name "autism spectrum disorder" (ASD) is commonly used to convey the associated clinical manifestations that vary in severity along a continuum of autistic traits. Most epidemiological records estimate the global prevalence of ASD at 1 in 160 individuals (Elsabbagh et al., 2012), with some studies reporting rates as high as 1 in 88 children (Centers for Disease Control and Prevention, 2008). Understanding the neurobiological bases of this pervasive developmental disorder, which highly impacts the societal integration and professional achievements of affected persons, is one of the main motivations driving the prolific research on the disorder.

Structural and functional neuroimaging studies on ASD are particularly abundant. Early morphometric studies reported increased brain volume, but decreased total volume thereafter, during the first years of life in patients with ASD compared to healthy controls (Courchesne et al., 2001; Courchesne, 2004). This pattern of early overgrowth followed by degenerative change has been explained by a failure to refine the cerebral circuitry through the adaptive, experience-driven processes normally occurring during childhood (Courchesne et al., 2011). Indeed, there is a large amount of evidence for disrupted organization of cerebral networks in children, adolescents and adults with autism. Structural brain imaging studies reported increased white matter volume in regions corresponding to local cortico-cortical connections, and only minor changes, or even sometimes decreased volumes, in regions corresponding to long-range or inter-hemispheric connections (reviewed in Minshew and Williams, 2007). Increased local connectivity and reduced distant connectivity was further corroborated by post-mortem examinations (Zikopoulos and Barbas, 2010) and by functional studies using EEG (Barttfeld et al., 2011). Finally, several fMRI studies measuring functional connectivity using resting-state paradigms observed decreased long-range functional connectivity in children or young adults with ASD (Kennedy and Courchesne, 2008; Assaf et al., 2010; Weng et al., 2010; von dem Hagen et al., 2013). Despite the plethora of evidence for disrupted structural and functional connectivity and a growing body of research demonstrating morphometric differences in the brains of patients with autism; there are surprisingly few integrated studies that show how differences in cerebral morphology and connectivity fit together. Adding to our knowledge of the relationships between different anatomical impairments should elucidate the mechanisms underlying brain alterations in autism.

It is accepted that cortical folding reflects a person's prenatal development (Regis et al., 2005) (as well as events from the first months of post-natal life (Schaer et al., 2009; Haukvik et al., 2011)). It follows that measuring the shape of the cortex, using three-dimensional cortical reconstructions, provides us with insight into early brain development. Although the processes underlying the creation of specific sulcal patterns are poorly understood, existing theories point to the determinants of early cortical folding. Initial hypotheses proposed that gyrification results from mechanical forces intrinsic to the cortex (Richman et al., 1975; Welker et al., 1990). However, more recent theories consider cortical shape as a product of underlying patterns of connectivity, implicating alterations to both connectivity and cortical folding, both of which are highly relevant in autism. The tension-based model of convolutional development (Van Essen, 1997) postulates that strongly interconnected cortical regions are pulled towards one another during embryological development, resulting in both compact and streamlined wiring of the nervous system. According to this model, disturbed gyrification in the adult human brain reflects abnormal patterns of white matter connectivity. Measuring gyrification abnormalities at any age may signal early adverse events and contribute to our understanding of both the timing and the nature of brain alterations in neurodevelopmental disorders.

Previous studies have noted alterations to cortical shape in autism (Levitt et al., 2003; Nordahl et al., 2007; Shokouhi et al., 2012), and some have used the Gyrification Index (GI; Hardan et al., 2004; Casanova et al., 2009; Kates et al., 2009; Jou et al., 2010; Meguid et al., 2010). Given that the cortex grows primarily through radial expansion (Rakic, 1988), the GI was specifically designed to identify early defects in cortical development. However, all but one (Wallace et al., 2013) existing studies quantifying GI in patients with ASD used two-dimensional or global approaches, which do not allow for the identification of focal differences. By contrast, the local Gyrification Index (*l*GI; Schaer et al., 2008) has been shown to provide reliable estimates of GI with fine-grained resolution in many conditions (Zhang et al., 2009; Juranek and Salman, 2010; Zhang et al., 2010; Palaniyappan and Liddle, 2012; Palaniyappan et al., 2011; Ronan et al., 2011; Thesen et al., 2011; Srivastava et al., 2012).

In the present study, we sought to combine advanced multimodal techniques in a small individually-matched group of ASD and healthy controls in order to simultaneously examine alterations in gyrification and structural connectivity. We first propose an exploratory analysis of the morphometry of gray and white matter structure, and of white matter connectivity. For that purpose, we use the T1-weighted imaging to quantify the total cerebral and cerebellar gray and white matter volumes, the regional cortical and white matter volumes, and to measure cortical thickness and *l*GI at thousands of points across the hemisphere. We also exploit Diffusion Tensor Imaging (DTI) to quantify voxel-wise alterations in white matter microstructure and use tractography to provide estimates of structural connectivity. In subsequent analyses, we aim at integrating the morphometric and the connectivity findings. In line with the Van Essen's tension-based morphogenesis hypothesis, we expect to observe that regions with altered gyrification in autism corresponds to areas with aberrant patterns of short- and long-range connectivity, as quantified using tractography.

MATERIALS AND METHODS

PARTICIPANTS

Patients with ASD

Eleven children and adolescents with ASD participated in the current study (8 males). The group had an average age of 12.9 ± 2.7 years (range 9.3–17.4) and an average full-scale IQ (using the Wechsler WISC-III (Wechsler, 1991)) score of 79.4 ± 18.1 (range 51–105). Participants were recruited with the help of local associations, therapeutic schools, and a local ASD diagnostic clinic. Once participants contacted us to express interest in the study, a detailed medical history, including details about their diagnosis were taken. Individuals with known genetic disorders, as well as malformations and birth defects, were excluded. An initial appointment was then set to reconfirm participants' diagnoses using the autism diagnostic interview-revised (ADI-R) interview with one or both parents. The group of patients with ASD had the following scores on the ADI-R (Le Couteur et al., 2007): social interaction: 15.7 ± 7.9, communication: 12.4 ± 6.6, restricted and repetitive behaviors: 5.7 ± 3.3. The ADI-R was followed by an autism diagnostic observation scale (ADOS; Lord et al., 2009), which was conducted by a research-reliable clinician from the institution's ASD diagnostic clinic. The parents of all participants also filled in the Social Communication Questionnaire (SCQ; Berument et al., 1999).

Control participants

The comparison group was comprised of 11 healthy controls, individually matched with each patient for gender and age. The control group had an average age of 12.7 ± 2.7 (range 8.7–16.8). There was no difference in mean age between patients and controls ($p = 0.897$). The average full-scale IQ of the control group was 110.5 ± 13.3 (range 88–129).

Written informed consent was received from all subjects and their parents in accordance with protocols approved by the local ethics committee.

IMAGE PROCESSING

Cerebral magnetic resonance images were acquired using a Siemens Trio 3T scanner at the Geneva Center for Biomedical Imaging (CIBM). A set of T1-weighted 3D volumetric images was acquired as a series of 192 contiguous coronal slices, with a voxel size of 0.86 × 0.86 × 1.1 mm (repetition time (TR) = 1200 ms, echo time (TE) = 3 ms, flip angle = 8°). DTI were acquired on the same day as a series of 64 axial slices with 30 directions, with a voxel size of 2 × 2 × 2 mm (b0 = 1000 ms, TR = 8300 ms, TE = 82 ms, flip angle = 90°).

Cortical reconstruction

The T1-weighted images were used to create cortical reconstruction and volumetric segmentation using the *FreeSurfer* package (Martinos Center for Biomedical Imaging, Massachusetts General Hospital, Boston[1]). Briefly, the processing was comprised of removing non-brain tissue, executing automatic segmentation of the subcortical gray matter structures, and extracting cortical surface (Dale et al., 1999; Fischl, 2012). Both intensity and continuity data from the entire three-dimensional MR volume are used in the segmentation procedures, thus producing accurate representations of cortical thickness and volumes. These procedures have been validated against histological studies (Rosas et al., 2002) and have been shown to be reliable across scanner models and field strengths (Han et al., 2006). At the end of the reconstruction process, the following volumes were available: total cerebral gray and white matter volumes, cerebellar gray and white matter volumes, corpus callosum volume, and the volumes of subcortical structures including thalamus, putamen, pallidum, caudate nucleus, as well as amygdala and hippocampus.

Regional cortical volumes

Subsequent to cortical reconstruction, the cortex was also subdivided into units based on gyral and sulcal structures (Desikan et al., 2006). This parcellation method has been shown to be both valid and reliable, with high intra-class correlation coefficients between the manual and automated procedures for both cortical volume estimates and region boundaries. The parcellation produces 34 cortical regions subdivided into 11 frontal regions, 9 temporal regions, 5 parietal regions, 4 occipital regions, 4 parts of the cingulate cortex, and one label for the insula.

Regional white matter volumes

The parcellation of the cortical gray matter was subsequently used to subdivide the underlying white matter as described in Salat et al. (2009), a Voronoi diagram was created in the white matter voxels based on the distance to the nearest parcellation label, using a distance constraint of 5 mm. As a result of this process, regional white matter volumes were available for each of the 34 regions corresponding to the aforementioned gyral labeling.

The corpus callosum was also identified and subdivided into 5 portions along its anteroposterior axis, according to procedures detailed in Rosas et al. (2010). The volume of the corpus callosum was measured for each of the 5 portions (anterior, mid-anterior, center, mid-posterior and posterior) on a 5 mm lateral extent centered on the mid-sagittal place.

Cortical thickness and cortical gyrification

Cortical thickness was measured in the native space of the images, as the shortest distance between the white (gray-white boundary) and the pial (gray-CSF interface) surfaces. As a result, cortical thickness values with submillimeter accuracy were available at more than 150,000 different points over each hemisphere resolution (Fischl and Dale, 2000). Finally, based on the outer cortical surface reconstruction (pial surface), *l*GI was measured at thousands of points across each hemisphere using previously validated algorithms (Schaer et al., 2008). *l*GI is a surface-based measurement of the degree of cortical folding that iteratively quantifies the amount of cortex buried within the sulcal folds in the surrounding circular region.

Inter-subject comparison of the cortical thickness and gyrification values is achieved through spherical registration of the surfaces that minimizes metric distortion and allows for a highly reliable point-to-point comparison of cortical thickness between groups (Fischl et al., 1999).

Tract-based spatial statistics of the white matter structure

The DTI images were used for voxelwise statistical analysis of the Fractional Anisotropy (FA) using Tract-Based Spatial Statistics (TBSS; Smith et al., 2006), which is part of FSL software.[2] First, FA images were created by fitting a tensor model to the raw diffusion data using algorithms embedded in the FDT toolbox, followed by skull stripping. As described in the original protocol (Smith et al., 2006, 2007), subjects' FA data were then aligned into a common space using nonlinear registration. Next, the mean FA image was created and thinned to create a mean FA skeleton that represents the centers of all tracts common to the group. Each subject's aligned FA data were then projected onto this skeleton and the resulting data were fed into voxelwise cross-subject statistics.

Tractography analyses

To relate the cortical anatomy with the underlying architecture of white matter fibers, we used tools embedded in the Connectome Mapping Toolkit (Daducci et al., 2012).[3] Briefly, registration between the T1-weighted and DTI images was completed using the *bbregister* function of FreeSurfer. The DTI images were processed with Diffusion Toolkit software[4] using the deterministic streamline algorithm (Mori et al., 1999) to obtain tractographic reconstruction of white matter bundles.

In the present study, we used the number of streamlines to quantify two different aspects of connectivity. First, we measured the amount of fibers connecting the homologous lobe between each hemisphere. The inter-hemispheric fibers obtained by this method represent a simple way to define long-range connectivity without having to define an arbitrary length threshold. To obtain the inter-hemispheric frontal fibers, we retained all streamlines connecting cortical regions comprised in the frontal lobe, as

[1] http://surfer.nmr.mgh.harvard.edu

[2] http://fsl.fmrib.ox.ac.uk/fsl/fslwiki/

[3] http://www.connectomics.org/connectomemapper/

[4] http://trackvis.org/dtk/

defined in the Desikan parcellation (Desikan et al., 2006). To select the streamlines corresponding to inter-hemispheric parietal streamlines, we repeated the process with cortical regions corresponding to the parietal lobe. Finally, streamlines connecting the temporal and occipital cortical regions were considered together for this analysis, given the small amount of inter-hemispheric fibers connecting these two lobes. As a result, three different variables summarizing one aspect of long-range connectivity were studied: the number of inter-hemispheric frontal, parietal, and temporo-occipital streamlines. Second, we measured the connectivity within each lobe (i.e., the number of streamlines connecting one lobe to itself) as an estimate of short-connectivity that also doesn't require any arbitrary length threshold.

STATISTICAL ANALYSES

Volumetric analyses

We used ANCOVA to compare cerebral, cerebellar and subcortical volumes between groups, including age and gender as covariates. To identify potential regional cortical alterations, we subsequently applied a MANCOVA on the 34 gyral regions in each hemisphere by entering diagnosis as the fixed factor, and both age and gender as covariates. Potential changes in regional white matter volumes were examined by doing a MANCOVA on the five corpus callosum regions, and another MANCOVA on the 34 regional white matter volume in each hemisphere. All the MANCOVA were performed with diagnosis as the fixed factor and both age and gender as covariates.

Cortical thickness and gyrification analyses

The comparisons of cortical thickness and gyrification over the whole brain used the *fsaverage* template included in the FreeSurfer distribution. Cortical thickness maps were smoothed using a full width at half maximum (FWHM) kernel of 10 mm. As *l*GI is already smooth (the degree of smoothness in our *l*GI data corresponds to a smoothing kernel of 10 mm), the data were not additionally smoothed prior to statistical analyses. Statistical analyses employed a General Linear Model (GLM) to estimate the effect of diagnosis, age and gender on thickness or gyrification at each cortical point. Cortical thickness or gyrification changes with age were fitted using a linear model. All results were corrected for multiple comparisons using the Monte Carlo simulation at the cluster level at the corrected significance threshold of $p < 0.05$.

Tract-Based Spatial Statistics of the white matter structure

TBSS voxel-wise analyses were carried out across subjects for each point of the common skeleton. As our population was comprised of children and adolescents, the mean FA volume provided by FMRIB software library (FSL) ("FMRIB58") based on 58 adult brains was not optimal. Therefore, we chose the recommended alternative, using the "most typical" subject in our sample, to process the statistics. Local FA differences between patients and controls were tested for significance using a GLM. The skeleton-based approach has the advantage of reducing the number of statistical tests performed by reducing the number of voxels being compared. Nevertheless, we performed a permutation-based approach to control for "Family-Wise Error" (FWE; Nichols and Holmes, 2002). The options we used in the statistic TBSS pipeline were the most recommended ones: the Threshold-Free Cluster Enhancement (TFCE) option and a number of permutations at 500 (see the TBSS user guide on http://fsl.fmrib.ox.ac.uk/fsl/fslwiki/TBSS). A post-hoc *t*-test was ultimately conducted, comparing individual measurements of axial and radial diffusivity in clusters of significant between-group FA differences.

Tractography analyses

We used ANCOVA to compare the total number of streamlines with the total number of inter-hemispheric streamlines between patients with ASD and controls, while correcting for age and gender. We then conducted two MANCOVA to quantify potential differences between groups for the number of inter-hemispheric streamlines (long-range connectivity) and the number of streamlines connecting each lobe with itself (short-range connectivity), with age, gender and the total number of streamlines as covariates.

Correlations between gyrification and connectivity

We conducted partial correlations between the average *l*GI in each cluster of between-group differences and measures of short- and long-range connectivity, while correcting for the effects of age, gender and total number of fibers. For long-range connectivity, we correlated *l*GI for each cluster with the inter-hemispheric fibers corresponding to the lobe where the largest part of the cluster was located. For the short-range connectivity, we correlated *l*GI with the number of intra-lobar fibers in the lobe where the largest part of the cluster was located. These partial correlations were conducted separately in ASD and control groups. Given that these correlations were based on our *a priori* hypothesis postulating a relationship between gyrification and underlying connectivity, we did not correct for multiple comparisons.

Correlations with the clinical phenotype

Finally, we explored how the neuroanatomical differences observed between the two groups may be related to the clinical outcome. For that purpose, we conducted partial correlations between neuroanatomical variables and the scores obtained at the ADI-R and in the SCQ, correcting for age and gender. In addition, variables measuring the number of streamlines between regions of interest were also corrected for the total number of streamlines. Correlations with clinical phenotype were not corrected for multiple comparisons.

RESULTS

VOLUMETRIC ANALYSES

We did not observe any significant differences between the cerebral, cerebellar and subcortical volumes of the groups (all $p > 0.386$). Upon further examination of the 34 cortical parcel volumes, we did not detect any significant patterns of change (left: Wilks Lambda: 0.042, $p = 0.612$; right: Wilks Lambda: 0.028, $p = 0.517$), nor did we detect pattern differences in the 34 subcortical white matter regions (left: Wilks Lambda: 0.001, $p = 0.087$; right: Wilks Lambda: 0.037, $p = 0.585$). Despite the trend for a significant pattern of between-group differences in the MANCOVA corresponding to the left white matter subregions, none of the individual subregions revealed any significant difference in the post-hoc analysis.

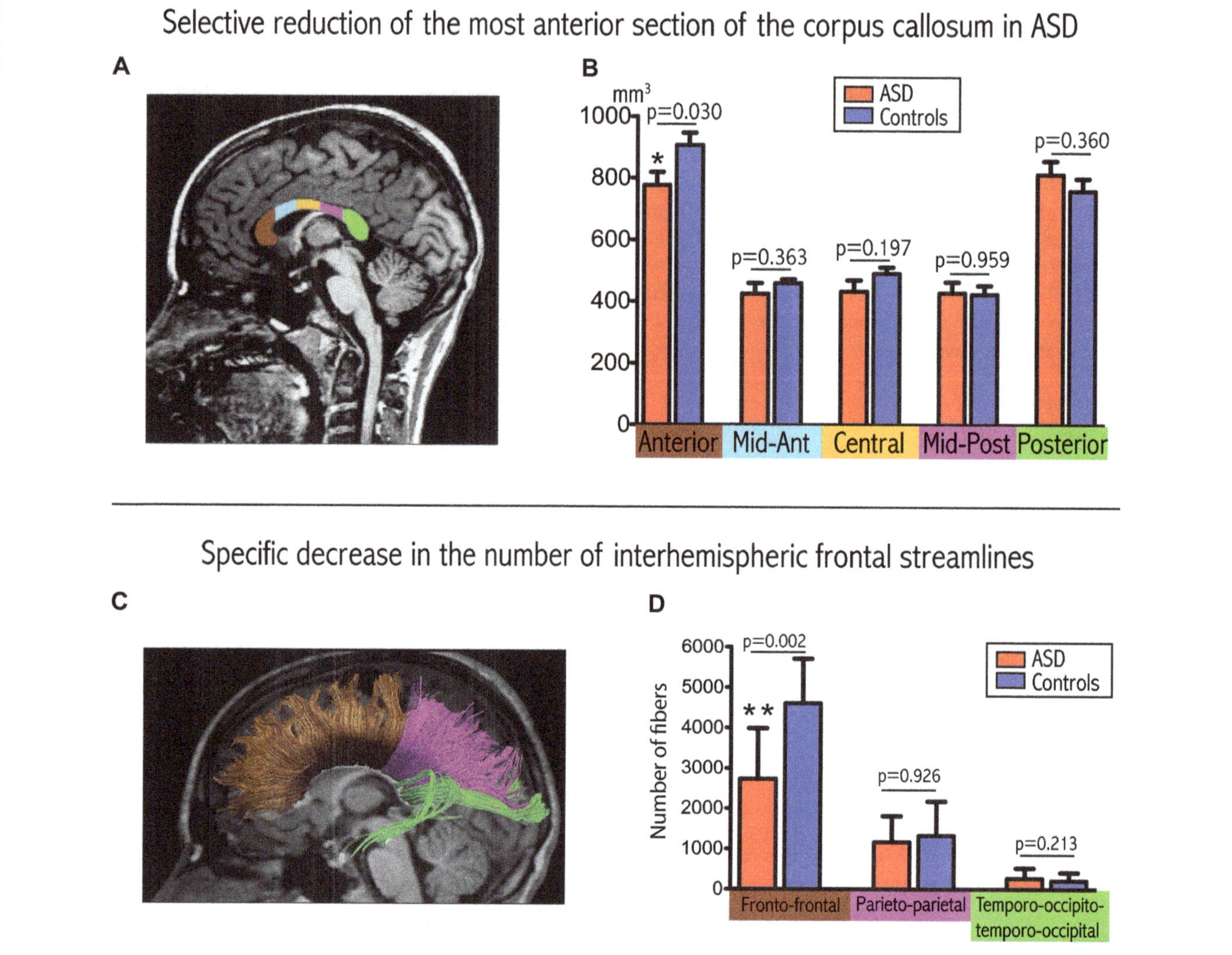

FIGURE 1 | Convergent evidence for disrupted connectivity at the level of inter-hemispheric frontal connectivity in ASD. **(A)** Example of subdivision of the five sections of the corpus callosum displayed on a mid-sagittal slice. **(B)** Boxplots depicting volumetric measurements for the five sections in the two groups. The *p*-values are extracted from the MANCOVA (with correction for age and gender). **(C)** Example of tractographic reconstruction where the inter-hemispheric fibers are subdivided into three groups according to the cortical regions that they connect. **(D)** Boxplots comparing the number of streamlines connecting homologous lobes. The *p*-values are extracted from the MANCOVA (correction for age, gender and total number of streamlines).

Results from the corpus callosum analysis are depicted in **Figures 1A, B**. We observed significant group differences among the five sub-regions of the corpus callosum (Wilks Lambda: 0.354, $p = 0.007$, $F = 5.11$), with a selective reduction in the most anterior part of the corpus callosum in the ASD group compared to controls ($p = 0.030$). These results remained significant when covarying for total intracranial volume or total white matter volume instead of age and gender, as well as for total white matter volume, age and gender.

VERTEX-WISE ANALYSES

We did not observe any significant differences in cortical thickness related to diagnosis. However, vertex-wise comparisons of gyrification revealed four clusters of significant *l*GI reduction in patients with ASD compared to controls that remained significant after correcting for multiple comparisons. As shown in **Figure 2**, the clusters were all located in the right hemisphere, in the inferior parietal region, the lower part of the precentral gyrus, the inferior frontal gyrus, and the medial parieto-occipital region (cuneus/precuneus).

TBSS ANALYSES

We found eight clusters of decreased FA in patients with ASD as compared to controls. The largest cluster of difference was located in the anterior part of the corpus callosum. The remaining seven clusters were located in the right hemisphere, no cluster of FA difference was seen in the left hemisphere. **Figure 3** further details the distribution, location and size of these clusters. When comparing axial and radial diffusivity measurements in the clusters where FA significantly differed between patients with ASD and controls, we observed a significant between-group difference for axial diffusivity in only one cluster (cluster H, patients: $9.44e^{-3} \pm 6.73e^{-5}$,

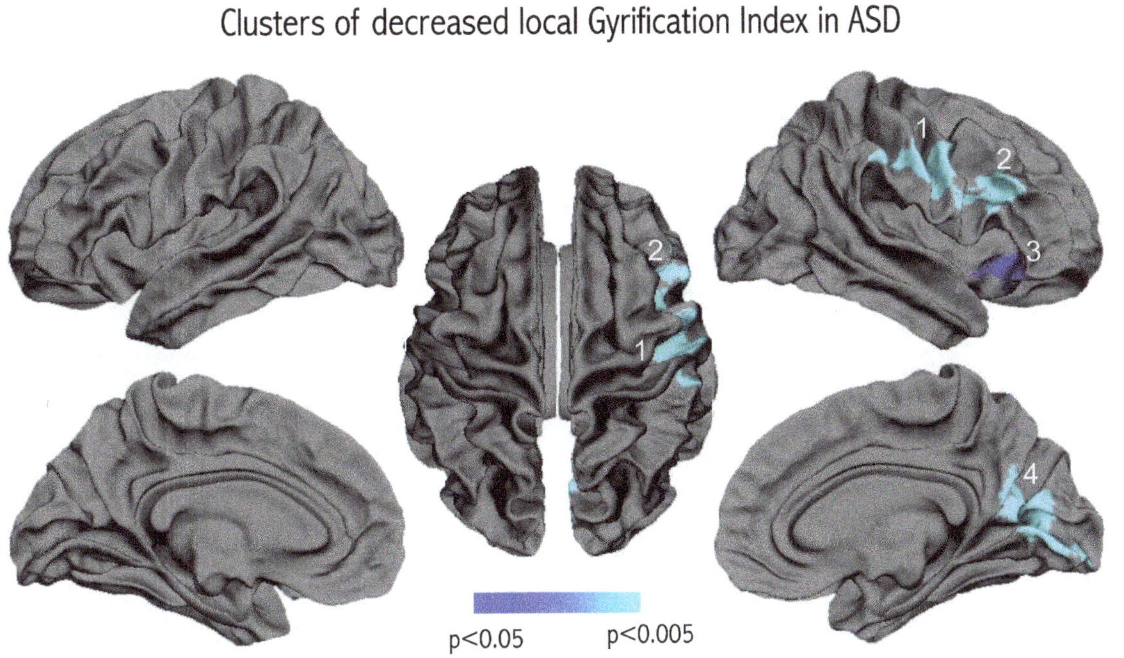

FIGURE 2 | Results of the vertex-wise comparison of *l*GI between groups. Four clusters of reduced *l*GI were observed in the group of children and adolescents with ASD compared to controls after correcting for multiple comparisons.

controls: $8.96e^{-3} \pm 4.59e^{-5}$, $p = 0.03$), whereas significantly decreased radial diffusivity was observed in all eight clusters in patients with ASD compared to controls (all $p < 0.003$).

TRACTOGRAPHIC ANALYSES

We did not observe any difference in the total number of streamlines reconstructed from the DTI images (ASD: 103021 ± 10883, controls: 107331 ± 12769, $p = 0.341$).

We observed a significant reduction in the total number of inter-hemispheric fibers in patients with ASD (ASD: 4293 ± 1834, controls: 6276 ± 1771; $p = 0.033$, $F = 5.405$). Furthermore, and as demonstrated in **Figures 1C, D**, we also observed a significant between-group difference in the regional pattern of inter-hemispheric fibers (MANCOVA covarying out the effect of age, gender and total number of fibers: Wilks Lambda: 0.478, $p = 0.010$, $F = 5.47$), showing a selective reduction in the number of inter-hemispheric frontal fibers ($p = 0.002$), with a selective reduction in the number of inter-hemispheric frontal fibers ($p = 0.002$), but no significant differences in the inter-hemispheric parietal and temporo-occipital fibers.

No difference in the pattern of short-range connectivity was observed between the group of patients with ASD and controls (Wilks Lambda: 0.600, $p = 0.594$).

CORRELATIONS BETWEEN GYRIFICATION AND CONNECTIVITY

Examining the relationship between gyrification and connectivity, we did not observe any significant relationships between the three clusters located in the frontal lobe and the number of inter-hemispheric frontal streamlines or in the occipital cluster and the number of inter-hemispheric occipital streamlines, in either diagnostic group. However, we found positive correlations between *l*GI and the variables measuring short-range connectivity, in the ASD group only. As depicted in **Figure 4**, we observed a significant positive correlation between *l*GI in all three right frontal clusters and the number of streamlines connecting the right frontal lobe to itself ($p = 0.043$, $p = 0.030$ and $p = 0.004$ for clusters 1, 2 and 3 respectively as numbered on **Figure 2**). We also observed a positive correlation between *l*GI in the right occipital cluster (cluster 4 on **Figure 2**) and the number of streamlines connecting the right occipital lobe to itself ($p = 0.010$, $R = 0.836$). The spatial correspondence of the positive correlation between gyrification and short-range connectivity is further supported by the absence of a significant correlation between the three frontal clusters of *l*GI differences and the occipital connectivity, and the absence of a significant correlation between the occipital *l*GI and the frontal connectivity (as depicted in **Figure 4** with dashed lines).

CORRELATIONS WITH THE CLINICAL PHENOTYPE WITHIN ASD

Results of the exploratory correlations between clinical scores at the ADI and SCQ and all variables that showed between-group differences are presented in **Table 1**. Briefly, *l*GI in the posterior cluster (number 4 in **Figure 2**) negatively correlated with the total score obtained on the ADI-R ($R = -0.737$, $p = 0.024$), and the reciprocal social interaction ($R = -0.726$, $p = 0.027$) and communication ($R = -0.773$, $p = 0.015$) domains from the ADI-R. Furthermore, the ADI-R scores in the domain of restrictive and stereotyped patterns of behaviors negative correlated negatively with the number of inter-hemispheric fibers ($R = -0.784$, $p = 0.021$) and with the number of inter-hemispheric frontal

Table 1 | Correlations between clinical scores and neuroanatomical variables with between-group differences in participants with ASD.

	ADI: Total score	ADI: Reciprocal social interactions score	ADI: Communication score	ADI: Restrictive and stereotyped patterns of behavior	ADI: Early anomalies in development	SCQ: Total score
Gyrification						
*l*GI in cluster 1	−.005 ($p = 0.989$)	−.216 ($p = 0.577$)	.030 ($p = 0.940$)	.497 ($p = 0.173$)	.056 ($p = 0.887$)	.076 ($p = 0.845$)
*l*GI in cluster 2	−.136 ($p = 0.728$)	−.386 ($p = 0.305$)	−.020 ($p = 0.959$)	.451 ($p = 0.223$)	.041 ($p = 0.917$)	−.181 ($p = 0.641$)
*l*GI in cluster 3	−.037 ($p = 0.925$)	−.292 ($p = 0.446$)	.045 ($p = 0.908$)	.494 ($p = 0.177$)	.146 ($p = 0.708$)	−.117 ($p = 0.764$)
*l*GI in cluster 4	**−.737 ($p = 0.024$)**	**−.726 ($p = 0.027$)**	**−.773 ($p = 0.015$)**	−.043 ($p = 0.912$)	.205 ($p = 0.597$)	−.541 ($p = 0.132$)
Volumetric measurements						
Anterior section of the corpus callosum	.482 ($p = 0.189$)	.537 ($p = 0.136$)	.649 ($p = 0.059$)	−.325 ($p = 0.394$)	−.419 ($p = 0.262$)	.315 ($p = 0.409$)
Tractographic measurements						
Number of inter-hemispheric streamlines	−.345 ($p = 0.402$)	−.165 ($p = 0.697$)	−.317 ($p = 0.445$)	**−.784 ($p = 0.021$)**	.544 ($p = 0.163$)	−.682 ($p = 0.063$)
Number of inter-hemispheric frontal streamlines	−.390 ($p = 0.339$)	−.241 ($p = 0.566$)	−.309 ($p = 0.457$)	**−.779 ($p = 0.023$)**	.392 ($p = 0.337$)	−.681 ($p = 0.063$)

This table provides R-values from partial correlations. Significance level is given in parentheses. Partial correlations accounted for an effect of age and gender on gyrification and volumetric measurements, as well as for an additional effect of total number of streamlines on tractographic measurements. Significant correlations at $p < 0.05$ (uncorrected) are highlighted in bold.

fibers ($R = -0.779$, $p = 0.023$). None of the neuroanatomical variables correlated with the total score obtained on the SCQ.

DISCUSSION

In this study, we applied neuroimaging techniques using T1-weighted and DTI images in the interest of quantifying morphometric and connectivity differences in a group of children and adolescents with ASD. We observed: (a) decreased gyrification in the right inferior frontal region extending into the inferior parietal region and in the medial parieto-occipital region of patients with ASD as compared to controls, the latter of which was related to the severity of social communications deficits in the group of ASD; (b) convergent evidence from three different analyses for altered long-range connectivity at the level of inter-hemispheric frontal fibers: volumetric reduction of the anterior corpus callosum, reduced FA in the anterior corpus callosum, and a decreased number of virtual streamlines connecting homologous frontal lobes which further correlated with the severity of restrictive/repetitive behaviors; (c) further reduced FA in seven clusters of the right hemisphere of patients with ASD compared to controls; and (d) a positive correlation between *l*GI in the clusters of between-group differences and short-range connectivity in the corresponding lobe.

DECREASED GYRIFICATION

We used a validated technique with exquisite resolution to measure local cortical gyrification across the hemispheres (Schaer et al., 2008), and observed four clusters of reduced GI in patients with ASD compared to controls, three of them located in the frontal lobe. This is in contrast with previous studies using GI in children, adolescents or adults with ASD, which report either an increased GI (Hardan et al., 2004; Jou et al., 2010), or an absence of significant difference (Casanova et al., 2009; Kates et al., 2009; Meguid et al., 2010). Lower intellectual abilities in our patient group may explain part of the divergence with previous results, given that both studies that reported increased GI comprised participants with higher full-scale IQ scores (means: 105 ± 16 for Hardan et al. (2004), 110 ± 15 for Jou et al. (2010) and 113 ± 15 for Wallace et al. (2013)). However, we believe part of the difference to relate to the way GI was calculated. Indeed, the two studies that reported higher GI in the frontal lobe of subjects with ASD used manual delineation on one single frontal slice. Aside from the fact that manual tracing may be less reliable than automated delineation, measuring GI on 2-D sections does not take into account the inherent 3-D nature of the cortical surface. 2-D measurement also can be biased by slice orientation (Zilles et al., 1997) and the presence of buried sulci (Magnotta et al., 1999), and it does not allow for precise localization of gyral anomalies in sublobar regions. Other studies that partly addressed these concerns did not report any significant differences in GI in patients with ASD compared to controls (Casanova et al., 2009; Kates et al., 2009; Meguid et al., 2010). Casanova et al. used manual delineation in 40 randomly selected slices; Kates et al. applied an automated technique for measuring global and lobar GI based on 2D sections; and Meguid et al. measured global GI using three-dimensional cortical reconstructions. The technique that we use in the present study to measure *l*GI is automated, unbiased by slice orientation, and allows the quantification of gyrification differences at thousands of points over the reconstructed cortical surface. As a result, by using *l*GI, we may have been able to detect gyrification differences in the frontal lobe of patients with ASD that had previously gone undetected. Studies using cortical reconstructions in autism corroborate this idea. They have detected focal changes to sulcal shape with alterations

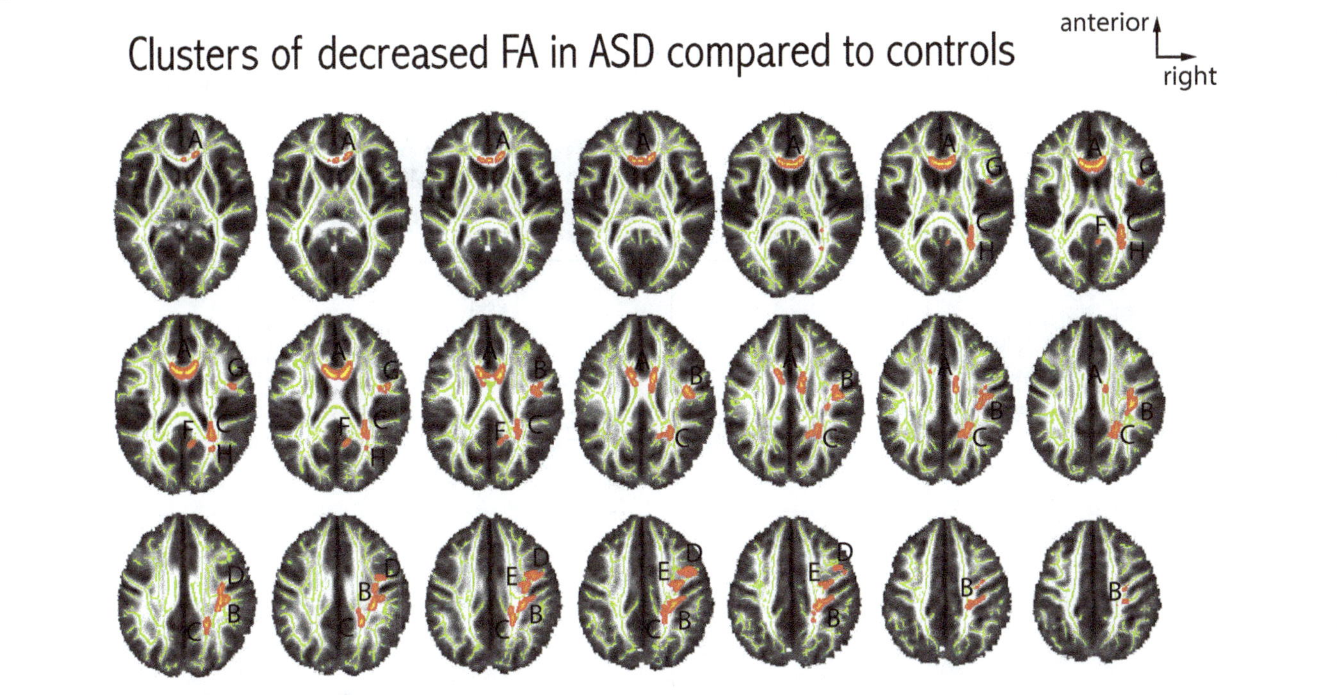

FIGURE 3 | Differences in FA between patients with ASD and controls. Eight clusters of decreased FA in patients with ASD were observed at $p < 0.05$ (corrected for multiple comparisons). Each cluster was attributed a letter according to decreasing size. The clusters were centered at the following MNI coordinates: A: $x = 81$, $y = 145$, $z = 90$ (939 voxels); B: $x = 52$, $y = 104$, $z = 104$ (725 voxels); C: $x = 66$, $y = 78$, $z = 101$ (470 voxels); D: $x = 57$, $y = 106$, $z = 129$ (186 voxels); E: $x = 46$, $y = 131$, $z = 112$ (137 voxels); F: $x = 82$, $y = 70$, $z = 93$ (70 voxels); G: $x = 43$, $y = 128$, $z = 90$ (42 voxels); H: $x = 60$, $y = 65$, $z = 88$ (23 voxels). We did not observe any clusters with increased FA in patients with ASD compared to controls.

to the sylvian fissure and inferior frontal sulcus (Levitt et al., 2003), left frontal operculum (Nordahl et al., 2007), and right intraparietal sulcus (Shokouhi et al., 2012). It is however worth noting that a recent study using the same technique as in the present study observed increased gyrification in different regions of the brain of 39 male adolescents with ASD as compared to 41 controls, namely in bilateral occipital areas as well as in the left superior precuneus (Wallace et al., 2013). This discrepancy in the location and direction of gyrification changes using the same technique suggest either that different developmental mechanisms take place in different regions of the brain of affected patients, or that that demographic characteristics (such as differences in age, gender, cognitive level, or symptom intensity) may have influenced the results. Indeed, it may be the case that the high clinical heterogeneity observed in patients affected with autism may be associated with different neurodevelopmental pathways.

Decreased gyrification, as observed in the present study, is highly suggestive of reduced cortical expansion during early brain development, a process that might differentially affect specific cortical regions. Neuropathological reports have pointed to abnormal cortical development in ASD, including a higher incidence of cortical dysgenesis, heterotopias and migration abnormalities (Avino and Hutsler, 2010; Wegiel et al., 2010). Further detailed examination revealed that one cell type affected by migration deficits in young children with ASD is von Economo neurons (Santos et al., 2011), which are spindle-shaped neurons thought to play a role in emotional function (Butti et al., 2013) that are located in the frontoinsular and cingulate cortices. The location of the von Economo neurons coincides with the location of cluster 3 in the present study (see **Figure 2**). This anterior fronto-insular region is attracting increased attention in autism because of its key role in the "salience network" (Menon and Uddin, 2010). The anterior insula may have a critical role in processing information relevant to social functioning (Uddin and Menon, 2009) as a sort of "hub" that mediates interactions between cerebral networks that are processing information related to an external or internal stimulus. Functional neuroimaging studies tend to confirm the hypothesis of hypoactivation of the right anterior insula in autism, as pointed out by a meta-analysis based on 24 functional neuroimaging studies examining social processes for a total of 276 patients with ASD and 291 controls (Di Martino et al., 2009).

Two other clusters, in the right inferior frontal gyrus (cluster 2) and in a region extending from the right inferior part of the precentral gyrus to the inferior parietal region (cluster 1), are also located in regions that have received attention in ASD. Indeed, these regions are striking in their correspondence to the location of the fronto-parietal mirror neuron system, implicated in action imitation (Rizzolatti and Craighero, 2004). Decreased gyrification in the inferior fronto-parietal region thus supports altered development of the mirror system in ASD during *in utero* life or the first months after birth, pointing to a potential mechanism for early-disrupted abilities to imitate action of others.

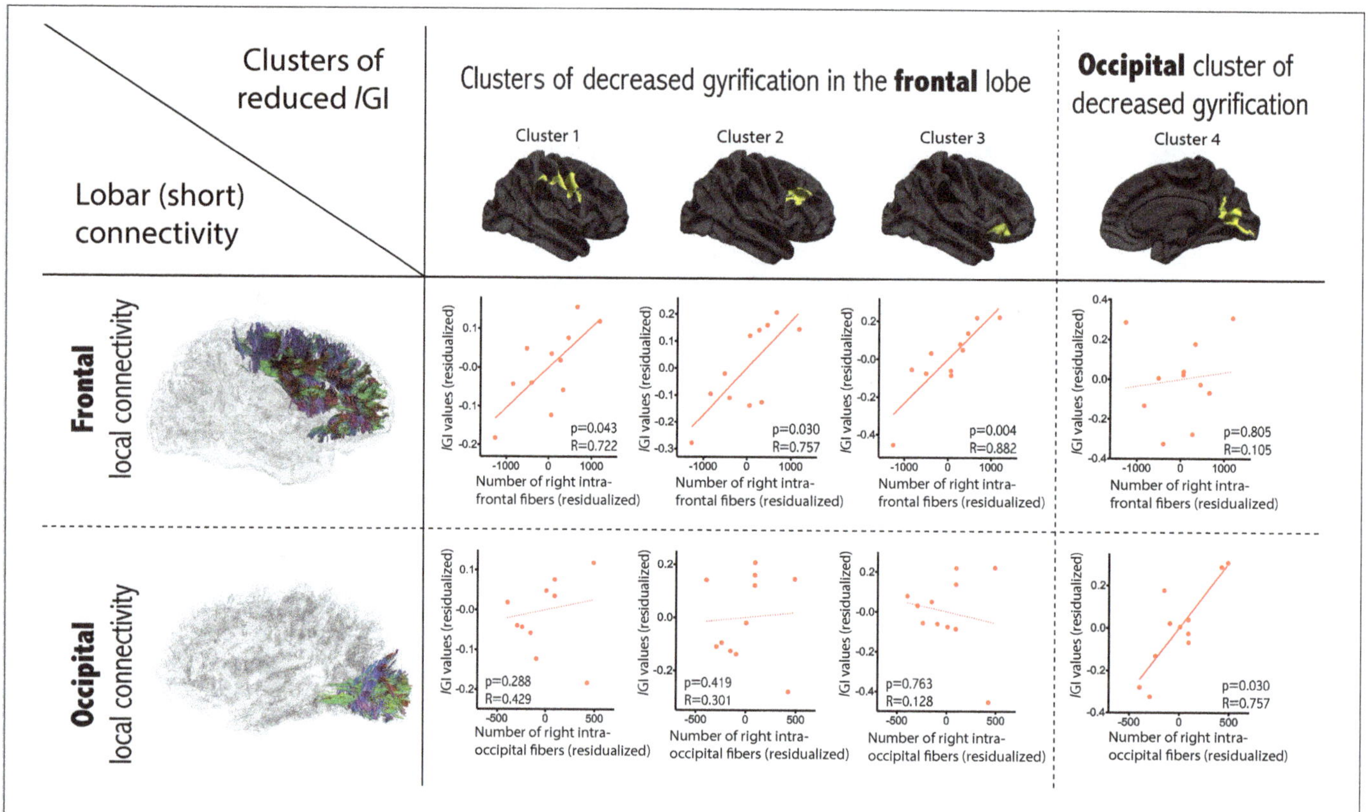

FIGURE 4 | Correlations between gyrification and short-range connectivity within the group of patients with ASD. Partial correlations accounting for age, gender and total number of streamlines were conducted between *l*GI in the cluster of between-group differences and the number of intra-lobar streamlines in the lobe where most of the cluster was located. Significant positive correlations were observed only in the corresponding lobe (dashed lines report non-significant relationships).

The final cluster of reduced gyrification (cluster 4) is centered in the occipital lobe, encompassing the cuneus and the pericalcarine sulcus, and further extending to the precuneus. Volumetric reductions have been consistently reported in the precuneus in structural neuroimaging studies of ASD (Cauda et al., 2011). The precuneus is a key part of the default mode network (DMN), which is thought to be concerned with self-referential and introspective activity, including the ability to understand others' intentions (Fair et al., 2008). Resting state paradigms have received increased recent interest in autism given the crucial role of the DMN in some aspects of social cognition. It is currently unclear to what extent the fronto-parietal mirror system (where we observed decreased *l*GI in clusters 1 and 2) interacts with other regions of the social brain, including regions of the DMN. In an attempt to integrate these different views of the social brain, (Uddin et al., 2007) postulated that the cortical midline structures of the DMN and the fronto-parietal mirror-neuron system may represent two interwoven parts of self-related processing and social cognition: the mirror neurons encode physical aspects of social understanding (motor simulation and imitation of behaviors) and the midline DMN structures are associated with sophisticated processing of social interactions. Accordingly, reduced gyrification in the mirror-neuron system may impair physical aspects of the self-other relationship, consequently altering the developmental cascade of the DMN responsible for more sophisticated social skills, such as empathy and theory of mind. The fact that cluster 4 extends into the precuneus may also point to an early defect, on top of which altered cortical maturation subsequently occurs. Indeed, the currently observed inverse relationship between gyrification and the level of autistic symptoms in the domains of reciprocal social interactions and communication points to the idea that early cortical development may determine the subsequent development of these more sophisticated social skills encoded in the precuneus.

ABSENCE OF CORTICAL THICKNESS OR VOLUME DIFFERENCE

We found reduced gyrification in the absence of differences in cortical thickness or volume. This absence contrasts with numerous studies that have reported altered cortical volume or thickness differences in ASD. Most studies have reported increased cortical volume or thickness in children with ASD (Hardan et al., 2006; Mak-Fan et al., 2012), whereas studies in adults have yielded more diverse results. Some studies in adults with ASD have reported mostly decreased cortical thickness (Hadjikhani et al., 2006; Jiao et al., 2010; Wallace et al., 2010), some have shown a co-occurrence of thickening together with thinning (Ecker et al., 2010, 2013), and at least one has shown mostly thickening (Dziobek et al., 2010). Volumetric studies have more consistently reported increased volume in children and reduced volume in adults, supporting the hypothesis of early brain overgrowth followed by neurodegenerative changes (Courchesne, 2004). Indeed, using a cross-sectional design with patients aged 1 to 50, the largest study published to date provides evidence for an aberrant trajectory of cortical volume changes with age, with a pattern of early overgrowth during the first years of life, followed by decreased volume around 7 or 8 years old (Courchesne et al., 2011). Longitudinal studies confirm this pattern of abnormal cortical development in toddlers with ASD (Schumann et al., 2010) and of higher rates of cortical loss with age (Hardan et al., 2009). It should be noted, however, that studies recording abnormal trajectories of cortical features require large sample sizes, a broad age range at inclusion, and preferably, a longitudinal design. By contrast, our small study sample does not have the power to detect subtle cortical thickness differences that may be further diluted by complex maturational changes.

CONVERGENT EVIDENCE FOR ALTERED LONG-RANGE CONNECTIVITY, MOST PROMINENT IN THE FRONTAL REGION

As the largest white matter bundle of the brain, the corpus callosum represents the most essential component of connectivity, and more specifically long-range connectivity. Several fMRI and EEG studies have reported decreased long-range connectivity (reviewed in Belmonte et al., 2004). Patients with ASD were also shown to perform poorly on tests of inter-hemispheric transfer for auditory, visual and motor tasks (Nyden et al., 2004). More generally, decreased abilities in associative (Nikolaenko, 2001a) and metaphoric thinking (Nikolaenko, 2001b) were thought to depend on decreased inter-hemispheric information transfer. Here, we observed decreased volume of the most anterior part of the corpus callosum, reduced inter-hemispheric frontal connections, and decreased FA in the anterior corpus callosum, providing strong multimodal evidence for altered inter-hemispheric frontal connections in ASD. Our volumetric finding is consistent with previous studies reporting reduced area of the entire corpus callosum, with greater magnitude of reduction in its anterior region (see the meta-analysis by Frazier and Hardan, 2009). Reduced FA in the corpus callosum is also consistent with many previous findings reported by others (Alexander et al., 2007; Noriuchi et al., 2010; Shukla et al., 2010). But, to the best of our knowledge, only one study reported a reduction in the number of inter-hemispheric frontal fibers using tractographic reconstructions in patients with ASD (Thomas et al., 2011). Thomas et al. observed decreased numbers of streamlines specific to the body in high-functioning adults with ASD, which further correlated with ADI scores in the domain of restricted, repetitive and stereotyped behaviors. The fact that we replicate this correlation (though we focus on a more anterior, but overlapping, region) provides strong support for a role for the corpus callosum in repetitive behaviors, across ages and across IQ.

REDUCED FA

In addition to multimodal evidence for altered inter-hemispheric connectivity, we also observed seven clusters of decreased FA in the right hemisphere of patients with ASD compared to controls. The direction of our results was consistent with most previously published studies, which show decreased FA, although a few studies do report increased FA (reviewed in Travers et al., 2012). Surprisingly, in our small sample of children and adolescents with ASD, we found reduced FA only in the right hemisphere and did not detect changes to FA in the left hemisphere. Exclusively right-sided alterations to gyrification in the same sample of participants provide initial support for a relationship between white matter connectivity and cortical folding. However, it was not possible to detect whether the observed FA differences were related to differences in the degree of myelinisation or to differences in the orientation or number of white matter bundles, using voxel-wise measurements of FA. The spatial correspondence of altered gyrification and white matter microstructure in the same hemisphere led us to further examine the relationship between cortical folding and connectivity using more sophisticated tractographic measurements.

CORRELATION BETWEEN GYRIFICATION AND CONNECTIVITY

We did not observe a relationship between long-range connectivity and gyrification, as may have been expected from Van Essen's hypothesis that mechanical tension exerted on long connections shapes cortical folds (Van Essen, 1997). However, three out of the four clusters with decreased gyrification were mostly located in the frontal region, i.e., the region where an important decrease in inter-hemispheric connectivity was observed. The co-occurrence of decreased long-range connections in regions of altered gyrification points to a possible relationship between these two anatomical variables, but the mechanisms governing their association is likely to be more complex than what a linear regression can capture.

We did, however, observe significant positive correlations between *l*GI and short-range connectivity in patients with ASD, but not in controls. This positive correlation means that higher *l*GI was observed in patients with higher intra-lobar (short-range) connectivity. According to Van Essen's theory, it may also be that short-range connections affect the creation of cortical folds during early brain development by reducing the distance between strongly interconnected regions from the two banks of one gyrus, thereby permitting compact wiring of the brain. Accordingly, the gyrification alterations observed in the present study may be a compensatory way of coping with altered connectivity in patients with ASD.

LIMITATIONS AND CONCLUSION

The main limitation of our study is its small sample size, restricting our ability to identify age-related maturational changes or subtle brain-behavior relationships. We realize that, in a heterogeneous disorder such as ASD, such small sample size may lead to observation of findings that may not be representative of the variability observed across the spectrum. However, despite the small sample size, we demonstrate the feasibility of multimodal studies in autism, bridging the gap between reports of altered cortical morphometry and findings of abnormal connectivity patterns. These preliminary results provide initial support for the idea that a higher degree of short-range connectivity alters the shape of the brain in patients with ASD during early neural development, and are an encouraging starting point for exploring this issue in larger samples of children, adolescents or adults with autism.

ACKNOWLEDGMENTS

We would like to thank the children, adolescents and families who participated in this study. The families were recruited as a part of a remediation study supported by the Eagle Foundation, the FHMS ("Fondation Handicap Mental and Société"), the Fondation Dora and the Fondation 1796. Further support for MRI acquisition was provided by the Center of Biomedical Imaging.[5] MS was supported by a grant from the National Center of Competence in Research (NCCR) "SYNAPSY—The Synaptic Bases of Mental Diseases" financed by the Swiss National Science Foundation, and then by a fellowship from the Swiss National Foundation of Science (#145760). The authors would like to extend a special thank you to Hilary Wood de Wilde and Sonia Martinez for their help with patients' assessment.

REFERENCES

Alexander, A. L., Lee, J. E., Lazar, M., Boudos, R., Dubray, M. B., Oakes, T. R., et al. (2007). Diffusion tensor imaging of the corpus callosum in Autism. Neuroimage 34, 61–73. doi: 10.1016/j.neuroimage.2006.08.032

Assaf, M., Jagannathan, K., Calhoun, V. D., Miller, L., Stevens, M. C., Sahl, R., et al. (2010). Abnormal functional connectivity of default mode sub-networks in autism spectrum disorder patients. Neuroimage 53, 247–256. doi: 10.1016/j. neuroimage.2010.05.067

Avino, T. A., and Hutsler, J. J. (2010). Abnormal cell patterning at the cortical gray- white matter boundary in autism spectrum disorders. Brain Res. 1360, 138–146. doi: 10.1016/j.brainres.2010.08.091

Barttfeld, P., Wicker, B., Cukier, S., Navarta, S., Lew, S., and Sigman, M. (2011). A big-world network in ASD: dynamical connectivity analysis reflects a deficit in long-range connections and an excess of short-range connections. Neuropsy-chologia 49, 254–263. doi: 10.1016/j.neuropsychologia.2010.11.024

Belmonte, M. K., Allen, G., Beckel-Mitchener, A., Boulanger, L. M., Carper, R. A., and Webb, S. J. (2004). Autism and abnormal development of brain connectivity. J. Neurosci. 24, 9228–9231. doi: 10.1523/jneurosci.3340-04.2004

Berument, S. K., Rutter, M., Lord, C., Pickles, A., and Bailey, A. (1999). Autism screening questionnaire: diagnostic validity. Br. J. Psychiatry 175, 444–451. doi: 10.1192/bjp.175.5.444

Butti, C., Santos, M., Uppal, N., and Hof, P. R. (2013). Von Economo neurons: clinical and evolutionary perspectives. Cortex 49, 312–326. doi: 10.1016/j.cortex. 2011.10.004

Casanova, M. F., El-Baz, A., Mott, M., Mannheim, G., Hassan, H., Fahmi, R., et al. (2009). Reduced gyral window and corpus callosum size in autism: possible macroscopic correlates of a minicolumnopathy. J. Autism Dev. Disord. 39, 751–764. doi: 10.1007/s10803-008-0681-4

Cauda, F., Geda, E., Sacco, K., D'agata, F., Duca, S., Geminiani, G., et al. (2011). Grey matter abnormality in autism spectrum disorder: an activation likelihood estimation meta-analysis study. J. Neurol. Neurosurg. Psychiatry 82, 1304–1313. doi: 10.1136/jnnp.2010.239111

Centers for Disease Control and Prevention (2008). "Prevalence of autism spectrum disorders - autism and developmental disabilities monitoring network, 14 sites, United States 2008" by Jon Baio. Centers for Disease Control and Prevention Morbidity and Mortality Weekly Report, Vol. 61, 1–19.

Courchesne, E. (2004). Brain development in autism: early overgrowth followed by premature arrest of growth. Ment. Retard. Dev. Disabil. Res. Rev. 10, 106–111. doi: 10.1002/mrdd.20020

Courchesne, E., Campbell, K., and Solso, S. (2011). Brain growth across the life span in autism: age-specific changes in anatomical pathology. Brain Res. 1380, 138–145. doi: 10.1016/j.brainres.2010.09.101

Courchesne, E., Karns, C. M., Davis, H. R., Ziccardi, R., Carper, R. A., Tigue, Z. D., et al. (2001). Unusual brain growth patterns in early life in patients with autistic disorder: an MRI study. Neurology 57, 245–254. doi: 10.1212/wnl.57.2.245

Daducci, A., Gerhard, S., Griffa, A., Lemkaddem, A., Cammoun, L., Gigandet, X., et al. (2012). The connectome mapper: an open-source processing pipeline to map connectomes with MRI. PLoS One 7:e48121. doi: 10.1371/journal.pone. 0048121

Dale, A. M., Fischl, B., and Sereno, M. I. (1999). Cortical surface-based analysis. I. Segmentation and surface reconstruction. Neuroimage 9, 179–194. doi: 10. 1006/nimg.1998.0395

Desikan, R. S., Segonne, F., Fischl, B., Quinn, B. T., Dickerson, B. C., Blacker, D., et al. (2006). An automated labeling system for subdividing the human cerebral cortex on MRI scans into gyral based regions of interest. Neuroimage 31, 968–980. doi: 10.1016/j.neuroimage.2006.01.021

Di Martino, A., Ross, K., Uddin, L. Q., Sklar, A. B., Castellanos, F. X., and Milham,

M. P. (2009). Functional brain correlates of social and nonsocial processes in autism spectrum disorders: an activation likelihood estimation meta-analysis. Biol. Psychiatry 65, 63–74. doi: 10.1016/j.biopsych.2008.09.022

Dziobek, I., Bahnemann, M., Convit, A., and Heekeren, H. R. (2010). The role of the fusiform-amygdala system in the pathophysiology of autism. Arch. Gen. Psychiatry 67, 397–405. doi: 10.1001/archgenpsychiatry.2010.31

Ecker, C., Ginestet, C., Feng, Y., Johnston, P., Lombardo, M. V., Lai, M. C., et al. (2013). Brain surface anatomy in adults with autism: the relationship between surface area, cortical thickness, and autistic symptoms. JAMA Psychiatry 70, 59–70. doi: 10.1001/jamapsychiatry.2013.265

Ecker, C., Marquand, A., Mourao-Miranda, J., Johnston, P., Daly, E. M., Brammer, M. J., et al. (2010). Describing the brain in autism in five dimensions–magnetic resonance imaging-assisted diagnosis of autism spectrum disorder using a multiparameter classification approach. J. Neurosci. 30, 10612–10623. doi: 10. 1523/jneurosci.5413-09.2010

Elsabbagh, M., Divan, G., Koh, Y. J., Kim, Y. S., Kauchali, S., Marcin, C., et al. (2012). Global prevalence of autism and other pervasive developmental disorders. Autism Res. 5, 160–179. doi: 10.1002/aur.239

Fair, D. A., Cohen, A. L., Dosenbach, N. U., Church, J. A., Miezin, F. M., Barch, D. M., et al. (2008). The maturing architecture of the brain's default network. Proc. Natl. Acad. Sci. U S A 105, 4028–4032. doi: 10.1073/pnas.0800376105

Fischl, B. (2012). FreeSurfer. Neuroimage 62, 774–781.

Fischl, B., and Dale, A. M. (2000). Measuring the thickness of the human cerebral cortex from magnetic resonance images. Proc. Natl. Acad. Sci. U S A 97, 11050– 11055. doi: 10.1073/pnas.200033797

Fischl, B., Sereno, M. I., and Dale, A. M. (1999). Cortical surface-based analysis. II: Inflation, flattening, and a surface-based coordinate system. Neuroimage 9, 195–207. doi: 10.1006/nimg.1998.0396

Frazier, T. W., and Hardan, A. Y. (2009). A meta-analysis of the corpus callosum in autism. Biol. Psychiatry 66, 935–941. doi: 10.1016/j.biopsych.2009. 07.022

Hadjikhani, N., Joseph, R. M., Snyder, J., and Tager-Flusberg, H. (2006). Anatom- ical differences in the mirror neuron system and social cognition network in autism. Cereb. Cortex 16, 1276–1282. doi: 10.1093/cercor/bhj069

Han, X., Jovicich, J., Salat, D., Van Der Kouwe, A., Quinn, B., Czanner, S., et al. (2006). Reliability of MRI-derived measurements of human cerebral cortical thickness: the effects of field strength, scanner upgrade and manufacturer. Neuroimage 32, 180–194. doi: 10.1016/j.neuroimage.2006.02.051

Hardan, A. Y., Jou, R. J., Keshavan, M. S., Varma, R., and Minshew, N. J. (2004). Increased frontal cortical folding in autism: a preliminary MRI study. Psychiatry Res. 131, 263–268. doi: 10.1016/j.pscychresns.2004.06.001

Hardan, A. Y., Libove, R. A., Keshavan, M. S., Melhem, N. M., and Minshew, N. J. (2009). A preliminary longitudinal magnetic resonance imaging study of brain volume and cortical thickness in autism. Biol. Psychiatry 66, 320–326. doi: 10. 1016/j.biopsych.2009.04.024

Hardan, A. Y., Muddasani, S., Vemulapalli, M., Keshavan, M. S., and Minshew, N. J. (2006). An MRI study of increased cortical thickness in autism. Am. J. Psychiatry 163, 1290–1292. doi: 10.1176/appi.ajp.163.7.1290

Haukvik, U. K., Schaer, M., Nesvag, R., Mcneil, T., Hartberg, C. B., Jonsson, E. G., et al. (2011). Cortical folding in Broca's area relates to obstetric complications in schizophrenia patients and healthy controls. Psychol. Med. 42, 1329–1337. doi: 10.1017/S0033291711002315

Jiao, Y., Chen, R., Ke, X., Chu, K., Lu, Z., and Herskovits, E. H. (2010).

Predictive models of autism spectrum disorder based on brain regional cortical thickness. Neuroimage 50, 589–599. doi: 10.1016/j.neuroimage.2009.12.047

Jou, R. J., Minshew, N. J., Keshavan, M. S., and Hardan, A. Y. (2010). Cortical gyri- fication in autistic and Asperger disorders: a preliminary magnetic resonance imaging study. J. Child Neurol. 25, 1462–1467. doi: 10.1177/0883073810368311

Juranek, J., and Salman, M. S. (2010). Anomalous development of brain structure and function in spina bifida myelomeningocele. Dev. Disabil. Res. Rev. 16, 23–30. doi: 10.1002/ddrr.88

Kates, W. R., Ikuta, I., and Burnette, C. P. (2009). Gyrification patterns in monozy- gotic twin pairs varying in discordance for autism. Autism Res. 2, 267–278. doi: 10.1002/aur.98

Kennedy, D. P., and Courchesne, E. (2008). The intrinsic functional organization of the brain is altered in autism. Neuroimage 39, 1877–1885. doi: 10.1016/j. neuroimage.2007.10.052

Le Couteur, A., Lord, C., and Rutter, M. L. (2007). Entretien pour le Diagnostic de l'Autisme - version révisée, adaptation française de Bernadette Rogé et collaborateurs. Editions Hogrefe France.

Levitt, J. G., Blanton, R. E., Smalley, S., Thompson, P. M., Guthrie, D., Mccracken, J. T., et al. (2003). Cortical sulcal maps in autism. Cereb. Cortex 13, 728–735. doi: 10.1093/cercor/13.7.728

Lord, C., Rutter, M. L., Dilavore, P. C., and Risi, S. (2009). ADOS: Echelle d'observation pour le diagnostic de l'autisme, adaptation française par Bernadette Rogé et collaborateurs. Editions Hogrefe France.

Magnotta, V. A., Andreasen, N. C., Schultz, S. K., Harris, G., Cizadlo, T., Heckel, D., et al. (1999). Quantitative in vivo measurement of gyrification in the human brain: changes associated with aging. Cereb. Cortex 9, 151–160. doi: 10. 1093/cercor/9.2.151

Mak-Fan, K. M., Taylor, M. J., Roberts, W., and Lerch, J. P. (2012). Measures of cortical grey matter structure and development in children with autism spectrum disorder. J. Autism Dev. Disord. 42, 419–427. doi: 10.1007/s10803-011- 1261-6

Meguid, N., Fahim, C., Yoon, U., Nashaat, N. H., Ibrahim, A. S., Mancini-Marie, A., et al. (2010). Brain morphology in autism and fragile X syndrome corre- lates with social IQ: first report from the Canadian-Swiss-Egyptian neurode- velopmental study. J. Child Neurol. 25, 599–608. doi: 10.1177/088307380934 1670

Menon, V., and Uddin, L. Q. (2010). Saliency, switching, attention and control: a network model of insula function. Brain Struct. Funct. 214, 655–667. doi: 10. 1007/s00429-010-0262-0

Minshew, N. J., and Williams, D. L. (2007). The new neurobiology of autism: cortex, connectivity, and neuronal organization. Arch. Neurol. 64, 945–950. doi: 10. 1001/archneur.64.10.1464

Mori, S., Crain, B. J., Chacko, V. P., and Van Zijl, P. C. (1999). Three-dimensional tracking of axonal projections in the brain by magnetic resonance imaging. Ann. Neurol. 45, 265–269. doi: 1531-8249(199902)45:2<265::aid-ana21> 3. 0.co;2-3

Nichols, T. E., and Holmes, A. P. (2002). Nonparametric permutation tests for functional neuroimaging: a primer with examples. Hum. Brain Mapp. 15, 1–25. doi: 10.1002/hbm.1058

Nikolaenko, N. N. (2001a). Associative process as an indicator of interhemispheric interaction in healthy children and children with autism. Dokl. Biol. Sci. 380, 430–432. doi: 10.1023/A:1012354801160

Nikolaenko, N. N. (2001b). Metaphorical thinking in healthy and autistic children as an index of interhemispheric interaction. Dokl. Biol. Sci. 379, 325–327. doi: 10. 1023/A:1011639927334

Nordahl, C. W., Dierker, D., Mostafavi, I., Schumann, C. M., Rivera, S. M., Amaral, D. G., et al. (2007). Cortical folding abnormalities in autism revealed by surface- based morphometry. J. Neurosci. 27, 11725–11735. doi: 10.1523/jneurosci.0777- 07.2007

Noriuchi, M., Kikuchi, Y., Yoshiura, T., Kira, R., Shigeto, H., Hara, T., et al. (2010). Altered white matter fractional anisotropy and social impairment in children with autism spectrum disorder. Brain Res. 1362, 141–149. doi: 10. 1016/j.brainres.2010.09.051

Nyden, A., Carlsson, M., Carlsson, A., and Gillberg, C. (2004). Interhemispheric transfer in high-functioning children and adolescents with autism spectrum disorders: a controlled pilot study. Dev. Med. Child Neurol. 46, 448–454. doi: 10. 1017/ s001216220400074x

Palaniyappan, L., and Liddle, P. F. (2012). Differential effects of surface area, gyrification and cortical thickness on voxel based morphometric deficits in schizophrenia. Neuroimage 60, 693–699.

Palaniyappan, L., Mallikarjun, P., Joseph, V., White, T. P., and Liddle, P. F. (2011). Folding of the prefrontal cortex in schizophrenia: regional differ- ences in gyrification. Biol. Psychiatry 69, 974–979. doi: 10.1016/j.biopsych.2010. 12.012

Rakic, P. (1988). Specification of cerebral cortical areas. Science 241, 170–176. doi: 10.1126/science.3291116

Regis, J., Mangin, J. F., Ochiai, T., Frouin, V., Riviere, D., Cachia, A., et al. (2005). "Sulcal root" generic model: a hypothesis to overcome the variability of the human cortex folding patterns. Neurol. Med. Chir. (Tokyo) 45, 1–17. doi: 10. 2176/nmc.45.1

Richman, D. P., Stewart, R. M., Hutchinson, J. W., and Caviness, Jr. V. S. (1975).

Mechanical model of brain convolutional development. Science 189, 18–21. doi: 10.1126/science.1135626

Rizzolatti, G., and Craighero, L. (2004). The mirror-neuron system. Annu. Rev. Neurosci. 27, 169–192. doi: 10.1146/annurev. neuro.27.070203.144230

Ronan, L., Scanlon, C., Murphy, K., Maguire, S., Delanty, N., Doherty, C. P., et al. (2011). Cortical curvature analysis in MRI-negative temporal lobe epilepsy: a surrogate marker for malformations of cortical development. Epilepsia 52, 28– 34. doi: 10.1111/j.1528-1167.2010.02895.x

Rosas, H. D., Lee, S. Y., Bender, A. C., Zaleta, A. K., Vangel, M., Yu, P., et al. (2010). Altered white matter microstructure in the corpus callosum in Huntington's disease: implications for cortical "disconnection". Neuroimage 49, 2995–3004. doi: 10.1016/j.neuroimage.2009.10.015

Rosas, H. D., Liu, A. K., Hersch, S., Glessner, M., Ferrante, R. J., Salat, D. H., et al. (2002). Regional and progressive thinning of the cortical ribbon in Huntington's disease. Neurology 58, 695–701. doi: 10.1212/wnl.58.5.695

Salat, D. H., Greve, D. N., Pacheco, J. L., Quinn, B. T., Helmer, K. G., Buckner, R. L.,

et al. (2009). Regional white matter volume differences in nondemented aging and Alzheimer's disease. Neuroimage 44, 1247–1258. doi: 10.1016/j.neuroimage. 2008.10.030

Santos, M., Uppal, N., Butti, C., Wicinski, B., Schmeidler, J., Giannakopoulos, P., et al. (2011). Von Economo neurons in autism: a stereologic study of the frontoinsular cortex in children. Brain Res. 1380, 206–217. doi: 10.1016/j. brainres.2010.08.067

Schaer, M., Cuadra, M. B., Tamarit, L., Lazeyras, F., Eliez, S., and Thiran, J. P.

(2008). A surface-based approach to quantify local cortical gyrification. IEEE Trans. Med. Imaging 27, 161–170. doi: 10.1109/ tmi.2007.903576

Schaer, M., Glaser, B., Cuadra, M. B., Debbane, M., Thiran, J. P., and Eliez, S. (2009). Congenital heart disease affects local gyrification in 22q11.2 deletion syndrome. Dev. Med. Child Neurol. 51, 746–753. doi: 10.1111/j.1469-8749.2009. 03281.x

Schumann, C. M., Bloss, C. S., Barnes, C. C., Wideman, G. M., Carper, R. A.,

Akshoomoff, N., et al. (2010). Longitudinal magnetic resonance imaging study of cortical development through early childhood in autism. J. Neurosci. 30, 4419–4427. doi: 10.1523/jneurosci.5714-09.2010

Shokouhi, M., Williams, J. H., Waiter, G. D., and Condon, B. (2012). Changes in the sulcal size associated with autism spectrum disorder revealed by sulcal morphometry. Autism Res. 5, 245–252. doi: 10.1002/aur.1232

Shukla, D. K., Keehn, B., Lincoln, A. J., and Muller, R. A. (2010). White matter compromise of callosal and subcortical fiber tracts in children with autism spectrum disorder: a diffusion tensor imaging study. J. Am. Acad. Child Adolesc. Psychiatry 49, 1269–1278, e1261–e1262. doi: 10.1016/j.jaac. 2010.08.018

Smith, S. M., Jenkinson, M., Johansen-Berg, H., Rueckert, D., Nichols, T. E., Mackay, C. E., et al. (2006). Tract-based spatial statistics: voxelwise analysis of multi-subject diffusion data. Neuroimage 31, 1487–1505. doi: 10.1016/j. neuroimage.2006.02.024

Smith, S. M., Johansen-Berg, H., Jenkinson, M., Rueckert, D., Nichols, T. E.,

Miller, K. L., et al. (2007). Acquisition and voxelwise analysis of multi-subject diffusion data with tract-based spatial statistics. Nat. Protoc. 2, 499–503. doi: 10. 1038/ nprot.2007.45

Srivastava, S., Buonocore, M. H., and Simon, T. J. (2012). Atypical developmental trajectory of functionally significant cortical areas in children with chromosome 22q11.2 deletion syndrome. Hum. Brain Mapp. 33, 213–223. doi: 10.1002/hbm. 21206

Thesen, T., Quinn, B. T., Carlson, C., Devinsky, O., Dubois, J., Mcdonald, C. R., et al. (2011). Detection of epileptogenic cortical malformations with surface- based

MRI morphometry. PLoS One 6:e16430. doi: 10.1371/journal. pone. 0016430

Thomas, C., Humphreys, K., Jung, K. J., Minshew, N., and Behrmann, M. (2011). The anatomy of the callosal and visual-association pathways in high-functioning autism: a DTI tractography study. Cortex 47, 863–873. doi: 10.1016/j.cortex. 2010.07.006

Travers, B. G., Adluru, N., Ennis, C., Tromp Do, P. M., Destiche, D., Doran, S., et al. (2012). Diffusion tensor imaging in autism spectrum disorder: a review. Autism Res. 5, 289–313. doi: 10.1002/ aur.1243

Uddin, L. Q., Iacoboni, M., Lange, C., and Keenan, J. P. (2007). The self and social cognition: the role of cortical midline structures and mirror neurons. Trends Cogn. Sci. 11, 153–157. doi: 10.1016/j. tics.2007.01.001

Uddin, L. Q., and Menon, V. (2009). The anterior insula in autism: under-connected and under-examined. Neurosci. Biobehav. Rev. 33, 1198–1203. doi: 10. 1016/j. neubiorev.2009.06.002

Van Essen, D. C. (1997). A tension-based theory of morphogenesis and com- pact wiring in the central nervous system. Nature 385, 313–318. doi: 10. 1038/385313a0 von dem Hagen, E. A., Stoyanova, R. S., Baron-Cohen, S., and Calder, A. J. (2013). Reduced functional connectivity within and between 'social' resting state networks in autism spectrum conditions. Soc. Cogn. Affect Neurosci. 8, 694–701.

Wallace, G. L., Dankner, N., Kenworthy, L., Giedd, J. N., and Martin, A. (2010). Age-related temporal and parietal cortical thinning in autism spectrum disor- ders. Brain 133, 3745–3754. doi: 10.1093/ brain/awq279

Wallace, G. L., Robustelli, B., Dankner, N., Kenworthy, L., Giedd, J. N., and Martin,

A. (2013). Increased gyrification, but comparable surface area in adolescents autism spectrum disorders. Brain 136, 1956–1967. doi: 10.1093/brain/awt106

Wechsler, D. (1991). Wechsler Intelligence Scale for Children - Third edition. Manual.

San Antonio, TX: The Psychological Corporation.

Wegiel, J., Kuchna, I., Nowicki, K., Imaki, H., Marchi, E., Ma, S. Y., et al. (2010). The neuropathology of autism: defects of neurogenesis and neuronal migration, and dysplastic changes. Acta Neuropathol. 119, 755–770. doi: 10.1007/s00401- 010-0655-4

Welker, W. (1990). "Why does cerebral cortex fissure and fold? A review of determinants of gyri and sulci," in Cerebral Cortex, eds E. G. Jones and A. Peters (New York: Plenum), 3–136.

Weng, S. J., Wiggins, J. L., Peltier, S. J., Carrasco, M., Risi, S., Lord, C., et al. (2010). Alterations of resting state functional connectivity in the default network in adolescents with autism spectrum disorders. Brain Res. 1313, 202–214. doi: 10. 1016/j.brainres.2009.11.057

Zhang, Y., Yu, C., Zhou, Y., Li, K., Li, C., and Jiang, T. (2009). Decreased gyrification in major depressive disorder. Neuroreport 20, 378–380. doi: 10.1097/wnr. 0b013e3283249b34

Zhang, Y., Zhou, Y., Yu, C., Lin, L., Li, C., and Jiang, T. (2010). Reduced cortical folding in mental retardation. AJNR Am. J. Neuroradiol. 31, 1063–1067. doi: 10. 3174/ajnr. a1984

Zikopoulos, B., and Barbas, H. (2010). Changes in prefrontal axons may disrupt the network in autism. J. Neurosci. 30, 14595–14609. doi: 10.1523/jneurosci.2257- 10.2010

Zilles, K., Schleicher, A., Langemann, C., Amunts, K., Morosan, P., Palomero-Gallagher, N., et al. (1997). Quantitative analysis of sulci in the human cerebral cortex: development, regional heterogeneity, gender difference, asymmetry, intersubject variability and cortical architecture. Hum. Brain Mapp. 5, 218–221. doi: 10.1002/(SICI)1097-0193(1997)5 :4<218::AID-HBM2>3.0.CO;2-6

7

Network efficiency in autism spectrum disorder and its relation to brain overgrowth

John D. Lewis[1]*, Rebecca J. Theilmann[2], Jeanne Townsend[3,4] and Alan C. Evans[1]

[1] *McConnell Brain Imaging Center, Montreal Neurological Institute, McGill University, Montreal, QC, Canada*
[2] *Department of Radiology, University of California, San Diego, La Jolla, CA, USA*
[3] *Department of Neuroscience, University of California, San Diego, La Jolla, CA, USA*
[4] *Research on Aging and Development Laboratory, University of California, San Diego, La Jolla, CA, USA*

Edited by:
Rajesh K. Kana, University of Alabama at Birmingham, USA

Reviewed by:
Alexandros Goulas, MPI Leipzig, Germany
Elizabeth J. Carter, Carnegie Mellon University, USA

****Correspondence:***
John D. Lewis, McConnell Brain Imaging Center, Montreal Neurological Institute, McGill University, 3801 University, WB208, Montreal, QC H3A 2B4, Canada
e-mail: jlewis@bic.mni.mcgill.ca

A substantial body of evidence links differences in brain size to differences in brain organization. We have hypothesized that the developmental aspect of this relation plays a role in autism spectrum disorder (ASD), a neurodevelopmental disorder which involves abnormalities in brain growth. Children with ASD have abnormally large brains by the second year of life, and for several years thereafter their brain size can be multiple standard deviations above the norm. The greater conduction delays and cellular costs presumably associated with the longer long-distance connections in these larger brains is thought to influence developmental processes, giving rise to an altered brain organization with less communication between spatially distant regions. This has been supported by computational models and by findings linking greater intra-cranial volume, an index of maximum brain-size during development, to reduced inter-hemispheric connectivity in individuals with ASD. In this paper, we further assess this hypothesis via a whole-brain analysis of network efficiency. We utilize diffusion tractography to estimate the strength and length of the connections between all pairs of cortical regions. We compute the efficiency of communication between each network node and all others, and within local neighborhoods; we then assess the relation of these measures to intra-cranial volume, and the differences in these measures between adults with autism and typical controls. Intra-cranial volume is shown to be inversely related to efficiency for wide-spread regions of cortex. Moreover, the spatial patterns of reductions in efficiency in autism bear a striking resemblance to the regional relationships between efficiency and intra-cranial volume, particularly for local efficiency. The results thus provide further support for the hypothesized link between brain overgrowth in children with autism and the efficiency of the organization of the brain in adults with autism.

Keywords: autism, brain size, network analysis, connectivity, tractography, optimal wiring, scaling

INTRODUCTION

Brains differ dramatically in both size and structure across species. These two dimensions of variation are not independent, but large brains are not big small brains. The organization of both gray- and white-matter varies with brain size, but not in a uniform manner. Larger brain size is associated with a greater white-matter to gray-matter ratio (Rilling and Insel, 1999b; Zhang and Sejnowski, 2000), but a reduced degree of long-distance connectivity (Ringo, 1991; Rilling and Insel, 1999a; Karbowski, 2003; Changizi, 2007), as well as with increased modular structure (Changizi and Shimojo, 2005), greater surface convolutedness (Jerison, 1982; Prothero and Sundsten, 1984; Hofman, 1985), and various other morphological and cellular aspects of neural organization. Scaling laws capture much of the variation in structure in terms of brain size (Jerison, 1982; Ringo, 1991; Karbowski, 2003; Changizi and Shimojo, 2005; Changizi, 2007). However, significant structural variability remains unaccounted for by these scaling laws.

The underpinnings of these scaling relationships are not well understood, but are thought to be related to a design principle originally postulated by Ramón y Cajal: that neural circuit design is under pressure to minimize cellular costs and conduction delays (Ramón y Cajal, 1995). Increased brain size provides increased computational power, but at hugely increased cost. Neural material is expensive to construct and to operate. The human brain makes up only about 2 percent of the total body weight, but its operation is responsible for approximately 15 percent of cardiac output, 20 percent of oxygen usage, and 25 percent of glucose usage (Magistretti, 1999). These metabolic costs are largely due to the cost of neural signaling, and maintaining the resting potentials needed for neural signaling. These costs increase with membrane surface area, which increases with the number and size of the axons. Larger brains have a larger number of axons, and the longest of these axons are both longer and slightly larger in diameter than are those of smaller brains; thus the total membrane surface area is increased. Axon diameter does not increase sufficiently with brain size, however, to compensate for the increased fiber lengths, so larger brains also have longer conduction delays (Olivares et al., 2001). These greater costs and conduction delays appear to be related to at least some of the aspects of organization that scale with brain size, e.g. the reduced degree of long-distance connectivity (Ringo, 1991; Rilling and Insel, 1999a; Karbowski, 2003; Changizi, 2007).

The focus on cross-species differences, where differences in brain size can be more than 1000-fold within classes, e.g., Mammalia, and 100-fold within orders, e.g., Primates, allows relationships between brain size and structure to be apparent despite differences in structure unrelated to brain size. But, it ignores potentially important differences in developmental brain growth trajectories. There are substantial inter-species differences in rate of brain growth, and developmental trajectories can even vary considerably between individuals, e.g., brain size may differ by as much as 50% in children of the same age (Giedd, 2008). Brain size differences between adults account for some of the differences in structure (Jäncke et al., 1997; Honey et al., 2009; Lewis et al., 2009); differences in brain growth trajectories likely account for additional structural variability.

Substantial neural reorganization occurs over development. Neural development is largely a combination of over-exuberance and competition-based elimination. Large numbers of transient projections are produced during cortical development (Rakic et al., 1986; LaMantia and Rakic, 1990), and which connections are retained is determined by their metabolic demands and their ability to compete for neurotrophins (Van Ooyen and Willshaw, 1999). Due to the lesser degree of myelination in the developing brain than in the mature brain, the differences in conduction delays and metabolic costs associated with differences in fiber length will be substantially greater (Chugani et al., 1987; Paus et al., 1999; Thatcher et al., 2008). Thus, to the extent that differences in brain size during development coincide with differences in brain size in mature individuals, normal developmental processes may underlie at least some portion of the scaling relationships seen across and within species; moreover, differences in brain size during development which do not coincide with differences in brain size in mature individuals may account for a portion of the structural variability that is not accounted for by scaling laws.

This conjecture is clearly relevant to developmental disorders showing abnormalities in brain growth trajectories. Autism spectrum disorder (ASD) is such a case. ASD is a disorder of neural developmental defined by impairments in reciprocal social interactions, impairments in verbal and non-verbal communication, and a restricted repertoire of activities and interests (American Psychiatric Association, 1994). The aetiology of ASD is unknown, but there is now consensus that brain size during development is increased. Infants who go on to a diagnosis of ASD show abnormally rapid brain growth during the first years of life (Lainhart et al., 1997; Redcay and Courchesne, 2005), and after the second or third year of life children with ASD show increased head size (Lainhart et al., 1997; Hazlett et al., 2005) and brain size (Piven et al., 1995; Courchesne et al., 2001; Hazlett et al., 2005). Early in development this size difference can be multiple standard deviations above the norm (Redcay and Courchesne, 2005).

Lewis and Elman (2008) have shown via computational modeling that the increased conduction delays presumably associated with the early brain overgrowth in ASD may lead to the later functional and structural long-range underconnectivity. Further, in adults with ASD, Lewis et al. (2012) have shown that callosal tract length adjusted for intra-cranial volume (ICV), an index of maximum brain-size during development (Whitwell et al., 2001; Aylward et al., 2002; Buckner et al., 2004), shows the typical inverse relation to relative corpus callosum size, and so the early brain overgrowth in autism appears to in fact account for some portion of the later observed long-range underconnectivity.

In the current paper we extended this work to assess the impact of the early brain overgrowth in ASD on overall brain organization. We performed a network analysis and assessed the relation between the network metrics and ICV. Network analysis methods have evolved over the past decade and a half, from straightforward applications of graph theory, which assess only network topology (Watts and Strogatz, 1998), to more sophisticated approaches which take account of the spatial aspects of connectivity to assess the efficiency of information transfer within the network (Latora and Marchiori, 2001, 2003; Achard and Bullmore, 2007; Bullmore and Sporns, 2012). Such approaches utilize measures of the length and strength of connections between all pairs of anatomical regions to estimate how efficiently information can be transferred between regions. We used probabilistic tractography to estimate the strength of connectivity between all pairs of regions, and the length of the connections between regions. We computed the efficiency of communication from all regions to all others, and within local neighborhoods. We then assessed the relation between both of these measures of efficiency and ICV, as well as group differences in efficiency. We predicted that there would be an inverse relation between ICV and both measures of efficiency, reflecting an adverse effect of brain overgrowth on overall brain organization, and that this would explain a portion of the group differences in efficiency.

METHODS

PARTICIPANTS

A total of 44 adult males participated in the study: 22 with ASD ranging between 19 and 51 years of age (mean 34.14; *SD* 10.67), and 22 typical adult males ranging between 20 and 45 years of age (mean 32.25; *SD* 9.98). All ASD participants met diagnostic criteria for ASD on the DSM-IV as confirmed by a licensed clinician. Eighteen of the twenty two ASD participants met the DSM diagnosis for autistic disorder (classic autism) and, based on absence of early language delay and no significant abnormality in communication, four of the twenty two subjects additionally met diagnostic criteria for Asperger's disorder. Autism Diagnostic Interview, Revised (ADI-R) scores were available for 16 of the ASD participants; Autism Diagnostic Observation Schedule (ADOS) scores were available for 18; and Childhood Autism Rating Scale (CARS) scores were available for 12. **Table 1** summarizes these data. In all but one case the ASD diagnosis was confirmed by all of the available additional assessments; the one exception was below the cutoff for the CARS, but above

Table 1 | The behavioral data.

	Cutoff	Range	Mean	*SD*
ADI-R Social	10	13–54	27.06	8.74
ADI-R Communication (Verbal)	8	6–25	18.75	4.43
ADI-R Repetitive behaviors	3	3–14	8.25	2.91
ADOS Social	6	4–20	10.50	3.60
ADOS Communication	3	2–9	6.39	1.85
ADOS Stereotyped behavior		0–13	2.29	2.97
CARS	30	23.5–51.5	36.46	7.46

Cutoff scores for the Autism Diagnostic Interview, Revised (ADI-R) and the Childhood Autism Rating Scale (CARS) are available only for autism; thus we also used the autism cutoffs for the Autism Diagnostic Observation Schedule (ADOS).

all cutoffs for the ADI-R and ADOS. General intellectual ability in the ASD participants was evaluated by the Wechsler Adult Intelligence Scale-Revised (WAIS-R) or the Wechsler Abbreviated Scale of Intelligence (WASI). Mean scores were: Verbal IQ, 88.48 ± 23.06; Performance IQ, 106.10 ± 15.91. Individuals with a history of significant medical or neurological disorders including seizures or with Fragile X syndrome were excluded from the sample. Typical participants with a first degree relative with a diagnosis of ASD were excluded from the sample. The participants were those from Lewis et al. (2012) augmented by new data from individuals with ASD. Those subjects who were capable gave informed consent; a caregiver gave informed consent for the others. The study was approved by the Human Research Protections Program at the University of California, San Diego.

IMAGING

All subjects were scanned at the UCSD Center for fMRI on a GE Signa EXCITE 3.0T short bore scanner with an eight-channel array head coil. Three types of images were acquired from each subject: (i) one set of 3D T_1-weighted images (Fast Gradient Echo, SPGR;$TE = 3.1$ ms; flip angle $= 12$; NEX $= 1$; FOV $=$ 25 cm; matrix $= 256 \times 256$); (ii) two sets of diffusion weighted images isotropically distributed along 15 directions (dual spin-echo,EPI; $TR = 15$ s; TE $= 89$ ms; 45 axial slices; NEX $= 2$; FOV$=$ 22 cm; matrix $= 128 \times 128$; resolution $= 1.875 \times 1.875 \times 3$ mm; 3 mm interleaved contiguous slices; b value $= 1400$ s/mm^2); and (iii) fieldmaps matched to the diffusion-weighted images. During acquisition scans were visually inspected to ensure that usable data were collected. Where motion introduced visible artifacts in multiple volumes, the scan sequence was aborted and reinitiated, or an additional scan was acquired. Note that at least two sets of diffusion weighted images were acquired, each with NEX $= 2$; thus each image was acquired at least four times. Fieldmaps were acquired before the first diffusion-weighted images were acquired, and, in cases where there was between scan motion, an additional set of fieldmaps was acquired after the second.

IMAGE PROCESSING

The T_1-volumes were processed with CIVET, a fully automated structural image analysis pipeline developed at the Montreal Neurological Institute. CIVET corrects intensity non-uniformities using N3 (Sled et al., 1998); aligns the input volumes to the Talairach-like ICBM-152-nl template (Collins et al., 1994); classifies the image into white matter, gray matter, cerebrospinal fluid, and background (Zijdenbos et al., 2002; Tohka et al., 2004); and extracts the white-matter and pial surfaces (Kim et al., 2005). ICV was calculated via the atlas based spatial normalization procedure described in Buckner et al. (2004). The CIVET results were visually inspected to ensure that surface construction was correct, and then used to construct the seed, stop, and target masks for use with FSL's *probtrackx* (Behrens et al., 2007). Seed masks control from which voxels tracts are seeded; seed masks were white-matter. Stop masks determine where tract propagation is halted; stop masks were voxels on the boundary of white-matter. Target masks determine the mapping from voxels of the stop masks to brain regions; target masks were the voxels at the boundary of white-matter and the cortex, and mapped these voxels to the Automatic Anatomical Labeling (AAL) atlas (Tzourio-Mazoyer et al., 2002), shown in **Figure 1**.

Each diffusion dataset was first corrected of distortions caused by inhomogeneities in the magnetic field using the fieldmaps. This was done using software developed by the UCSD Center for fMRI. The resulting diffusion-weighted volumes were then subjected to a quantitative quality control evaluation using *DTIprep* (Liu et al., 2010). *DTIprep* corrects motion artifacts where possible, and excludes directions from the data when correction is not possible. For each subject, the two diffusion-weighted volumes with the fewest number of excluded directions were chosen for further processing. The *b*0 volumes of both diffusion scans were then affine registered to the T_1-volume in stereotaxic space using the Oxford University FMRIB Software Library's (FSL) *flirt* (Jenkinson and Smith, 2001), and the resultant transforms used to align the two 4D volumes; the rotational component was applied to the directional vectors. The two were then merged using FSL's *fslmerge*. The merged volume was then preprocessed for probablistic tractography with FSL's *bedpostx* (Behrens et al., 2007). Probabilistic tractography, utilizing FSL's *probtrackx* with distance-bias correction (Behrens et al., 2003, 2007), was then seeded from 10,000 random locations within each voxel of the seed masks to generate the number of tracts connecting voxels in the target mask. A native-scale 4D diffusion volume was generated using the same procedure, but with the scaling component removed from the transforms; this was processed in the same way to generate the lengths of the connections between voxels in the target mask. These results were then compiled for each AAL region generating matrices of the total number of connections between each pair of AAL regions, and the mean length of those connections. The total number of connections between each pair of AAL regions was then divided by the mean size of the two AAL regions to provide an index of the strength of connectivity between pairs of regions.

ANALYSIS

The efficiency of communication was calculated for all regions, based on the definition provided by Latora and Marchiori (2001, 2003). The relation of ICV to efficiency was assessed with statistical linear models, as well as group differences in efficiency. Correction for multiple comparisons was done using the false discovery rate method (Benjamini and Hochberg, 1995).

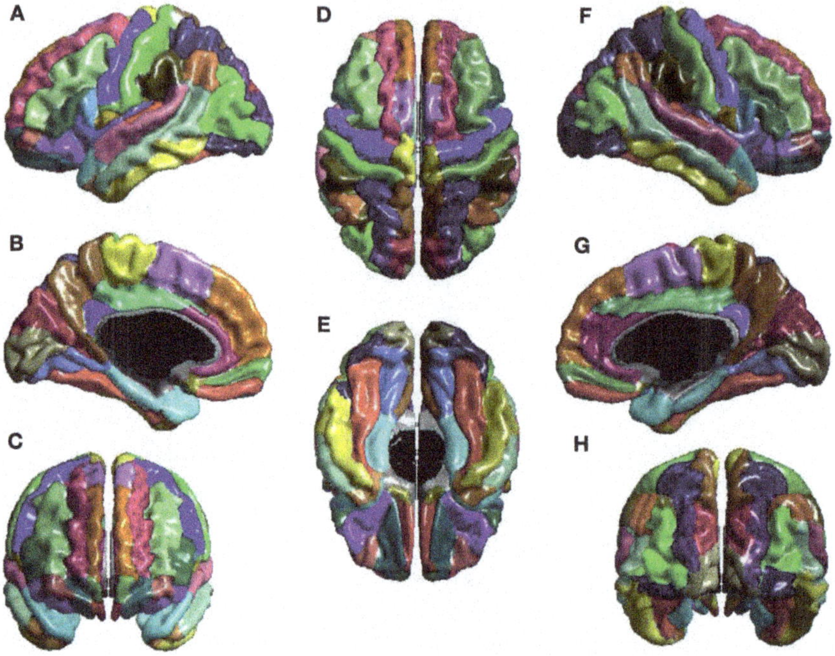

FIGURE 1 | The AAL atlas views: (A) left lateral, (B) left medial, (C) anterior, (D) superior, (E) inferior, (F) right lateral, (G) right medial, and (H) posterior. The regions are colored to identify region boundaries. Similarity of colors between spatially separated regions is not meaningful; all regions are spatially contiguous. The cortical parcellation is based on anatomical landmarks, e.g., sulci. There are 78 cortical regions. These cortical regions serve as the nodes of the network.

Latora and Marchiori (2001) defined the efficiency ε_{ij} in the communication between nodes i and j to be inversely proportional to the shortest path length d_{ij} between nodes i and j. They take the shortest path length d_{ij} to be the smallest sum of the physical distances throughout all of the possible paths from i to j in the graph, i.e., the travel distance, not the number of edges nor the Euclidean distance. The efficiency of a network, G, is then

$$E(G) = \frac{\sum_{i \neq j \in G} \varepsilon_{ij}}{N(N-1)} = \frac{1}{N(N-1)} \sum_{i \neq j \in G} \frac{1}{d_{ij}}$$

where N is the number of nodes in the network graph G; ε_{ij} is the efficiency of the connection between nodes i and j; and d_{ij} is the length of the shortest path, in terms of physical distances, between nodes i and j. This measure is normalized by $E(G_{IDEAL})$, the fully connected network. Note that the measures of efficiency take into account the physical distances involved in information transfer, and so relate more closely to the neurobiological substrates than do purely topological measures (Watts and Strogatz, 1998; Achard and Bullmore, 2007; Rubinov and Sporns, 2010).

Latora and Marchiori (2001) apply this formulation to both the entire network, which they refer to as *global efficiency*, and to the subnetworks of the immediate neighbors of each node; they define *local efficiency* as the mean of $E(G_i)$, for all nodes i, where G_i is the subgraph of all the neighbors of node i. These definitions give a single measure of *local efficiency* and of *global efficiency* for the entire network. But, the definitions can be given straightforward translations to provide measures of efficiency for each node, or for collections of nodes. Achard and Bullmore (2007) define *nodal efficiency*, which we will refer to as *nodal global efficiency*, as the inverse of the harmonic mean of the minimum number of edges between a node, i, and all other nodes in the network. Utilizing the physical distances, as per Latora and Marchiori (2001), the *nodal global efficiency* of node i is thus

$$E_{nodal\,global}(G, i) = \frac{\sum_{j \in G, i \neq j} \varepsilon_{ij}}{(N-1)} = \frac{1}{(N-1)} \sum_{j \in G, i \neq j} \frac{1}{d_{ij}}$$

where N is the number of nodes in the network graph G; ε_{ij} is the efficiency of the connection between nodes i and j; and d_{ij} is the length of the shortest path, in terms of physical distances, between nodes i and j. The definition of *local efficiency* can likewise be parsed to provide a measure of *nodal local efficiency*; recall that the *local efficiency* of a network is the mean of $E(G_i)$, for all nodes i, where G_i is the subgraph of all the neighbors of node i. Thus, the *nodal local efficiency* of node i is simply

$$E_{nodal\,local}(G, i) = \frac{\sum_{j \neq k \in G_i} \varepsilon_{jk}}{N_{G_i}(N_{G_i} - 1)} = \frac{1}{N_{G_i}(N_{G_i} - 1)} \sum_{j \neq k \in G_i} \frac{1}{d_{jk}}$$

where N_{Gi} is the number of nodes in the subgraph G_i consisting of all of the neighbors of i; ε_{jk} is the efficiency of the connection between nodes j and k; and d_{jk} is the length of the shortest path, in terms of physical distances, between nodes j and k.

These definitions treat connections in a binarized fashion, i.e., as either existing or not. But, the strengths of the connections reflect, albeit poorly, biophysical properties of the underlying axons that are related to conduction velocity and metabolic costs, e.g., myelination. Moreover, weak long-range connections between strongly connected modules have been argued to provide the shortcuts that make the brain an efficient small-world architecture (Gallos et al., 2012). The strengths of the connections in the brain may thus be critical to an accurate assessment of its efficiency. Therefore, we utilize a version of these measures that incorporates connection weight, i.e., the total number of tracts connecting two regions, corrected for the distance-bias and region size. Based on Rubinov and Sporns (2010), we define the *weighted distance* between nodes *i* and *j* as

$$d_{ij}^{w} = \sum_{\forall e \in S} \frac{l_e}{w_e}$$

where *S* is the set of edges in the shortest path between nodes *i* and *j*; l_e is the length of edge *e*; and w_e is the connection weight for edge *e*. Also based on Rubinov and Sporns (2010), our weighted formulations of *nodal global efficiency* and *nodal local efficiency* are

$$E_{nodal\ global}^{weighted}(G, i) = \frac{1}{(N-1)} \sum_{j \in G, i \neq j} \left(d_{ij}^{w}\right)^{-1}$$

where *N* is the number of nodes in the network graph *G*; and d_{ij}^{w} is the shortest path, in terms of *weighted distance*, between nodes *i* and *j*; and

$$E_{nodal\ local}^{weighted}(G, i) = \frac{1}{N_{G_i}(N_{G_i}-1)} \sum_{j \neq k \in G_i} \left(\left(d_{jk}^{w}\right)^{-1} w_{ij} w_{ik} \right)^{1/3}$$

where N_{Gi} is the number of nodes in the subgraph G_i consisting of all of the neighbors of *i*; is the shortest path, in terms of *weighted distance*, between nodes *j* and *k*; and w_{ij} and w_{ik} are the connection weights between nodes *i* and *j*, and *i* and *k*, respectively. As per Latora and Marchiori (2001), these measures are normalized by considering the fully connected network.

The impact of maximum brain size during development on efficiency was assessed, as well as the group differences in efficiency. As per Lewis et al. (2012), we used ICV as an index of maximum brain size during development (Whitwell et al., 2001; Aylward et al., 2002; Buckner et al., 2004). The relation between ICV and efficiency was assessed via statistical linear models, controlling for age and total brain volume. Group differences in efficiency were assessed via statistical linear models, controlling for age. Potential group differences in the relationships between ICV and measures of efficiency were assessed by considering the group x ICV interaction term in models with both terms. In all cases, correction for multiple comparisons was done using the false discovery rate method (Benjamini and Hochberg, 1995).

RESULTS

The relation between ICV and *nodal local efficiency* is shown in **Figure 2**. The *t*-statistic is negative over the entire cortex, thus for all regions this is an inverse relation: larger ICV is associated with less *nodal local efficiency*. This inverse relation is significant over almost the entirety of the posterior of the brain, and also the right hemisphere frontal lobe. The relation is conspicuously less negative over left dorsal lateral frontal cortex, and does not reach significance over much of left hemisphere dorsal lateral cortex; the inverse relation is stronger over the medial surface, and is significant over much of the medial surface of either hemisphere.

The ICV * group interaction term was non-significant in all regions, thus this inverse relation between ICV and *nodal local efficiency* does not differ between individuals with ASD and typical controls.

The group differences in *nodal local efficiency* are shown in **Figure 3**. The *t*-statistic is negative over the entire cortex, thus for all regions *nodal local efficiency* is reduced in individuals with ASD. This reduction is significant over almost the entirety of the posterior of the brain, and also the right hemisphere frontal lobe. The *t*-statistic is conspicuously less negative over left lateral frontal cortex, and the group difference does not reach significance over much of the left lateral frontal cortex; the difference is significant over much of the left medial surface. The group difference is non-significant for most of the right medial surface anterior to the cuneus. Note that the pattern of group differences in *nodal local efficiency* parallels that of the inverse relation between ICV and *nodal local efficiency*. The cosine similarity of the two *t*-statistic vectors is 0.9848.

The relation between ICV and *nodal global efficiency* is shown in **Figure 4**. The *t*-statistic is negative over most of the cortex, thus this is again generally an inverse relation: larger ICV is associated with less *nodal global efficiency*. Significant inverse relations are seen in the left hemisphere in all lobes, notably in visual cortex, the pre- and post-central gyri, and in primary auditory cortex; significant inverse relations are seen in the right hemisphere in the temporal lobe, the precuneus, and the paracentral lobule; and significant inverse relations are seen bilaterally in the cingulate and orbitofrontal cortex.

The ICV * group interaction term was non-significant in all regions, thus this inverse relation between ICV and *nodal global efficiency* does not differ between individuals with ASD and typical controls.

The group differences in *nodal global efficiency* are shown in **Figure 5**. The *t*-statistic is negative over the entire cortex, thus for all regions *nodal global efficiency* is reduced in individuals with ASD. This reduction is significant over regions of all lobes in both hemispheres. Note that these reductions overlap with those of the relation of ICV and *nodal global efficiency* but are more extensive, particularly in the right hemisphere. The cosine similarity of the two *t*-statistic vectors is 0.9584.

Thus, both *nodal local efficiency* and *nodal global efficiency* showed an inverse relation to ICV, and in neither case was the ICV * group interaction significant. Moreover, for both measures, the pattern of results for the inverse relation between ICV and efficiency was similar to the pattern of reductions in efficiency in ASD.

DISCUSSION

Networks with a high degree of spatially local connectivity, but with few long-range connections, i.e., shortcuts, have high local efficiency and low global efficiency; networks with a high degree

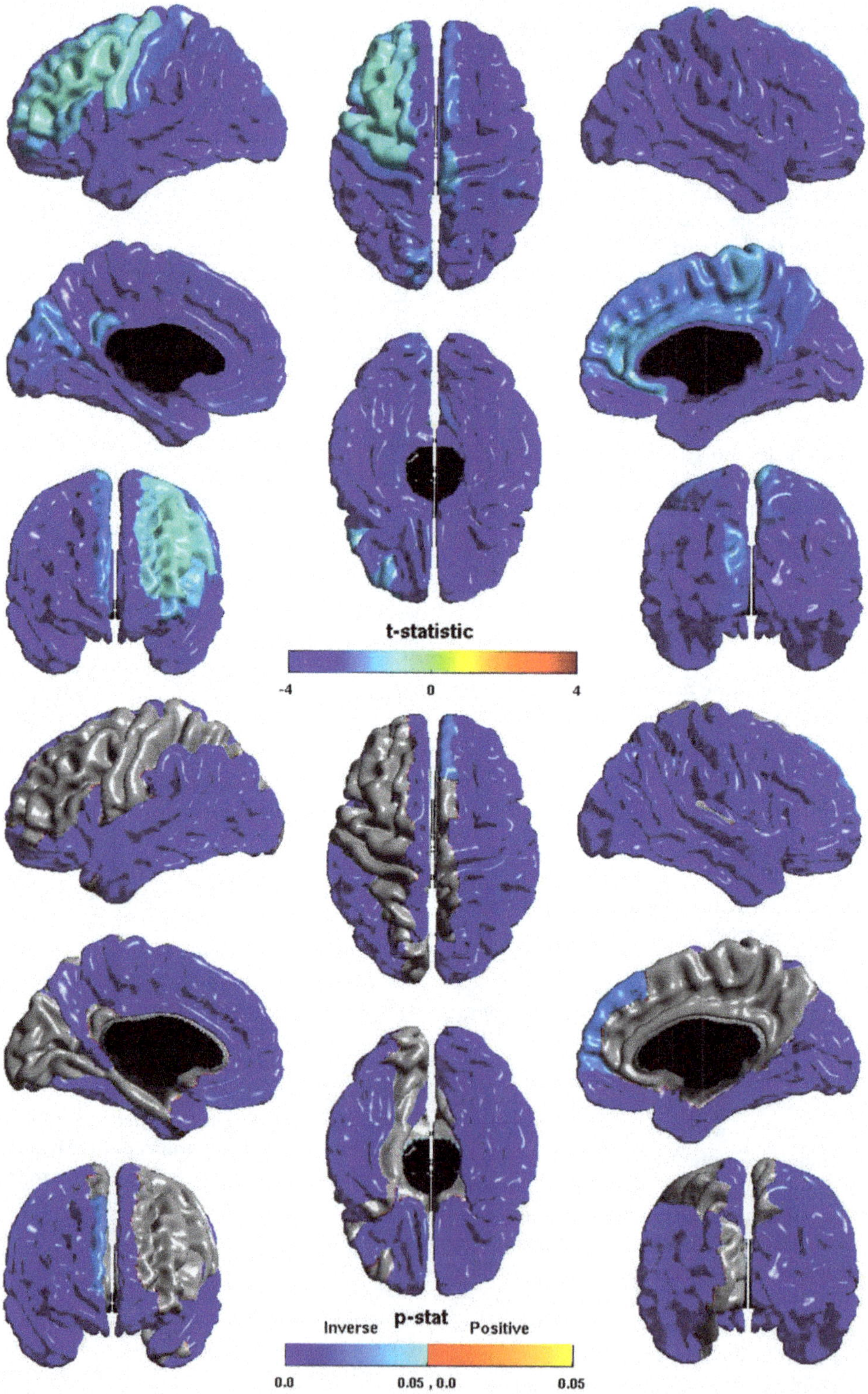

FIGURE 2 | Nodal Local Efficiency and ICV. The *t*-statistic **(top)** and the *p*-statistic **(bottom)** for the relation between ICV and *nodal local efficiency* in each region of the AAL atlas. A negative *t*-statistic represents decreasing *nodal local efficiency* with increasing ICV. The *t*-statistic is overwhelmingly negative. The *p*-statistic is FDR-corrected, and is blue where the inverse relation is significant, and orange where a positive relation is significant. No regions show a significant positive relation. Significant inverse relations are seen bilaterally over the temporal lobes, the angular and supramarginal gyri, the pars opercularis, orbital frontal cortex, and the superior frontal gyrus; the right hemisphere shows this inverse relation more extensively over the frontal and parietal lobe; the left hemisphere shows the relation more extensively on the medial surface.

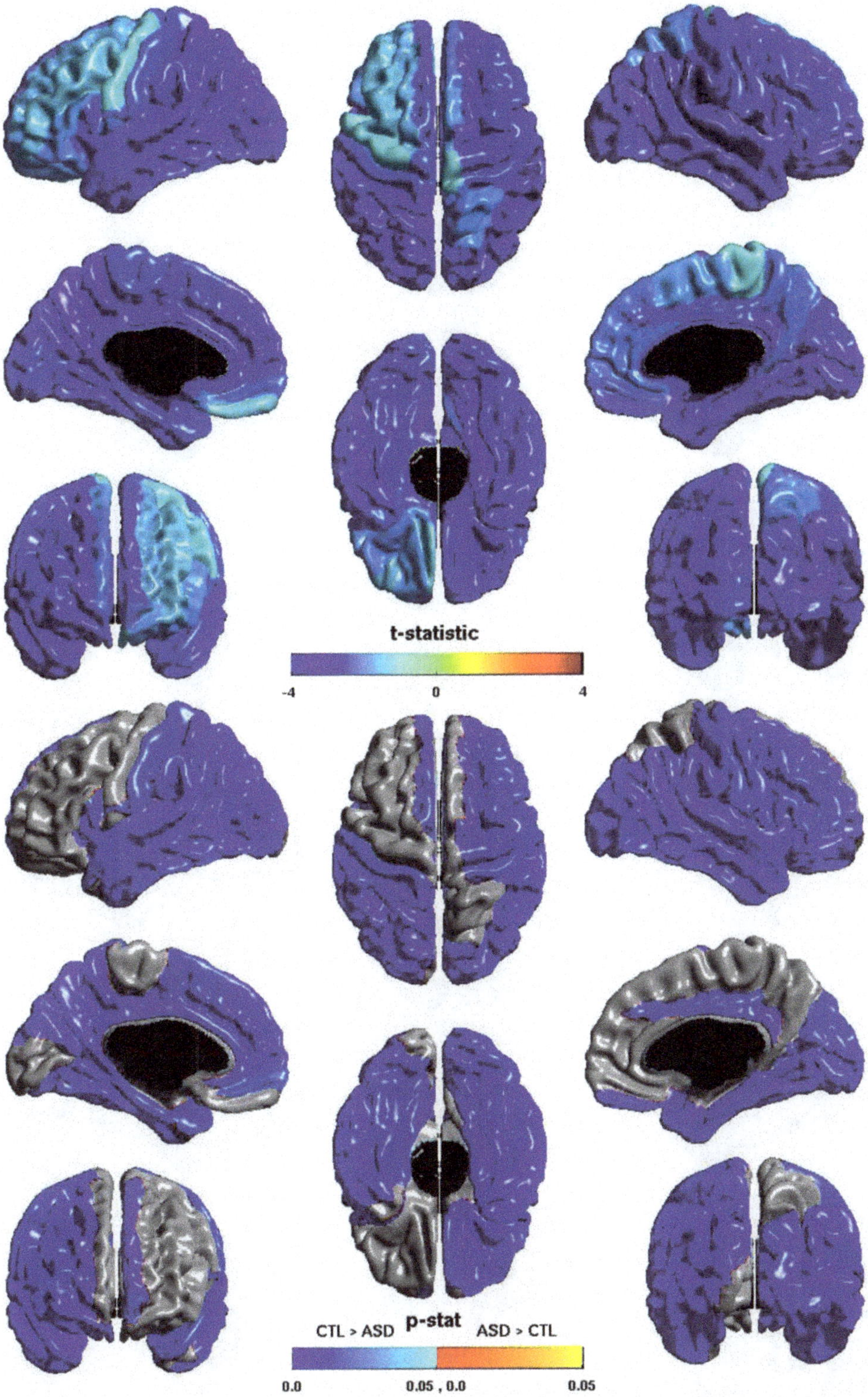

FIGURE 3 | Nodal Local Efficiency and Group. The *t*-statistic **(top)** and the *p*-statistic **(bottom)** for the group difference in *nodal local efficiency* in each region of the AAL atlas. A negative *t*-statistic represents reduced efficiency in ASD. The *t*-statistic is negative everywhere. The *p*-statistic is FDR-corrected, and is blue where there is a significant reduction in *nodal local efficiency* in ASD, and orange where there is a significant increase in ASD. No regions show significantly increased nodal local efficiency in ASD. Significant reductions are seen bilaterally in the temporal, occipital, and parietal lobes, and in the pars opercularis; the right hemisphere additionally shows reductions over lateral regions of the frontal lobe; the left hemisphere shows more extensive reductions over the medial surface. Note the similarities to the relation of *nodal local efficiency* and ICV.

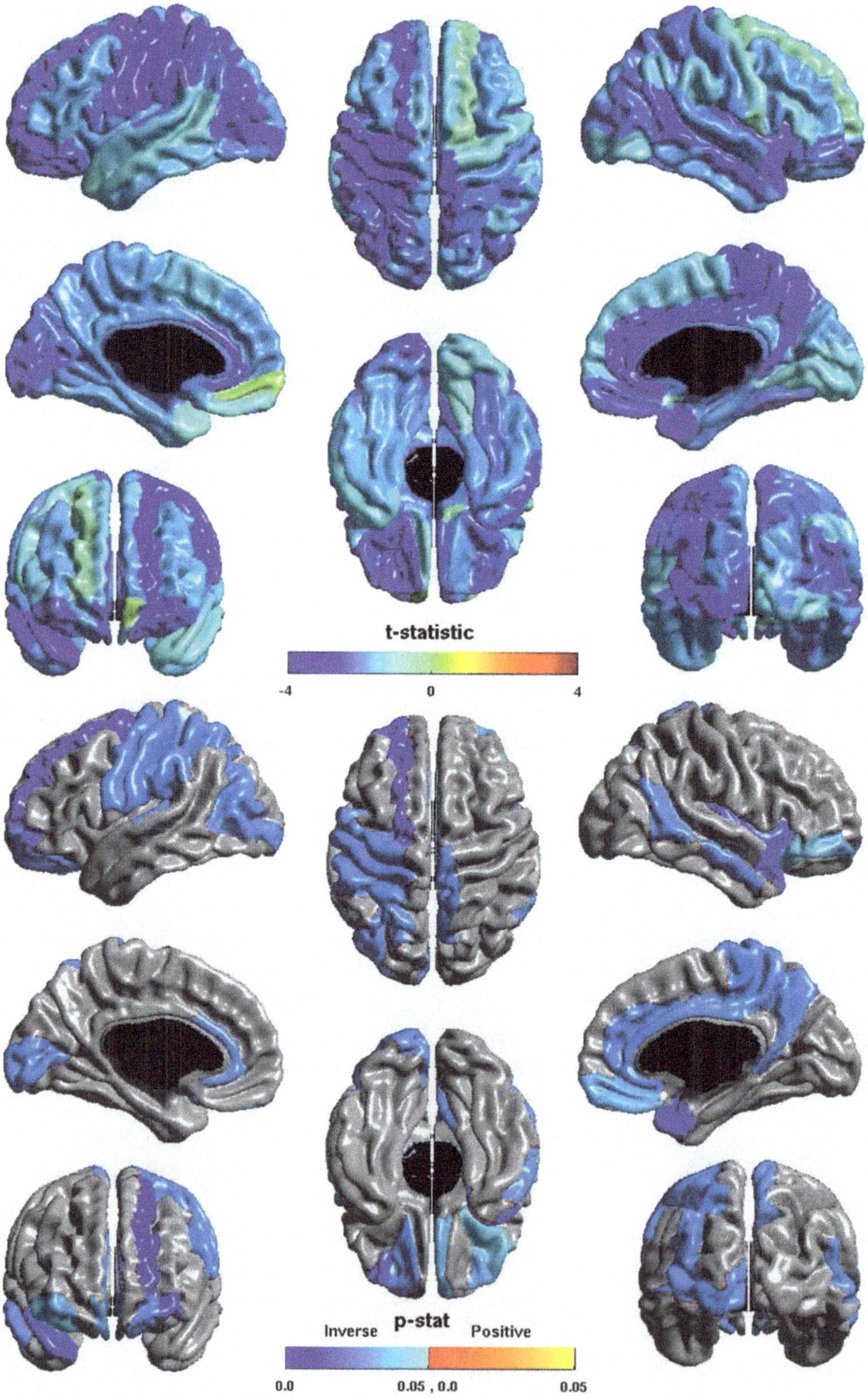

FIGURE 4 | Nodal Global Efficiency and ICV. The *t*-statistic **(top)** and the *p*-statistic **(bottom)** for the relation between ICV and *nodal global efficiency* in each region of the AAL atlas. A negative *t*-statistic represents decreasing *nodal global efficiency* with increasing ICV. The *t*-statistic is predominately negative. The *p*-statistic is FDR-corrected, and is blue where the inverse relation is significant and orange where a positive relation is significant. No regions show a significant positive relation. Significant inverse relations are seen in the left occipital, parietal, and frontal lobes, and in primary auditory cortex; in the right temporal lobe, precuneus, and paracentral lobule; and bilaterally in the cingulate and orbitofrontal cortex.

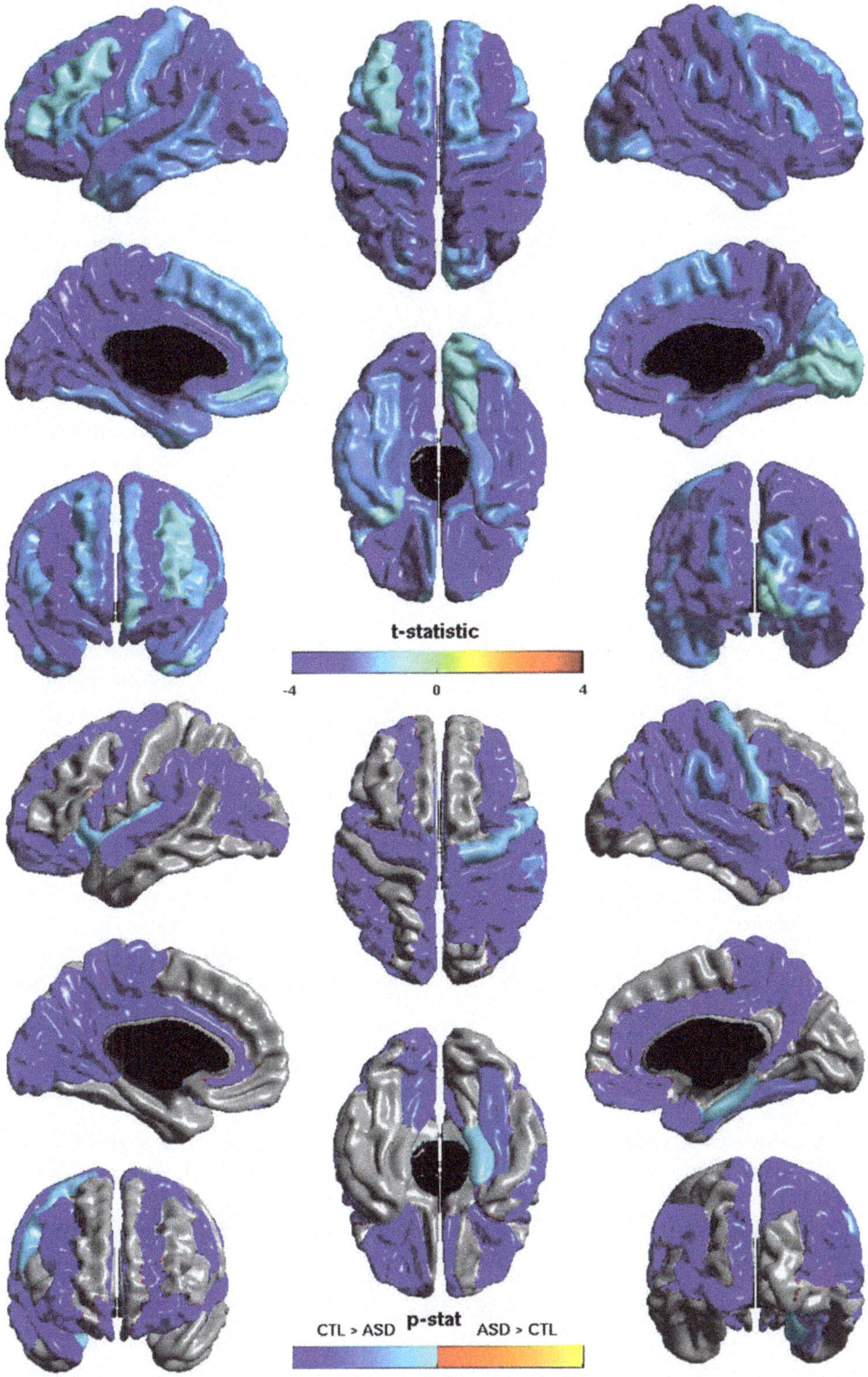

FIGURE 5 | Nodal Global Efficiency and Group. The *t*-statistic **(top)** and the *p*-statistic **(bottom)** for the group difference in *nodal global efficiency* in each region of the AAL atlas. A negative *t*-statistic represents reduced efficiency in ASD. The *t*-statistic is negative everywhere. The *p*-statistic is FDR-corrected, and is blue where there is a significant reduction in *nodal global efficiency* in ASD, and orange where there is a significant increase in ASD. No regions show significantly increased *nodal global efficiency* in ASD. Significant reductions are seen bilaterally in all lobes. Note the similarities to the relation of *nodal global efficiency* and ICV.

of long-range connectivity, but which lack spatially local clustering, have high global efficiency and low local efficiency. Biological systems in general, and neural networks in particular, tend to balance global efficiency with local efficiency, having strong local clustering mixed with sufficient long-range connectivity to allow rapid communication between distant nodes; these have been dubbed "small-world" properties (Watts and Strogatz, 1998; Latora and Marchiori, 2001, 2003). The inverse relation shown here between ICV and both *nodal local* and *nodal global efficiency* suggests that deviation in brain growth trajectories impacts both long-range communication and within-neighborhood communication, and impacts both similarly. The absence of a group $*$ ICV interaction in either case indicates that the same is true in both typical adults and adults with ASD. The reductions in both *nodal local* and *nodal global efficiency* seen in individuals with ASD align with this inverse relation, in combination with the brain overgrowth that occurs in ASD, to suggest that the brain overgrowth may explain at least part of the reductions in efficiency; and the similarity of the spatial pattern of reductions in efficiency with the pattern of the relations between ICV and efficiency further supports this conclusion.

These results complement our previous work showing an inverse relation between the ICV-adjusted length of callosal fibers and degree of inter-hemispheric connectivity in ASD (Lewis et al., 2012), and our computational modeling work showing that the early brain overgrowth in ASD may cause the later reductions in long-range connectivity (Lewis and Elman, 2008). Those studies suggested that the brain overgrowth that occurs in ASD may underlie the reductions in long-range connectivity seen in adolescents and adults with ASD (Horwitz et al., 1988; Just et al., 2004, 2007; Kana et al., 2007). The current study extends that work to network analysis, relating the brain overgrowth in ASD to overall network organization.

The measures of efficiency utilized here do not directly correspond to connectivity; efficiency is defined in terms of paths through a network, not the strengths of individual connections. The network measures capture more complex aspects of brain organization. The inefficiencies in ASD shown here suggest a more random network organization, providing less well-segregated local processing and a reduced capacity to integrate information across the network. Reductions in *nodal global efficiency* might stem from either generally weaker connections, longer paths between nodes, or both. Topological measures show shorter characteristic path length in ASD (Rudie et al., 2013), meaning that communication between pairs of nodes is more direct. Together with the reductions in *nodal global efficiency* shown here this implies a more random configuration, with more but weaker shortcuts. The reductions in *nodal local efficiency* support this interpretation. Since the degree to which a node is a neighbor of another is determined by the strength of the direct connection between them, the neighbors of a node may be spatially distant. The local efficiency of a node thus reflects the spatial clustering of its neighbors, as well as the strength of the connections between them. Topological measures show reductions in modularity in ASD (Rudie et al., 2013), thus the reductions in *nodal local efficiency* in ASD should not be interpreted as short-distance under-connectivity, but as indicative of a more random configuration with more diffuse processing clusters. The inefficiencies in ASD thus suggest both less segregation and less integration. The inverse relation between the measures of efficiency and ICV suggests that these aspects of network organization are impacted by differences in brain growth trajectories.

This study complements the substantial body of research showing strong relationships between brain size and brain structure (Tower, 1954; Jerison, 1982; Ringo, 1991; Prothero, 1997; Zhang and Sejnowski, 2000; Karbowski, 2003; Changizi, 2007; Lewis et al., 2009). That research leaves unanswered the question of the aetiology of these scaling relationships. We have hypothesized that at least some of these scaling relationships come about over development as a consequence of the impact on normal developmental mechanisms of differences in metabolic costs and conduction delays associated with differences in brain size (Lewis and Elman, 2008; Lewis et al., 2012). Our hypothesis applies both to individual variability in growth trajectories in typical development, including gender differences, and to the atypical variations that are generally present in developmental disorders. The current results lend support to this conjecture.

ICV, however, is a very crude index of a very complex phenomenon. In typically developing infants the brain increases from approximately 25 percent of adult size at birth to approximately 75 percent of adult size by 2 years of age with substantial individual variability in rate of growth as well as mature brain size (Blinkov and Glezer, 1968; Dobbing and Sands, 1973; Courchesne et al., 2000). Multiple parameters are required to capture even the most basic aspects of such trajectories. ICV provides only an index of maximum brain size during development. Likewise, true efficiency of communication is determined by conduction delays and metabolic costs, and the measures used here serve as only crude proxies for such properties. The biophysical properties that determine conduction delays and metabolic costs, such as the density of fibers, axon diameters, and the degree of myelination, are only weakly related to the probabilistic tractography results used here as connection strengths. Further, the extent to which the results reported here are robust to the variety of factors that influence tractography-based estimates of connectivity, e.g., scan protocols, tractography parameters, and target parcellation (Jones et al., 2012), remains to be explored. The inverse relations between ICV and efficiency thus suggest that brain growth trajectories may account for a substantial part of the individual differences in brain organization both in typical adults as well as those with ASD, but the conjecture must be further tested utilizing methods which can provide more accurate estimates of brain growth trajectories, metabolic costs, and conduction delays.

ACKNOWLEDGMENTS

This research was supported by grant NIH/NINDS R01 NS42639, awarded to Jeanne Townsend. Computations were performed on the guillimin supercomputer at the CLUMEQ HPC Consortium (http://www.clumeq.ca). Under the auspices of Compute Canada, CLUMEQ is funded by the Canada Foundation for Innovation (CFI), the Government of Québec, the National Science and Engineering Research Council (NSERC), and the Fonds Québécois de Recherche sur la Nature et les Technologies (FQRNT).

REFERENCES

Achard, S., and Bullmore, E. (2007). Efficiency and cost of economical brain functional networks. PLoS Comput. Biol. 3:e17. doi: 10.1371/journal.pcbi.0030017 American Psychiatric Association. (1994). Diagnostic and Statistical Manual of Mental Disorders: DSM-IV. Washington, DC: Amer Psychiatric Pub Inc.

Aylward, E. H., Minshew, N. J., Field, K., Sparks, B. F., and Singh, N. (2002). Effects of age on brain volume and head circumference in autism. Neurology 59, 175–183. doi: 10.1212/WNL.59.2.175

Behrens, T., Berg, H. J., Jbabdi, S., Rushworth, M., and Woolrich, M. (2007). Probabilistic diffusion tractography with multiple fibre orientations: what can we gain? Neuroimage 34, 144–155. doi: 10.1016/j.neuroimage.2006.09.018

Behrens, T., Johansen-Berg, H., Woolrich, M., Smith, S., Wheeler-Kingshott, C., Boulby, P., et al. (2003). Non-invasive mapping of connections between human thalamus and cortex using diffusion imaging. Nat. Neurosci. 6, 750–757. doi: 10.1038/nn1075

Benjamini, Y., and Hochberg, Y. (1995). Controlling the false discovery rate: a practical and powerful approach to multiple testing. J. R. Stat. Soc. B Methodol. 57, 289–300.

Blinkov, S. M., and Glezer, I. I. (1968). The Human Brain in Figures and Tables: a Quantitative Handbook. New York, NY: Basic Books.

Buckner, R. L., Head, D., Parker, J., Fotenos, A. F., Marcus, D., Morris, J. C., et al. (2004). A unified approach for morphometric and functional data analysis in young, old, and demented adults using automated atlas-based head size normalization: reliability and validation against manual measurement of total intracranial volume. Neuroimage 23, 724–738. doi: 10.1016/j.neuroimage.2004.06.018

Bullmore, E., and Sporns, O. (2012). The economy of brain network organization. Nat. Rev. Neurosci. 13, 336–349. doi: 10.1038/nrn3214

Changizi, M. (2007). "Scaling the brain and its connections," in Evolution of Nervous Systems. A Comprehensive Reference, Vol. 3, eds J. H. Kaas and L. Krubitzer (Amsterdam, Oxford: Academic Press; Elsevier), 167–180. doi: 10.1016/B0-12-370878-8/00061-6

Changizi, M. A., and Shimojo, S. (2005). Parcellation and area-area connectivity as a function of neocortex size. Brain Behav. Evol. 66, 88–98. doi: 10.1159/000085942

Chugani, H. T., Phelps, M. E., and Mazziotta, J. C. (1987). Positron emission tomography study of human brain functional development. Ann. Neurol. 22, 487–497. doi: 10.1002/ana.410220408

Collins, D., Neelin, P., Peters, T., and Evans, A. (1994). Automatic 3D intersubject registration of MR volumetric data in standardized Talairach space. J. Comput. Assist. Tomogr. 18, 192. doi: 10.1097/00004728-199403000-00005

Courchesne, E., Chisum, H. J., Townsend, J., Cowles, A., Covington, J., Egaas, B., et al. (2000). Normal brain development and aging: quantitative analysis at in vivo MR imaging in healthy Volunteers1. Radiology 216, 672–682. doi: 10.1148/radiology.216.3.r00au37672

Courchesne, E., Karns, C. M., Davis, H. R., Ziccardi, R., Carper, R. A., Tigue, Z. D., et al. (2001). Unusual brain growth patterns in early life in patients with autistic disorder: an MRI study. Neurology 57, 245–254. doi: 10.1212/WNL. 57.2.245

Dobbing, J., and Sands, J. (1973). Quantitative growth and development of human brain. Arch. Dis. Child. 48, 757–767. doi: 10.1136/adc.48.10.757 Gallos, L. K., Makse, H. A., and Sigman, M. (2012). A small world of weak ties provides optimal global integration of self-similar modules in functional brain networks. Proc. Natl. Acad. Sci. U.S.A. 109, 2825–2830. doi: 10.1073/pnas.1106612109

Giedd, J. N. (2008). The teen brain: insights from neuroimaging. J. Adoles. Health 42, 335–343. doi: 10.1016/j.jadohealth.2008.01.007

Hazlett, H. C., Poe, M., Gerig, G., Smith, R. G., Provenzale, J., Ross, A., et al. (2005). Magnetic resonance imaging and head circumference study of brain size in autism: birth through age 2 years. Arch. Gen. Psychiatry 62, 1366–1376. doi: 10.1001/archpsyc.62.12.1366

Hofman, M. A. (1985). Size and shape of the cerebral cortex in mammals. I. The cortical surface. Brain Behav. Evol. 27, 28–40. doi: 10.1159/000 118718

Honey, C., Sporns, O., Cammoun, L., Gigandet, X., Thiran, J.-P., Meuli, R., et al. (2009). Predicting human resting-state functional connectivity from structural connectivity. Proc. Natl. Acad. Sci. U.S.A. 106, 2035–2040. doi: 10.1073/pnas.0811168106

Horwitz, B., Rumsey, J. M., Grady, C. L., and Rapoport, S. I. (1988). The cerebral metabolic landscape in autism: intercorrelations of regional glucose utilization. Arch. Neurol. 45, 749–755. doi: 10.1001/archneur.1988.0052031 0055018

Jäncke, L., Staiger, J. F., Schlaug, G., Huang, Y., and Steinmetz, H. (1997). The rela- tion between corpus callosum size and forebrain volume. Cereb. Cortex 7, 48–56. doi: 10.1093/cercor/7.1.48

Jenkinson, M., and Smith, S. (2001). A global optimisation method for robust affine registration of brain images. Med. Image Anal. 5, 143–156. doi: 10.1016/S1361-8415(01)00036-6

Jerison, H. J. (1982). "Allometry, brain size, cortical surface, and convolutedness," in Primate Brain Evolution, eds E. Armstrong and D. Falk (New York, NY: Plenum Press), 77–84.

Jones, D. K., Knösche, T. R., and Turner, R. (2012). White matter integrity, fiber count, and other fallacies: the do's and don'ts of diffusion MRI. Neuroimage.

Just, M. A., Cherkassky, V. L., Keller, T. A., and Minshew, N. J. (2004). Cortical activation and synchronization during sentence comprehension in high- functioning autism: evidence of underconnectivity. Brain 127, 1811–1821. doi: 10.1093/brain/awh199

Just, M., Cherkassky, V., Keller, T., Kana, R., and Minshew, N. (2007). Functional and anatomical cortical underconnectivity in autism: evidence from an fMRI study of an executive function task and corpus callosum morphometry. Cereb. Cortex 17, 951. doi: 10.1093/cercor/bhl006

Kana, R. K., Keller, T. A., Minshew, N. J., and Just, M. A. (2007). Inhibitory control in high-functioning autism: decreased activation and underconnectivity in inhibition networks. Biol. Psychiatry 62, 198–206. doi: 10.1016/j.biopsych.2006.08.004

Karbowski, J. (2003). How does connectivity between cortical areas depend on brain size? Implications for efficient computation. J. Comput. Neurosci. 15, 347–356. doi: 10.1023/A:1027467911225

Kim, J., Singh, V., Lee, J., Lerch, J., Ad-Dab'bagh, Y., MacDonald, D., et al. (2005). Automated 3-D extraction and evaluation of the inner and outer cortical sur- faces using a Laplacian map and partial volume effect classification. Neuroimage 27, 210–221. doi: 10.1016/j.neuroimage.2005.03.036

Lainhart, J. E., Piven, J., Wzorek, M., Landa, R., Santangelo, S. L., Coon, H., et al. (1997). Macrocephaly in children and adults with autism. J. Am. Acad. Child Adolesc. Psychiatry 36, 282–290. doi: 10.1097/00004583-199702000-00019

LaMantia, A. S., and Rakic, P. (1990). Axon overproduction and elimination in the corpus callosum of the developing Rhesus monkey. Neuroscience 10, 2156–2175. Latora, V., and Marchiori, M. (2001). Efficient behavior of small-world networks. Phys. Rev. Lett. 87, 198701. doi: 10.1103/PhysRevLett.87. 198701

Latora, V., and Marchiori, M. (2003). Economic small-world behavior in weighted networks. Eur. Phys. J. B-Condensed Matt. Complex Syst. 32, 249–263. doi: 10.1140/epjb/e2003-00095-5

Lewis, J. D., and Elman, J. L. (2008). Growth-related neural reorganization and the autism phenotype: a test of the hypothesis that altered brain growth leads to altered connectivity. Dev. Sci. 11, 135–155. doi: 10.1111/j.1467-7687.2007.00634.x

Lewis, J. D., Theilmann, R. J., Fonov, V., Bellec, P., Lincoln, A., Evans, A. C., et al. (2012). Callosal fiber length and interhemispheric connectivity in adults with autism: brain overgrowth and underconnectivity. Hum. Brain Mapp. 34, 1685–1695. doi: 10.1002/hbm.22018

Lewis, J. D., Theilmann, R. J., Sereno, M. I., and Townsend, J. (2009). The relation between connection length and degree of connectivity in young adults: a DTI analysis. Cereb. Cortex 19, 554–562. doi: 10.1093/cercor/bhn105

Liu, Z., Wang, Y., Gerig, G., Gouttard, S., Tao, R., Fletcher, T., et al. (2010). Quality control of diffusion weighted images. Proc. SPIE, Med. Imaging 7628:844748. doi: 10.1117/12.844748

Magistretti, P. (1999). Brain energy metabolism. Fundam. Neurosci. 3, 271–293.

Olivares, R., Montiel, J., and Aboitiz, F. (2001). Species differences and similarities in the fine structure of the mammalian corpus callosum. Brain Behav. Evol. 57, 98–105. doi: 10.1159/000047229

Paus, T., Zijdenbos, A., Worsley, K., Collins, D. L., Blumenthal, J., Giedd, J. N., et al. (1999). Structural maturation of neural pathways in children and adolescents: in vivo study. Science 283, 1908. doi: 10.1126/science.283.5409.1908

Piven, J., Arndt, S., Bailey, J., Havercamp, S., Andreasen, N. C., and Palmer, P. (1995). An MRI study of brain size in autism. Am. J. Psychiatry 12, 1145–1149. Prothero, J. W. (1997). Cortical scaling in mammals: a repeating units model. J. Hirnforsch. 38, 195–207.

Prothero, J. W., and Sundsten, J. W. (1984). Folding of the cerebral cortex in mammals. A scaling model. Brain Behav. Evol. 24, 152–167. doi: 10.1159/ 000121313

Rakic, P., Bourgeois, J. P., Eckenhoff, M. F., Zecevic, N., and Goldman-Rakic, P. S. (1986). Concurrent overproduction of synapses in diverse regions of the primate cerebral cortex. Science 232, 232–235. doi: 10.1126/science. 3952506

Ramón y Cajal, S. (1995). Histology of the Nervous System of Man and Vertebrates. New York, NY: Oxford University Press.

Redcay, E., and Courchesne, E. (2005). When is the brain enlarged in autism? A meta-analysis of all brain size reports. Biol. Psychiatry 58, 1–9. doi: 10.1016/j. biopsych.2005.03.026

Rilling, J. K., and Insel, T. R. (1999a). Differential expansion of neural projection systems in primate brain evolution. Neuroreport 10, 1453–1459. doi: 10.1097/00001756-199905140-00012

Rilling, J. K., and Insel, T. R. (1999b). The primate neocortex in comparative per- spective using magnetic resonance imaging. J. Hum. Evol. 37, 191–223. doi: 10.1006/ jhev.1999.0313

Ringo, J. L. (1991). Neuronal interconnection as a function of brain size. Brain Behav. Evol. 38, 1–6. doi: 10.1159/000114375

Rubinov, M., and Sporns, O. (2010). Complex network measures of brain connectivity: uses and interpretations. Neuroimage 52, 1059–1069. doi: 10.1016/j.neuroimage.2009.10.003

Rudie, J., Brown, J., Beck-Pancer, D., Hernandez, L., Dennis, E., Thompson, P., et al. (2013). Altered functional and structural brain network organization in autism. Neuroimage Clin. 2, 79–94. doi: 10.1016/j.nicl.2012.11.006

Sled, J., Zijdenbos, A., and Evans, A. (1998). A nonparametric method for automatic correction of intensity nonuniformity in MRI data. IEEE Trans. Med. Imaging 17, 87–97. doi: 10.1109/42.668698

Thatcher, R. W., North, D. M., Biver, C. J., Petersburg, F., To, S. R. R., and Thatcher, R. W. (2008). Development of cortical connections as measured by EEG coherence and phase delays. Hum. Brain Mapp. 29, 1400–1415. doi: 10.1002/ hbm.20474

Tohka, J., Zijdenbos, A., and Evans, A. (2004). Fast and robust parameter estimation for statistical partial volume models in brain MRI. Neuroimage 23, 84–97. doi: 10.1016/j.neuroimage.2004.05.007

Tower, D. B. (1954). Structural and functional organization of mammalian cerebral cortex: the correlation of neuron density with brain size. J. Comp. Neurol. 101, 9–52. doi: 10.1002/cne.901010103

Tzourio-Mazoyer, N., Landeau, B., Papathanassiou, D., Crivello, F., Etard, O., Delcroix, N., et al. (2002). Automated anatomical labeling of activations in SPM using a macroscopic anatomical parcellation of the MNI MRI single-subject brain. Neuroimage 15, 273–289. doi: 10.1006/nimg. 2001.0978

Van Ooyen, A., and Willshaw, D. J. (1999). Competition for neurotrophic factor in the development of nerve connections. Proc. R. Soc. Lond. B Biol. Sci. 266, 883–892. doi: 10.1098/rspb.1999.0719

Watts, D. J., and Strogatz, S. H. (1998). Collective dynamics of 'small-world' networks. Nature 393, 440–442. doi: 10.1038/30918

Whitwell, J. L., Crum, W. R., Watt, H. C., and Fox, N. C. (2001). Normalization of cerebral volumes by use of intracranial volume: implications for longitudinal quantitative MR imaging. Am J. Neuroradiol. 22, 1483.

Zhang, K., and Sejnowski, T. J. (2000). A universal scaling law between gray matter and white matter of cerebral cortex. Proc. Natl. Acad. Sci. U.S.A. 97, 5621–5626. doi: 10.1073/pnas.090504197

Zijdenbos, A., Forghani, R., and Evans, A. (2002). Automatic "pipeline" analysis of 3-D MRI data for clinical trials: application to multiple sclerosis. IEEE Trans. Med. Imaging 21, 1280–1291. doi: 10.1109/TMI.2002. 806283

8

Altered oscillation patterns and connectivity during picture naming in autism

Isabelle Buard[1], Sally J. Rogers[2], Susan Hepburn[3], Eugene Kronberg[1] and Donald C. Rojas[1]*

[1] UCD Magnetoencephalography Lab, Department of Psychiatry, University of Colorado at Denver – Anschutz Medical Campus, Aurora, CO, USA
[2] Psychiatry and Behavioral Sciences, UC Davis MIND Institute, Sacramento, CA, USA
[3] University of Colorado/JFK Partners, Aurora, CO, USA

Edited by:
Tal Kenet, Massachusetts General Hospital, USA

Reviewed by:
Manfred G. Kitzbichler, Harvard Medical School, USA
Guillaume Dumas, Florida Atlantic University, USA
Sheraz Khan, Massachusetts General Hospital, USA

***Correspondence:**
Donald C. Rojas, UCD Magnetoencephalography Lab, Department of Psychiatry, University of Colorado at Denver – Anschutz Medical Campus, 13001 East 17th Pl F546, Aurora, CO 80045, USA
e-mail: don.rojas@ucdenver.edu

Similar behavioral deficits are shared between individuals with autism spectrum disorders (ASD) and their first-degree relatives, such as impaired face memory, object recognition, and some language aspects. Functional neuroimaging studies have reported abnormalities in ASD in at least one brain area implicated in those functions, the fusiform gyrus (FG). High frequency oscillations have also been described as abnormal in ASD in a separate line of research. The present study examined whether low- and high-frequency oscillatory power, localized in part to FG and other language-related regions, differs in ASD subjects and first-degree relatives. Twelve individuals with ASD, 16 parents of children with ASD, and 35 healthy controls participated in a picture-naming task using magnetoencephalography (MEG) to assess oscillatory power and connectivity. Relative to controls, we observed reduced evoked high-gamma activity in the right superior temporal gyrus (STG) and reduced high-beta/low-gamma evoked power in the left inferior frontal gyrus (IFG) in the ASD group. Finally, reductions in phase-locked beta-band were also seen in the ASD group relative to controls, especially in the occipital lobes (OCC). First degree relatives, in contrast, exhibited higher high-gamma band power in the left STG compared with controls, as well as increased high-beta/low-gamma evoked power in the left FG. In the left hemisphere, beta- and gamma-band functional connectivity between the IFG and FG and between STG and OCC were higher in the autism group than in controls. This suggests that, contrary to what has been previously described, reduced connectivity is not observed across all scales of observation in autism. The lack of behavioral correlation for the findings warrants some caution in interpreting the relevance of such changes for language function in ASD. Our findings in parents implicates the gamma- and beta-band ranges as potential compensatory phenomena in autism relatives.

Keywords: magnetoencephalography, gamma-band, beta-band, oscillations, functional connectivity, Granger causality, fusiform gyrus, endophenotype

INTRODUCTION

High-frequency brain activities have a central role in various normal functions (Buzsaki and Draguhn, 2004), including sensory binding (Rodriguez et al., 1999), temporal regulation of neuronal activity during synaptic plasticity (Traub et al., 1998), memory processing (Fell et al., 2001), and large-scale integration (Varela et al., 2001). Several suggestions have been proposed to define the role of gamma-band oscillations (30 Hz and higher) as a correlate of auditory awareness (Makeig and Jung, 1996; Yordanova et al., 2002) or encoding mental representations (Tallon-Baudry and Bertrand, 1999). Moreover, the correlation between gamma synchronization and hemodynamic responses reconciles common findings in fMRI and brain electrophysiology (Niessing et al., 2005). Particularly, gamma-band has been associated with face processing, notably in the fusiform gyrus (FG; Zion-Golumbic and Bentin, 2007; Gao et al., 2013). In autism spectrum disorders (ASD), impairments of gamma oscillations have been previously described in auditory (Wilson et al., 2007; Gandal et al., 2010) and visual domains (Grice et al., 2001; Brown et al., 2005; Milne et al., 2009; Isler et al., 2010; Stroganova et al., 2012), suggesting a link between high-frequency oscillations and perceptual dysfunction. We have also established that these deficits are seen in adult first-degree relatives, suggesting that such impairment constitutes an autism endophenotype (Rojas et al., 2008, 2011; McFadden et al., 2012). Lower frequency oscillatory activity has also been described as affected in autism, such as impaired mu wave suppression during action observation (Oberman et al., 2005).

Autism is defined by a triad of core impairments in social interaction, communication, and behavioral flexibility (American Psychiatric Association, 2000). Communication deficits include individual with autism's difficulty using spoken language and gestures, inability to initiate and sustain appropriate conversation and use of inappropriate, repetitive language (Lord et al., 2000). The severity of language impairment is highly variable in autism, ranging from highly verbal to essentially non-verbal (Tager-Flusberg et al., 2009), and it remains the best-known indicator of prognosis in affected individuals (Venter et al., 1992). Within the language domain, problematic pragmatic language use has been repeatedly documented among relatives (Losh et al., 2008). Among language impairments, word processing is particularly affected in ASD (Walenski et al., 2008). To examine the prediction of altered lexical processing, we tested subjects with autism on a picture-naming task, in which subjects named pictures of objects. Two major areas in the human brain are responsible for language (Binder et al., 1997): Broca's area (localized to left inferior frontal gyrus, or IFG) which is involved in language production, and Wernicke's area (localized in the superior temporal gyrus, STG) which is thought to be implicated in language processing. Other brain structures may also play a role in language. Among them, the FG has been initially studied as being a part of the visual system specialized in facial recognition (Fusiform Face Area; Kanwisher et al., 1997) because of the importance of face processing to successful social functioning. Its additional role in language processing, called the visual word form area (McCandliss et al., 2003), highlights its relevance for language studies. Interestingly, individuals with ASDs show atypical functional lateralization, with reduced left hemisphere and/or reversed patterns of cortical activation in linguistic experiments (Just et al., 2004; Flagg et al., 2005; Wang et al., 2006; Frye and Beauchamp, 2009).

Hypoactivity in the FG (Schultz et al., 2000) and IFG (Groen et al., 2010) areas has been reported in individuals with autism, suggesting that there should be physiological signatures underlying autism-related language impairments. The objective of this study was to compare gamma-band oscillations in the FG, STG, and IFG, language-related areas of control participants to patients with autism and first-degree relative of persons with ASD during a picture-naming task. Based on prior findings from simple auditory and visual processing experiments, as well as face perception experiments, we expected to observe reduced phase-locked, or evoked gamma-band activity in both the autism group and in parents of individuals with autism compared to controls. Increases in non-phase-locked, or induced gamma-band activity have also been reported in autism (e.g., see Brown et al., 2005; Rojas et al., 2008). We therefore separately analyzed the evoked and induced gamma-band activity in the study.

Building upon previous studies, we found some differential activation in the gamma- and beta-band range in people with autism compared to their first-degree relatives. Patterns of activation were opposite, as parent brains were over-activated while autistic brains showed under-activation. The connectivity analyses and results add to the existing literature by extension to an object naming task and examination of both individuals with autism and first-degree relatives.

MATERIALS AND METHODS

SUBJECTS

Participants were 12 persons with ASD, 16 parents of a child with ASD (PASD), and 35 controls (**Table 1**). One-way ANOVAs were used to examine demographic variables (age) for significant differences. No significant group differences were present at $p > 0.05$ for any of these group characteristics. For ASD subjects, diagnosis was based on convergence of clinical judgment by experimenters using DSM-IV criteria (American Psychiatric Association, 2000), and research reliability trained on the Autism Diagnostic Interview, Revised (ADI-R; Lord et al., 1994), and the Autism Diagnostic Observation Schedule (ADOS; Lord et al., 2000). Each of the 16 PASD group subjects had a single child who met the same criteria for ASD as the ASD group participants. The PASD group subjects were not biologically related to the study participants in the ASD group. The healthy comparison subjects had no personal history of developmental, psychiatric, or neurologic disorders, and no family history of developmental disorders. All subjects signed informed consent to participate in the study consistent with the guidelines of the Colorado Multiple Institution Review Board.

Table 1 | Participants characteristics.

Measure	Controls	ASD	Parents	*p*-value
Age (mean years ± SD)	34.2 ± 11.9	28.3 ± 13.3	37.9 ± 5.9	0.082
Handedness score	0.62 ± 0.53	0.35 ± 0.79	0.74 ± 0.41	0.202

Handedness was assessed in all subjects using the Annett Handedness Questionnaire (Annett, 1985). Handedness score means were 0.62 ± 0.53, 0.35 ± 0.79, and 0.74 ± 0.41 for healthy controls, ASD subjects and PASD, respectively (**Table 1**). One-way ANOVA (SPSS version 21 – IBM Corp, Armonk, NY, USA) revealed no difference among groups: $F(2, 54) = 1.65$, $p = 0.202$.

STIMULI AND EXPERIMENTAL DESIGN

The stimuli consisted of 192 black and white line art images from the International Picture Naming Project database[1], which includes items from the Peabody Picture Vocabulary Test (PPVT; Dunn, 1997), Snodgrass and Vanderwart (1980) and other sources. The pictures represent simple objects such as a shovel or an airplane. Trials consisted of periods of picture stimuli lasting for 1200 ms, followed by a central fixation cross for a random inter-stimulus interval between 3000 and 5000 ms. Picture stimuli were presented by an LCD projector onto a screen located 45 cm in front of the subject and subtended an average of 7.27° horizontal visual angle and 6.02° vertical visual angle. Subjects were instructed to sub-vocalize (whisper) the name of the object depicted in the image they had just seen as soon as the fixation cross appeared (i.e., after the picture was removed) and received practice trials until they understood the instructions. Sub-vocalization was used instead of overt naming to reduce motion and muscle artifact in the MEG data. The entire recording session lasted approximately 16 min.

MEG DATA ACQUISITION AND PRE-PROCESSING

We employed a Magnes 3600 WH whole-head MEG device (4-D Neuroimaging, San Diego, CA, USA), which comprises 248 first-order axial-gradiometer sensors in a helmet-shaped array. Five head position indicator coils attached to the subject's scalp were used to determine the head position with respect to the sensor array. The locations of the coils with respect to three anatomical landmarks (nasion and pre-auricular points) and two extra

[1] http://crl.ucsd.edu/experiments/ipnp/

non-fiducial points, as well as the scalp surface were determined with a 3D digitizer (Polhemus, Colchester, VT, USA). Identifying the three fiducial points on an SPM standard head model established the coordinate transformation between MEG and the standard MRI template used for the volume conductor in source modeling.

The MEG signals were acquired in a 0.1–200 Hz bandwidth and sampled continuously at 508 Hz and 24-bit quantization. MEG data pre-processing was conducted using the 4-D Neuroimaging software, Fieldtrip[2] and Statistical Parametric Mapping SPM8 (Wellcome Trust Centre for Neuroimaging, London, UK) implemented in Matlab (2009b; MathWorks, Inc., Natick, MA, USA). Eye movement and blink artifacts were corrected using independent components analysis using the FastICA algorithm (Hyvarinen, 1999). Epochs were then defined of 1200 ms duration, with a baseline of −200 to 0 ms pre-stimulus onset and 1000 ms post-stimulus. Epochs were baseline corrected to remove any DC offset and those trials contaminated by excessively large MEG amplitudes (±3000 fT) were rejected from further analysis. An average of 119 (±25) artifact free epochs was obtained for source analysis.

MEG SOURCE ANALYSIS AND SOURCE SPACE STATISTICS

Source analysis was performed in Matlab (2009b; MathWorks, Inc., Natick, MA, USA) using the SPM8 toolbox (Statistical Parametric Mapping; Wellcome Department of Cognitive Neurology, London, UK). Following co-registration of the MEG fiducials with the SPM8 standard template, leadfields were computed using a single shell volume conductor model. Source localization was then performed using a cortically constrained group minimum norm inversion with multiple sparse priors (Litvak et al., 2011), on all subjects' data pooled together from the three groups, which resulted in a common source space images across subjects. The cortical surface used was a standard MNI space surface with 20484 vertices supplied within SPM8. Source analysis was performed on the 35–120 Hz passband between 100 and 250 ms.

Source space images were submitted to GLM-based statistical analysis using a one-sample t-test across subjects in all three groups to find a common set of activated regions for subsequent spectral analyses. Several active brain regions were obtained (**Table 2**), where activity during the task survived multiple comparison correction, using a false discovery rate (FDR) of $q < 0.05$. Among all active regions, we focused on the FG, the inferior frontal gyrus, the STG, and the occipital lobe (OCC) for further ROI-based analyses for three reasons: (1) their relevance to language function, (2) the engagement of visual structures in this specific task, and (3) leadfield correlation is high among closely spaced regions and induces artificial correlation in source waveforms derived from such locations. A limited set of widely spaced ROI is therefore more appropriate given these correlations.

SOURCE WAVEFORMS, SPECTRAL ANALYSES, AND FUNCTIONAL CONNECTIVITY

Regional time-courses were created via source-space projection (Tesche et al., 1995) from dipoles within each region of interest: left and right FG, IFG, STG, and OCC. We computed the lead field and its pseudoinverse and then we created current source waveform (Ross et al., 2000). Montreal Neurological Institute (MNI) coordinates described in **Table 2** were used for this step. Afterward, from those source-space projections were computed time-frequency transforms using a Morlet wavelet decomposition with wave number linearly increasing from 3 to 12 across the frequency range of 10–110 Hz, on the epochs from −200 to 800 ms. For each subject, evoked and induced power, relative to the 200 ms pre-stimulus baseline, were calculated, along with the phase-locking factor (PLF; Tallon-Baudry et al., 1996), a measure of inter-trial phase-consistency (also sometimes referred to as intertrial coherence). Mass univariate, non-parametric statistical analyses were performed across the entire time-frequency space, corrected for multiple comparisons using cluster size metrics at FWE < 0.01. Fieldtrip's cluster-based correction for multiple comparisons uses Monte Carlo randomization to compute a sampling distribution for cluster sizes. Our threshold for cluster formation was set to $p = 0.01$ and the number of permutations set to 1000 (Maris and Oostenveld, 2007).

In order to evaluate directional functional connectivity between our regions of interest in the frequency domain, we computed frequency domain Granger causality using the Fieldtrip connectivity analysis functions (Oostenveld et al., 2011), which first involved an autoregressive model fit to the data using the bsmart matlab toolbox (Cui et al., 2008). For these analyses, we downsampled

Table 2 | List of brain regions that were significantly active (FDR $q < 0.05$) from source analyses of the 35–120 Hz band between 100 and 250 ms post-stimulus.

Region	Side	MNI coordinates			*T* value
Pre-cuneus	R	4	−70	36	32.78
	L	−7	−74	42	32.12
Cuneus	R	10	76	38	32.62
	L	−10	−68	42	31.25
Inferior temporal gyrus area (includes **fusiform gyrus**)	R	54	−34	−26	11.18
	L	−48	−56	−14	18.78
Pre-central gyrus	R	42	−14	48	15.81
Post-central gyrus	R	44	−26	46	13.96
Superior temporal gyrus	R	50	−44	16	11.18
	L	−50	−44	18	16.92
Basal forebrain	R	22	10	−18	12.87
	L	−24	8	−18	12.87
Inferior frontal gyrus	R	42	28	16	12.18
	L	−42	24	18	12.24
Inferior frontal orbital	L	−34	40	−14	9.71
Lobe occipital Superior	R	22	−80	40	26.90
	L	−18	−80	34	25.88
Superior frontal gyrus	R	20	−8	64	6.69
	L	−20	−6	66	6.70

Regions in bold print were selected for ROI based analyses.

[2]http://fieldtrip.fcdonders.nl

the data to 250 Hz for better model order estimation and submit the data to detrenting, differencing, and pre-whitening. Then, we estimated the model order to be 15 (60 ms) using ARfit toolbox for Matlab (Schneider and Neumaier, 2001). Group comparisons of Granger spectra were analyzed between regions of interest and between the two hemispheres, and corrected for multiple comparisons using the FDR method on the overall set of comparisons, $q < 0.1$.

BEHAVIORAL TESTING

Since we did not measure spoken responses due to concern over excessive motion, the PPVT was performed and scored independently outside of the scanner, on a separate day following the MEG session, as a proxy indication of picture naming performance. The 192 items presented in the scanner contained 62 pictures from the PPVT items. A Kruskal–Wallis one-way analysis of variance was applied to test for statistical differences between groups.

RESULTS

SOURCE ANALYSIS RESULTS

Table 2 presents the regions that were significantly active from the source analyses of the 35–120 Hz band between 100 and 250 ms. Indeed, those brain regions included mainly visual and language areas. Among them, the four cortical regions of interest to us during this task (FG, STG, IFG, and OCC) that were selected for source space projections and time-frequency analyses are depicted in **Figure 1**.

TIME-FREQUENCY RESULTS

Fusiform gyrus

For the left FG, the evoked power was significantly higher in the PASD group, relative to the controls, for high beta/low gamma-band activity centered around 35 Hz and from around 580–700 ms post-stimulus onset (**Figure 2**). No differences in PLF or induced power were observed for the FG. No difference between the ASD group and both other ones were found in either left or right FG.

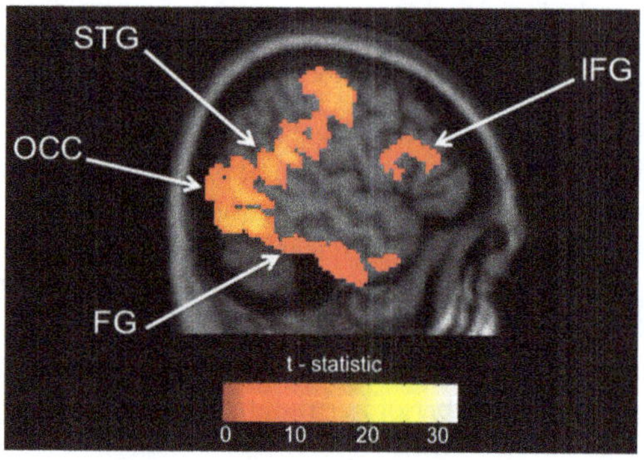

FIGURE 1 | Regions of interest from within source analysis results. Gamma (35–120 Hz) activation maps 100–250 ms after stimulus presentation (FWE, $p < 0.05$) across all participants. FG, fusiform gyrus; STG, superior temporal gyrus; IFG, inferior frontal gyrus; OCC, occipital lobe. All four clusters used to define our ROIs are depicted in this slice, but the exact location of the MNI coordinate used is listed in **Table 2**.

Superior temporal gyrus

In the left STG, no significant differences were observed between the HC and ASD groups, but there was a significant increase in high-gamma evoked power for the PASD group relative to controls between 570 and 630 ms post-stimulus (**Figure 3**). No differences in PLF or induced power were seen for the left STG. In the right hemisphere STG, there was a significant decrease in high-gamma evoked power peaking at 900 ms in the ASD group compared to controls. No differences in PLF or induced power were observed in the right STG between groups.

Inferior frontal gyrus

For left IFG, there was a significant decrease in evoked power of the high beta/low gamma-band between 630 and 720 ms post-stimulus in the control group compared to the autism group (**Figure 4**). No other significant differences were observed, for any measures within the right IFG and for PLF or induced power in the left IFG.

Occipital lobe

In both left and right OCC (**Figure 5**), PLF but not evoked/induced power was significantly reduced in the ASD group in the beta band around 200 (for the right) and 300–400 ms (left). No difference between the parents and controls was found in any measures and any hemispheres.

BEHAVIORAL RESULTS

All participants were asked to complete the PPVT language test. **Figure 6** shows the scores for each group. Comparison between groups did not yield any statistical difference, according to a Kruskall–Wallis test ($p = 0.50$). There were no significant correlations between PPVT performance and either early or late high-gamma-band PLF, evoked or induced power, or those measures in the beta-band, even at uncorrected $p < 0.05$.

ALTERED FUNCTIONAL CONNECTIVITY IN THE AUTISM GROUP

Left inferior frontal gyrus to left fusiform

Increased directional connectivity was observed between the left IFG to the left FG (**Figure 7**, top and horizontal slice) for the autism group compared to the control group. This increase was significant across the high-beta and low gamma frequencies after correction for multiple comparisons (FDR, $q < 0.1$).

Left superior temporal gyrus to left occipital lobe

As found between left IFG and FG, there was stronger connectivity in the group of autism participants compared to the controls from the left STG to the left OCC (**Figure 7**, bottom and right horizontal slice). This was statistically significant within the full beta-and gamma-band ranges.

No other significant differences in connectivity within or between hemispheres, for any frequency, were found among groups. We also observed no significant correlations between the connectivity data and the PPVT.

DISCUSSION

Our results, if replicated, suggest that altered high- and low-frequency brain oscillations in regions involved in object and

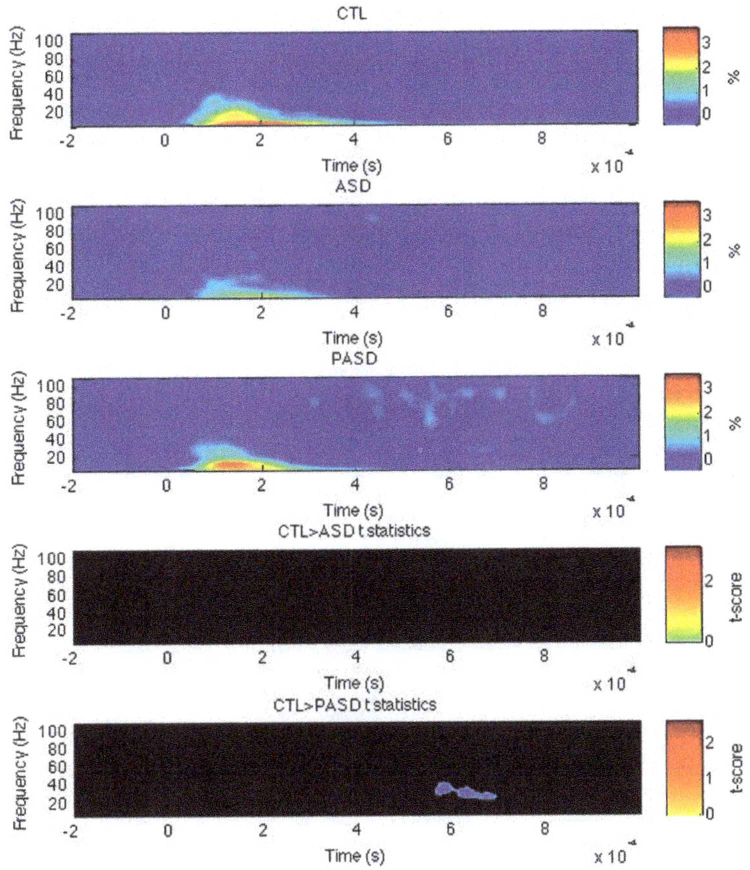

FIGURE 2 | Fusiform gyrus evoked power time-frequency results. Grand average evoked power is shown for each group (three top rows) for the left fusiform gyrus (FG). *T*-statistic maps are shown in the two bottom rows that illustrate contrasts between controls (CTL) and ASD (row 4) and CTL and parents (PASD; row 5). Masked *t*-score results represent cluster-corrected findings at $p < 0.01$.

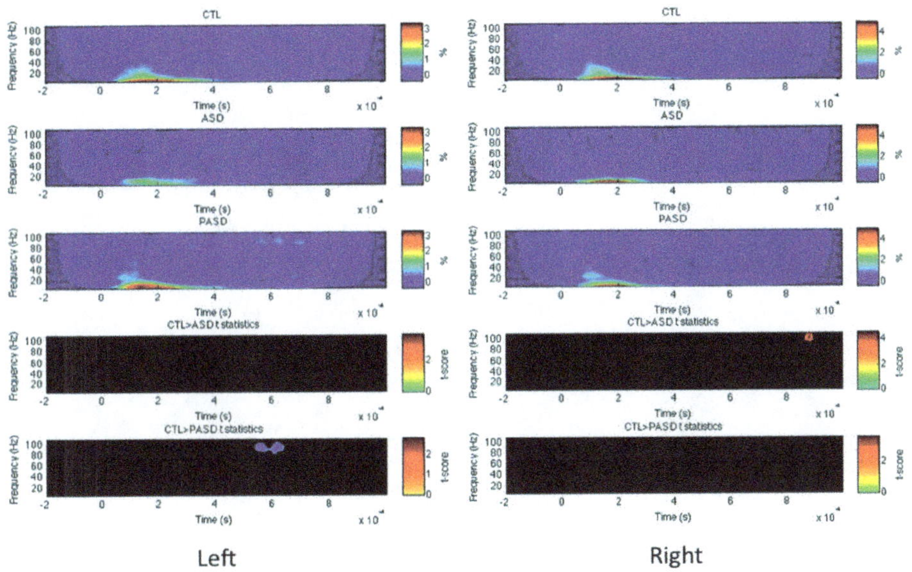

FIGURE 3 | Superior temporal gyrus evoked power time-frequency results. Grand average evoked power is shown for each group (three top rows) for the left and right superior temporal gyrus (STG). *T*-statistic maps are shown in the two bottom rows that illustrate contrasts between controls (CTL) and ASD (row 4) and CTL and parents (PASD; row 5). Masked *t*-score results represent cluster-corrected findings at $p < 0.01$.

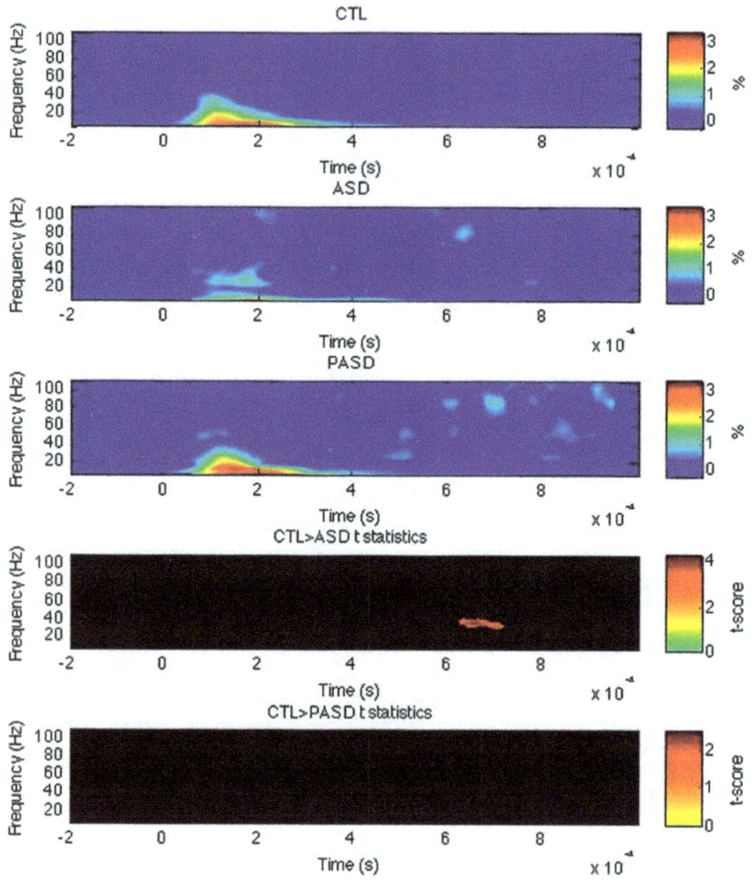

FIGURE 4 | Inferior frontal gyrus evoked power time-frequency results. Grand average evoked power is shown for each group (three top rows) for the left inferior frontal gyrus (IFG). *T*-statistic maps are shown in the two bottom rows that illustrate contrasts between controls (CTL) and ASD (row 4) and CTL and parents (PASD; row 5). Masked *t*-score results represent cluster-corrected findings at $p < 0.01$.

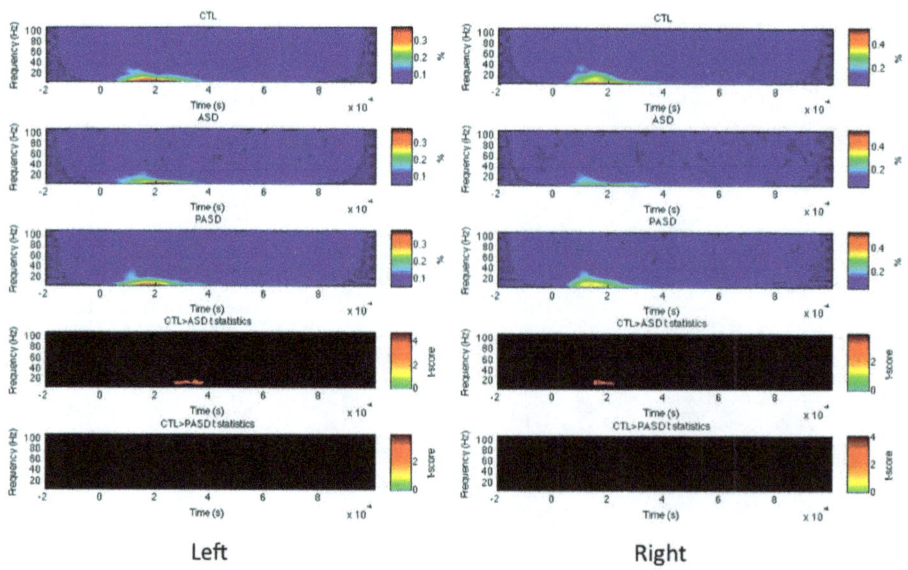

FIGURE 5 | Occipital lobe PLF time-frequency results. Grand average PLF are shown for each group (three top rows) for the left and right occipital lobe (OCC). *T*-statistic maps are shown in the two bottom rows that illustrate contrasts between controls (CTL) and ASD (row 4) and CTL and parents (PASD; row 5). Masked *t*-score results represent cluster-corrected findings at $p < 0.01$.

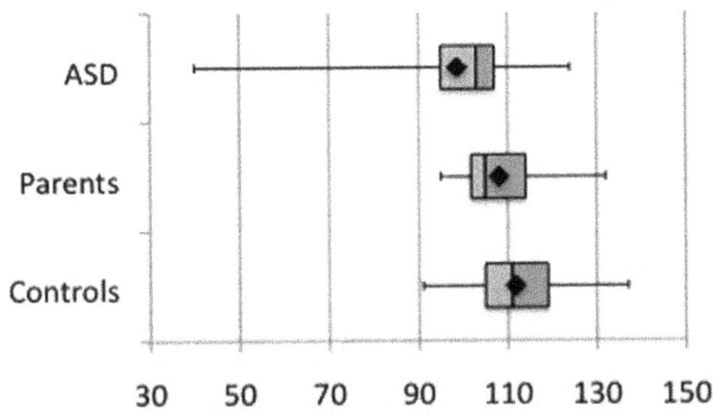

FIGURE 6 | Comparison of PPVT performance scores across group subjects. No significant difference was observed ($p = 0.50$).

language-related processes are a notable characteristic of autism, and that first-degree relatives share some of those differences. The findings appeared to be regionally and temporally specific in the context of the current task and sample.

CHANGES IN OSCILLATORY POWER AND OVER-CONNECTIVITY IN AUTISM

Converging evidence from across many studies and a variety of experimental paradigms suggests a gamma-band deficit in ASD (Grice et al., 2001; Brown et al., 2005; Wilson et al., 2007; Rojas et al., 2008, 2011; Gandal et al., 2010; McFadden et al., 2012; Wright et al., 2012; Gao et al., 2013), which has been proposed as a biomarker of autism (Uhlhaas et al., 2010).

In the STG, decreased high-gamma band activity was found. Using auditory-verbal stimulus material, we have already reported similar STG activation trends within autism (Wilson et al., 2007) albeit at a lower gamma-band frequency range of 30–50 Hz. In a language context, both structural and functional differences in the STG have been described in previous autism studies (Herbert et al., 2002; Harris et al., 2006; Hubbard et al., 2012). Altered gamma-band responses have also previously been reported in the STG of children with autism in response to simple, pure tone auditory stimulation (Gandal et al., 2010). In the left IFG, we also found decreased evoked power in the low-gamma band in autism compared to controls. Alterations in oscillations patterns in those language-network structures may be related to language impairments observed in people with autism.

We also note that the low gamma-band findings extended to the beta-range. Indeed, impaired beta-band oscillations have previously been observed in children with ASD compared to healthy controls (Stroganova et al., 2007, 2012). The delineation between the end of one band and beginning of the next is relatively arbitrary, so it is not unexpected to find that high beta and low gamma changes would be present. Additionally, beta-band oscillatory activity is independently known to be responsive to language stimuli (Hirata et al., 2004).

In the OCC, reduced beta PLF was found in both left and right sides of subjects with autism. The presence of those abnormalities in early visual responses is consistent with previous neurophysiological research on face processing (Dawson et al., 2005). Using MEG (Kylliainen et al., 2006), also reported differences in the processing of faces and other complex objects (motorbikes) at 100 ms in ASD children matched with typically developing controls. Those results and our study showing an impaired oscillation pattern related to object naming in autism suggest that visual brain activity may partly reflect general visual processing differences observed in this population (Jemel et al., 2006).

The observed changes in the STG and IFG occurred later in the post-stimulus window than the early phase-locked changes observed for the OCC. This is in accordance with the involvement of the occipital areas in visual functions, whereas the left FG (Binder et al., 1997; Balsamo et al., 2006) and the STG (Heath et al., 2012) have been reported as active during semantic processing at latter stages in the process of picture naming. A previous MEG study on picture naming reported visual and semantic processing around 0–150 and 275–400 ms after stimulus presentation (Levelt et al., 1998). Our differences were found between 600 and 900 ms, the timing of which suggests a role in early semantic or covert speech processes.

The autism group exhibited stronger functional connectivity from anterior to posterior language and visual areas compared with the control and parent groups, which may partially explain the impaired activation we found in that group in those regions. This finding is suggestive of differences in long-range neural synchronization present in our patient group. Alteration of long-range connectivity is an often reported finding in autism (Courchesne and Pierce, 2005). For example, reduced non-directional functional connectivity between anterior and posterior speech areas has been reported previously (Just et al., 2004). Our current result, however, does not support the underconnectivity theory. It should be noted that, apart from our finding of overconnectivity, other evidence also suggest overconnectivity in autism, such as a recent study showing enhanced functional excitation from occipital to frontal areas (Dominguez et al., 2013). In another recent paper, individuals with Asperger syndrome had higher, not lower, fractional anisotropy than controls in a diffusion tensor study of white matter (Roine et al., 2013). Together, these findings suggest that both underconnectivity and overconnectivity can be observed in autism relative to control subjects.

The range of oscillations where ASD people exhibited higher connectivity included both beta and gamma frequencies. Literature reports that gamma rhythms are prevalent in local visual response synchronization, but more distant coherence occurring during multimodal integration between parietal and temporal cortices uses rhythms in the beta range (Roelfsema et al., 1997). Since gamma-band activity is phase-amplitude coupled to lower frequency alpha- and theta-band oscillations, it is possible that the higher connectivity we observe in the gamma-range is a direct effect of the increased connectivity in the beta band between the same regions. A recent MEG paper reported that reduced high-gamma connectivity between the FG and other brain areas was related to decreased local connectivity, as assessed by phase-amplitude coupling to low frequency oscillations in those areas (Khan et al., 2013). One difference between this study and ours

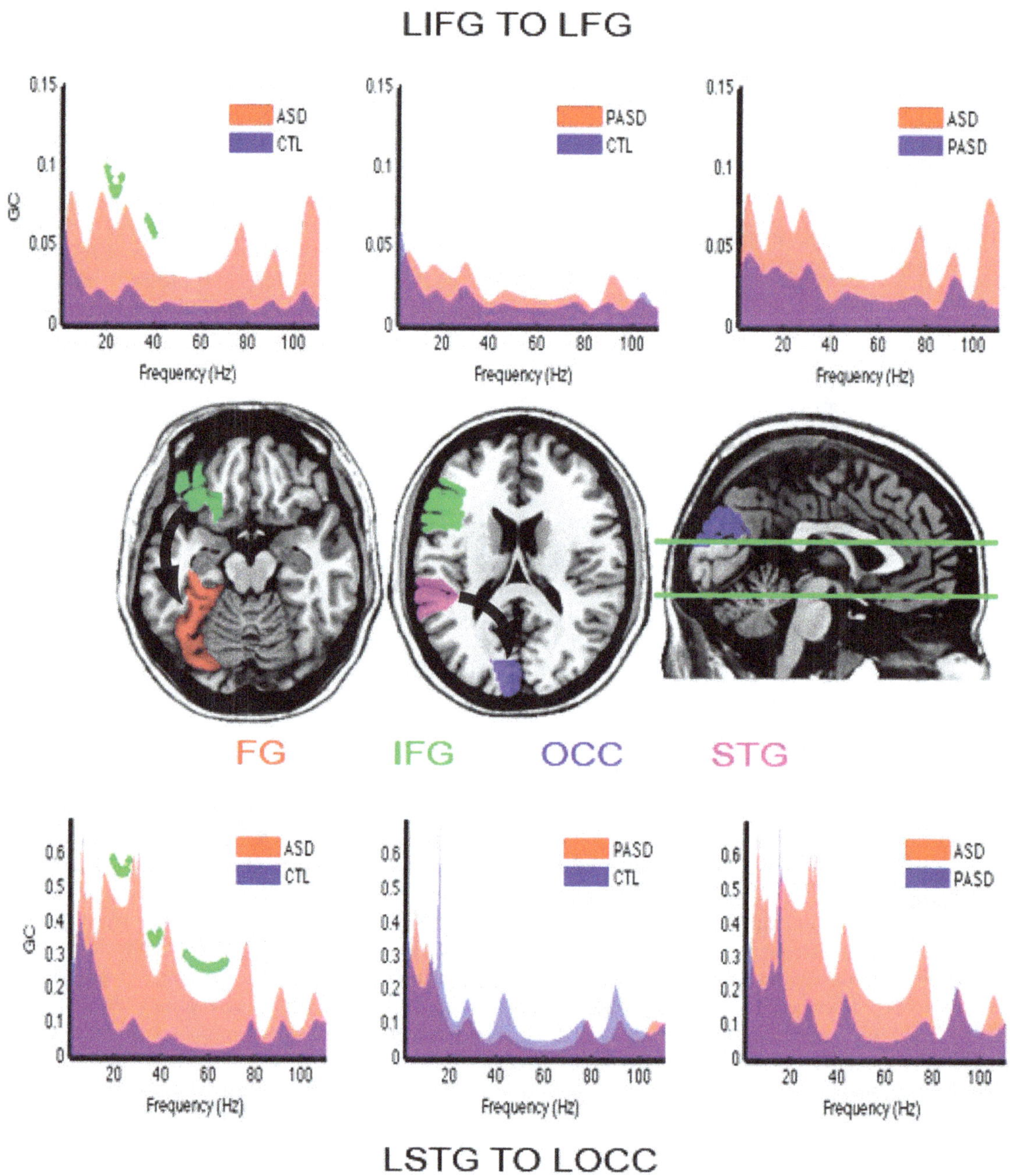

FIGURE 7 | Granger causality results. Granger spectra show functional connectivity between regions of interest with significant differences between the ASD and control groups. GC, Granger causality; FG, fusiform gyrus; STG, superior temporal gyrus; IFG, inferior frontal gyrus; OCC, occipital lobe. The title reading from left to right (e.g., IFG–FG) indicates the direction of causation. Significant group differences are shown with green asterisks (FDR, $q < 0.1$). Brain slices in the middle row illustrate location of those brain areas and flux of information (arrows) between them.

was the involvement of the FG relative to the task. In the paper reporting underconnectivity (Khan et al., 2013), the stimuli were faces; in ours, all of the stimuli were non-face objects. Thus, FG might be differentially affected in autism in a task specific manner.

The PPVT scores were not significantly different between the ASD and control groups. Together with the oscillatory and connectivity changes, this might suggest that the increase in communication between language and visual areas could provide a compensatory mechanism for coping with language and/or object naming difficulties. We also did not find any significant relationships between our groups' performance on the behavioral language task and on their gamma-related results. This indicates that this paradigm might not well-suited to study language processes per se in autism, but is perhaps more relevant to issues in early visual perception and object recognition. Consistent with this, for example, a previous study reported FG activation during color naming (Price and Devlin, 2003). Finally, we note that although we have speculated concerning language deficits in autism, there is no behavioral evidence for such deficits in our sample. A more severely affected sample might be necessary to establish a relationship, if any, between oscillatory power changes, connectivity, and language deficits in people with autism.

A POTENTIAL COMPENSATORY/PROTECTIVE MECHANISM IN FIRST-DEGREE RELATIVES

In the FG, evoked power revealed an increase in late high-beta/low-gamma band activity in the PASD group compared to controls. Similarly, we recently published evidence of gamma-band over-activation in the FG in autism first-degree relatives using language stimuli delivered in the auditory modality (McFadden et al., 2012). This increase also extended to the beta-band. Indeed, parents of children with autism show evidence of several areas of difference in common with persons with ASD, such as face memory and object recognition (Wallace et al., 2010), social cognition and working memory (Gokcen et al., 2009), and executive function, the latter being also shared by unaffected siblings (Wong et al., 2006). At the functional level, our group has recently published the evidence of differences in neural patterns associated with phonological processing in first-degree relatives (Wilson et al., 2012).

In the STG, increased activation in the high-gamma band was found in the left hemisphere of parents. Here again, we have already reported similar STG activation trends within autism relatives (McFadden et al., 2012) albeit at a lower gamma-band frequency range of 30–50 Hz. This finding is opposite to what we found in the ASD group. Such differential findings have been reported previously in autism subjects and relatives, such as intact verbal IQ in relatives while probands generally exhibit lower levels relative to performance IQ (Schmidt et al., 2008). In this context, it is possible that the observed over-activity in language-related regions is either a compensatory or protective mechanism.

ACKNOWLEDGMENTS

This work was funded by NIH RO1 MH082820 and Cure Autism Now (currently Autism Speaks). The authors of the manuscript declare that they have no conflict of interest to report regarding this manuscript.

CONCLUSION

Our findings of altered beta and gamma oscillations in people with ASD is consistent with a change in neural synchrony, which adds to a growing literature on gamma-band deficits across a number of simple sensory and complex cognitive tasks. The findings suggest that such oscillatory changes may also be relevant to higher order visual object processing and possibly to some language functions, at least in the context of object naming. The lack of similarity between the probands and the parents represents a challenge to the endophenotype interpretation. Alternative explanations include a compensatory or protective mechanism in the first-degree relatives. Impaired connections between posterior and anterior regions of the brain may be a marker of language and/or visual processing differences in autism, but future studies of language impaired individuals with autism will be needed to clarify a specific role, if any, for altered intra-hemispheric connectivity in the language processing deficits observed in the disorder.

REFERENCES

Annett, M. (1985). Left, Right, Hand, and Brain: The Right Shift Theory. Hove: Cambridge University Press.

American Psychiatric Association. (2000). Diagnostic and Statistical Manual of Mental Disorders, 4th ed. DSM-IV-TR. USA: American Psychiatric Association.

Balsamo, L. M., Xu, B., and Gaillard, W. D. (2006). Language lateralization and the role of the fusiform gyrus in semantic processing in young children. Neuroimage 31, 1306–1314. doi: 10.1016/j.neuroimage.2006.01.027

Binder, J. R., Frost, J. A., Hammeke, T. A., Cox, R. W., Rao, S. M., and Prieto, T. (1997). Human brain language areas identified by functional magnetic resonance imaging. J. Neurosci. 17, 353–362.

Brown, C., Gruber, T., Boucher, J., Rippon, G., and Brock, J. (2005). Gamma abnormalities during perception of illusory figures in autism. Cortex 41, 364–376. doi: 10.1016/S0010-9452(08)70273-9

Buzsaki, G., and Draguhn, A. (2004). Neuronal oscillations in cortical networks. Science 304, 1926–1929. doi: 10.1126/science.1099745

Courchesne, E., and Pierce, K. (2005). Why the frontal cortex in autism might be talking only to itself: local over-connectivity but long-distance disconnection. Curr. Opin. Neurobiol. 15, 225–230. doi: 10.1016/j.conb.2005.03.001

Cui, J., Xu, L., Bressler, S. L., Ding, M., and Liang, H. (2008). BSMART: a Matlab/C toolbox for analysis of multichannel neural time series. Neural Netw. 21, 1094–1104. doi: 10.1016/j.neunet.2008.05.007

Dawson, G., Webb, S. J., and McPartland, J. (2005). Understanding the nature of face processing impairment in autism: insights from behavioral and electrophysiolog- ical studies. Dev. Neuropsychol. 27, 403–424. doi: 10.1207/s15326942dn2703_6

Dominguez, L. G., Velazquez, J. L., and Galan, R. F. (2013). A model of functional brain connectivity and background noise as a biomarker for cognitive phenotypes: application to autism. PLoS ONE 8:e61493. doi: 10.1371/journal.pone.0061493

Dunn, L. M. (1997). PPVT-III: Peabody Picture Vocabulary Test-Third Edition. Circle Pines, MN: American Guidance Service, Inc.

Fell, J., Klaver, P., Lehnertz, K., Grunwald, T., Schaller, C., Elger, C. E., et al. (2001). Human memory formation is accompanied by rhinal-hippocampal coupling and decoupling. Nat. Neurosci. 4, 1259–1264. doi: 10.1038/nn759

Flagg, E. J., Cardy, J. E., Roberts, W., and Roberts, T. P. (2005). Language lateralization development in children with autism: insights from the late field magnetoen-cephalogram. Neurosci. Lett. 386, 82–87. doi: 10.1016/j.neulet.2005.05.037

Frye, R. E., and Beauchamp, M. S. (2009). Receptive language organization in high-functioning autism. J. Child Neurol. 24, 231–236. doi: 10.1177/0883073808329572

Gandal, M. J., Edgar, J. C., Ehrlichman, R. S., Mehta, M., Roberts, T. P., and Siegel, S. J. (2010). Validating gamma oscillations and delayed auditory responses as translational biomarkers of autism. Biol. Psychiatry 68, 1100–1106. doi: 10.1016/j.biopsych.2010.09.031

Gao, Z., Goldstein, A., Harpaz, Y., Hansel, M., Zion-Golumbic, E., and Bentin, S. (2013). A magnetoencephalographic study of face processing: M170, gamma-band oscillations and source localization. Hum. Brain Mapp. 34, 1783–95 doi: 10.1002/hbm.22028

Gokcen, S., Bora, E., Erermis, S., Kesikci, H., and Aydin, C. (2009). Theory of mind and verbal working memory deficits in parents of autistic children. Psychiatry Res. 166, 46–53. doi: 10.1016/j.psychres.2007.11.016

Grice, S. J., Spratling, M. W., Karmiloff-Smith, A., Halit, H., Csibra, G., De Haan, M., et al. (2001). Disordered visual processing and oscillatory brain activity in

autism and Williams syndrome. Neuroreport 12, 2697–2700. doi: 10.1097/00001756- 200108280-00021
Groen, W. B., Tesink, C., Petersson, K. M., Van Berkum, J., Van Der Gaag, R. J., Hagoort, P., et al. (2010). Semantic, factual, and social language comprehension in adolescents with autism: an FMRI study. Cereb. Cortex 20, 1937–1945. doi: 10.1093/cercor/bhp264
Harris, G. J., Chabris, C. F., Clark, J., Urban, T., Aharon, I., Steele, S., et al. (2006). Brain activation during semantic processing in autism spectrum disorders via functional magnetic resonance imaging. Brain Cogn. 61, 54–68. doi: 10.1016/j.bandc.2005.12.015
Heath, S., McMahon, K., Nickels, L., Angwin, A., MacDonald, A., Van Hees, S., et al. (2012). Priming picture naming with a semantic task: an fMRI investigation. PLoS ONE 7:e32809. doi: 10.1371/journal.pone.0032809
Herbert, M. R., Harris, G. J., Adrien, K. T., Ziegler, D. A., Makris, N., Kennedy, D. N., et al. (2002). Abnormal asymmetry in language association cortex in autism. Ann. Neurol. 52, 588–596. doi: 10.1002/ana.10349
Hirata, M., Kato, A., Taniguchi, M., Saitoh, Y., Ninomiya, H., Ihara, A., et al. (2004). Determination of language dominance with synthetic aperture magnetometry: comparison with the Wada test. Neuroimage 23, 46–53. doi: 10.1016/j.neuroimage.2004.05.009
Hubbard, A. L., McNealy, K., Scott-Van Zeeland, A. A., Callan, D. E., Bookheimer, S. Y., and Dapretto, M. (2012). Altered integration of speech and gesture in children with autism spectrum disorders. Brain Behav. 2, 606–619. doi: 10.1002/brb3.81
Hyvarinen, A. (1999). Fast and robust fixed-point algorithms for independent component analysis. IEEE Trans. Neural Netw. 10, 626–634. doi: 10.1109/72.761722
Isler, J. R., Martien, K. M., Grieve, P. G., Stark, R. I., and Herbert, M. R. (2010). Reduced functional connectivity in visual evoked potentials in children with autism spectrum disorder. Clin. Neurophysiol. 121, 2035–2043. doi: 10.1016/j.clinph.2010.05.004
Jemel, B., Mottron, L., and Dawson, M. (2006). Impaired face processing in autism: fact or artifact? J. Autism Dev. Disord. 36, 91–106. doi: 10.1007/s10803-005- 0050-5
Just, M. A., Cherkassky, V. L., Keller, T. A., and Minshew, N. J. (2004). Cortical activation and synchronization during sentence comprehension in high- functioning autism: evidence of underconnectivity. Brain 127, 1811–1821. doi: 10.1093/brain/awh199
Kanwisher, N., McDermott, J., and Chun, M. M. (1997). The fusiform face area: a module in human extrastriate cortex specialized for face perception. J. Neurosci. 17, 4302–4311.
Khan, S., Gramfort, A., Shetty, N. R., Kitzbichler, M. G., Ganesan, S., Moran, J. M., et al. (2013). Local and long-range functional connectivity is reduced in concert in autism spectrum disorders. Proc. Natl. Acad. Sci. U.S.A. 110, 3107–3112. doi: 10.1073/pnas.1214533110
Kylliainen, A., Braeutigam, S., Hietanen, J. K., Swithenby, S. J., and Bai- ley, A. J. (2006). Face- and gaze-sensitive neural responses in children with autism: a magnetoencephalographic study. Eur. J. Neurosci. 24, 2679–2690. doi: 10.1111/j.1460-9568.2006.05132.x
Levelt, W. J., Praamstra, P., Meyer, A. S., Helenius, P., and Salmelin, R. (1998). An MEG study of picture naming. J. Cogn. Neurosci. 10, 553–567. doi: 10.1162/089892998562960
Litvak, V., Mattout, J., Kiebel, S., Phillips, C., Henson, R., Kilner, J., et al. (2011). EEG and MEG data analysis in SPM8. Comput. Intell. Neurosci. 2011, 852961. doi: 10.1155/2011/852961
Lord, C., Risi, S., Lambrecht, L., Cook, E. H. Jr., Leventhal, B. L., Dilavore, P. C., et al. (2000). The autism diagnostic observation schedule-generic: a standard measure of social and communication deficits associated with the spectrum of autism. J. Autism Dev. Disord. 30, 205–223. doi: 10.1023/A:1005592401947
Lord, C., Rutter, M., and Le Couteur, A. (1994). Autism diagnostic interview-revised: a revised version of a diagnostic interview for caregivers of individuals with possible pervasive developmental disorders. J. Autism Dev. Disord. 24, 659–685. doi: 10.1007/BF02172145
Losh, M., Childress, D., Lam, K., and Piven, J. (2008). Defining key features of the broad autism phenotype: a comparison across parents of multiple- and single- incidence autism families. Am. J. Med. Genet. B Neuropsychiatr. Genet. 147B, 424–433. doi: 10.1002/ajmg.b.30612
Makeig, S., and Jung, T. P. (1996). Tonic, phasic, and transient EEG correlates of auditory awareness in drowsiness. Brain Res. Cogn. Brain Res. 4, 15–25. doi: 10.1016/0926-6410(95)00042-9
Maris, E., and Oostenveld, R. (2007). Nonparametric statistical test- ing of EEG- and MEG-data. J. Neurosci. Methods 164, 177–190. doi: 10.1016/j.jneumeth.2007.03.024
McCandliss, B. D., Cohen, L., and Dehaene, S. (2003). The visual word form area: expertise for reading in the fusiform gyrus. Trends Cogn. Sci. 7, 293–299. doi: 10.1016/S1364-6613(03)00134-7
McFadden, K. L., Hepburn, S., Winterrowd, E., Schmidt, G. L., and Rojas, D. C. (2012). Abnormalities in gamma-band responses to language stimuli in first- degree relatives of children with autism spectrum disorder: an MEG study. BMC Psychiatry 12:213. doi: 10.1186/1471-244X-12-213
Milne, E., Scope, A., Pascalis, O., Buckley, D., and Makeig, S. (2009). Independent component analysis reveals atypical electroencephalographic activity during visual perception in individuals with autism. Biol. Psychiatry 65, 22–30. doi: 10.1016/j.biopsych.2008.07.017
Niessing, J., Ebisch, B., Schmidt, K. E., Niessing, M., Singer, W., and Galuske, R. A. (2005). Hemodynamic signals correlate tightly with synchronized gamma oscillations. Science 309, 948–951. doi: 10.1126/science.1110948
Oberman, L. M., Hubbard, E. M., McCleery, J. P., Altschuler, E. L., Ramachandran, V. S., and Pineda, J. A. (2005). EEG evidence for mirror neuron dysfunction in autism spectrum disorders. Brain Res. Cogn. Brain Res. 24, 190–198. doi: 10.1016/j.cogbrainres.2005.01.014
Oostenveld, R., Fries, P., Maris, E., and Schoffelen, J. M. (2011). FieldTrip: open source software for advanced analysis of MEG, EEG, and invasive electrophysio- logical data. Comput. Intell. Neurosci. 2011, 156869. doi: 10.1155/2011/156869
Price, C. J., and Devlin, J. T. (2003). The myth of the visual word form area. Neuroimage 19, 473–481. doi: 10.1016/S1053-8119(03)00084-3
Rodriguez, E., George, N., Lachaux, J. P., Martinerie, J., Renault, B., and Varela, F. J. (1999). Perception's shadow: long-distance synchronization of human brain activity. Nature 397, 430–433. doi: 10.1038/17120
Roelfsema, P. R., Engel, A. K., Konig, P., and Singer, W. (1997). Visuomotor integration is associated with zero time-lag synchronization among cortical areas. Nature 385, 157–161. doi: 10.1038/385157a0
Roine, U., Roine, T., Salmi, J., Nieminen-Von Wendt, T., Leppamaki, S., Rintahaka, P., et al. (2013). Increased coherence of white matter fiber tract organization in adults with Asperger syndrome: a diffusion tensor imaging study. Autism Res. doi: 10.1002/aur.1332 [Epub ahead of print].
Rojas, D. C., Maharajh, K., Teale, P., and Rogers, S. J. (2008). Reduced neural synchronization of gamma-band MEG oscillations in first-degree relatives of children with autism. BMC Psychiatry 8:66. doi: 10.1186/1471- 244X-8-66
Rojas, D. C., Teale, P. D., Maharajh, K., Kronberg, E., Youngpeter, K., Wilson, L. B., et al. (2011). Transient and steady-state auditory gamma-band responses in first-degree relatives of people with autism spectrum disorder. Mol. Autism 2, 11. doi: 10.1186/2040-2392-2-11
Ross, B., Borgmann, C., Draganova, R., Roberts, L. E., and Pantev, C. (2000). A high-precision magnetoencephalographic study of human auditory steady-state responses to amplitude-modulated tones. J. Acoust. Soc. Am. 108, 679–691. doi: 10.1121/1.429600
Schmidt, G. L., Kimel, L. K., Winterrowd, E., Pennington, B. F., Hepburn, S. L., and Rojas, D. C. (2008). Impairments in phonological processing and nonverbal intellectual function in parents of children with autism. J. Clin. Exp. Neuropsychol. 30, 557–567. doi: 10.1080/13803390701551225
Schneider, T., and Neumaier, A. (2001). Algorithm 808: ARfit – a Matlab package for the estimation of parameters and eigenmodes of multivariate autoregressive models. ACM Trans. Math. Softw. 27, 58–65. doi: 10.1145/382043.382316
Schultz, R. T., Gauthier, I., Klin, A., Fulbright, R. K., Anderson, A. W., Volkmar, F., et al. (2000). Abnormal ventral temporal cortical activity during face discrimination among individuals with autism and Asperger syndrome. Arch. Gen. Psychiatry 57, 331–340. doi: 10.1001/archpsyc.57.4.331
Snodgrass, J. G., and Vanderwart, M. (1980). A standardized set of 260 pictures: norms for name agreement, image agreement, familiarity and visual complexity. J. Exp. Psychol. Hum. Learn. 6, 174–215. doi: 10.1037/0278-7393.6.2.174
Stroganova, T. A., Orekhova, E. V., Prokofyev, A. O., Posikera, I. N., Morozov, A. A., Obukhov, Y. V., et al. (2007). Inverted event-related potentials response to illusory contour in boys with autism. Neuroreport 18, 931–935. doi: 10.1097/WNR.0b013e32811e151b

Stroganova, T. A., Orekhova, E. V., Prokofyev, A. O., Tsetlin, M. M., Gratchev, V. V., Morozov, A. A., et al. (2012). High-frequency oscillatory response to illusory contour in typically developing boys and boys with autism spectrum disorders. Cortex 48, 701–717. doi: 10.1016/j.cortex.2011.02.016

Tager-Flusberg, H., Rogers, S., Cooper, J., Landa, R., Lord, C., Paul, R., et al. (2009). Defining spoken language benchmarks and selecting measures of expressive language development for young children with autism spectrum disorders. J. Speech Lang. Hear. Res. 52, 643–652. doi: 10.1044/1092-4388(2009/08- 0136)

Tallon-Baudry, C., and Bertrand, O. (1999). Oscillatory gamma activity in humans and its role in object representation. Trends Cogn. Sci. 3, 151–162. doi: 10.1016/S1364-6613(99)01299-1

Tallon-Baudry, C., Bertrand, O., Delpuech, C., and Pernier, J. (1996). Stimulus specificity of phase-locked and non-phase-locked 40 Hz visual responses in human. J. Neurosci. 16, 4240–4249.

Tesche, C. D., Uusitalo, M. A., Ilmoniemi, R. J., Huotilainen, M., Kajola, M., and Salonen, O. (1995). Signal-space projections of MEG data characterize both distributed and well-localized neuronal sources. Electroencephalogr. Clin. Neurophysiol. 95, 189–200. doi: 10.1016/0013-4694(95)00064-6

Traub, R. D., Spruston, N., Soltesz, I., Konnerth, A., Whittington, M. A., and Jefferys, G. R. (1998). Gamma-frequency oscillations: a neuronal popula- tion phenomenon, regulated by synaptic and intrinsic cellular processes, and inducing synaptic plasticity. Prog. Neurobiol. 55, 563–575. doi: 10.1016/S0301- 0082(98)00020-3

Uhlhaas, P. J., Roux, F., Rodriguez, E., Rotarska-Jagiela, A., and Singer, W. (2010). Neural synchrony and the development of cortical networks. Trends Cogn. Sci. 14, 72–80. doi: 10.1016/j.tics.2009.12.002

Varela, F., Lachaux, J. P., Rodriguez, E., and Martinerie, J. (2001). The brainweb: phase synchronization and large-scale integration. Nat. Rev. Neurosci. 2, 229–239. doi: 10.1038/35067550

Venter, A., Lord, C., and Schopler, E. (1992). A follow-up study of high-functioning autistic children. J. Child Psychol. Psychiatry 33, 489–507. doi: 10.1111/j.1469-7610.1992.tb00887.x

Walenski, M., Mostofsky, S. H., Gidley-Larson, J. C., and Ullman, M. T. (2008). Brief report: enhanced picture naming in autism. J. Autism Dev. Disord. 38, 1395–1399. doi: 10.1007/s10803-007-0513-y

Wallace, S., Sebastian, C., Pellicano, E., Parr, J., and Bailey, A. (2010). Face processing abilities in relatives of individuals with ASD. Autism Res. 3, 345–349. doi: 10.1002/aur.161

Wang, A. T., Lee, S. S., Sigman, M., and Dapretto, M. (2006). Neural basis of irony comprehension in children with autism: the role of prosody and context. Brain 129, 932–943. doi: 10.1093/brain/awl032

Wilson, L. B., Tregellas, J. R., Slason, E., Pasko, B. E., Hepburn, S., and Rojas, D. C. (2012). Phonological processing in first-degree relatives of indi- viduals with autism: an fMRI study. Hum. Brain Mapp. 34, 1447–1463. doi: 10.1002/hbm.22001

Wilson, T. W., Rojas, D. C., Reite, M. L., Teale, P. D., and Rogers, S. J. (2007). Children and adolescents with autism exhibit reduced MEG steady-state gamma responses. Biol. Psychiatry 62, 192–197. doi: 10.1016/j.biopsych.2006.07.002

Wong, D., Maybery, M., Bishop, D. V., Maley, A., and Hallmayer, J. (2006). Profiles of executive function in parents and siblings of individuals with autism spectrum disorders. Genes Brain Behav. 5, 561–576. doi: 10.1111/j.1601-183X.2005.00199.x Wright, B., Alderson-Day, B., Prendergast, G., Bennett, S., Jordan, J., Whitton, C., et al. (2012). Gamma activation in young people with autism spectrum disorders and typically-developing controls when viewing emotions on faces. PLoS ONE 7:e41326. doi: 10.1371/journal.pone.0041326

Yordanova, J., Kolev, V., Heinrich, H., Woerner, W., Banaschewski, T., and Rothenberger, A. (2002). Developmental event-related gamma oscillations: effects of auditory attention. Eur. J. Neurosci. 16, 2214–2224. doi: 10.1046/j.1460-9568.2002.02286.x

Zion-Golumbic, E., and Bentin, S. (2007). Dissociated neural mechanisms for face detection and configural encoding: evidence from N170 and induced gamma- band oscillation effects. Cereb. Cortex 17, 1741–1749. doi: 10.1093/cercor/bhl100

9

Functional and structural connectivity of frontostriatal circuitry in Autism Spectrum Disorder

Sonja Delmonte[1,2], Louise Gallagher[1]*, Erik O'Hanlon[3], Jane McGrath[1,2] and Joshua H. Balsters[2,4]

[1] Department of Psychiatry, Trinity College Dublin, Dublin, Ireland
[2] Trinity College Institute of Neuroscience, Trinity College Dublin, Dublin, Ireland
[3] Department of Psychiatry, Royal College of Surgeons, Dublin, Ireland
[4] Neural Control of Movement Lab, Department of Health Sciences and Technology, ETH Zurich, Zurich, Switzerland

Edited by:
Ralph-Axel Müller, San Diego State University, USA

Reviewed by:
Xiaobo Li, Albert Einstein College of Medicine, USA
Adriana Di Martino, New York University Langone Medical Center, USA

***Correspondence:**
Louise Gallagher, Department of Psychiatry, Trinity College Dublin, College Green, Dublin 2, Ireland
e-mail: lgallagh@tcd.ie

Abnormalities in frontostriatal circuitry potentially underlie the two core deficits in Autism Spectrum Disorder (ASD); social interaction and communication difficulties and restricted interests and repetitive behaviors. Whilst a few studies have examined connectivity within this circuitry in ASD, no previous study has examined both functional and structural connectivity within the same population. The present study provides the first exploration of both functional and structural frontostriatal connectivity in ASD. Twenty-eight right-handed Caucasian male ASD (17.28 ± 3.57 years) and 27 right-handed male, age and IQ matched controls (17.15 ± 3.64 years) took part in the study. Resting state functional connectivity was carried out on 21 ASD and control participants, and tractography was carried out on 22 ASD and 24 control participants, after excluding subjects for excessive motion and poor data quality. Functional connectivity analysis was carried out between the frontal cortex and striatum after which tractography was performed between regions that showed significant group differences in functional connectivity. The ASD group showed increased functional connectivity between regions in the frontal cortex [anterior cingulate cortex (ACC), middle frontal gyrus (MFG), paracingulate gyrus (Pcg) and orbitofrontal cortex (OFC)], and striatum [nucleus accumbens (NAcc) and caudate]. Increased functional connectivity between ACC and caudate was associated with deactivation to social rewards in the caudate, as previously reported in the same participants. Greater connectivity between the right MFG and caudate was associated with higher restricted interests and repetitive behaviors and connectivity between the bilateral Pcg and NAcc, and the right OFC and NAcc, was negatively associated with social and communicative deficits. Although tracts were reliably constructed for each subject, there were no group differences in structural connectivity. Results are in keeping with previously reported increased corticostriatal functional connectivity in ASD.

Keywords: Autism Spectrum Disorder, connectivity, frontostriatal, striatum, fMRI, DTI, social reward

INTRODUCTION

Frontostriatal circuitry plays an important role in social motivation, which is postulated to underlie deficits in social interaction and communication in Autism Spectrum Disorder (ASD) (Dawson et al., 2005, 2012; Chevallier et al., 2012). Aberrant BOLD responses to social rewards have been reported in a number of studies of social reward processing in ASD, providing support for this hypothesis (Scott-Van Zeeland et al., 2010; Dichter et al., 2011; Delmonte et al., 2012; Kohls et al., 2012a,b). Studies of reward and executive function also implicate frontostriatal circuitry in repetitive behavior symptoms (Langen et al., 2011a,b; Dichter et al., 2012). Additionally, functional abnormalities in frontostriatal circuitry have been reported during higher-order cognitive and sensorimotor tasks (Schmitz et al., 2006; Takarae et al., 2007; Scott-Van Zeeland et al., 2010). Therefore, abnormalities in frontostriatal circuitry may underlie the two core deficits in ASD; social interaction and communication, and restricted interests and repetitive behaviors (Langen et al., 2011a,b; Chevallier et al., 2012; Dichter et al., 2012), as well as other cognitive and motor impairments that are associated with ASD.

Frontostriatal circuitry plays a key role in a number of different processes such as emotion, motivation, cognition, and the control of movement, which work in tandem to execute goal directed behaviors (Haber, 2003). The functional variety of frontostriatal circuits can be explained to some extent by examining its cortical inputs. Frontostriatal circuits have a looped structure with cortical inputs feeding information to the striatum which in turn projects back to the cortex via the thalamus (Alexander et al., 1986, 1990). Primate studies have shown that frontostriatal projections are arranged into a number of parallel, integrative loops, with each loop comprising discrete regions of striatum, cortex, globus pallidus, substantia nigra and thalamus, and subserving specific motor, cognitive, or affective function (Groenewegen et al., 1999, 2003; Haber and Knutson, 2009). Information is primarily channelled from ventral limbic, to more dorsal cognitive and motor loops such that action decision-making is influenced by motivation and cognition (Middleton and Strick, 2000; Haber, 2003). Diffusion tensor imaging (DTI) studies indicate that corticostriatal circuitry is similarly organized into segregated and converging loops in humans (Lehéricy et al., 2004; Leh et al., 2007; Draganski et al., 2008; Verstynen et al., 2012) and resting state functional connectivity analysis of the human striatum has shown functional organization of corticostriatal loops into affective, cognitive, and motor components (Di Martino et al., 2008; Choi et al., 2012).

ASD is characterized by abnormal functional and structural connectivity (Just et al., 2004; Cherkassky et al., 2006; Alexander et al., 2007; Keller et al., 2007; Kleinhans et al., 2008; Di Martino et al., 2010; Weng et al., 2010; Langen et al., 2011a,b; Müller et al., 2011; Sato et al., 2012; Von dem Hagen et al., 2012). Despite the growing evidence implicating frontostriatal circuitry in ASD pathology, few studies have specifically examined connectivity within this circuit. In a resting state study of corticostriatal connectivity, children with ASD showed increased connectivity between the caudate and putamen and a number of cortical and subcortical regions (Di Martino et al., 2010). Only one previous DTI tractography study has examined frontostriatal structural connectivity in ASD. The ASD group showed lower fractional anisotropy (FA) in tracts connecting the putamen to the frontal cortex, and increased mean diffusivity (MD) in tracts connecting the NAcc to the frontal cortex (Langen et al., 2011a,b).

To date, no previous study has combined functional and structural MRI data from the same participants to examine the connectivity of frontostriatal circuitry in ASD. In the present study, we investigated functional connectivity between frontostriatal regions and potential white matter differences underlying group differences in functional connectivity. Group differences in connectivity were examined in relation to behavioral impairments and striatal deactivation to social rewards as previously reported in the same particpants (Delmonte et al., 2012).

METHODS

PARTICIPANTS

Twenty-eight right-handed Caucasian male ASD [mean age (*SD*) = 17.28 (3.57) years] and 27 right-handed male, age and IQ matched controls [mean age (*SD*) = 17.15 (3.64) years] took part in the MRI study. Twenty-one ASD and control participants were retained for the fMRI analysis and 22 ASD and 24 control participants were included in the DTI analysis after excluding subjects for excessive motion (movements >3 mm) or poor data quality. ASD participants were recruited through an associated genetics research programme, clinical services, schools and advocacy groups. Controls were recruited through schools, the university and volunteer websites. Ethical approval was obtained from the St. James's Hospital/AMNCH (ref: 2010/09/07) and the Linn Dara CAMHS Ethics Committees (ref: 2010/12/07). Written informed consents/assents were obtained from all participants and their parents (where under 18 years of age).

Exclusion criteria included a Full Scale IQ (FSIQ) <70, known psychiatric, neurological, or genetic disorders, a history of a loss of consciousness for more than 5 min and those currently taking psychoactive medication. Four subjects in the ASD group had a secondary diagnosis of Attention Deficit Disorder (ADD) or Attention Deficit Hyperactivity Disorder (ADHD). Controls were excluded if they had a first degree relative with ASD or scored above 50 on the Social Responsiveness Scale (SRS) (Constantino et al., 2003) or above 10 on the Social Communication Questionnaire (SCQ) (Rutter et al., 2003). The Adult prepublication version of the SRS was used with permission in cases 18 years or older (Constantino and Todd, 2005). All participants had normal, or corrected to normal, vision.

DIAGNOSTIC ASSESSMENTS AND COGNITIVE MEASURES

ASD diagnosis was confirmed using the Autism Diagnostic Observation Schedule (ADOS) (Lord et al., 1994) and the Autism Diagnostic Interview Revised (ADI-R; Lord et al., 2000). Clinical consensus diagnosis was established using DSM-IV-TR criteria and expert clinician (Louise Gallagher). FSIQ was measured using the four subtest version of the Wechsler Abbreviated Scale of Intelligence (WASI; Wechsler, 1999) or the Wechsler Intelligence scale for Children-Fourth Edition (WISC-IV; Wechsler, 2003). Performance IQ (PIQ) score was based on the Matrix Reasoning and Block Design subtests and Verbal IQ (VIQ) score on the Vocabulary and Similarities subtests.

MRI DATA ACQUISITION

A high-resolution 3D T_1-weighted MPRAGE image was acquired for each participant ($FOV = 256 \times 256 \times 160$ mm; $TR = 8.5$ ms; $TE = 3.9$ ms; acquisition time = 7.3 min; voxel size = $1 \times 1 \times 1$ mm). One hundred and fifty resting state (eyes shut) functional scans were acquired using a using a T_2^* weighted gradient echo sequence to visualize changes in the BOLD signal ($TR = 2000$ ms, $TE = 28$ ms; flip angle = 90°; $FOV = 240 \times 240$ mm; voxel size: $3 \times 3 \times 3.5$ mm, slice gap 0.35 mm; 38 slices; acquisition time = 5.06 min). Diffusion weighted data were encoded along 32 independent directions, with one non-diffusion weighted image, using a single-shot echo-planar imaging (EPI) sequence with SENSE parallel imaging scheme (SENSivitiy Encoding; $TR = 12052$ ms; $TE = 55$ ms; *B*-value 1000; slice thickness/gap FOV; slice number = 70; voxel dimensions $2 \times 2 \times 2$ mm; acquisition time 8.08 min).

STATISTICAL ANALYSIS OF BEHAVIORAL DATA

Behavioral data were analysed using SPSSv16. Two sample *t*-tests were used to examine group differences in age and IQ measures. Correlations were performed to examine relationships between structural and functional connectivity, between connectivity values and ADI-R scores and between connectivity values and striatal activation to social rewards. For correlations with the ADI-R, the DSM-5 model, which classifies ASD symptoms into social and communicative deficits (SCD) and restricted and repetitive behaviors (RRB), was used. The two factor model has been supported by a number of factor analytic studies (Boomsma et al., 2008; Frazier et al., 2008; Georgiades et al., 2012; Mandy et al., 2012). Item level data were classified into SCD or RRB symptom domains according to the two factor model reported by Georgiades et al. (2012) to create a quantitative score on each factor. Pearsons's and Spearman's rank-order correlations were used where appropriate.

FUNCTIONAL CONNECTIVITY ANALYSIS

fMRI preprocessing was carried out in SPM8 (www.fil.ion.ucl.ac.uk/spm) in Matlab, 2009a (MathWorks Inc., United Kingdom). Before preprocessing, the origin was set to the anterior commisure for both T_1-weighted and EPI Images. The images were slice-time corrected, realigned to correct for motion artifacts and co-registered to the skull stripped T_1-weighted image. Normalization to standard stereotaxic space (Montreal Neurological Institute; MNI) was performed using the ICBM EPI template and the unified segmentation approach (Ashburner and Friston, 2005). The data were then re-sliced to a voxel size of $2 \times 2 \times 2\,mm^3$. Finally, the images were smoothed using a 5 mm full-width-half-maximum (FWHM) Gaussian kernel to conform to assumptions of statistical inference using Gaussian Random Field Theory (Friston et al., 1995a,b). Given recent evidence that resting-state networks are particularly susceptible to head motion (Power et al., 2012; Van Dijk et al., 2012) independent samples t-tests were performed to ensure that groups did not differ on rotation or translation parameters [translation: mean $ASD = 0.0401$ ($SD = 0.016$), mean control $= 0.0331$ ($SD = 0.0157$) $p = 0.136$; rotation: mean ASD $= 0.0006$ ($SD = 0.00002$), mean control $= 0.0005$ ($SD = 0.00002$) $p = 0.122$] and average frame-wise displacements (see **Figure 1**) were included as covariates of no interest in the analyses as findings from a recent resting-state study indicate that this yields similar results to removing high-movement time-points (scrubbing) (Fair et al., 2012; Di Martino et al., 2013; Satterthwaite et al., 2013; Yan et al., 2013).

Functional connectivity analysis was carried out using the CONN toolbox (http://www.nitrc.org/projects/conn/) (Whitfield-Gabrieli and Nieto-Castanon, 2012). Normalized bias corrected T_1 images were generated in SPM (http://www.fil.ion.ucl.ac.uk/spm/) and segmented into gray matter, white matter, and CSF. The principle eigenvariate of the BOLD time-courses from white matter and CSF, as well as the 6 motion correction parameters were included as regressors in the analysis to remove signals associated with these factors. The data were then band pass filtered between 0.008 and 0.2 Hz as recommended by Baria et al. (2011). A hanning window was used to weight down the initial and end scans within the resting state period. Seed regions were defined within the left and right frontal cortex [including the frontal medial and orbital cortices, inferior frontal gyrus, pars opercularis and pars triangularis, frontal pole, middle, superior frontal gyrus, subcallosal cortex, cingulate gyrus-anterior division, the paracingulate gyrus, precentral gyrus, and juxtapositional lobule cortex/supplementary motor area (see **Figure 2**)]. As the amygdala provides important inputs to the striatum (Haber, 2003; Groenewegen et al., 2003; Haber and Knutson, 2009) and has been implicated in functional and structural MRI studies of ASD (Baron-Cohen et al., 2000; Schultz, 2005; Verhoeven et al., 2009; Groen et al., 2010; Greimel et al., 2012a,b; Sato et al., 2012), it was also included as a seed region in this analysis (see **Figure 3**). Target regions included the left and right caudate, putamen, and NAcc (see **Figure 3**). Masks for these regions were generated using the Harvard-Oxford probabilistic atlas in FSL (http://fsl.fmrib.ox.ac.uk/fsl/fslwiki/) and thresholded at 20%. The ROI time series were defined as the principle eigenvariate of the time series within the ROI voxels using principle component decomposition. ROI-to-ROI correlational analyses were performed between each of the seed regions in the frontal cortex and amygdala and the target regions in the striatum. Second level random effects analyses were computed to examine group differences in connectivity using a t-test with age, IQ, and frame-wise displacements included as covariates to control for the effects of these factors. Results were corrected for multiple comparisons for the target regions at the FDR threshold ($p < 0.05$).

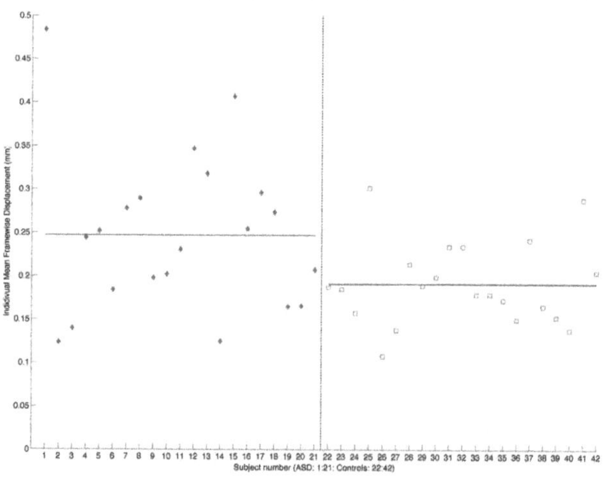

FIGURE 1 | Scatterplot showing individual mean framewise displacement. Individual subjects are shown on the x-axis and framewise displacement (mm) on the y-axis. ASD subjects are shown as gray diamonds and controls as white squares. The dashed vertical line divides the two groups. Solid horizontal lines across the ASD and Control values show the group mean.

DIFFUSION TENSOR TRACTOGRAPHY

Preprocessing of diffusion weighted data was carried out using Explore DTI (Leemans et al., 2009). The data were first screened by looping through each subjects' image to ensure that there were no gross artifacts such as signal dropout. Data were then corrected for eddy current distortions and subject motion with b-matrix rotation to preserve orientational information (Leemans and Jones, 2009). First, the diffusion-weighted images were realigned to the non-diffusion weighed (B0) image using a full affine transformation and cubic interpolation. Motion tensor values were estimated using robust estimation of tensors by outlier rejection (RESTORE; Chang et al., 2005). The RESTORE method improves tensor estimation compared to the linear and non-linear least squares methods, correcting for distortions due to fat suppression and cardiac pulsation. The final preprocessing step involved correcting for physically implausible signals. The data were then visually inspected to ensure that the gradient components were in the correct orientation. Finally, participants were excluded for excessive motion (>3 mm), with 22 ASD and 24 control participants retained for further analysis.

Tractography analyses were confined to intra-hemispheric tracts between regions that showed significant group differences in functional connectivity. Whole brain tractography was carried

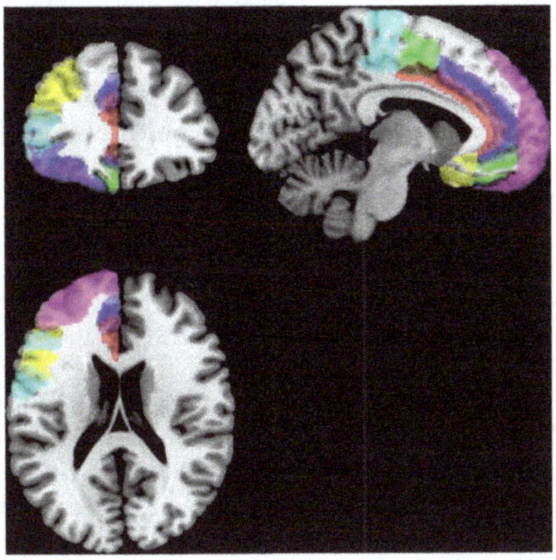

FIGURE 2 | Masks for the frontal cortex (only the left hemisphere is shown). ACC is shown in red, the OFC in blue, the MPFC in green, frontal pole in violet, IFG opercularis in yellow, IFG triangularis in cyan, juxapositional lobe in green, MFG in yellow, paracingulate in blue, precentral gyrus in light blue, SFG in grayscale and the subcallosal gyrus in yellow, displayed on the left hemisphere of a standard brain in neurological convention (left is left and right is right).

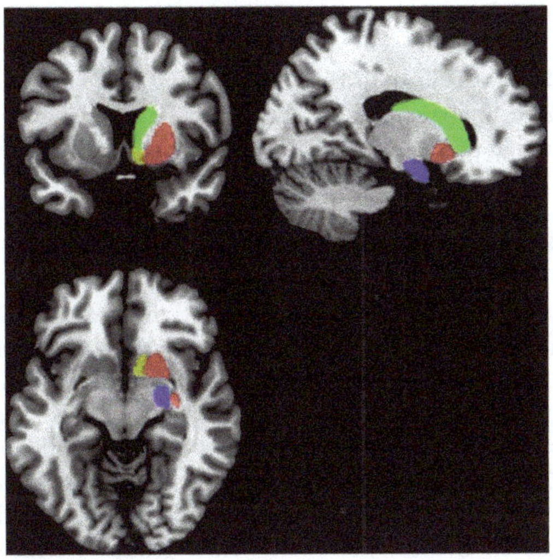

FIGURE 3 | Masks for the striatum and amygdala. The NAcc is shown in yellow, the caudate in green, the putamen in red and the amygdala in blue displayed on the right hemisphere of a standard brain in neurological convention (left is left).

out using the deterministic streamline algorithm (Basser et al., 2000) as implemented in Explore DTI (Leemans et al., 2009). Tractography was carried out in each subjects' native space using a 2 mm seed point resolution, a 1 mm step size, an angle threshold of 30° and an FA tract termination threshold of 0.2. Specific tracts of interest were then isolated using regions of interest (ROIs) with inclusive Boolean logical "AND" operators used to include tracts passing through a specific regions and exclusion "NOT"

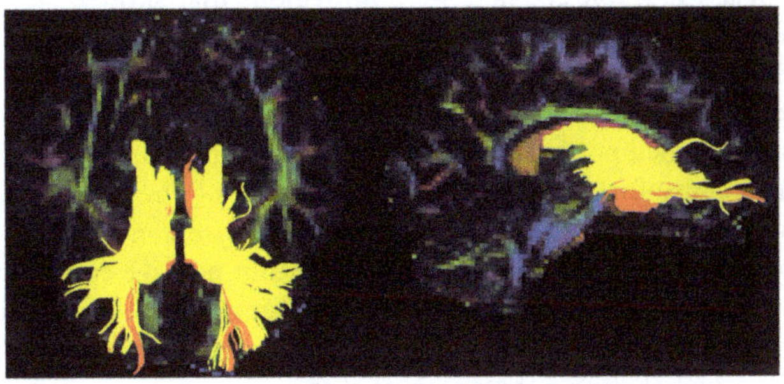

FIGURE 4 | Caudate and NAcc tracts for the template subject. Tracts are shown in the axial (left) and sagittal (right) planes in neurological convention (left is left). The caudate-prefrontal tracts are shown in yellow and NAcc-prefrontal tracts are shown in red.

operators used to exclude tracts passing through other regions. The atlas based segmentation approach was used to define ROIs in a template subject's native space (Lebel et al., 2008). These ROIs were then transformed to each subjects' native space for tractography analysis. A template subject was chosen at random as in Lebel et al. (2008). Masks of the caudate and NAcc from the Harvard-Oxford atlas, and a mask of the frontal cortex from the MNI atlas were created in FSL and thresholded at 20% in SPM8. These masks were then transformed to the template subjects native space by (i) co-registering the subjects T1 image to the subject's motion distortion corrected FA map (ii) multiplying the masks by the inverse transform parameters (MNI->Native space) generated using the segmentation option in SPM, (iii) re-slicing the masks to the same dimensions as the FA map and binarising them using the "imcalc" option in SPM. These masks were then visually inspected to ensure that they provided a good fit to the anatomical structure. Tractography analysis was carried out in the template subject using these inclusion masks (see **Figure 4**). "AND" gates were then placed at the caudate and NAcc to include only the regions from which tracts projected to the PFC. NOT gates were drawn in the planes across the midline and the posterior commisure, and to exclude motor tracts, cortico-spinal tracts, tracts from the corpus callosum and tracts to the temporal lobe. The atlas based segmentation tool was used to carry out tractography analysis in each subject's native space using the ROIs transformed into the subject specific space for each tract as this method has been successfully applied to improve tract delineation (Verhoeven et al., 2010). An upper limit of 100 mm was placed on the tract length. Outliers were excluded for each group separately for FA, MD, RD and AD values that were greater than 1.5 box lengths from the inter-quartile range. Multivariate analyses were computed to compare groups in terms of FA, MD, RD, and AD.

RESULTS

Groups did not differ in terms of age or IQ (see **Table 1**).

STRIATAL FUNCTIONAL CONNECTIVITY

Group-wise comparisons

Regions showing significantly increased functional connectivity between the frontal cortex and the striatum in the ASD group are listed in **Table 2**. There were no regions that showed significantly reduced connectivity between the frontal cortex and the striatum and there were no significant group differences in connectivity between the amygdala and striatum. Bar charts showing z-transformed r-values, adjusted for age, IQ and frame-wise displacements, for connectivity between each of the regions for which there was a significant group difference can be seen in **Figure 5**. The ASD group showed significant positive connectivity between regions for which there were significant connectivity differences between groups, whereas controls showed negative connectivity between these regions at rest, when adjusting for age, IQ and frame-wise displacements. With the exception of right MFG to NAcc connectivity, negative connectivity was no longer apparent between frontostriatal regions in controls when covariates were not included in the analysis. Within group values for regions showing significant group differences in connectivity can be seen in **Table 3**.

Correlations with social reward processing

The same participants previously completed an fMRI study of social and monetary reward processing (Delmonte et al., 2012), the results of which indicated that the ASD group showed deactivation to social rewards in the left caudate. We therefore explored whether increased connectivity between the right ACC and the left caudate in ASD was associated with deactivation to social rewards. There was a negative correlation between connectivity and SID activation in ASD but not controls (*ASD*: $r = -0.576$, $p = 0.006$; CON: $r = 0.234$; $p = 0.307$), see **Figure 6**. In the ASD group, deactivation to social rewards in the left caudate was associated with increased connectivity between the left caudate and the anterior cingulate.

Correlations with behavior

There was a positive correlation between connectivity in the right MFG and the right caudate and RRB in the ASD group ($r = 0.573$, $p = 0.008$); greater connectivity was associated with greater impairment. Connectivity between the right and left Pcg and the right NAcc was negatively correlated with SCD in the ASD group ($r = -0.511$, $p = 0.012$; $r = -0.572$; $p = 0.008$); greater connectivity was associated with less impairment. Similarly, there was a negative correlation between connectivity between the right OFC and right NAcc and SCD score in the ASD group ($r = -0.519$; $p = 0.019$). Associations between connectivity values and behavioral measures can be seen in **Figure 7**. These correlations did not withstand correction for multiple comparisons at the bonferroni level [$p_{(0.05/24)} = 0.002$]. Twenty-four correlations were performed as there were twelve regions showing significant group differences in functional connectivity and 2 behavioral measures. **Figure 7** shows plots of the correlations between connectivity values and behavioral measures in the ASD group.

Table 1 | Mean age and IQ scores.

	Autism	Controls	*P*
Age	17.28 (3.57)	17.15 (3.64)	0.545
WASI			
Full Scale IQ	109.25 (15.04)	111.85 (12.32)	0.889
Verbal IQ	108.54 (14.22)	110.52 (13.59)	0.967
Performance IQ	107.52 (14.68)	110.81 (11.11)	0.660

Standard deviations are shown in parenthesis.

Table 2 | T-scores and *p*-values for regions showing significantly increased connectivity in the ASD group, controlling for age, IQ and frame-wise displacements.

Source	Target	*T*-Value	*P*-Unc	*P*-FDR
Right cingulate gyrus, anterior division	Right accumbens	2.52	0.016	0.032
	Right caudate	2.72	0.009	0.029
	Left caudate	2.98	0.005	0.029
Right middle frontal gyrus	Right accumbens	2.68	0.011	0.044
	Right caudate	2.56	0.015	0.044
Right paracingulate gyrus	Right accumbens	3.24	0.003	0.014
	Right caudate	3.01	0.005	0.014
Right frontal orbital gyrus	Right accumbens	2.67	0.011	0.048
	Left accumbens	2.53	0.016	0.048
Left paracingulate gyrus	Right accumbens	2.92	0.006	0.018
	Right caudate	3.04	0.004	0.018
	Left caudate	2.38	0.023	0.045

STRIATAL STRUCTURAL CONNECTIVITY

Multivariate analyses with age, I.Q. and TIV entered as covariates indicated that there were no significant between group differences in FA, MD, RD, or AD in the tracts of interest.

CORRELATIONS BETWEEN STRUCTURAL AND FUNCTIONAL CONNECTIVITY

There was a significant positive correlation between AD in the right caudate to prefrontal tract and functional connectivity (raw z-scores) between the right MFG and the right caudate across the group as a whole ($r = 0.414$, $p = 0.010$), however, a within group analysis showed only a trend in the ASD group ($r = 0.445$, $p = 0.056$) and no relationship with control participants ($r = 0.214$, $p = 0.380$) indicating that the significant correlation was largely driven by variance in the ASD group. There were no other significant correlations between functional and structural connectivity.

DISCUSSION

The ASD group showed increased functional connectivity between the ACC, Pcg, OFC, and the MFG in the prefrontal cortex and the caudate and NAcc in the striatum, with group differences primarily in the right hemisphere. Increased functional connectivity between frontostriatal regions in ASD was associated BOLD deactivation to social rewards (Delmonte et al., 2012) and behavioral measures of SCD and RRB. There were no significant group differences in the structure of frontostriatal tracts. This suggests that group differences in functional connectivity, reported in the present study, may not be due to alterations in

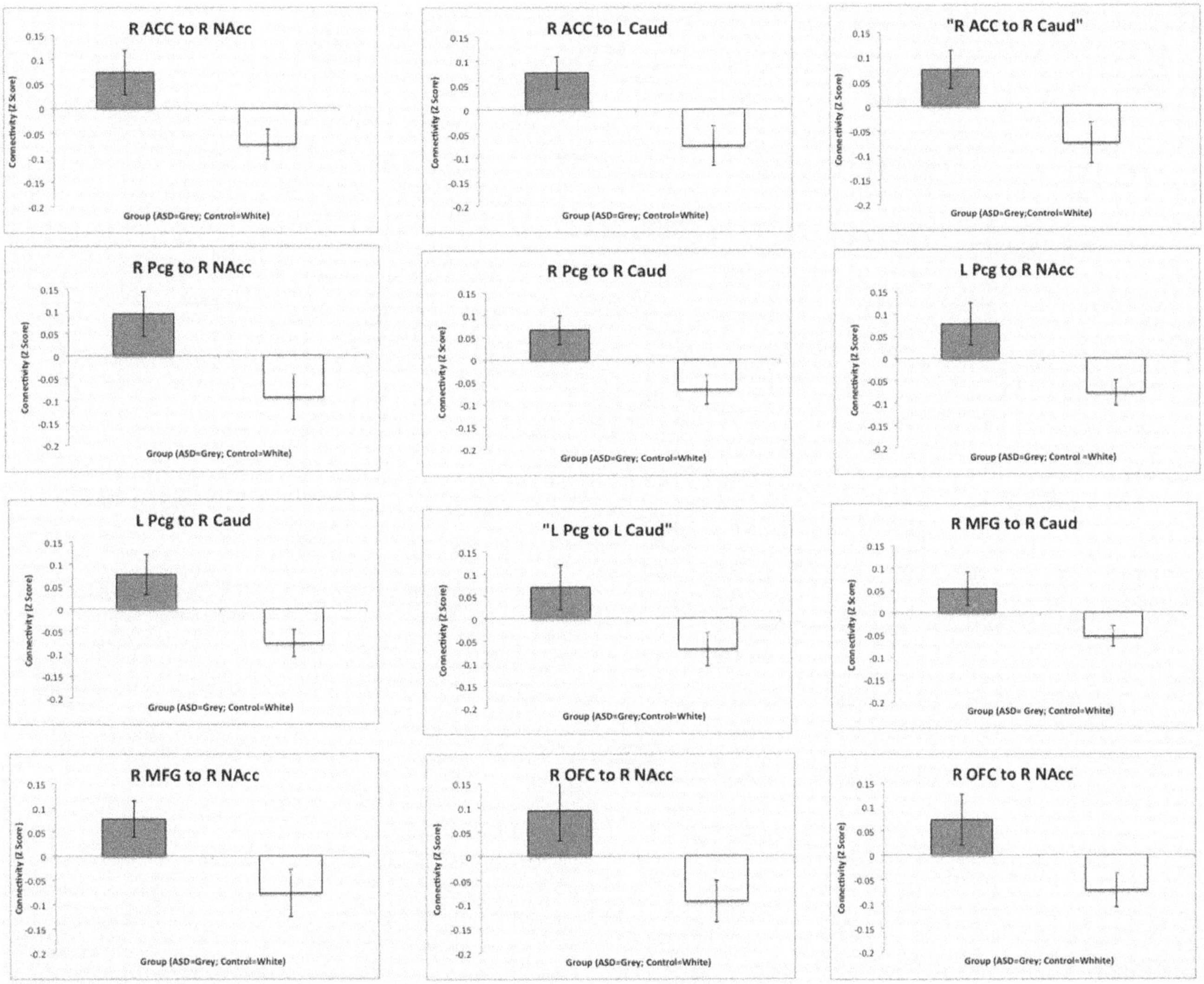

FIGURE 5 | Group differences in functional connectivity between the frontal cortex and the striatum. Bar charts show Z-transformed *R*-Values for connectivity between each of the regions for which there was a significant group difference, adjusting for age, IQ and frame-wise displacements. The ASD group is shown in gray and the controls in white with standard error of the mean displayed. R, Right; L, Left; ACC, Anterior Cingulate Cortex; MFG, Middle Frontal Gyrus; Pcg, Paracingulate Gyrus; NAcc, Nucleus Accumbens; Caud, Caudate.

frontostriatal structural connectivity in ASD, though these findings could also reflect methodological issues associated with DTI tractography.

GROUP DIFFERENCES IN FUNCTIONAL CONNECTIVITY

Hyperconnectivity between the anterior cingulate cortex (ACC) and striatum in ASD

Neuranatomical connections between the ACC and the striatum are organized in functionally distinct loops. The ventral ACC is connected to the ventral and dorsal striatum (VS and DS) and the dorsal ACC to the DS (Beckmann et al., 2009). ACC regions connected to the VS are involved in emotion, reward and pain whereas regions connected to the DS are mostly involved in motor functions, conflict/error detection and reward (Beckmann et al., 2009). The dorsal cognitive division of the ACC is connected to other regions involved in attention including the dorsolateral prefrontal cortex (dlPFC) and parietal attention regions. The rostral-ventral affective division is connected to limbic regions including the OFC, amygdala, and periaqueductal gray (PAG) (Bush et al., 2000).

Previous findings, together with the present results, suggest that hyperconnectivity between the ACC and caudate may be specific to adolescents/adults with ASD. Increased bilateral connectivity between the ACC and caudate has been reported during visuomotor performance among adults with ASD (Turner et al., 2006) but not resting state among children with ASD (Di Martino et al., 2010). ACC pathology has also been implicated more generally in functional and structural neuroimaging studies of ASD.

Table 3 | Within-groups t-scores and p-values for regions showing group differences in functional connectivity controlling for age, IQ and frame-wise displacements.

Source	Target	*T*-value	P-FDR
Right cingulate gyrus, anterior division	Right accumbens	ASD = 2.53	ASD = 0.0314
		Control = −2.35	Control = −0.0486
	Left caudate	ASD = 2.98	ASD = 0.0299
		Control = −2.76	Control = 0.0486
	Right caudate	ASD = 2.67	ASD = 0.0314
		Control = −2.36	Control = 0.049
Right middle frontal gyrus	Right accumbens	ASD = 2.73	ASD = 0.0378
		Control = −2.68	Control = 0.0355
	Right caudate	ASD = 2.62	ASD = 0.0378
		Control = −2.64	Control = 0.0355
Right paracingulate gyrus	Right accumbens	ASD = 3.29	ASD = 0.0118
		Control = −3.55	Control = 0.0006
	Right caudate	ASD = 3.07	ASD = 0.0118
		Control = −3.14	Control = 0.0009
Right frontal orbital gyrus	Right accumbens	ASD = 2.67	ASD = 0.0484
		Control = −2.47	Control = 0.07
	Left accumbens	ASD = 2.38	ASD = 0.0484
		Control = −1.91	Control = 0.09
Left paracingulate gyrus	Right accumbens	ASD = 2.98	ASD = 0.0149
		Control = −3.05	Control = 0.0247
	Right caudate	ASD = 0.3.00	ASD = 0.0149
		Control = −2.68	Control = 0.0328
	Left caudate	ASD = 2.39	ASD = 0.0436
		Control = −2.25	Control = 0.06

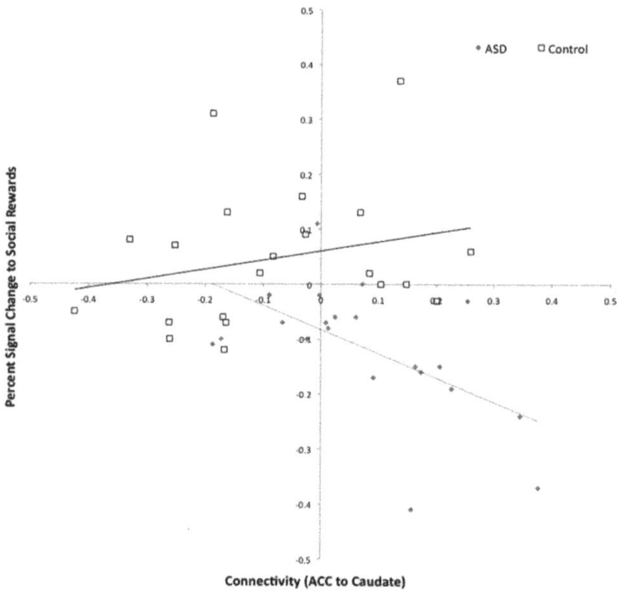

FIGURE 6 | Connectivity between the left caudate and right anterior cingulate and activation to social rewards in the left caudate. Connectivity values are shown on the *x*-axis and percent signal change for social reward feedback is shown on the *y*-axis. The ASD group is shown in gray (with dashed trend-line) and the controls in white (with solid black trend-line).

In a meta-analysis of functional neuroimaging studies, hypoactivation was reported in the perigenual ACC in ASD during social tasks and in the dorsal ACC for non-social tasks (Di Martino et al., 2009). Reduced ACC gray matter volume (Haznedar et al., 2000; Greimel et al., 2012a,b) and surface area (Hadjikhani et al., 2006; Doyle-Thomas et al., 2012), primarily in the right hemisphere, have also been reported.

Hyperconnectivity between the right ACC and the left caudate was associated with deactivation to social rewards in ASD as reported in a previous study among the same participants (Delmonte et al., 2012). This is in keeping with the role of the ACC in social perception and social cognition deficits in ASD (Di Martino et al., 2009) and with recent evidence of abnormal ACC activation during social and non-social reward processing (Dichter et al., 2011; Kohls et al., 2012a,b)—although we did not observe the latter in our previous study. Taken together these results suggest that abnormal activation in the left caudate during social reward feedback may have been due to abnormal top–down processes governed by the ACC.

Hyperconnectivity between the paracingulate (Pcg) and striatum in ASD

The Pcg is often thought of as part of the ACC (Gallagher and Frith, 2003; Walter et al., 2005), though it is anatomically, and perhaps functionally, distinct from the ACC (Gallagher and Frith, 2003). Diffusion MRI data in humans indicates that it is connected to the VS and DS and the dorsal prefrontal cortex (Beckmann et al., 2009). The Pcg is involved in emotion, social interaction, reward and decision-making, conflict monitoring and error detection (Vogt, 2005; Amodio and Frith, 2006; Beckmann et al., 2009). The anterior Pcg, along with the superior temporal sulci and the temporal poles, plays an important role in theory of mind (Gallagher and Frith, 2003; Walter et al., 2005) with activation modulated by the amount of social interaction involved in the task (Walter et al., 2004). The Pcg and striatum are thought to be involved in separate phases of decision-making, with the Pcg involved in action selection and the VS responding to positive outcomes (Rogers et al., 2004).

Previous functional connectivity studies of the striatum in ASD have not implicated the Pcg (Turner et al., 2006; Di Martino et al., 2010), however, reduced connectivity between the Pcg and the intraparietal sulcus during working memory task performance (Koshino et al., 2005) and reduced connectivity with the IFG during sentence comprehension have been reported in ASD (Just et al., 2004). Additionally, reduced Pcg activation during theory of mind tasks (Kana et al., 2009) and reduced gray matter volume in the right Pcg (Abell et al., 1999) have been reported. In the present study increased connectivity between the Pcg and the NAcc was negatively associated with SCD deficits, suggesting that increased connectivity between these regions in people with high functioning ASD could reflect a compensatory mechanism.

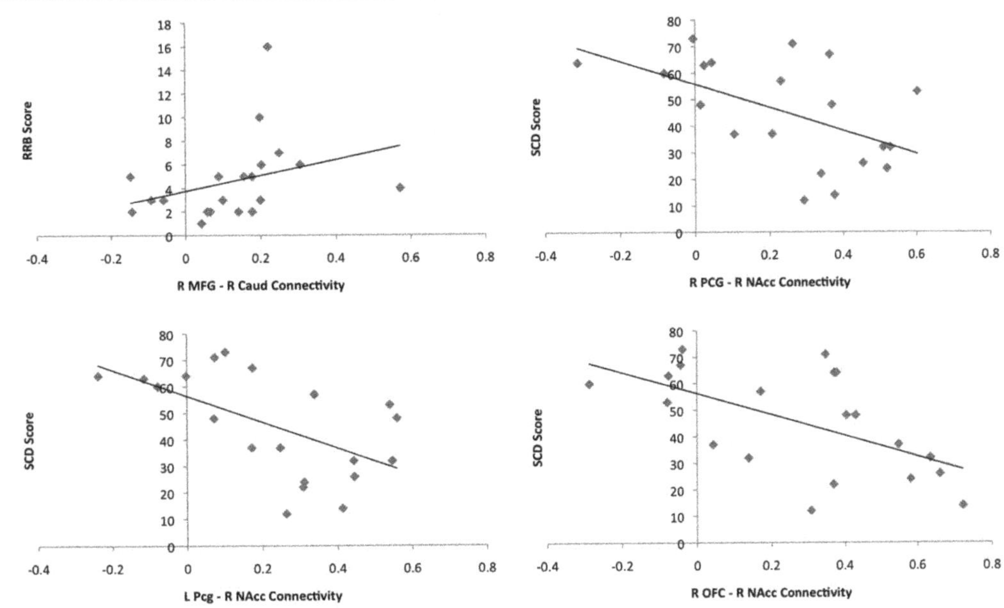

FIGURE 7 | Plots of the correlations between connectivity values and behavioral measures for the ASD group. Connectivity values are shown on the x-axes and scores on the behavioral measures on the y-axes. ASD single subjects are represented as gray diamonds (solid black trend-line).

Hyperconnectivity between the middle frontal gyrus (MFG) and striatum in ASD

The MFG, along with part of the SFG, comprises the dlPFC (Barbas and Pandya, 1989; Badre and D'Esposito, 2009; Yeterian et al., 2012), which is connected to the rostral dorsolateral caudate as well as the OFC and medial prefrontal cortex (mPFC) (Haber, 2003; Lehéricy et al., 2004; Leh et al., 2007; Draganski et al., 2008). The dlPFC is involved in a host of executive functions including working memory, set-shifting, rule learning, and planning (Goldman-Rakic et al., 1996; Leung et al., 2002; Badre and D'Esposito, 2009) and is thought to work together with the caudate to mediate these functions (Haber, 2003; Pasupathy and Miller, 2005). In terms of rule-learning, rewarded associations are thought to be identified in the striatum, which trains slower learning mechanisms in the dlPFC (Pasupathy and Miller, 2005). The dlPFC is involved in rule-learning via reinforcement; once the rule has been acquired, the dlPFC is no longer required and action execution is controlled by the premotor cortex (Badre and D'Esposito, 2009).

As in previous studies of striatal connectivity (Turner et al., 2006; Di Martino et al., 2010), there was a significant increase in connectivity between the caudate and MFG in ASD. In addition, the ASD group showed hyperconnectivity between the MFG and the NAcc. This is in keeping with a body of evidence implicating the MFG/dlPFC in ASD. Decreased functional connectivity has been reported between the dlPFC and the visuospatial regions in the occipital and parietal lobes during visuospatial processing (Damarla et al., 2010). ASD subjects also show less negative correlation between the dlPFC and amygdala during passive viewing of emotional facial expressions (Rudie et al., 2011) and increased regional homogeneity (local synchronization of the BOLD signal) in the right MFG during rest (Paakki et al., 2010). Reduced activation in the dlPFC during social and non-social information processing, including spatial working memory (Luna et al., 2002), sustained attention (Christakou et al., 2012) and memory encoding of social information have been recorded (Greimel et al., 2012a,b) as well as abnormal involvement in tasks such as gaze perception (Vaidya et al., 2011). In addition, increased gray matter volume (Ecker et al., 2012) and neuronal number (Courchesne et al., 2011) indicate structural abnormalities in the dlPFC in ASD.

Connectivity between the right MFG and right caudate was associated with increased RRB. This in keeping with previous literature implicating the frontostriatal circuitry, particularly the caudate and MFG/dlPFC, in executive function and repetitive behavior deficits in ASD (Hollander et al., 2005; Rojas et al., 2006; Estes et al., 2011; Langen et al., 2011a; Ecker et al., 2012) and suggests that cognitive as opposed to sensorimotor circuitry is implicated in repetitive behaviors in high functioning ASD.

Hyperconnectivity between the orbitofrontal cortex (OFC) and striatum in ASD

The OFC is involved emotion, motivation and reward, and is the region of prefrontal cortex most often associated with reward-guided decision-making, subserving both sensory and abstract reward processing (Haber, 2003; Haber and Knutson, 2009; Rushworth et al., 2011). Specifically, OFC activity is thought to reflect signal valuation, for both rewards and punishments, tracking expected reward value prior to decision-making and the received reward value after a choice has been made (Rushworth et al., 2011). Efferent connections from the OFC provide input to the VS, with the VS also receiving input from the amygdala and hypothalamus (Haber, 2003; Draganski et al., 2008). The OFC, together with the VS and amygdala, is thought to compute the salience value of social stimuli, with this circuitry playing a potential role in social motivation deficits in ASD (Chevallier et al., 2012; Kohls et al., 2012a,b).

Previous fMRI studies have indicated abnormal activation of the OFC, VS and amygdala during both social and non-social reward processing in ASD (Scott-Van Zeeland et al., 2010; Dichter et al., 2011, 2012; Kohls et al., 2012a,b), providing support for the hypothesized role of these regions in social motivation difficulties in ASD. Additionally, structural alterations have been recorded in the OFC in ASD, including decreased gray matter volume (Ecker et al., 2012), increased cortical thickness (Hyde et al., 2010) and altered sulcogyral morphology (Watanabe et al., 2013). Previous examinations of frontostriatal functional connectivity in ASD have not specifically implicated abnormal OFC—VS connectivity (Turner et al., 2006; Di Martino et al., 2010). The results of the present study indicated that increased connectivity between the OFC and NAcc was associated with fewer SCD deficits, suggesting that increased connectivity between these regions may function to reduce social difficulties among adolescents/young adults with high-functioning ASD.

FRONTOSTRIATAL STRUCTURAL CONNECTIVITY

There were no significant group differences in white matter microstructure (FA, MD, RD, AD) in tracts connecting the caudate or NAcc to the prefrontal cortex. Only one previous study has specifically examined microstructural integrity of frontostriatal circuits. Greater MD was reported in projections between the right NAcc and prefrontal cortex but not in projections between the caudate and prefrontal cortex among adults with ASD (Langen et al., 2011a,b). The disparity between the present findings and those of Langen et al. (2011a,b) could be due to age differences between the samples, with the sample in the present study being younger than those previously examined. The difference between structural and functional connectivity findings in the present study, with significant group differences for functional data but not structural data, may be due to several factors. Resting state connectivity analysis is not anatomically constrained therefore differences in connections between the striatum and PFC could potentially arise from structural alterations in another part of the circuit, for example in fiber pathways connecting the striatum and pallidum, pallidum and thalamus, or thalamus and cortex. Frontostriatal connections may be characterized by topographical reorganization of fiber pathways in ASD rather than microstructural alterations. This could be explored using connectivity based classification methods (Behrens et al., 2007). Another potential explanation is that structural data may be less sensitive to group differences than functional data (Finger et al., 2012) or that subtle white matter differences may remain undetected by the typical "tract averaged" approach used in most tractography studies and may require the use of "tract resampling" techniques to capture more subtle variations over the length of a tract (Colby et al., 2012). Finally, with the exception of a significant correlation between functional connectivity between the right caudate and MFG, and AD in the right caudate to prefrontal tract, measures of functional connectivity were unrelated to structural metrics in the present study. Greater concordance between functional and structural connectivity metrics may be obtained by examining specific loops (i.e., cingulo-striatal loops or dlPFC-striatal loops) in frontostriatal circuitry rather than connections between the striatum and the entire frontal cortex. It is likely that such analyses would require high-resolution diffusion imaging (HARDI) data and advanced modeling techniques such as constrained spherical deconvolution (CSD) rather than the tensor model used here.

LIMITATIONS AND FUTURE DIRECTIONS

The results of the present study should be interpreted in the light of several methodological issues. We did not replicate previous findings showing positive functional connectivity between frontostriatal regions, for example between the MFG and the caudate, in our control group (Di Martino et al., 2008). This is perhaps due to developmental factors related to the age range of the participants in the present study. Indeed negative connectivity between frontostriatal regions in controls was no longer apparent when covariates were not included in the analyses. Another potential explanation is that Di Martino et al. (2008) divided the caudate into ventral and dorsal regions, which showed distinct patterns of connectivity with sub-regions of the ACC and dlPFC, whereas we examined connectivity using gross morphological boundaries. Examining connectivity across entire structures in the current study may have obscured functional relationships between sub-regions of these structures. This can be circumvented to some extent by using a seed-to-voxel approach rather than the ROI-to-ROI approach taken in this study. However, the seed-to-voxel approach also requires a significantly greater number of statistical comparisons, which can potentially lead to Type II errors (false negatives). Given that ASD is a functionally heterogeneous population and this study has a relatively small sample size ($N = 21$), the ROI-to-ROI approach used in the present study is likely to have been more sensitive to group differences. Recent studies have shed light on the topography of functional and structural connections within the striatum (Robinson et al., 2012; Verstynen et al., 2012; Tziortzi et al., 2013) which may be useful in defining seed regions for future studies of functional and anatomical connections in frontostriatal circuitry in ASD.

A limitation of functional connectivity methods used in the present study is that one cannot infer the source of differences in functional connectivity. Frontostriatal loops are part of larger circuitry which also involve thalamo-cortical connections (Haber and Knutson, 2009). Increased connectivity between the thalamus and frontal cortical regions has been reported in ASD (Mizuno et al., 2006), indicating that thalamo-cortical circuitry is also abnormal in ASD, which could impact on frontostriatal circuitry. Given the looped structure of cortico-striatal-thalamo-cortical connections (Alexander et al., 1986, 1990), and various regulatory influences on this circuitry (Haber and Knutson, 2009), it is difficult to infer at what point dysregulation occurs, i.e., in the frontal cortex, the thalamus, the striatum, other regulatory subcortical structures, or in specific connections between these structures. We did not examine the connectivity of the midbrain—which provides important dopaminergic input to the striatum (Schultz et al., 1997; Haber and Knutson, 2009)—due to the fact that the midbrain is particularly susceptible to artifacts from cardiac (Greitz et al., 1992; Dagli et al., 1999) and respiratory (Raj et al., 2001) signals. Future studies could examine midbrain function in ASD using optimized fMRI methods (Limbrick-Oldfield et al., 2012), could include additional ROIs in regions such as the midbrain and thalamus, and could use effective connectivity modeling techniques to more fully characterize connectivity within frontostriatal circuitry (and potentially shed light on the source of hyperconnectivity in this circuit) in ASD.

The lack of group differences in structural connectivity should be interpreted in the light of several factors. Firstly, DTI is associated with a number of confounds (Jones, 2010). The tensor model cannot characterize diffusion in regions of complex fiber architecture, or "crossing fibers" where fibers kiss, twist, splay kink, or bend (Basser et al., 2000; Frank, 2001; Tuch, 2004; Jones, 2010). This is an important issue given that crossing fibers are thought to make up to 90% of white matter (Jeurissen et al., 2012). Tensor derived metrics are also influenced by acquisition parameters, such as the *b*-value (Vos et al., 2012), which may further confound results. Improved understanding of brain structural connectivity in ASD will therefore require the use of HARDI methods such as CSD tractography. Another potential concern is that the presence of subtle differences along white matter fiber tract may remain undetected as the diffusion metrics are typically averaged along the entire tract segment under investiagtion, thus masking subtle and highly localized regions of effect. Emerging tractography techniques that assess variations in the diffuison meteric along the tract using a "tract resampling mechanism" have been shown to potentially increase the sensitivity of analyses to the presence of very subtle but important white matter fiber differences (Colby et al., 2012). Again the use of HARDI methods may provide futher insight into more subtle stuctural differences in ASD. Another potential methodological issue is that the age range of the participants in the present study may have introduced heterogeneity in the data due to ongoing developmental processes, which could have reduced power to detect group differences. Previous studies suggest that both gray and white matter undergo different developmental trajectories in ASD (Carper et al., 2002; Keller et al., 2007; Langen et al., 2009; Cheng et al., 2010; Mak-Fan et al., 2012), therefore future studies should use tighter age ranges to limit heterogeneity for group-wise comparisons. Finally, the size of the sample in the present study may have reduced power to detect potential group differences in structural connectivity.

Interestingly, hyperconnectivity between the PFC and the striatum was primarily lateralized to the right hemisphere in the present study. This is in keeping with evidence that differences in the structure and function of the ACC are largely lateralized to the right hemisphere (Haznedar et al., 2000; Bejjani et al., 2012; Dichter et al., 2012; Joshi et al., 2012), that increased gray and white matter volume asymmetries are lateralized to the right hemisphere (Herbert et al., 2005) and that regional homoegeneity, a measure of functional connectivity thought to index local synchrony in the BOLD signal, is primarily lateralized to the right hemisphere in ASD (Liu et al., 2008; Paakki et al., 2010). Future studies may wish to further examine potential hemispheric asymmetries in functional and structural connectivity in ASD.

CONCLUSIONS

These results are in line with previous reports of increased functional connectivity between the striatum and frontal, temporal and parietal lobes as well as the pons in ASD (Turner et al., 2006; Di Martino et al., 2010). In the present study, hyperconnectivity was confined to limbic and associative frontostriatal circuits. Unlike previous studies (Di Martino et al., 2010), there were no group differences in sensorimotor loops. These findings add to a growing body of literature indicating significant increases as well as decreases in functional connectivity in ASD and do not support general under-connectivity accounts (Just et al., 2007), but suggest that ASD is characterized by complex functional re-organization which also involves hyperconnectivity within certain circuits. Increased functional connectivity in frontostriatal circuitry was associated with behavioral characteristics of ASD in terms of social interaction and communication and restricted interests/repetitive behaviors, as well as deactivation to social rewards in the striatum. There were no differences in structural connectivity as measured by DTI. This suggests that differences in functional connectivity were not detectable by DTI tractography in frontostriatal white matter but further research using advanced CSD based tractography is needed to clarify if subtle structural abnormalities exist in this region.

ACKNOWLEDGMENTS

We would like to thank all of the participants and their families who kindly took part in this study.

REFERENCES

Abell, F., Krams, M., Ashburner, J., Passingham, R., Friston, K., Frackowiak, R., et al. (1999). The neuroanatomy of autism: a voxel-based whole brain analysis of structural scans. *Neuroreport* 10, 1647–1651. doi: 10.1097/00001756-199906030-00005

Alexander, A., Lee, J. E., Lazar, M., Boudos, R., DuBray, M. B., Oakes, T. R., et al. (2007). Diffusion tensor imaging of the corpus callosum in autism. *Neuroimage* 34, 61–73. doi: 10.1016/j.neuroimage.2006.08.032

Alexander, E. G., Crutcher, M. D., and DeLong, M. R. (1990). Basal ganglia-thalamocortical circuits: parallel substrates for motor, oculomotor, 'prefrontal' and 'limbic' functions. *Prog. Brain Res.* 85, 119–146. doi: 10.1016/S0079-6123(08)62678-3

Alexander, E. G., DeLong, M. R., and Strick, P. L. (1986). Parallel organization of functionally segregated circuits linking basal ganglia and cortex. *Annu. Rev. Neurosci.* 9, 357–381. doi: 10.1146/annurev.ne.09.030186.002041

Amodio, D. M., and Frith, C. D. (2006). Meeting of minds: the medial frontal cortex and social cognition. *Nat. Rev. Neurosci.* 7, 268–277. doi: 10.1038/nrn1884

Ashburner, J., and Friston, K. J. (2005). Unified Segmentation. *Neuroimage* 26, 839–851. doi: 10.1016/j.neuroimage.2005.02.018

Badre, D., and D'Esposito, M. (2009). Is the rostro-caudal axis of the frontal lobe hierarchical? *Nat. Rev. Neurosci.* 10, 659–669.

Barbas, H., and Pandya, D. N. (1989). Architecture and intrinsic connections of the prefrontal cortex in the rhesus monkey.

J. Comp. Neurol. 286, 353–375. doi: 10.1002/cne.902860306

Baria, A. T., Baliki, M. N., Parrish, T., and Apkarian, A. V. (2011). Anatomical and functional assemblies of brain BOLD oscillations. *J. Neurosci.* 31, 7910–7919. doi: 10.1523/JNEUROSCI.1296-11.2011

Baron-Cohen, S., Ring, H. A., Bullmore, E. T., Wheelwright, S., Ashwin, C., and Williams, S. C. R. (2000). The amygdala theory of autism. *Neurosci. Biobehav. Rev.* 24, 355–364. doi: 10.1016/S0149-7634(00)00011-7

Basser, J. P., Pajevic, S., Pierpaoli, C., Duda, J., and Aldroubi, A. (2000). *In vivo* fiber tractography using DT-MRI data. *Magn. Reson. Med.* 44, 625–632.

Beckmann, M., Johansen-Berg, H., and Rushworth, M. F. S. (2009). Connectivity-based parcellation of human cingulate cortex and its relation to functional specialization. *J. Neurosci.* 29, 1175–1190. doi: 10.1523/JNEUROSCI.3328-08.2009

Behrens, J. T. E., Berg, J. H., Jbabdi, S., Rushworth, M. F. S., and Woolrich, M. W. (2007). Probabilistic diffusion tractography with multiple fibre orientations: what can we gain? *Neuroimage* 34, 144–155.

Bejjani, A., O'Neill, J., Kim, J. A., Frew, A. J., Yee, V. W., Ly, R., et al. (2012). Elevated glutamatergic compounds in pregenual anterior cingulate in pediatric autism spectrum disorder demonstrated by 1H MRS and 1H MRSI. *PLoS ONE* 7:e38786. doi: 10.1371/journal.pone.0038786

Boomsma, A., Van Lang, N. D. J., De Jonge, M. V., De Bildt, A. A., Van Engeland, H., and Minderaa, R. B. (2008). A new symptom model for autism cross-validated in an independent sample. *J. Child Psychol. Psychiatry* 49, 809–816. doi: 10.1111/j.1469-7610.2008.01897.x

Bush, G., Luu, P., and Posner, M. I. (2000). Cognitive and emotional influences in anterior cingulate cortex. *Trends Cogn. Sci.* 4, 215–222. doi: 10.1016/S1364-6613(00)01483-2

Carper, R. A., Moses, P., Tigue, Z. D., and Courchesnes, E. (2002). Cerebral lobes in autism: early hyperplasia and abnormal age effects. *Neuroimage* 16, 1038–1051. doi: 10.1006/nimg.2002.1099

Chang, L.-C., Jones, D. K., and Pierpaoli, C. (2005). RESTORE: robust estimation of tensors by outlier rejection. *Magn. Reson. Med.* 53, 1088–1095. doi: 10.1002/mrm.20426

Cheng, Y., Chou, K.-H., Chen, I.-Y., Fan, Y.-T., Decety, J., and Lin, C.-P. (2010). Atypical development of white matter microstructure in adolescents with autism spectrum disorders. *Neuroimage* 50, 873–882. doi: 10.1016/j.neuroimage.2010.01.011

Cherkassky, V. L., Kana, R. K., Keller, T. A., and Just, M. A. (2006). Functional connectivity in a baseline resting-state network in autism. *Neuroreport* 17, 1687–1690. doi: 10.1097/01.wnr.0000239956.45448.4c

Chevallier, C., Kohls, G., Troiani, V., Brodkin, E. S., and Schultz, R. T. (2012). The social motivation theory of autism. *Trends Cogn. Sci.* 16, 231–239. doi: 10.1016/j.tics.2012.02.007

Choi, E. Y., Yeo, B. T. T., and Buckner, R. L. (2012). The organization of the human striatum estimated by intrinsic functional connectivity. *J. Neurophysiol.* 108, 2242–2263. doi: 10.1152/jn.00270.2012

Christakou, A., Murphy, C. M., Chantiluke, K., Cubillo, A. I., Smith, A. B., Giampietro, V., et al. (2012). Disorder-specific functional abnormalities during sustained attention in youth with attention deficit hyperactivity disorder (ADHD) and with autism. *Mol. Psychiatry* 18, 236–244. doi: 10.1038/mp.2011.185

Colby, J. B., Soderberg, L., Lebel, C., Dinov, I. D., Thompson, P. M., and Sowell, E. R. (2012). Along-tract statistics allow for enhanced tractography analysis. *Neuroimage* 59, 3227–3242. doi: 10.1016/j.neuroimage.2011.11.004

Constantino, J. N., Davis, S. A., Todd, R. D., Schindler, M. K., Gross, M. M., Brophy, S. L., et al. (2003). Validation of a brief quantitative measure of autistic traits: comparison of the social responsiveness scale with the autism diagnostic interview-revised. *J. Autism Dev. Disord.* 33, 427–433. doi: 10.1023/A:1025014929212

Constantino, J. N., and Todd, R. D. (2005). Intergenerational transmission of subthreshold autistic traits in the general population. *Biol. Psychiatry* 57, 655–660. doi: 10.1016/j.biopsych.2004.12.014

Courchesne, E., Mouton, P. R., Calhoun, M. E., Semendeferi, K., Ahrens-Barbeau, C., Hallet, M. J., et al. (2011). Neuron number and size in prefrontal cortex of children with autism. *JAMA* 306, 2001–2010. doi: 10.1001/jama.2011.1638

Dagli, M. S., Ingeholm, J. E., and Haxby, J. V. (1999). Localization of cardiac-induced signal change in fMRI. *Neuroimage* 9, 407–415. doi: 10.1006/nimg.1998.0424

Damarla, S. R., Keller, T. A., Kana, R. K., Cherkassky, V. L., Williams, D. L., Minshew, N. J., et al. (2010). Cortical underconnectivity coupled with preserved visuospatial cognition in autism: evidence from an fMRI study of an embedded figures task. *Autism Res.* 3, 273–279. doi: 10.1002/aur.153

Dawson, G., Bernier, R., and Ring, R. H. (2012). Social attention: a possible early indicator of efficacy in autism clinical trials. *J. Neurodev. Disord.* 4, 11.

Dawson, G., Webb, S. J., and McPartland, J. (2005). Understanding the nature of face processing impairment in autism: insights from behavioral and electrophysiological studies. *Dev. Neuropsychol.* 27, 403–424. doi: 10.1207/s15326942dn2703_6

Delmonte, S., Balsters, J. H., McGrath, J., Fitzgerald, J., Brennan, S., Fagan, A. J., et al. (2012). Social and monetary reward processing in autism spectrum disorders. *Mol. Autism* 3, 7.

Dichter, S., Felder, J. N., Green, S. R., Rittenberg, A. M., Sasson, N. J., and Bodfish, J. W. (2012). Reward circuitry function in autism spectrum disorders. *Soc. Cogn. Affect. Neurosci.* 7, 160–172. doi: 10.1093/scan/nsq095

Dichter, S., Richey, J. A., Rittenberg, A. M., Sabatino, A., and Bodfish, J. W. (2011). Reward circuitry function in autism during face anticipation and outcomes. *J. Autism Dev. Disord.* 42, 147–160. doi: 10.1007/s10803-011-1221-1

Di Martino, A., Kelly, C., Grzadzinski, R., Zuo, X.-N., Mennes, M., Angeles Mairena, M., et al. (2010). Aberrant striatal functional connectivity in children with autism. *Biol. Psychiatry* 69, 847–857. doi: 10.1016/j.biopsych.2010.10.029

Di Martino, A., Scheres, A., Margulies, D. S., Kelly, A. M. C., Uddin, L. Q., Shehzad, Z., et al. (2008). Functional connectivity of human striatum: a resting state fMRI study. *Cereb. Cortex* 18, 2735–2747. doi: 10.1093/cercor/bhn041

Di Martino, A., Yan, C.-G., Li, Q., Denio, E., Castellanos, F. X., Alaerts, K., et al. (2013). The autism brain imaging data exchange: towards large-scale evaluation of the intrinsic brain architecture in autism. *Mol. Psychiatry.* doi: 10.1038/mp.2013.78. [Epub ahead of print].

Di Martino, A., Ross, K., Uddin, L. Q., Sklar, A. B., Castellanos, F. X., and Milham, M. P. (2009). Functional brain correlates of social and nonsocial processes in autism spectrum disorders: an activation likelihood estimation meta-analysis. *Biol. Psychiatry* 65, 63–74. doi: 10.1016/j.biopsych.2008.09.022

Doyle-Thomas, K. A. R., Kushki, A., Duerden, E. G., Taylor, M. J., Lerch, J. P., Soorya, L. V., et al. (2012). The effect of diagnosis, age, and symptom severity on cortical surface area in the cingulate cortex and insula in autism spectrum disorders. *J. Child Neurol.* 28, 729–736. doi: 10.1177/0883073812451496

Draganski, B., Kherif, F., Klöppel, S., Cook, P. A., Alexander, D. C., Parker, G. J. M., et al. (2008). Evidence for segregated and integrative connectivity patterns in the human basal ganglia. *J. Neurosci.* 28, 7143–7152. doi: 10.1523/JNEUROSCI.1486-08.2008

Ecker, C., Suckling, J., Deoni, S. C., Lombardo, M. V., Bullmore, E. T., Baron-Cohen, S., et al. (2012). Brain anatomy and its relationship to behavior in adults with autism spectrum disorder: a multicenter magnetic resonance imaging study. *Arch. Gen. Psychiatry* 69, 195–209. doi: 10.1001/archgenpsychiatry.2011.1251

Estes, A., Shaw, D. W. W., Sparks, B. F., Friedman, S., Giedd, J. N., Dawson, G., et al. (2011). Basal ganglia morphometry and repetitive behavior in young children with autism spectrum disorder. *Autism Res.* 4, 212–220. doi: 10.1002/aur.193

Fair, D. A., Nigg, J. T., Iyer, S., Bathula, D., Mills, K. L., Dosenbach, N. U., et al. (2012). Distinct neural signatures detected for ADHD subtypes after controlling for micro-movements in resting state functional connectivity MRI data. *Front Syst. Neurosci.* 6:80. doi: 10.3389/fnsys.2012.00080

Finger, C. E., Marsh, A., Blair, K. S., Majestic, C., Evangelou, I., Gupta, K., et al. (2012). Impaired functional but preserved structural connectivity in limbic white matter tracts in youth with conduct disorder or oppositional defiant disorder plus psychopathic traits. *Psychiatry Res.* 202, 239–244. doi: 10.1016/j.pscychresns.2011.11.002

Frank, L. R. (2001). Anisotropy in high angular resolution diffusion-weighted MRI. *Magn. Reson. Med.* 45, 935–939. doi: 10.1002/mrm.1125

Frazier, W. T., Youngstrom, E. A., Kubu, C. S., Sinclair, L., and Rezai, A. (2008). Exploratory and confirmatory factor analysis of the autism diagnostic interview-revised.

J. Autism Dev. Disord. 38, 474–480. doi: 10.1007/s10803-007-0415-z

Friston, K. J., Frith, C. D., Frackowiak, R. S., and Turner, R. (1995a). Characterizing dynamic brain responses with fMRI: a multivariate approach. *Neuroimage* 2, 166–172.

Friston, K. J., Frith, C. D., Turner, R., and Frackowiak, R. S. J. (1995b). Characterizing evoked hemodynamics with fMRI. *Neuroimage* 2, 157–165.

Gallagher, H. L., and Frith, C. D. (2003). Functional imaging of 'Theory of Mind'. *Trends Cogn. Sci.* 7, 77–83. doi: 10.1016/S1364-6613(02)00025-6

Georgiades, S., Szatmari, P., Boyle, M., Hanna, S., Duku, E., Zwaigenbaum, L., et al. (2012). Investigating phenotypic heterogeneity in children with autism spectrum disorder: a factor mixture modeling approach. *J. Child Psychol. Psychiatry* 54, 206–215. doi: 10.1111/j.1469-7610.2012.02588.x

Goldman-Rakic, P. S., Cools, A. R., and Srivastava, K. (1996). The prefrontal landscape: implications of functional architecture for understanding human mentation and the central executive [and discussion]. *Philos. Trans. R. Soc. Lond. B Biol. Sci.* 351, 1445–1453. doi: 10.1098/rstb.1996.0129

Greimel, E., Nehrkorn, B., Fink, G. R., Kukolja, J., Kohls, G., Müller, K., et al. (2012a). Neural mechanisms of encoding social and Non-social context information in autism spectrum disorder. *Neuropsychologia* 50, 3440–3449. doi: 10.1016/j.neuropsychologia.2012.09.029

Greimel, E., Nehrkorn, B., Schulte-Rüther, M., Fink, G. R., Nickl-Jockschat, T., Herpertz-Dahlmann, B., et al. (2012b). Changes in grey matter development in autism spectrum disorder. *Brain Struct. Funct.* 18, 929–942. doi: 10.1007/s00429-012-0439-9

Greitz, D., Wirestam, R., Franck, A., Nordell, B., Thomsen, C., and Ståhlberg, F. (1992). Pulsatile brain movement and associated hydrodynamics studied by magnetic resonance phase imaging. The Monro-Kellie Doctrine revisited. *Neuroradiology* 34, 370–380. doi: 10.1007/BF00596493

Groen, W., Teluij, M., Buitelaar, J., and Tendolkar, I. (2010). Amygdala and hippocampus enlargement during adolescence in autism. *J. Am. Acad. Child Adolesc. Psychiatry* 49, 552–560.

Groenewegen, J. H., van den Heuvel, O. A., Cath, D. C., Voorn, P., and Veltman, D. J. (2003). Does an imbalance between the dorsal and ventral striatopallidal systems play a role in tourette's syndrome? A neuronal circuit approach. *Brain Dev.* 25(Suppl. 1), S3–S14. doi: 10.1016/S0387-7604(03)90001-5

Groenewegen, J. H., Wright, C. I., Beijer, A. V., and Voorn, P. (1999). Convergence and segregation of ventral striatal inputs and outputs. *Ann. N.Y. Acad. Sci.* 877, 49–63. doi: 10.1111/j.1749-6632.1999.tb09260.x

Haber, S. N. (2003). The primate basal ganglia: parallel and integrative networks. *J. Chem. Neuroanat.* 26, 317–330. doi: 10.1016/j.jchemneu.2003.10.003

Haber, S. N., and Knutson, B. (2009). The reward circuit: linking primate anatomy and human imaging. *Neuropsychopharmacology* 35, 4–26. doi: 10.1038/npp.2009.129

Hadjikhani, N., Joseph, R. M., Snyder, J., and Tager-Flusberg, H. (2006). Anatomical differences in the mirror neuron system and social cognition network in autism. *Cereb. Cortex* 16, 1276–1282. doi: 10.1093/cercor/bhj069

Haznedar, M. M., Buchsbaum, M. S., Wei, T. C., Hof, P. R., Cartwright, C., Bienstock, C. A., et al. (2000). Limbic circuitry in patients with autism spectrum disorders studied with positron emission tomography and magnetic resonance imaging. *Am. J. Psychiatry* 157, 1994–2001. doi: 10.1176/appi.ajp.157.12.1994

Herbert, M. R., Ziegler, D. A., Deutsch, C. K., O'Brien, L. M., Kennedy, D. N., Filipek, P. A., et al. (2005). Brain asymmetries in autism and developmental language disorder: a nested whole-brain analysis. *Brain* 128, 213–226.

Hollander, E., Anagnostou, E., Chaplin, W., Esposito, K., Mehmet Haznedar, M., Licalzi, E., et al. (2005). Striatal volume on magnetic resonance imaging and repetitive behaviors in autism. *Biol. Psychiatry* 58, 226–232. doi: 10.1016/j.biopsych.2005.03.040

Hyde, L. K., Samson, F., Evans, A. C., and Mottron, L. (2010). Neuroanatomical Differences in brain areas implicated in perceptual and other core features of autism revealed by cortical thickness analysis and voxel-based morphometry. *Hum. Brain Mapp.* 31, 556–566.

Jeurissen, B., Leemans, A., Tournier, J.-.D., Jones, D. K., and Sijbers, J. (2012). Investigating the prevalence of complex fiber configurations in white matter tissue with diffusion magnetic resonance imaging. *Hum. Brain Mapp.* doi: 10.1002/hbm.22099. [Epub ahead of print].

Jones, D. K. (2010). Challenges and limitations of quantifying brain connectivity *in vivo* with diffusion MRI. *Imaging* 2, 341–355. doi: 10.2217/iim.10.21

Joshi, G., Biederman, J., Wozniak, J., Goldin, R. L., Crowley, D., Furtak, S., et al. (2012). Magnetic resonance spectroscopy study of the glutamatergic system in adolescent males with high-functioning autistic disorder: a pilot study at 4T. *Eur. Arch. Psychiatry Clin. Neurosci.* doi: 10.1007/s00406-012-0369-9. [Epub ahead of print].

Just, M. A., Cherkassky, V. L., Keller, T. A., Kana, R. K., and Minshew, N. J. (2007). Functional and anatomical cortical underconnectivity in autism: evidence from an fmri study of an executive function task and corpus callosum morphometry. *Cereb. Cortex* 17, 951–961. doi: 10.1093/cercor/bhl006

Just, M. A., Cherkassky, V. L., Keller, T. A., and Minshew, N. J. (2004). Cortical activation and synchronization during sentence comprehension in high-functioning autism: evidence of underconnectivity. *Brain J. Neurol.* 127(Pt 8), 1811–1821. doi: 10.1093/brain/awh199

Kana, R. K., Keller, T. A., Cherkassky, V. L., Minshew, N. J., and Just, M. A. (2009). Atypical frontal-posterior synchronization of theory of mind regions in autism during mental state attribution. *Soc. Neurosci.* 4, 135–152. doi: 10.1080/17470910802198510

Keller, T. A., Kana, R. K., and Just, M. A. (2007). A developmental study of the structural integrity of white matter in autism. *Neuroreport* 18, 23–27. doi: 10.1097/01.wnr.0000239965.21685.99

Kleinhans, N. M., Richards, T., Sterling, L., Stegbauer, K. C., Mahurin, R., Johnson, L. C., et al. (2008). Abnormal functional connectivity in autism spectrum disorders during face processing. *Brain* 131, 1000–1012. doi: 10.1093/brain/awm334

Kohls, G., Chevallier, C., Troiani, V., and Schultz, R. T. (2012a). Social 'Wanting' dysfunction in autism: neurobiological underpinnings and treatment implications. *J. Neurodev. Disord.* 4, 10.

Kohls, G., Schulte-Rüther, M., Nehrkorn, B., Müller, K., Fink, G. R., Kamp-Becker, I., et al. (2012b). Reward system dysfunction in autism spectrum disorders. *Soc. Cogn. Affect. Neurosci.* 8, 565–572. doi: 10.1093/scan/nss033

Koshino, H., Carpenter, P. A., Minshew, N. J., Cherkassky, V. L., Keller, T. A., and Just, M. A. (2005). Functional connectivity in an fMRI working memory task in high-functioning autism. *Neuroimage* 24, 810–821. doi: 10.1016/j.neuroimage.2004.09.028

Langen, M., Durston, S., Kas, M. J. H., van Engeland, H., and Staal, W. G. (2011a). The neurobiology of repetitive behavior: ...and men. *Neurosci. Biobehav. Rev.* 35, 356–365.

Langen, M., Leemans, A., Johnston, P., Ecker, C., Daly, E., Murphy, C. M., et al. (2011b). Fronto-striatal circuitry and inhibitory control in autism: findings from diffusion tensor imaging tractography. *Cortex* 48, 183–193. doi: 10.1016/j.cortex.2011.05.018

Langen, M., Schnack, H. G., Nederveen, H., Bos, D., Lahuis, B. E., de Jonge, M. V., et al. (2009). Changes in the developmental trajectories of striatum in autism. *Biol. Psychiatry* 66, 327–333. doi: 10.1016/j.biopsych.2009.03.017

Lebel, C., Walker, L., Leemans, A., Phillips, L., and Beaulieu, C. (2008). Microstructural maturation of the human brain from childhood to adulthood. *Neuroimage* 40, 1044–1055. doi: 10.1016/j.neuroimage.2007.12.053

Leemans, A., Jeurissen, B., Sijbers, J., and Jones, D. K. (2009). "ExploreDTI: A graphical toolbox for processing, analyzing, and visualizing diffusion MR Data." in *Presented at the Proceedings 17th Scientific Meeting, International Society for Magnetic Resonance in Medicine* (Honolulu, HI).

Leemans, A., and Jones, D. K. (2009). The B−matrix must be rotated when correcting for subject motion in DTI data. *Magn. Reson. Med.* 61, 1336–1349. doi: 10.1002/mrm.21890

Leh, S. E., Ptito, A., Chakravarty, M. M., and Strafella, A. P. (2007). Fronto-striatal connections in the human brain: a probabilistic diffusion tractography study. *Neurosci. Lett.* 419, 113–118. doi: 10.1016/j.neulet.2007.04.049

Lehéricy, S., Ducros, M., Van De Moortele, P. F., Francois, C., Thivard, L., Poupon, C., et al. (2004). Diffusion tensor fiber tracking shows distinct corticostriatal circuits in humans. *Ann. Neurol.* 55, 522–529. doi: 10.1002/ana.20030

Leung, H.-C., Gore, J. C., and Goldman-Rakic, P. S. (2002). Sustained mnemonic response in the human middle frontal gyrus during on-line storage of spatial memoranda. *J. Cogn. Neurosci.* 14, 659–671. doi: 10.1162/08989290260045882

Limbrick-Oldfield, E. H., Brooks, J. C. W., Wise, R. J. S., Padormo, F., Hajnal, J. V., Beckmann, C. F., et al. (2012). Identification and characterisation of midbrain nuclei using optimised functional magnetic resonance imaging. *Neuroimage* 59, 1230–1238. doi: 10.1016/j.neuroimage.2011.08.016

Liu, Y., Wang, K., Yu, C., He, Y., Zhou, Y., Liang, M., et al. (2008). Regional homogeneity, functional connectivity and imaging markers of Alzheimer's disease: a. review of resting-state fMRI studies. *Neuropsychologia* 46, 1648–1656. doi: 10.1016/j.neuropsychologia.2008.01.027

Lord, C., Rutter, M., DiLavore, P. C., and Risi, S. (2000). Autism diagnostic observation schedule (ADOS). *J. Autism Dev. Disord.* 30, 205–233. doi: 10.1023/A:1005592401947

Lord, C., Rutter, M., and Le Couteur, A. (1994). Autism diagnostic interview[mdash]revised: a revised version of a diagnostic interview for caregivers of individuals with possible pervasive developmental disorders. *J. Autism Dev Disord* 24, 659–685. doi: 10.1007/BF02172145

Luna, B., Minshew, N. J., Garver, K. E., Lazar, N. A., Thulborn, K. R., Eddy, W. F., et al. (2002). Neocortical system abnormalities in autism an fMRI study of spatial working memory. *Neurology* 59, 834–840. doi: 10.1212/WNL.59.6.834

Mak-Fan, K. M., Morris, D., Vidal, J., Anagnostou, E., Roberts, W., and Taylor, M. J. (2012). White matter and development in children with an autism spectrum disorder. *Autism.* doi: 10.1177/1362361312442596. [Epub ahead of print].

Mandy, L. W. P., Charman, T., and Skuse, D. H. (2012). Testing the construct validity of proposed criteria for DSM-5 autism spectrum disorder. *J. Am. Acad. Child Adolesc. Psychiatry* 51, 41–50. doi: 10.1016/j.jaac.2011.10.013

Middleton, A. F., and Strick, P. L. (2000). Basal ganglia and cerebellar loops: motor and cognitive circuits. *Brain Res. Brain Res. Rev.* 31, 236–250. doi: 10.1016/S0165-0173(99)00040-5

Mizuno, A., Villalobos, M. E., Davies, M. M., Dahl, B. C., and Müller, R. (2006). Partially enhanced thalamocortical functional connectivity in autism. *Brain Res.* 1104, 160–174. doi: 10.1016/j.brainres.2006.05.064

Müller, R., Shih, P., Keehn, B., Deyoe, J. R., Leyden, K. M., and Shukla, D. K. (2011). Underconnected, but How? A survey of functional connectivity MRI studies in autism spectrum disorders. *Cereb. Cortex* 21, 2233–2243. doi: 10.1093/cercor/bhq296

Paakki, J., Rahko, J., Long, X., Moilanen, I., Tervonen, O., Nikkinen, J., et al. (2010). Alterations in regional homogeneity of resting-state brain activity in autism spectrum disorders. *Brain Res.* 1321, 169–179. doi: 10.1016/j.brainres.2009.12.081

Pasupathy, A., and Miller, E. K. (2005). Different time courses of learning-related activity in the prefrontal cortex and striatum. *Nature* 433, 873–876. doi: 10.1038/nature03287

Power, D. J., Barnes, K. A., Snyder, A. Z., Schlaggar, B. L., and Petersen, S. E. (2012). Spurious but systematic correlations in functional connectivity MRI networks arise from subject motion. *Neuroimage* 59, 2142–2154. doi: 10.1016/j.neuroimage.2011.10.018

Raj, D. A., Anderson, W., and Gore, J. C. (2001). Respiratory effects in human functional magnetic resonance imaging due to bulk susceptibility changes. *Phys. Med. Biol.* 46, 3331–3340. doi: 10.1088/0031-9155/46/12/318

Robinson, J. L., Laird, A. R., Glahn, D. C., Blangero, J., Sanghera, M. K., Pessoa, L., et al. (2012). The functional connectivity of the human caudate: an application of meta-analytic connectivity modeling with behavioral filtering. *Neuroimage* 60, 117–129. doi: 10.1016/j.neuroimage.2011.12.010

Rogers, D. R., Ramnani, N., Mackay, C., Wilson, J. L., Jezzard, P., Carter, C. S., et al. (2004). Distinct portions of anterior cingulate cortex and medial prefrontal cortex are activated by reward processing in separable phases of decision-making cognition. *Biol. Psychiatry* 55, 594–602. doi: 10.1016/j.biopsych.2003.11.012

Rojas, D., Peterson, E., Winterrowd, E., Reite, M., Rogers, S., and Tregellas, J. (2006). Regional gray matter volumetric changes in autism associated with social and repetitive behavior symptoms. *BMC Psychiatry* 6:56. doi: 10.1186/1471-244X-6-56

Rudie, J. D., Shehzad, Z., Hernandez, L. M., Colich, N. L., Bookheimer, S. Y., Iacoboni, M., et al. (2011). Reduced functional integration and segregation of distributed neural systems underlying social and emotional information processing in autism spectrum disorders. *Cereb. Cortex* 22, 1025–1037. doi: 10.1093/cercor/bhr171

Rushworth, M. F. S., Noonan, M. P., Boorman, E. D., Walton, M. E., and Behrens, T. E. (2011). Frontal cortex and reward-guided learning and decision-making. *Neuron* 70, 1054–1069. doi: 10.1016/j.neuron.2011.05.014

Rutter, M., Bailey, A., and Lord, C. (2003). *Social Communication Questionnaire.* Los Angeles, CA: Western Psychological Services.

Sato, W., Toichi, M., Uono, S., and Kochiyama, T. (2012). Impaired social brain network for processing dynamic facial expressions in autism spectrum disorders. *BMC Neurosci.* 13:99. doi: 10.1186/1471-2202-13-99

Satterthwaite, T. D., Elliott, M. A., Gerraty, R. T., Ruparel, K., Loughead, J., Calkins, M. E., et al. (2013). An improved framework for confound regression and filtering for control of motion artifact in the preprocessing of resting-state functional connectivity data. *Neuroimage* 64, 240–256. doi: 10.1016/j.neuroimage.2012.08.052

Schmitz, N., Rubia, K., Daly, E., Smith, A., Williams, S., and Murphy, D. G. M. (2006). Neural correlates of executive function in autistic spectrum disorders. *Biol. Psychiatry* 59, 7–16. doi: 10.1016/j.biopsych.2005.06.007

Schultz, R. T. (2005). Developmental deficits in social perception in autism: the role of the amygdala and fusiform face area. *Int. J. Dev. Neurosci.* 23, 125–141. doi: 10.1016/j.ijdevneu.2004.12.012

Schultz, W., Dayan, P., and Montague, P. R. (1997). A neural substrate of prediction and reward. *Science* 275, 1593–1599. doi: 10.1126/science.275.5306.1593

Takarae, Y., Minshew, N. J., Luna, B., and Sweeney, J. A. (2007). Atypical involvement of frontostriatal systems during sensorimotor control in autism. *Psychiatry Res.* 156, 117–127. doi: 10.1016/j.pscychresns.2007.03.008

Tuch, D. S. (2004). Q-ball Imaging. *Magn. Reson. Med.* 52, 1358–1372. doi: 10.1002/mrm.20279

Turner, K. C., Frost, L., Linsenbardt, D., McIlroy, J. R., and Müller, R. (2006). Atypically diffuse functional connectivity between caudate nuclei and cerebral cortex in autism. *Behav. Brain Funct.* 2, 34.

Tziortzi, A. C., Haber, S. N., Searle, G. E., Tsoumpas, C., Long, C. J., Shotbolt, P., et al. (2013). Connectivity-based functional analysis of dopamine release in the striatum using diffusion-weighted MRI and positron emission tomography. *Cereb. Cortex.* doi: 10.1093/cercor/bhs397. [Epub ahead of print].

Van Dijk, A. K. R., Sabuncu, M. R., and Buckner, R. L. (2012). The influence of head motion on intrinsic functional connectivity MRI. *Neuroimage* 59, 431–438. doi: 10.1016/j.neuroimage.2011.07.044

Scott-Van Zeeland, K., McNealy, K., Wang, A. T., Sigman, M., Bookheimer, S. Y., and Dapretto, M. (2010). No neural evidence of statistical learning during exposure to artificial languages in children with autism spectrum disorders. *Biol. Psychiatry* 68, 345–351. doi: 10.1016/j.biopsych.2010.01.011

Vaidya, J. C., Foss-Feig, J., Shook, D., Kaplan, L., Kenworthy, L., and Gaillard, W. D. (2011). Controlling attention to gaze and arrows in childhood: an fMRI. study of typical development and autism spectrum disorders. *Dev. Sci.* 14, 911–924. doi: 10.1111/j.1467-7687.2011.01041.x

Verhoeven, J., De Cock, P., Lagae, L., and Sunaert, S. (2009). Neuroimaging of autism. *Neuroradiology* 52, 3–14. doi: 10.1007/s00234-009-0583-y

Verhoeven, S. J., Sage, C. A., Leemans, A., Van Hecke, W., Callaert, D., Peeters, R., et al. (2010). Construction of a stereotaxic DTI atlas with full diffusion tensor information for studying white matter maturation from childhood to adolescence using tractography-based segmentations. *Hum. Brain Mapp.* 31, 470–486.

Verstynen, D. T., Badre, D., Jarbo, K., and Schneider, W. (2012). Microstructural organizational patterns in the human corticostriatal system. *J. Neurophysiol.* 107, 2984–2995. doi: 10.1152/jn.00995.2011

Vogt, B. A. (2005). Pain and emotion interactions in subregions of the cingulate gyrus. *Nature Rev. Neurosci.* 6, 533–544. doi: 10.1038/nrn1704

Von dem Hagen, E. A., Stoyanova, R. S., Baron-Cohen, S., and Calder, A. J. (2012). Reduced functional connectivity within and between 'social' resting state networks in autism spectrum conditions. *Soc. Cogn. Affect. Neurosci.* doi: 10.1093/scan/nss053. [Epub ahead of print].

Vos, B. S., Jones, D. K., Jeurissen, B., Viergever, M. A., and Leemans, A. (2012). The influence of complex white matter architecture on the mean diffusivity in diffusion tensor MRI of the human brain. *Neuroimage* 59, 2208–2216. doi: 10.1016/j.neuroimage.2011.09.086

Walter, H., Abler, B., Ciaramidaro, A., and Erk, S. (2005). Motivating forces of human actions. Neuroimaging reward and social interaction. *Brain Res. Bull.* 67, 368–381. doi: 10.1016/j.brainresbull.2005.06.016

Walter, H., Adenzato, M., Ciaramidaro, A., Enrici, I., Pia, L., and Bara, B. G. (2004). Understanding intentions in social interaction: the role of the anterior paracingulate cortex. *J. Cogn. Neurosci.* 16, 1854–1863. doi: 10.1162/0898929042947838

Watanabe, H., Nakamura, M., Ohno, T., Itahashi, T., Tanaka, E., Ohta, H., et al. (2013). Altered orbitofrontal sulcogyral patterns in adult males with high-functioning autism spectrum disorders. *Soc. Cogn. Affect. Neurosci.* doi: 10.1093/scan/nst016. [Epub ahead of print].

Wechsler, D. (1999). *Wechsler Abbreviated Scale of Intelligence.* San Antonio, TX: The Psychological Corporation.

Wechsler, D. (2003). *Wechsler Intelligence Scale for Children, 4th Edn (WISC-IV).* San antonio, TX: The Psychological Corporation.

Weng, S. J., Wiggins, J. L., Peltier, S. J., Carrasco, M., Risi, S., Lord, C., et al. (2010). Alterations of resting state functional connectivity in the default network in adolescents with autism spectrum disorders. *Brain Res.* 1313, 202–214. doi: 10.1016/j.brainres.2009.11.057

Whitfield-Gabrieli, S., and Nieto-Castanon, A. (2012). Conn: a functional connectivity toolbox for correlated and anticorrelated brain networks. *Brain Connect.* 2, 125–141. doi: 10.1089/brain.2012.0073

Yan, C. G., Cheung, B., Kelly, C., Colcombe, S., Craddock, R. C., Di Martino, A., et al. (2013). A comprehensive assessment of regional variation in the impact of head micromovements on functional connectomics. *Neuroimage* 76, 183–201. doi: 10.1016/j.neuroimage.2013.03.004

Yeterian, E. H., Pandya, D. N., Tomaiuolo, F., and Petrides, M. (2012). The cortical connectivity of the prefrontal cortex in the monkey brain. *Cortex* 48, 58–81. doi: 10.1016/j.cortex.2011.03.004

10

The perils of global signal regression for group comparisons: a case study of Autism Spectrum Disorders

Stephen J. Gotts[1]*, Ziad S. Saad[2], Hang Joon Jo[2], Gregory L. Wallace[1], Robert W. Cox[2] and Alex Martin[1]

[1] Section on Cognitive Neuropsychology, Laboratory of Brain and Cognition, National Institute of Mental Health, National Institutes of Health, Bethesda, MD, USA
[2] Scientific and Statistical Computing Core, National Institute of Mental Health, National Institutes of Health, Bethesda, MD, USA

Edited by:
Ralph-Axel Müller, San Diego State University, USA

Reviewed by:
Michael Milham, Child Mind Institute, USA
Jeff Anderson, University of Utah, USA

***Correspondence:**
Stephen J. Gotts, Laboratory of Brain and Cognition, National Institute of Mental Health, National Institutes of Health, Bldg. 10, Rm. 4C-217, Bethesda, MD 20892-1366, USA
e-mail: gottss@mail.nih.gov

We have previously argued from a theoretical basis that the standard practice of regression of the Global Signal from the fMRI time series in functional connectivity studies is ill advised, particularly when comparing groups of participants. Here, we demonstrate in resting-state data from participants with an Autism Spectrum Disorder and matched controls that these concerns are also well founded in real data. Using the prior theoretical work to formulate predictions, we show: (1) rather than simply altering the mean or range of correlation values amongst pairs of brain regions, Global Signal Regression systematically alters the rank ordering of values in addition to introducing negative values, (2) it leads to a reversal in the direction of group correlation differences relative to other preprocessing approaches, with a higher incidence of both long-range and local correlation differences that favor the Autism Spectrum Disorder group, (3) the strongest group differences under other preprocessing approaches are the ones most altered by Global Signal Regression, and (4) locations showing group differences no longer agree with those showing correlations with behavioral symptoms within the Autism Spectrum Disorder group. The correlation matrices of both participant groups under Global Signal Regression were well predicted by our previous mathematical analyses, demonstrating that there is nothing mysterious about these results. Finally, when independent physiological nuisance measures are lacking, we provide a simple alternative approach for assessing and lessening the influence of global correlations on group comparisons that replicates our previous findings. While this alternative performs less well for symptom correlations than our favored preprocessing approach that includes removal of independent physiological measures, it is preferable to the use of Global Signal Regression, which prevents unequivocal conclusions about the direction or location of group differences.

Keywords: functional connectivity, typically developing, artifact, resting-state fMRI, GCOR, global correlation

INTRODUCTION

Interest in the functional organization of large-scale brain circuitry in normal and disordered populations has exploded in recent years. Out of the variety of methods and techniques in use to study this organization, much effort has been focused on studies of very slow fluctuations of brain activity during rest using BOLD fMRI (see Fox and Raichle, 2007, for review). In part, resting-state studies of inter-regional brain correlations, also referred to as "functional connectivity," have proliferated because of the ease of acquiring the data. However, there are also promising potential benefits of the method for studying participant groups that are less able to perform complex behavioral tasks, including clinical populations (e.g., Fox and Greicius, 2010), human infants (e.g., Fransson et al., 2007), and animals (e.g., Vincent et al., 2007; Margulies et al., 2009).

The study of Autism Spectrum Disorders (ASD), in particular, has benefited from these methods, with a growing number of studies evaluating the hypothesis that the behavioral impairments in ASD result from abnormal brain connectivity (e.g., Castelli et al., 2002; Belmonte et al., 2004; Just et al., 2004; see Müller et al., 2011,for review). To date, most resting-state (as well as task-based) fMRI studies of ASD have found evidence of decreased correlations throughout a variety of brain regions involved in social processing (e.g., Kennedy and Courchesne, 2008; Monk et al., 2009; Assaf et al., 2010; Weng et al., 2010; Anderson et al., 2011b; Ebisch et al., 2011; Gotts et al., 2012; von dem Hagen et al., 2012). However, not all studies have found this pattern. A recent resting-state study with a relatively large participant sample ($N \approx 40$ per group) reported a mixture of increased and decreased correlations in ASD relative to typically developing (TD) control participants (Rudie et al., 2013). Another recent study, given the well-publicized concern about residual head-motion artifacts in functional connectivity studies (e.g., Deen and Pelphrey, 2012; Power et al., 2012; Van Dijk et al., 2012), carefully examined head motion artifacts and failed to find large group differences in connectivity between ASD and TD participants (Tyszka et al., 2013).

Indeed, time-varying artifacts are a large source of concern in functional connectivity studies. Major sources of artifact include head motion (e.g., Power et al., 2012; Satterthwaite et al., 2012,

2013; Jo et al., 2013; Yan et al., 2013), non-neural physiological variation resulting from cardiac and respiration cycles (e.g., Glover et al., 2000; Birn et al., 2006, 2008; Shmueli et al., 2007; Chang and Glover, 2009; Chang et al., 2009), as well as hardware artifacts (e.g., Cordes et al., 2002; Jo et al., 2010). Much recent attention has been given in the literature to the confounding impact of head motion on group differences in correlation, while much less has been given to physiological and hardware artifacts, perhaps because many researchers still do not collect the independent cardiac and respiration measures and/or utilize the analysis tools that would permit more direct examination. The goal of preprocessing steps in resting-state fMRI studies is to remove as much nuisance or "noise" variation from the time series as possible in order to allow observed correlation patterns (and group differences) to reflect the underlying neural interactions rather than non-neural artifacts. Not all preprocessing recipes are as comprehensive or direct in addressing the myriad of noise sources as others, and there is no currently accepted standard in the field for these critical noise cleaning procedures. A principal difficulty is to remove noise/artifact components of the time series data without removing neurally-derived components.

The goal of the current paper is to draw attention to the detrimental effects of the still common practice of removing the Global Signal (GS), the average time series in a whole-brain mask, from the data prior to comparing groups of participants. Multiple motivations for including the GS as a nuisance regressor have been articulated, including that it helps to remove uninteresting global fluctuations that mask circuit-level organization, that it captures global physiological artifacts that other tissue-derived measures from the ventricles or white matter fail to capture, and that it enhances the strength and reliability of experimental results (e.g., Fox et al., 2009; Keller et al., 2013). Most recently, the GS has been argued to provide additional aid in attenuating residual motion artifacts that can confound group comparisons (Satterthwaite et al., 2013; Yan et al., 2013). However, including the GS as a nuisance regressor can also have a number of undesirable effects. Its role in introducing negative correlations that are otherwise largely absent from fMRI correlations has been widely discussed (Fox et al., 2009; Murphy et al., 2009; Anderson et al., 2011a). It has also been demonstrated in monkeys that the GS in fMRI is tightly coupled with electrical neural activity (local field potential recordings) across a range of frequencies (Schölvinck et al., 2010). Removing it will therefore be expected to alter the actual pattern of neural interactions that one desires to measure, a point recently acknowledged by some of the originators of the practice (Snyder and Raichle, 2012).

Less widely discussed to date are the detrimental effects for interpreting group comparisons. In a recent paper (Saad et al., 2012), we used simulation and mathematical analyses to show the impact of GS regression on correlation patterns and group comparisons, a summary of which is provided graphically in **Figure 1**. We simulated two groups of participants, A and B, for which the circuit-level structure differed in a simple way. In Group A, three simulated patches of voxels had positive correlations within but not across patches (correlations of zero). In Group B, correlations within patches were identical to A, with the

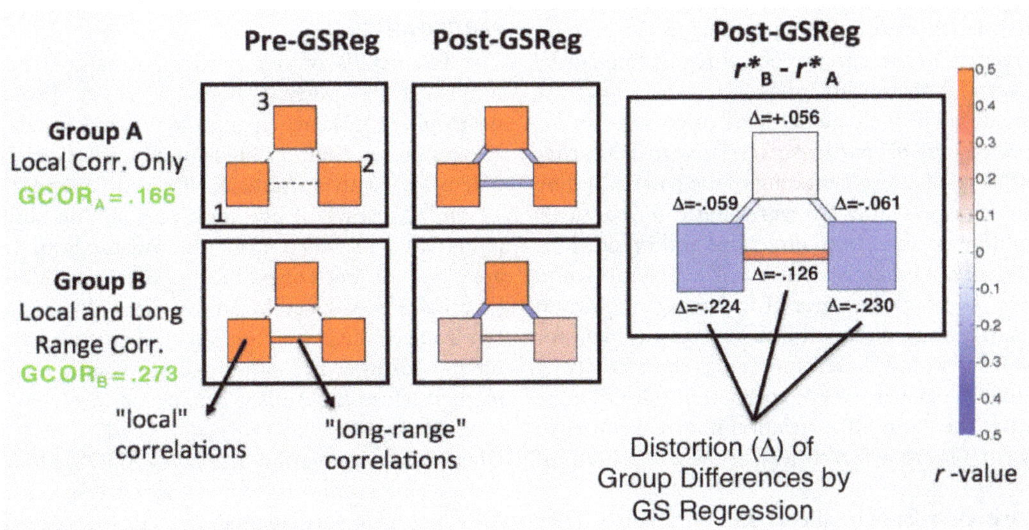

FIGURE 1 | Distortion of simulated group differences in correlation by GS regression. Adapted from Figure 4 in Saad et al. (2012), patterns of correlation are shown for two simulated groups of participants, Group A and B ($N = 30$ in each). Pre-GS regression (**left panels**), both groups have three patches of simulated voxels (counter-clockwise from lower left: patches 1, 2, and 3) that have average within-patch correlations of 0.5 (see color bar to the right). Group B also has a correlation across patches 1 and 2, with all other inter-patch correlations in both groups set to be approximately 0. The presence of the across-patch correlation in Group B leads to an overall larger level of global correlation (GCOR values shown to left in green). After GS regression (**middle panels**), negative correlations are introduced among many of the patches and a larger amount of global variation is removed from patches 1 and 2 in Group B. Significant group correlation differences (**right panel**) are then found at all locations instead of at the one appropriate location (correlation between, not within, patches 1 and 2). The appropriate group differences are most distorted (Δ) by GS regression in and between patches 1 and 2, the locations involved in the largest true differences.

only difference between groups being a positive correlation of 0.5 between patches 1 and 2. After GS regression (middle column of **Figure 1**), negative correlations were inappropriately introduced between patches for Group A, and the within-patch correlations were slightly reduced. For Group B, the presence of correlations among patches 1 and 2 led these time series to contribute relatively more to the GS than the time series in patch 3 (since they will weight into the global average more). Correspondingly, GS regression led more shared variation to be removed in patches 1 and 2, decreasing the related "local" and "long-range" correlations. In all, this procedure led to significant group differences being expressed at every location, rather than just at the single appropriate location (between patches 1 and 2) (rightmost column of **Figure 1**). The virtue of this demonstration is that the true statistics are known in all of their details, so it is clear that the effects one would observe after GS regression are artifactual. While the complexity of real data (and the absence of perfect knowledge about what patterns of data to expect) make these kinds of artifacts harder to examine, it is possible to derive three main predictions from this simulation and from a more comprehensive mathematical understanding of how GS regression should affect correlation matrices:

(1) The equations that describe the influence of GS regression on any given correlation matrix show that the new matrix will depend in a complex manner on the initial matrix, with *all of the values* being "warped" to varying degrees (Saad et al., 2012, 2013). The prediction for real data is that rather than simply re-centering or re-scaling correlation values around a new mean value in an all-to-all matrix (0 after GS regression: Fox et al., 2009), the rank ordering of these values should also be altered. Furthermore, the alterations to the correlation matrix relative to the absence of GS regression can be predicted in a straightforward manner;

(2) If two groups differ in their global level of correlation (as might be expected for ASD participants relative to TD participants), then the resultant re-centering of the corresponding correlation matrices to 0 after GS regression will necessarily lead to group differences in both directions and in locations where they should not occur, both in "local" correlations and in "long-range" correlations—even if the underlying group differences go in a single direction (see Jones et al., 2010, for an example of this in task-based functional connectivity of ASD). Note that the global level of correlation (GCOR), the grand average of the all-to-all correlation matrix, is lower in Group A than in Group B (green text in the left column of **Figure 1**);

(3) Group comparisons will not be altered indiscriminately. They will tend to be altered most in locations that exhibit the largest underlying group differences - differences that are large enough and coherent enough over the spatial extent of the brain that they affect the GS measure. This is shown in the rightmost column of **Figure 1**, with the magnitudes of distortion (Δ) from the underlying group differences being the largest within and across patches 1 and 2. There is a simple mathematical explanation for this phenomenon. Whole-brain "connectedness" measures have been used in a number of studies to find locations of high connectivity with the rest of the brain (i.e., "hubs": Buckner et al., 2009; Cole et al., 2010) and locations that differ between two groups in their interaction with the rest of the brain (e.g., Salomon et al., 2011; Gotts et al., 2012). The primary difference between whole-brain connectedness and correlation with the GS is simply whether whole-brain averaging is done before or after the correlation calculation. Indeed, if the time series are first transformed to *z*-scores with unit variance (allowing each voxel to contribute equally to the GS), whole-brain connectedness using Pearson correlation is directly proportional to both correlation and regression with the GS, with the effect of GS removal being greater removal of the largest connectedness differences.

In the remainder of this paper, we systematically vary the preprocessing procedures in order to evaluate these predictions in our own previously published ASD and TD resting-state data (Gotts et al., 2012). In addition to the GS and our preferred ANATICOR de-noising approach, which more explicitly models physiological and hardware artifacts (Jo et al., 2010), we evaluate a simple alternative to GS regression when independent cardiac and respiration measures are not available. The alternative, referred to as GCOR (for Global Correlation, Saad et al., 2013), treats the level of global correlation amongst all brain voxels as a nuisance covariate at the group-level of analysis, after the relevant correlation measures have already been calculated for each individual participant without the use of GS regression.

MATERIALS AND METHODS

PARTICIPANTS

The full details of our participant sample have already been published previously (Gotts et al., 2012). Twenty-nine typically developing (TD) participants (28 males, 1 female) between 12 and 23 years of age and 31 high-functioning participants (29 males, 2 females) with an autism spectrum disorder (ASD) between 12 and 23 years of age took part in the study. ASD participants were recruited from the Washington, DC metropolitan area, and all met *Diagnostic and Statistical Manual-IV* diagnostic criteria as assessed by an experienced clinician (20 Asperger's syndrome, 7 high-functioning autism, and 4 pervasive developmental disorder-not otherwise specified). Thirty ASD participants received the Autism Diagnostic Interview (ADI or ADI-R) (Le Couteur et al., 1989; Lord et al., 1994) and the Autism Diagnostic Observation Schedule (ADOS, Modules 3 or 4; Lord et al., 2000), administered by a trained, research-reliable clinician. All scores from participants with ASD met cut-off for the category designated as 'broad autism spectrum disorders' according to criteria established by the National Institute of Child Health and Human Development/National Institute on Deafness and Other Communication Disorders Collaborative Programs for Excellence in Autism (see Lainhart et al., 2006). Because the ADI and ADOS do not provide an algorithm for Asperger's syndrome, Lainhart and colleagues developed criteria that include an individual on the broad autism spectrum if s/he meets the ADI cut-off for "autism" in the social domain and at least one other domain or meets the ADOS cut-off for the combined social and communication score. Scores on the Social Responsiveness Scale (SRS) (Constantino, 2002), an informant-based rating scale used to assess ASD social and communication traits quantitatively over the full range of severity, were obtained from parents for 29 ASD participants. IQ scores were obtained for all participants, and all full-scale IQ scores were $\geq$ 85 as measured by the Wechsler Abbreviated Scale of Intelligence (26 ASD, 29 TD), the Wechsler Adult Intelligence Scale-III (3 ASD), or the Wechsler Intelligence Scale for Children-IV (2 ASD). Participant groups did not differ in terms of full-scale IQ, age, or sex ratio (see Gotts et al., 2012, Table 1). Informed assent and consent were obtained from all participants and/or their parent/guardian when appropriate in accordance with a National Institutes of Health Institutional Review Board-approved protocol.

fMRI IMAGING METHODS

fMRI data were collected using a GE Signa 3 Tesla whole-body MRI scanner at the NIH Clinical Center NMR Research Facility using standard imaging procedures. For each participant, a high-resolution T_1-weighted anatomical image (MPRAGE) was obtained (124 axial slices, 1.2-mm slice thickness, Field of View = 24 cm, 224 × 224 acquisition matrix). Spontaneous, slowly-fluctuating brain activity was measured during fMRI using a gradient-echo echo-planar series with whole-brain coverage while participants maintained fixation on a central cross and were instructed to lie still and rest quietly (TR = 3500 ms, TE = 27 ms, flip angle = 90°, 42 axial contiguous interleaved slices per volume, 3.0-mm slice thickness, FOV = 22 cm, 128 × 128 acquisition matrix, single-voxel volume = 1.7 × 1.7 × 3.0 mm). Each resting scan lasted 8 min and 10 s for a total of 140 consecutive whole-brain volumes. Independent measures of nuisance physiological variables (cardiac and respiration) were recorded during the resting scan for later removal in the majority of participants (24 ASD, 22 TD). Seven additional participants without these measures were included in each group after comparing descriptive statistics of the whole-brain-averaged EPI time series post-preprocessing to those calculated for the participants with measures present (see Gotts et al., 2012, Supplementary Materials and Methods, for full description). A GE 8-channel send-receive head coil was used for all scans, with a SENSE factor of 2 used to reduce gradient coil heating during the session.

fMRI PREPROCESSING

Four preprocessing models were compared in the current study. All preprocessing conditions utilized the AFNI software package (Cox, 1996) and had the following series of steps in common. The first 4 EPI volumes were removed from the resting scan, and large transients in the remaining volumes were removed by constraining values to be within 4 standard deviation units of the mean (using AFNI's 3dDespike). Volumes were then slice-time corrected, co-registered to the anatomical scan, resampled to 2.0-mm isotropic voxels, smoothed with an isometric 6-mm full width half maximum Gaussian kernel, normalized by the mean signal intensity in each voxel to reflect percent signal change, and transformed into the standardized Talairach and Tournoux (1988) volume for the purposes of group analyses. Tissue-based nuisance regressors were created by segmenting the anatomical scan into tissue compartments using Freesurfer (Fischl et al., 2002). Ventricle and white-matter masks were created, eroding the outer voxels of the masks to prevent partial volume effects with grey matter. Eroded masks were then applied to the volume-registered EPI data (prior to smoothing) in order to yield nuisance time series with minimal contribution from gray matter signals for the ventricles, as well as a local average, at each voxel, of the EPI signal from the (eroded mask) white matter voxels within a 15 mm radius of the central voxel.

Basic Model: Motion + Ventricles + Local WM

The "basic model" is a reduced version of our full ANATICOR model without the independent physiological measures. It is common to the other three preprocessing models considered in this study. As indicated by the label above, nuisance variables for each voxel included the 6 head motion parameters (3 translation, 3 rotation) derived from the volume registration step, one average time series from the eroded ventricle mask, and the "local" average white matter time series. Throughout the remainder of the paper, the shorthand label "Basic" model refers exclusively to this preprocessing pipeline. The Basic model has two essential virtues that convey to the remaining preprocessing models: (1) it virtually eliminates the distance-dependent artifacts that result from transient head motion, even for the high movement cohorts such as the children cohort reported in Power et al. (2012) (Jo et al., 2013; see also Gotts et al., 2012, Supplementary Figures 5–11), and (2) the local white matter regressor (Local WM) markedly attenuates transient hardware artifacts that result from faulty channels in send/receive head coils and that generate spatially restricted signals in adjacent white and gray matter voxels (Jo et al., 2010). Indeed, TD participants from our study served as examples of the artifact in Jo et al. (2010). The EPI time series and all nuisance time series were detrended with fourth-order polynomials prior to least-squares model fitting to each voxel's time series. No further temporal filtering was applied to the Basic model, since cardiac and respiratory cycles (frequencies above the Nyquist frequency of $0.5 * 1/\text{TR} \approx 0.14286$ Hz) are aliased to lower frequencies, preventing a bandpass filter from removing them appropriately.

Basic Model + GCOR

The temporal preprocessing steps in the +GCOR model are identical to the Basic model. The only addition is the use of the Global Correlation (or GCOR) measure as a nuisance covariate in the group analyses, after the correlation values of interest have already been calculated. This is explained in full in the section fMRI Analyses.

Basic Model + GS regression

In the +GS Regression model, the GS has been added to the list of nuisance regressors in the Basic model. The GS is calculated by applying a whole-brain mask for each participant to the volume-registered EPI time series to yield one average time series. As with the other nuisance regressors and the BOLD time series, the GS was detrended with fourth-order polynomials prior to least-squares model fitting.

ANATICOR

This is the preprocessing model used in our prior study (Gotts et al., 2012). It consists of the Basic model plus regressors for RETROICOR (Glover et al., 2000; estimated for slice time 0) and Respiration Volume Per Time (RVT) (Birn et al., 2008), created from independently acquired cardiac and respiration measures during the EPI scan (sampling rate 50 Hz). These physiological regressors are intended to estimate: (1) aliased cardiac and respiration cycles, and (2) slower, BOLD-like effects of respiration (end-tidal CO_2) that are typically below 0.1 Hz. These influences are not small for data in the current study, accounting for approximately 10–20% of variance in the EPI/BOLD signal and leading to Type II statistical errors if they are not removed (Gotts et al., 2012, Supplementary Figure 1).

fMRI ANALYSES

In Gotts et al. (2012), we developed an analysis approach to identifying resting-state correlation differences between ASD and TD participants throughout the entire brain (see also Anderson et al., 2011b; Salomon et al., 2011). In the current paper, we adopt a mixture of approaches intended to illustrate the impact of preprocessing steps on correlation differences calculated between pairs of regions that are sampled throughout the brain, as well as to estimate correspondences with our previously reported results.

Large-scale sampling of whole-brain mask with 1880 ROIs

As one relatively comprehensive approach, we uniformly sampled spherical ROIs (6 mm radius) within our previous group brain mask (each voxel present in >85% of participants in each group). ROI centers were chosen by down-sampling the original voxel grid in Talairach coordinates to a new 4 × 4 × 4 grid of the original voxels (a new volume of 8 × 8× 8 mm^3), resulting in a total of 1880 ROIs (from 119,751 original voxels). Example ROI centers (each of which represents a 6 mm-radius sphere) are shown in **Figure 2** in red, overlaid on the group brain mask in green. Note that the mask excludes ventricles, white matter, and the sagittal sinus, focusing on signals from the gray matter and subcortical structures. Correlations of the preprocessed average time series from each ROI for each participant were calculated in an all-to-all fashion and transformed to approximately normally distributed values (Fisher's z transform). Average group ROI-ROI correlation matrices were then calculated across participants within the ASD and TD groups and compared with two-sample t-tests. The relative rank ordering of correlation values within the ROI-ROI matrix was compared across preprocessing models using the Spearman rank correlation.

Assessing agreement with previous results using Gotts et al. (2012) ROIs

The 27 ROIs identified in Gotts et al. (2012) as showing greater correlation in TD than in ASD participants were also applied to the de-noised data from each preprocessing model in order to evaluate consistency with our previously reported group comparisons, as well as with our previous ASD symptom correlations using the SRS total score (Constantino, 2002). These ROIs are shown in **Figure 3**, with each ROI assigned a unique color. As with the analyses using 1880 ROIs, the all-to-all ROI correlation matrix

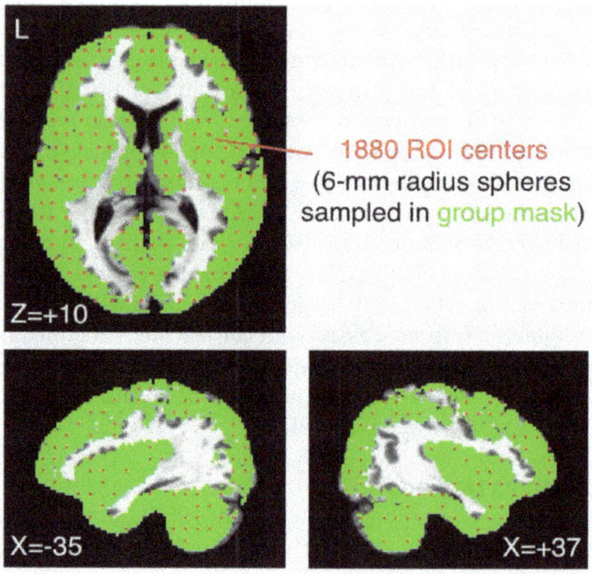

FIGURE 2 | Sampling the group brain mask with 1880 ROIs. The original group brain mask from Gotts et al. (2012) (voxels shared in >85% of participants in both ASD and TD groups; shown in green) was sampled by choosing every fourth voxel from the original voxel grid (in X,Y,Z directions in Talairach coordinates). Each chosen voxel (red voxels) served as the center for a 6-mm radius sphere, totaling 1880 ROIs. The original group brain mask excluded voxels in white matter, the ventricles, and the sagittal sinus.

was calculated for each participant, comparing groups using two-sample t-tests after first transforming to normally distributed values (Fisher's z). In analyses of correlation with SRS total score, partial correlations were calculated across participants using the values in the ASD group at each ROI-ROI combination, removing the shared variation with Age and Full Scale IQ. Predictions regarding the influence of preprocessing model on "short-range" correlations were also assessed for these 27 ROIs. For these analyses, the average voxel-to-voxel Pearson correlation within each ROI was calculated for each ASD and TD participant, these values were then transformed using Fisher's z, and then they were compared across groups in each ROI using two-sample t-tests. The Pearson correlation was chosen for ease of implementation, and the results are not expected to depart markedly from those using canonical correlation and other similar methods (e.g., Regional Homogeneity or "ReHo": Zang et al., 2004; Paakki et al., 2010; Shukla et al., 2010; see also Jiang et al., 2013).

GCOR preprocessing model and analyses

The +GCOR model, as discussed above in the section Basic Model + GCOR, involves the same preprocessing steps as the Basic model. After the calculation of correlation coefficients between a pair of ROIs(/voxels) and the application of the Fisher's z transform, the GCOR method involves partialling out the influence of the global level of correlation (grand mean correlation of all voxels with all voxels in a whole-brain mask) on the group comparison of correlation values using an Analysis of Covariance (ANCOVA) approach (Saad et al., 2013). The top panel of **Figure 4** provides a simplified illustration of the

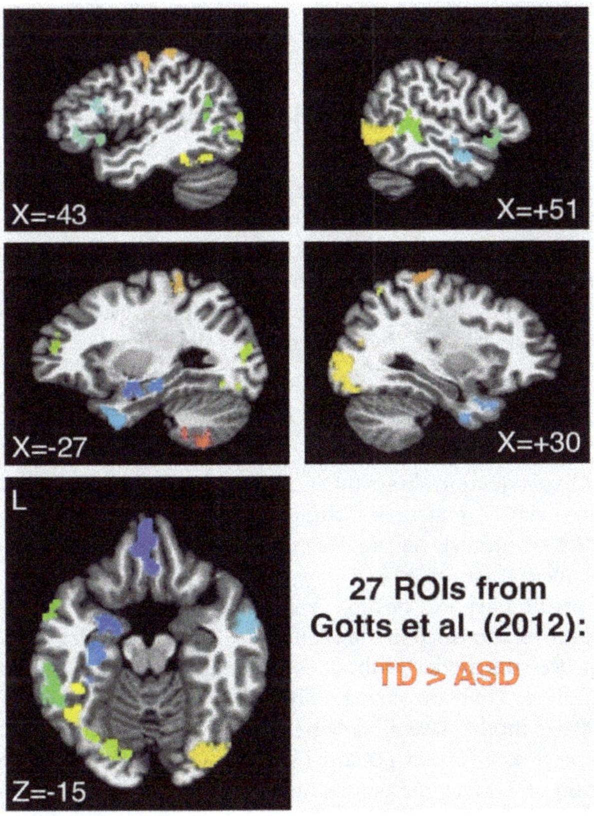

FIGURE 3 | ROIs showing the largest group differences (TD > ASD) in Gotts et al. (2012). ROIs 1–27 are shown using a distinct color for each ROI, ranging from cool colors (blue = 1) up to hot colors (red = 27).

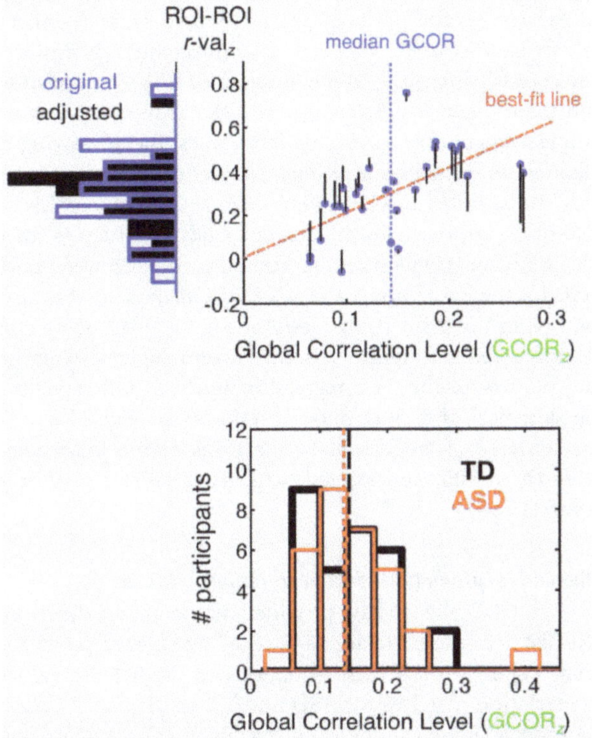

FIGURE 4 | GCOR method of removing global correlations. (top panel) The x-axis shows the global level of Pearson correlation (GCOR) for each of the 29 TD participants, calculated among all possible voxel combinations in a whole brain mask and then transformed with Fisher's z. The y-axis shows the Fisher's z-transformed correlation value between two example ROIs for each participant, with frequency histograms across participants shown to the left of the y-axis. The blue dots are the original values of GCOR and ROI-ROI correlation for each participant under the Basic preprocessing model. Covariate removal is illustrated here for a single-group of participants, but appropriate removal for group comparisons is more complicated, carried out using Analysis of Covariance (ANCOVA), which is implemented in AFNI with the program 3dttest++ for two-level grouping variables. For a single group, the best-fit regression line (dashed red) is used to adjust y-values as a function of the distance from the median x-value (dashed blue vertical line). The adjusted values are shown relative to the blue dots using black vertical lines, with the new values at the endpoints. The adjusted values have a reduced standard deviation on the y-axis relative to the original distribution (see histogram of solid black bars on the left). **(bottom panel)** Frequency histograms of GCOR values are shown for TD (black) and ASD (red) participants. Distributions are overlapping and skewed for both groups, which motivated the choice of median rather than mean for re-centering.

partialling process for a single participant group (the 29 TD participants) using an example pair of ROIs. The blue dots form a scatterplot of the Fisher's z GCOR value on the x-axis and the Fisher z-transformed ROI-ROI r-value on the y-axis across the TD participants. A frequency histogram of the y-axis values prior to GCOR removal ("original") is shown to the left of the plot using blue-outlined bars. For this single-group example, the y-values are adjusted (vertical black lines leading away from the blue dots) using the slope of the best-fit line and the distance of the GCOR value from the group median GCOR value (shown with a vertical dashed blue line). The actual ANCOVA is more complex in implementation (program 3dttest++ in AFNI), involving the full model of grouping variable (2 levels: ASD and TD) and the continuous covariate (GCOR). The choice of mean or median for centering should depend on whether the distribution is approximately symmetrical or skewed, respectively (the GCOR distributions are skewed for both ASD and TD populations, shown in the bottom panel of **Figure 4**). The effect of covariate removal is to yield a more narrow distribution with reduced variance (frequency histogram of solid black bars to the left of the y-axis). This will tend to have the impact of increasing the amplitude of corresponding t-values when comparing groups if correlations in both groups strongly depend on the level of global correlation. For the analyses in the current paper, separate medians are used for centering each group, permitting differential levels of average correlation between the groups (as in **Figure 1**). If a single grand-mean or median is desired for centering both groups (depending on the study and hypotheses), then it is critical to verify that the groups being compared have similar overall ranges of GCOR. Otherwise, distortions similar to GS regression are expected to occur to a certain extent (see Saad et al., 2013, for further discussion).

Comparisons of whole-brain "connectedness"

In our prior study (Gotts et al., 2012), we compared functional connectivity levels between ASD and TD groups in a whole-brain manner by first finding the average correlation of each voxel with the rest of the brain mask (i.e., whole-brain "connectedness"; see also Salomon et al., 2011). Connectedness is similar, but not necessarily identical, to the measure of "degree centrality" in graph theory, and it is related to GCOR through calculation of a simple average over connectedness values. By comparing connectedness maps between groups, we identified good candidate "seeds" to be tested in subsequent analyses. We utilize this same whole-brain approach in the current study in order to identify the locations of strongest correlation differences between groups. Results for the Basic model and ANATICOR models were already presented in the prior study (see Gotts et al., 2012, Figures 2, 3, and Supplementary Figure 1). In the current paper, we conducted these analyses for the +GS regression and +GCOR models. The same statistical and cluster-size thresholds were used as in the prior study to afford direct comparisons of the preprocessing models ($p < 0.05$, uncorrected, with a spatial extent of at least 100 voxels).

Mathematical prediction of GS correlation matrices

Saad et al. (2012, 2013) have provided mathematical descriptions of the distortion in correlations induced by GS regression. In the current paper, we use these equations to predict the values of the correlation matrices for ASD and TD participants under the +GS preprocessing model using the time series data under the Basic model (without GS regression). These equations would be exact (i.e., equivalent to carrying out GS regression) if we were to use all voxel time series in a whole-brain mask. Here, we will use only data from the 1880 ROIs sampled from the group brain mask, excluding time series from white matter, ventricles and the sinuses. Therefore, the equations will only serve as predictive estimates, and these predictions will be accurate to the extent that the effects of GS regression depend primarily on gray matter signals and do not depend on signals in the excluded "non-neural" tissue compartments.

The equations used for these analyses are derived in detail in Saad et al. (2013), but we repeat them briefly here for convenience:

$$Z = \left(I - g\left(g^{\mathrm{T}}g\right)^{-1}g^{\mathrm{T}}\right)Y$$

where Z is the data matrix after GS regression (N time points x M voxels), I is the identity matrix, g is the GS of the NxM data matrix Y prior to GS regression. The time series in Y are presumed to have been de-meaned (i.e., means set to 0). Then:

$$P = 1/N\, Y^{\mathrm{T}}Y$$

$$Q = 1/N\, Z^{\mathrm{T}}Z = P - \left(P11^{\mathrm{T}}P\right)/(1^{\mathrm{T}}P1)$$

$$R = P * \sigma_P \sigma_P^{\mathrm{T}}$$

where P and Q are the MxM covariance matrices of the Y and Z data matrices, R is the full correlation matrix based on Y, $*$ is the Hadamard element-wise matrix product, σ_P is the reciprocal square root (1/sqrt) of the diagonal elements (variances) of P. Next,

$$S = Q * \sigma_Q \sigma_Q^{\mathrm{T}}$$
$$= \left(P - \left(P11^{\mathrm{T}}P\right)/\left(1^{\mathrm{T}}P1\right)\right) * \sigma_Q \sigma_Q^{\mathrm{T}}$$

where S is the correlation matrix after GS regression, 1 is an Mx1 vector of ones, and σ_Q is the reciprocal square root of the diagonal elements of Q. From this equation, it is clear that S is a function of the covariance matrix P of the data prior to GS regression. The "warping" effect of GS regression on the original correlation matrix R can then be seen by examining the difference S-R:

$$S - R = \left(P - \left(P11^{\mathrm{T}}P\right)/\left(1^{\mathrm{T}}P1\right)\right) * \sigma_Q \sigma_Q^{\mathrm{T}} - P * \sigma_P \sigma_P^{\mathrm{T}}$$

This final equation shows that GS regression warps every value of the correlation matrix in a complex manner that depends solely on the covariance matrix P (the variance terms of Q are also dependent solely on P).

For the purposes of the current analyses, we use the average time series calculated in the 1880 ROIs (**Figure 2**) under the Basic preprocessing model (without GS regression). This is tantamount to applying GS regression serially after the nuisance regressors in the Basic model have already been removed. This simplification will serve as a further potential source of inaccuracy in the estimation of S, since the regression in the +GS model removes all nuisance variables simultaneously.

RESULTS

As discussed above, the main goal of the current paper is to evaluate three central theoretical predictions about the distorting effects of GS regression on group comparisons of functional connectivity in real data. To this end, we re-analyze resting-state data from 31 ASD and 29 TD participants that were originally reported in Gotts et al. (2012) using four different preprocessing models: (1) the Basic model (Motion + Ventricles + Local WM), (2) the Basic model +GCOR, (3) the Basic model +GS regression, and (4) our preferred ANATICOR model (Basic model + RETROICOR and RVT physiological regressors).

PREDICTION 1: CORRELATION MATRICES ARE "WARPED" UNDER GS REGRESSION

We begin by evaluating the first prediction articulated in the introduction, namely that the effect of GS regression is not simply to re-center (alter the mean) or re-scale (alter the standard deviation) the correlations amongst a collection of voxel time series. Rather, the values are also "warped" as a function of the initial data covariance matrix, altering the rank orderings of the values within the all-to-all matrix. Correlations were calculated among all combinations of the 1880 ROIs (**Figure 2**) for the 31 ASD and 29 TD participants using the four preprocessing models. These results are shown averaged within each group in **Figure 5** by preprocessing model. Also shown are the two-sample t-tests by ROI-ROI combination and thresholded t-maps ($p < 0.05$, uncorrected), with corresponding colorbars shown to the right of each plot. Few if any negative correlations were observed in either

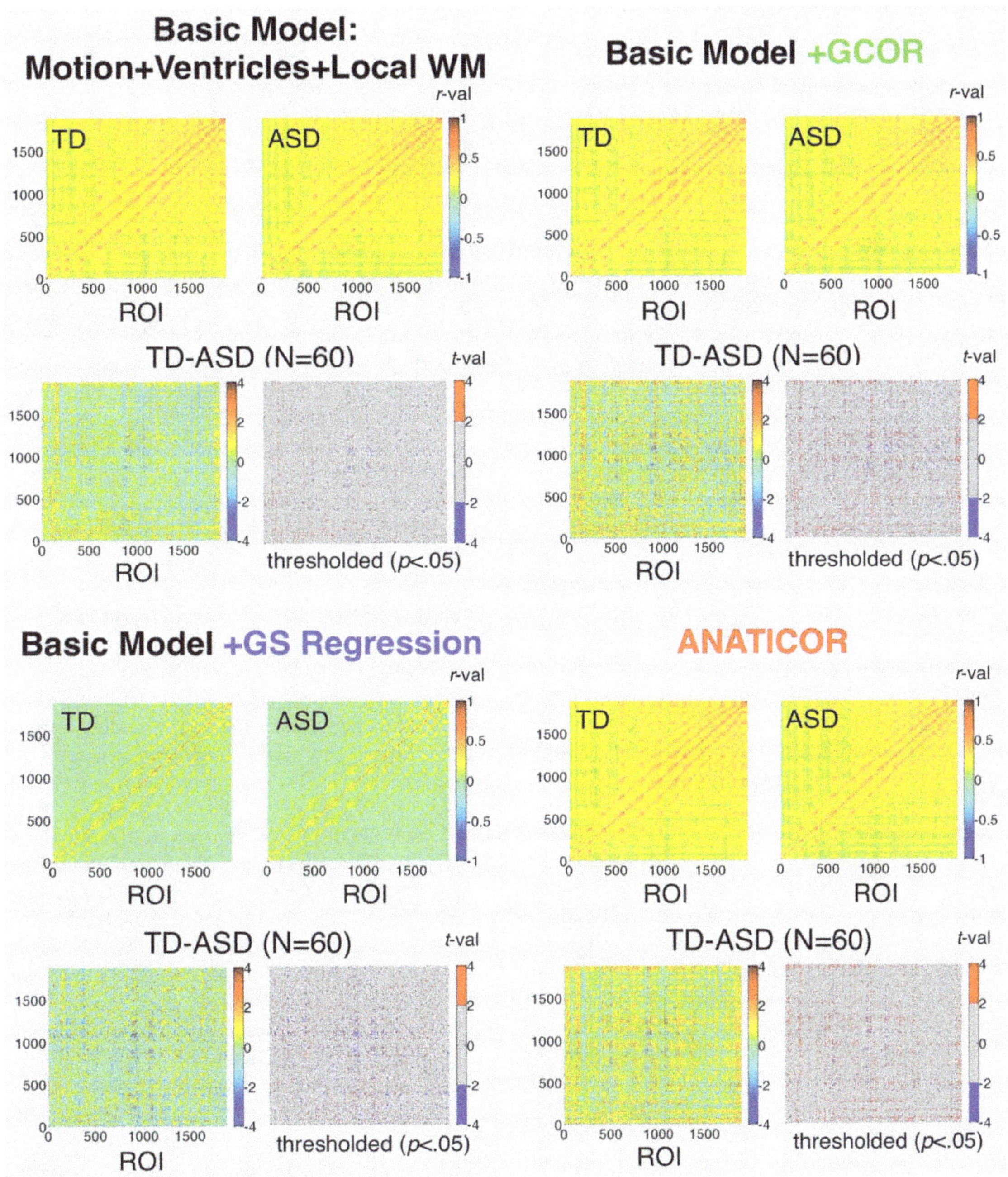

FIGURE 5 | Effect of preprocessing model on ROI-ROI correlations and group differences. Correlation matrices for the TD and ASD groups and the corresponding group comparisons are shown for each of the four preprocessing models using 1880 ROIs sampled from the group brain mask. Results for the "Basic" model (Motion+Ventricles+Local WM) are shown in the upper left, the Basic+GCOR model in the upper right, the Basic+GS regression model in the lower left, and the full ANATICOR model in the lower right. The upper two plots of each model show the average ROI-ROI correlation matrices for the TD and ASD groups (see corresponding colorbars for scale), the lower left plot of each model shows the unthresholded t-values, and the lower right plot of each model shows the t-values thresholded at $p < 0.05$ (uncorrected). ROIs are ordered by scanner coordinates (ranked by Inferior-Superior, then by Anterior-Posterior, then by Right-Left).

participant group for the Basic, +GCOR or ANATICOR models, whereas negative correlations were common in both groups under the +GS Regression model, yielding an average correlation value of approximately 0 for both groups. For both groups, the average correlation matrices are quite similar, both in scale and in rank-order for the Basic, +GCOR, and ANATICOR models. The grand mean (and standard deviation) of the correlation matrices for the ASD group were 0.2138 (0.1105), 0.2155 (0.1128), and 0.2028 (0.1111) for the Basic, +GCOR, and ANATICOR models, respectively. These same numbers for the TD group were

0.2222 (0.1133), 0.2275 (0.1160), 0.2240 (0.1166). Note that the TD group had an average correlation greater than the ASD group of approximately 0.01–0.02 across these three models. In contrast, for the +GS model the means (standard deviations) of the ASD and TD groups were 0.0155 (0.1165) and 0.0146 (0.1215), with the average correlation slightly larger for the ASD group. As with the mean correlations, the rank orderings of values within the ROI-ROI matrices were highly similar for the Basic, +GCOR, and ANATICOR models. Spearman rank correlations among these models were 0.9885 or larger for the ASD matrices and 0.9844 or larger for the TD matrices. In contrast, the Spearman rank correlation of the +GS model with the Basic, +GCOR, and ANATICOR models was 0.6896,0.6963, and 0.7125 for the ASD group and 0.6976,0.6930, and 0.6794 for the TD group. In other words, while better than 96.9% of the variance (R^2 values) was shared in the rank orderings of group-average correlation values among the Basic, +GCOR, and ANATICOR models for both groups, approximately 50% of the variance was shared between the correlation matrices under the +GS model and those of the other models for both groups.

While it is difficult to compare these numbers statistically for the group-average matrices (there are statistical dependencies amongst the rows and columns), deriving the same measures for the ASD and TD individuals allowed comparisons and assessment of reliability across participants. Paired t-tests across participants within both the ASD and TD groups showed that the Spearman rank correlations of the +GS correlation matrices with the Basic and ANATICOR models were significantly reduced relative to the Spearman rank correlations between the Basic and ANATICOR models (+GCOR is applicable only to group-level analyses and was not part of these analyses). For the 31 ASD participants, average Spearman rank correlations of the +GS model with Basic and ANATICOR models were 0.7535 and 0.7261, respectively, whereas the average rank correlation between the Basic and ANATICOR models was 0.9362 [paired $t_{(30)} > 8.50, p < 1.0\text{e-}08$, for both; Bonferroni-corrected P-value = 0.05/3 = 0.0167]. For the 29 TD participants, Spearman rank correlations of the +GS model with the Basic and ANATICOR models were 0.7494 and 0.6971, respectively, whereas the rank correlations between the Basic and ANATICOR models was 0.9329 [paired $t_{(28)} > 8.61$, $p < 1.0\text{e-}08$, for both]. In summary, the rank ordering of the ROI-ROI correlation values for both ASD and TD participants is significantly altered or "warped" by GS regression, consistent with Prediction 1.

PREDICTION 2: GS REGRESSION WILL ALTER THE DIRECTION OF GROUP COMPARISONS

The second prediction articulated in the introduction is that GS regression should alter the direction of group comparisons. In the case of Autism Spectrum Disorders, the prediction is that GS regression should lead to a higher incidence of ROI-ROI pairs for which ASD correlations are greater than TD correlations. This can occur for at least two reasons in the current context. First, if the average level of correlation differs between groups prior to GS regression (as shown in the previous section: TD > ASD), the re-centering of the average correlation (to approximately 0) will be differential in magnitude for the two groups, with a larger subtraction of correlation values from the TD group than from the ASD group. This will necessarily lead to reverse group differences (with ASD>TD) in some locations that did not differ prior to GS regression (possible Type I errors). Differential re-centering should also lead to the attenuation of real group differences in locations where they should be found (possible Type II errors). The second reason that correlation differences can become reversed after GS regression has to do with differential warping of the correlations in the two groups. A clear example of this phenomenon is shown in **Figure 1**, where larger shared variation is removed from patches 1 and 2 in Group B after GS regression compared to Group A. In either case, the expectation for real data is that the incidence of ASD>TD group differences should increase for the +GS model relative to the other models. For a previous task-based study (verbal fluency) of functional connectivity of ASD and TD participants in our lab, this phenomenon has already been demonstrated (Jones et al., 2010). In this section, we evaluate the effects of preprocessing model on the warping of the entire matrix of t-values, as well as on the relative incidence of significant group differences in both directions (TD > ASD and ASD > TD).

Warping of group comparisons by GS regression

As with the average group correlation values for the ASD and TD groups among the 1880 ROIs (section Prediction 1: Correlation matrices are "warped" under GS regression), it was possible to evaluate the alteration of the corresponding t-values by preprocessing model. The means (standard deviations) of the t-values of the Basic, +GCOR, +GS regression, and ANATICOR models were 0.0593 (0.9438), 0.3127 (1.1015), −0.0327 (1.1015), and 0.4606 (1.0081) (see **Figure 5** and summary histograms in **Figure 6A**). The Spearman rank correlations for the t-values among the Basic, +GCOR, and ANATICOR models were 0.8989 and greater (Basic with +GCOR:0.9899; Basic with ANATICOR: 0.8989; +GCOR with ANATICOR:0.9057). In contrast, the Spearman rank correlations of the +GS model with the others were 0.7504, 0.7604, and 0.6662 with the Basic, +GCOR, and ANATICOR models. In summary, the contrast t-values were most positive under the +GCOR and ANATICOR models, slightly positive for the Basic model, and slightly negative for the +GS model (i.e., greater correlations for the ASD participants). The rank orderings of the t-values were similar for the Basic, +GCOR, and ANATICOR models, despite differences in the mean values, sharing at least 80% of the variance among any combination of these models. In contrast, the rank orderings under the +GS model shared between 44 and 58% of the variance with those under the remaining models. All of these distributions are highly discriminable from one another, with t-values from paired t-tests well above 100 for all comparisons due to the diminishing standard error values for these very large sample sizes (N = 1766260 values in each).

Incidence of group differences in both directions as a function of preprocessing model

Both differential re-centering and warping of the correlation values by participant group predict a relatively higher incidence of group differences favoring the ASD group under the +GS

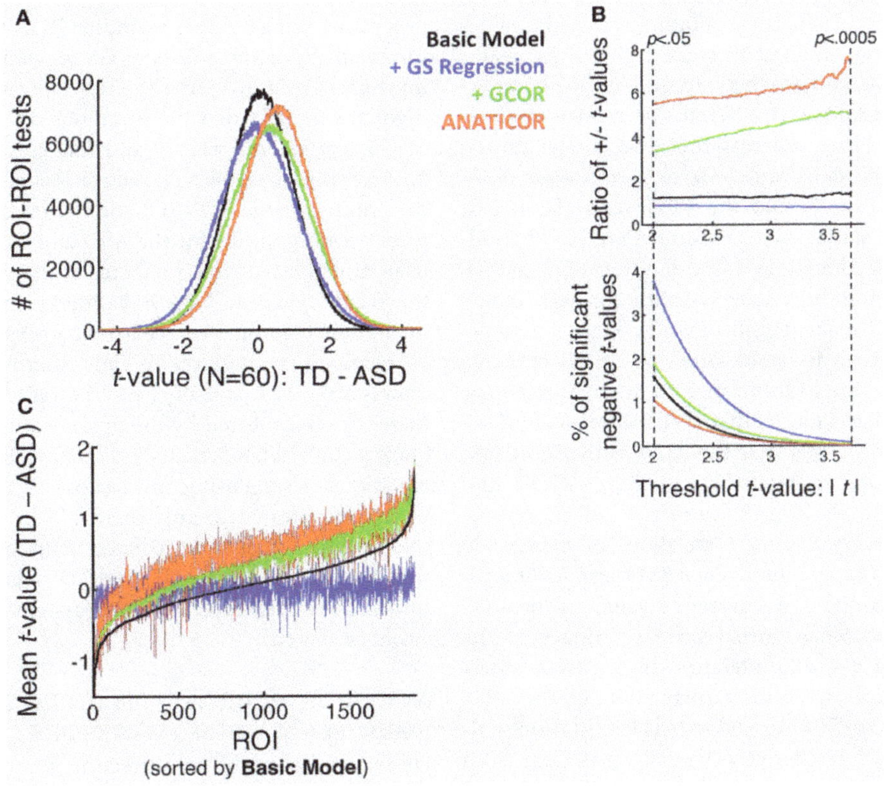

FIGURE 6 | Effect of preprocessing model on the distributions of group differences. (A) Full distributions of t-values (TD-ASD) over all unique combinations of the 1880 ROIs ($N = 1766260$) under all four preprocessing models. **(B)** (top panel) Ratio of positive to negative t-values that survive the threshold t-value, shown as a function of the threshold on the x-axis (ranging from $p < 0.05$ to $p < 0.0005$, uncorrected). (bottom panel) Percentage of tests that yield significant negative t-values (i.e., favoring the ASD group) as a function of threshold t-value and preprocessing model. These values serve as the denominator in the ratios of the top panel. **(C)** Mean t-value across all 1880 ROI for each ROI as the seed (i.e., averaging across the rows of the full, unthresholded t-matrix of each model), rank-ordered from small to large by the mean t-values in the Basic model. These curves demonstrate that the largest alterations to the group comparisons by GS regression are for ROIs that elicit the largest average t-values under the +GCOR and ANATICOR models.

model (the other models favor the TD group to varying degrees). Information about the relative likelihood of TD > ASD and ASD > TD group differences is present in graphical form in **Figures 5, 6**. The full matrices of t-values in **Figure 5** show that the +GS model yields the most blue colors, indicating greater correlations for the ASD group. This is apparent both in the unthresholded and thresholded plots (lower left and right for each of the four models). In contrast, the +GCOR and ANATICOR models yielded the most positive (yellow/red) t-values, and the Basic model yielded fewer significant values in either direction (upper left panels of **Figure 5**). This can be quantified by counting the number of significant positive and negative t-values for a given significance threshold. Using $p < 0.05$ (uncorrected), out of 1766260 unique ROI-ROI combinations (1880 ROIs), the Basic model yielded 1.9155% significant positive t's and 1.5759% negative t's (+/−ratio: 1.2154), the +GCOR model yielded 6.1231% positive t's and 1.8582% negative t's (+/−ratio: 3.2952), the ANATICOR model yielded 5.6807% positive t's and 1.035% negative t's (+/−ratio: 5.4888). In contrast, the +GS model yielded 3.2192% positive t's and 3.7507% negative t's (+/−ratio: 0.8583). As the P-value threshold is lowered (down to $p < 0.0005$), ratios of positive to negative counts increase slightly for the +GCOR and ANATICOR models whereas they decrease for the +GS model (see **Figure 6B**). Combined with the information from section Warping of group comparisons by GS regression that the overall distributions of t-values are significantly shifted to more negative values for the +GS model relative to the other three models, it is clear that Prediction 2 (greater incidence of ASD>TD group differences) holds for this dataset across choice of statistical threshold (see also Jones et al., 2010). Indeed, the average TD-ASD t-value over all ROI-ROI combinations is significantly less than 0 under GS regression, a notable departure from the other models [mean = −0.0327, median = −0.0301, $SD = 1.1015$; one-sample t-test: $t_{(1766259)} = -39.44$, $p < 1.0e\text{-}10$].

PREDICTION 3: GS REGRESSION WILL MOST ALTER THE STRONGEST GROUP DIFFERENCES UNDER OTHER PREPROCESSING MODELS

The third prediction articulated in the introduction is that GS regression will not alter group comparisons indiscriminately. Rather, it will tend to alter results most in locations that exhibit the largest underlying group differences. One relatively simple way to evaluate this prediction for the current dataset is to first find regions out of the 1880 that yield the largest average group differences. This was done by averaging the t-values across the rows of the 1880 × 1880 *t*-matrices in **Figure 5** for each preprocessing model. Then, these column-averaged *t*-values can be rank ordered from smallest to largest. Given the results in the section on Prediction 2, one expects the rank orderings of the Basic, +GCOR, and ANATICOR models to have quite similar rank orderings, whereas the +GS model should differ—at least relatively—in its rank orderings from these models. The critical prediction is that the ROIs with the largest average *t*-values for the Basic, +GCOR, and ANATICOR models should be the most altered in value for the +GS model. Rather than rank ordering the average *t*-values for each model separately (which would make it difficult to evaluate the agreement of particular ROIs in the rank ordering across models), we chose to rank order the ROIs relative to a single reference model, in this case the Basic model that is common to all of the other models. **Figure 6C** shows that the ROIs with the largest average *t*-values are quite similar for the Basic, +GCOR, and ANATICOR models (the black, green, and red curves, respectively). Indeed, the Spearman rank correlations of these 1880 column-averaged values ranged between 0.8848 and 0.9863 for these three models. In contrast, the average *t*-values of the +GS model are relatively flat when sorted by the *t*-values of the Basic model, indicating a strong alteration in the rank ordering. Accordingly, the Spearman rank correlation of the +GS model with the Basic, +GCOR, and ANATICOR models is 0.255, 0.2678, and 0.2623 respectively. Visually, it is clear from **Figure 6C** that the average *t*-values under the +GS model are most different from the +GCOR and ANATICOR models at the highest average *t*-values. In order to evaluate this phenomenon statistically, we compared the slopes of the best-fit regression lines to these curves. The slopes of the best-fit lines to the +GCOR and ANATICOR curves were 8.1509e-04 and 7.3080e-04, respectively, while the best-fit slope to the +GS curve was 0.73161e-04. The 99% confidence intervals calculated for the slope estimates were non-overlapping for the +GS model and those of the +GCOR and ANATICOR curves, demonstrating that they are significantly different from each other. The larger positive slopes for the +GCOR and ANATICOR models guarantees that they will differ most from the +GS model at their largest *t*-values.

MATHEMATICAL PREDICTION OF ASD AND TD CORRELATION MATRICES UNDER THE +GS MODEL

In the sections above, we evaluated and confirmed three main predictions about effect of GS regression on group comparisons in real data. The purpose of the current section is to evaluate the extent to which the distorting effect of GS regression on a matrix of correlation values is captured by the equations of Saad et al. (2012, 2013). As described in section Mathematical prediction of GS correlation matrices, if we were to use all voxel time series in a whole brain mask, these equations would be exact (i.e., equivalent to performing GS regression). What makes this analysis more interesting is that only time series from the 1880 ROIs sampled from the group brain mask (**Figure 2**) were used for the estimation. Since the group brain mask excluded the brain tissue types that have been argued to contain the largest global nuisance signals (white matter, ventricles, and sinuses), successful prediction of +GS model correlations using only data from the Basic preprocessing model in these sampled ROIs would demonstrate that the main distorting effects of GS regression derive from averaging signals in gray matter voxels. Successful prediction will also highlight the fact that the equations describe the warping effect of GS regression correctly and that the reported distortions of group comparisons should not come as a surprise. **Figure 7** shows the group-average ROI-ROI correlation matrices under the +GS preprocessing model for the ASD and TD groups in the left column and the matrices predicted from the sampled ROIs using the Basic model and the equations from Saad et al. (2013) in the middle column. Both Pearson correlation and Spearman rank correlations (scatterplots in right column) reveal that approximately 95% or better of the variation (R^2 values) in the actual matrices are captured by the predicted matrices for both participant groups. These results indicate excellent performance of the equations, despite using only a subset of the voxel time series that were concentrated in gray matter. Note further that the agreement of the actual and predicted matrices is substantially higher than that between the +GS model correlation matrices and those under the other three models (approximately 50–55% of the variance shared).

ANATOMICAL LOCATIONS OF THE STRONGEST GROUP DIFFERENCES UNDER THE +GS VERSUS +GCOR MODELS

Under one method of correcting for global correlations, GS regression, correlation matrices and group comparisons are distorted. Under another, GCOR, results appear to be qualitatively similar in many respects to our previously published results using ANATICOR. In order to facilitate more direct comparisons with the anatomical locations of our previous results in Gotts et al. (2012) (the 27 ROIs shown in **Figure 3**), we calculated whole-brain connectedness measures for each participant using both the +GS and +GCOR models and compared across groups using two-sample *t*-tests (see also Salomon et al., 2011). Using the same statistical and cluster-size thresholds as in the previous study, the results are shown for both models in **Figure 8**. The results for the +GCOR model are in good accord with our previous results, with greater connectedness values in the TD relative to the ASD group being observed throughout social brain areas, particularly in limbic-related brain regions (compare to **Figure 3**). In contrast, the +GS model yielded many more locations for which connectedness values were greater for the ASD group (note the results in cerebellum and striatum) and with relatively weak overall agreement with either the +GCOR or ANATICOR results.

EFFECT OF GS REGRESSION AND OTHER PREPROCESSING MODELS ON "LOCAL" CORRELATIONS

In **Figure 1**, we highlighted the inter-dependence of long- and short-range correlations under GS regression. "Long-range" differences between groups that are large enough to manifest in the GS measure will have a tendency to be aliased into the "short-range" correlations involving the same voxels, although in the opposite direction as the long-range differences (note the reverse within-patch group differences in patches 1 and 2 after GS regression). In the current paper, we evaluated whether this same

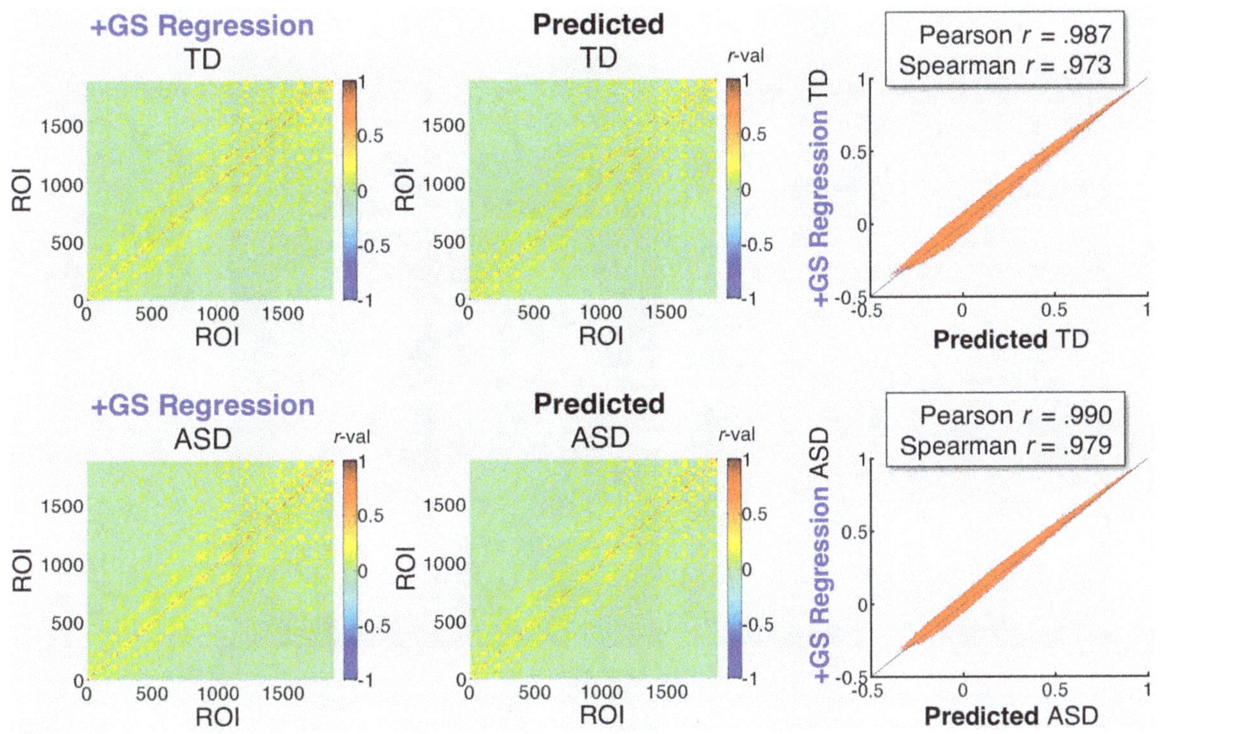

FIGURE 7 | Mathematical prediction of correlation matrices under GS regression. The left two panels show the group average ROI-ROI correlation matrices for the TD and ASD groups under the +GS preprocessing model (shown also in **Figure 5**). The middle two panels show the matrices predicted by the equations developed by Saad et al. (2013) when applied to the time series data under the Basic preprocessing model (for equations used, see section Mathematical prediction of GS correlation matrices). Scatterplots of the agreement between the left and middle panels are shown in the rightmost panels, with Pearson and Spearman rank correlations shown to quantify the level of agreement. The predictions are accurate despite only estimating the distortions under GS regression from 1880 ROIs sampled in the group brain mask (excluding nuisance tissue signals such as white matter, ventricles, and sinuses).

phenomenon occurs in our ASD/TD data by calculating "local" correlations among voxel time series within each of the 27 ROIs that we have shown exhibit greater long-range correlations for the TD group (Gotts et al., 2012; see **Figure 3**). If the groups exhibited equal levels of local correlation prior to GS regression, then there should be a tendency for significantly greater local correlations in the ASD group after GS regression. If the TD group exhibits larger local correlations prior to GS regression, then these differences should be attenuated or reversed after GS regression. In the event that the ASD group exhibits greater local correlations than the TD group prior to GS regression, then these differences should become enhanced after GS regression. In summary, since the long-range differences in these 27 ROIs favor the TD group, the influence of GS regression should be to shift the local correlations in these regions toward favoring the ASD group regardless of the initial direction of these differences. The results for the four preprocessing models, shown in **Figure 9**, are presented left-to-right from ROIs 1 to 27 (listed in the same order as Table 1 from Gotts et al., 2012). The Basic, +GCOR, and ANATICOR models all show a tendency for greater local correlations in the TD group, with results significant at $p < 0.05$ for 3, 6, and 6 ROIs out of the 27, respectively, and no ROIs showing significant differences favoring the ASD group. In contrast, the +GS model yielded results in 17/27 ROIs that numerically favored the ASD group (compared to 5, 4, and 3 out of 27 for the Basic, +GCOR, and ANATICOR models), with 2/27 ROIs showing significant differences (ROIs 4 and 16: the right ventromedial anterior temporal ROI and the left anterior superior frontal ROI). The +GS model also yielded results favoring the TD group in 2/27 ROIs, although with smaller t-values than for the +GCOR and ANATICOR models. The distributions of these t-values across ROIs did not differ from normality for any of the models, permitting their comparison with t-tests. The only two models that failed to show significant differences with each other are the +GCOR and ANATICOR models ($p < 0.1$). The +GS model yielded t-values that were significantly more negative than all of the other models [vs. Basic: paired $t_{(26)} = -8.7585$, $p <$ 3.1055e-09; vs. +GCOR: paired $t_{(26)} = -13.2229$, $p <$ 4.7379e-13; vs. ANATICOR: paired $t_{(26)} = -11.8368$, $p <$ 5.6743e-12]. In accordance with the predictions articulated above, these results establish that the same aliasing of long-range correlation differences into reversed local correlations (as in **Figure 1**) occurs in our ASD/TD data. They also provide additional new evidence that local correlation differences between ASD and TD participants have a tendency to occur in the same direction as the long-range correlation differences when GS regression is not applied (i.e., favoring the TD participants; e.g., Khan et al., 2013; for further discussion, see Belmonte et al., 2004; Müller et al., 2011).

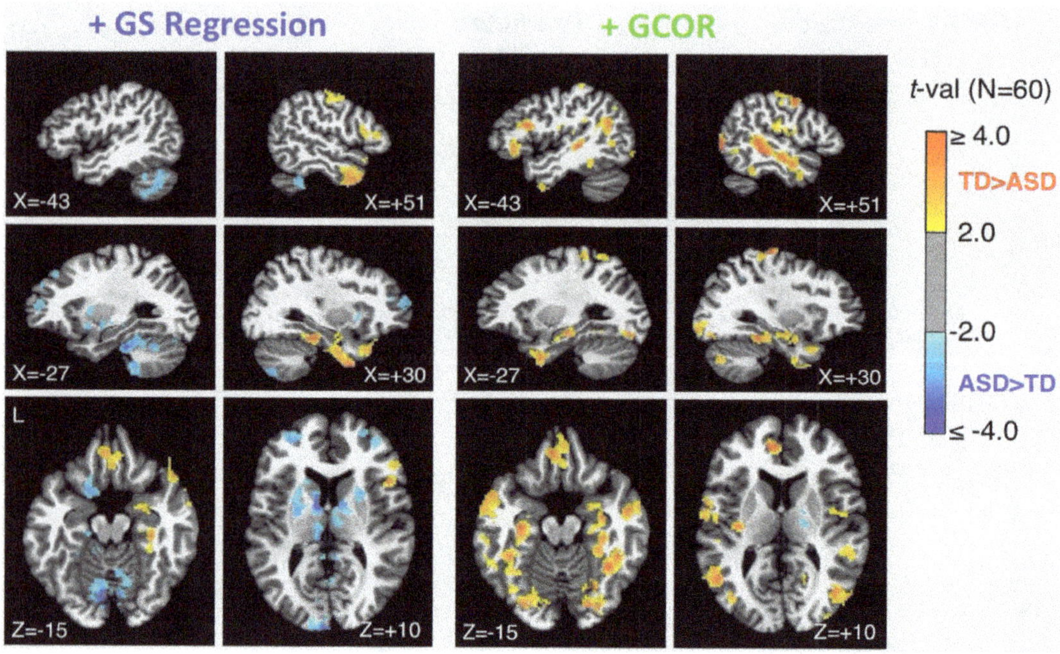

FIGURE 8 | Group comparisons of whole-brain connectedness for the +GS and +GCOR preprocessing models. Whole-brain connectedness (i.e., the average correlation of each voxel time series with the rest of the voxels in the brain mask) was compared separately for the +GS regression and the +GCOR models. The +GS regression model, shown in the left plots, led to a larger number of locations with ASD connectedness values larger than TD values, as well as the absence of TD > ASD effects in locations found previously using ANATICOR. In contrast, the +GCOR method of removing global correlations, shown in the right plots, largely replicated the results found with ANATICOR (compare to ROIs in **Figure 3** from the same sagittal and axial views). See text for full description.

ANATOMICAL ALIGNMENT OF GROUP DIFFERENCES AND CORRELATIONS WITH ASD SOCIAL SYMPTOMS

One critical demonstration of our prior study (Gotts et al., 2012) is that the brain locations showing the largest group differences between ASD and TD groups are also those that exhibit the largest associations between correlation level and the severity of social impairment within the ASD group (indexed by SRS total score). In particular, among the 3 clusters of ROIs that we examined, the largest effects of both types (group differences and SRS correlations) occurred between the limbic-related ROIs of Cluster 1 (ROIs 1–7) and the remaining social brain regions in Clusters 2 and 3 (ROIs 8–27). In the current study, we evaluated the agreement of the group differences and SRS correlations for the four preprocessing models using these same 27 ROIs (see **Figure 3**). Results are presented in **Figure 10**, with group differences (t-tests: TD-ASD) shown in the top row and correlation with SRS total score, partialling Age and IQ (as in our previous study), shown in the bottom row. Symptom correlations in the case of the +GCOR model were conducted using the participant-specific correlation matrices under the Basic model, partialling the GCOR value for each participant along with Age and IQ. Yellow/red colors for the group comparisons indicate greater correlations for the TD group, blue colors indicate greater correlations for the ASD group, and light green indicates t-values that fail to reach a two-tailed significance level of $p < 0.05$. For the correlations with SRS within the ASD group, blue colors indicate that low ROI-ROI correlation levels predict high SRS total scores (i.e., lower correlation → higher social impairment), whereas yellow/red colors indicate the opposite relationship. **Figure 10** shows that the locations of the strongest group differences (TD > ASD) are quite similar for the Basic, +GCOR, and ANATICOR models (between ROIs 1–7 and ROIs 8–27), while the +GS model shows weak or non-significant differences in these same locations. The relative lack of results in these locations is in agreement with the earlier results reported for Prediction 3 and shown in **Figures 6C, 8.**

On visual examination, the only preprocessing model of the four that exhibited good agreement between the group comparisons and symptom correlations was the ANATICOR model. This was examined in more detail statistically with the use of permutation tests (e.g., Maris and Oostenveld, 2007), as the column/row interdependencies of the matrices prevented easy estimation of the appropriate degrees of freedom. The quantitative agreement between the matrices in the top and bottom rows for each model was first assessed using Pearson correlation. Rather than using the t-values in the top row directly for these analyses, the group mean difference of the correlation values (TD-ASD) was used so that the same type of measure (with the same numerical scale/distribution) was being associated in both matrix types. After calculation of the r-values for the group difference and behavioral correlation matrices using the original data, P-values were estimated empirically by randomly re-labeling participants as either ASD or TD. The group

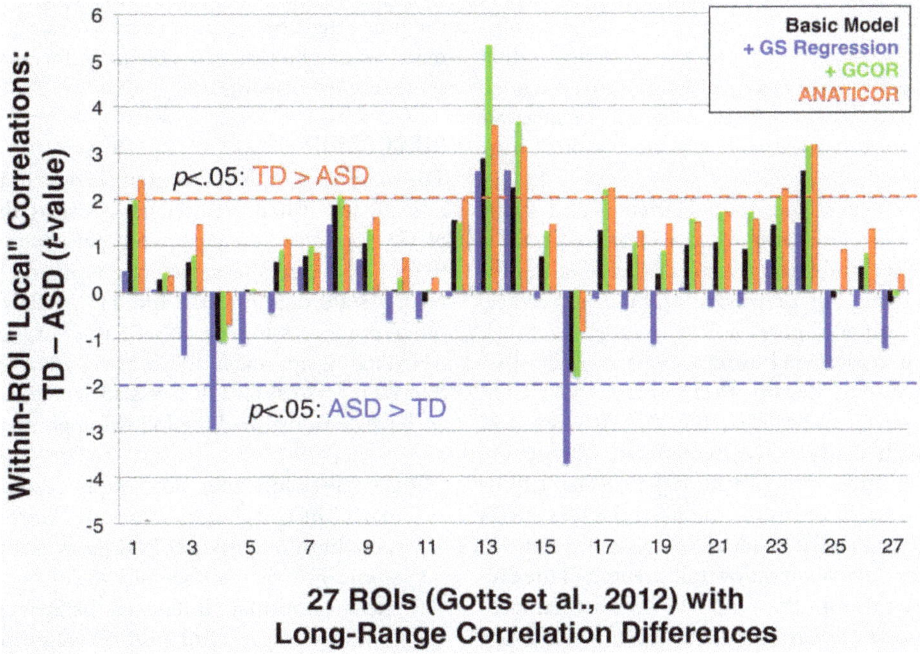

FIGURE 9 | Effect of preprocessing model on group comparisons of local correlation. Group t-tests of local correlation (TD-ASD) under the four preprocessing models are shown for regions in Gotts et al. (2012) that exhibited greater long-range correlations for TD participants (ROIs 1-27; see **Figure 3**). Dashed red (TD > ASD) and blue horizontal lines (ASD > TD) mark the $p < 0.05$ significance level for individual tests. On average, the +GS model yielded more negative t-values (favoring the ASD participants) relative to the other three models.

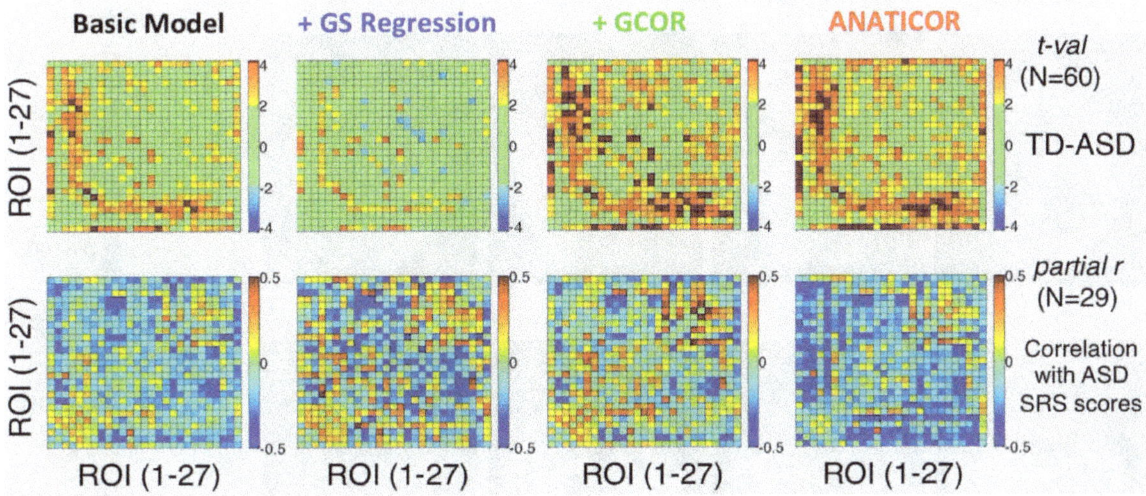

FIGURE 10 | Effect of preprocessing model on the agreement of group differences and social symptom correlations within the ASD group. Group t-tests are shown for the four preprocessing models in the top row using ROIs 1–27 (**Figure 3**) (see colorbar for scale of t-values to the right). Partial correlations of SRS total score with ROI-ROI correlation level within the ASD group, removing shared variation with Age and full scale IQ, are shown in the bottom row (see colorbar for scale of partial r-values to the right). Only the ANATICOR model produced significant correspondence between the group differences and behavioral correlations solely within the ASD group (see text for details). The +GS model also failed to exhibit strong group differences using these ROIs, consistent with the results of **Figure 6C**.

comparisons and behavioral correlations were re-calculated for these randomly formed groups along with the corresponding Pearson r-value between matrices, and the entire randomization process was repeated 1000 times. The P-value (Type I error) for the original matrix agreement measures corresponded to the percentage of random iterations with an agreement value stronger than that observed for the original data. The Pearson r-values (and P-values) for the Basic, +GS, +GCOR, and ANATICOR models were -0.0477 ($p > 0.3$), -0.0198 ($p > 0.4$), -0.1051 ($p > 0.1$), and -0.2777 ($p < 0.027$), respectively. The significant negative r-value for the ANATICOR model indicates that ROI pairs with group differences favoring the TD group tended to be the same ROI pairs as those with a significant negative correlation with SRS score, as originally reported (Gotts et al., 2012).

The anatomical agreement of the group differences and symptom correlations could also be examined in a whole-brain fashion using the voxel-wise whole-brain connectedness values for each participant under the four preprocessing models (see also **Figure 8** in the current paper; Figures 2, 5 in Gotts et al., 2012). These results are shown in **Figure 11** using a single axial slice that captures the largest overlap of the two effects for the ANATICOR model ($z = -14$). As previously reported, the ANATICOR model shows a good agreement between the two effects, with spatial overlap of the results in three out of seven of the Cluster 1 ROIs (ROIs 1–7). Isolated locations of overlap between the two effects also exist for the Basic and +GCOR models (e.g., in the ventromedial prefrontal cortex), although the overall strength of the SRS correlations is notably weaker for these models. Group differences and SRS correlations were both robust when using whole-brain connectedness with the +GS model. However, they had little or no spatial overlap with one another. Furthermore, it was not just the group comparisons that were altered by GS regression relative to the other models: the SRS correlations solely within the ASD group were also strongly altered. This last effect underscores the point that the warping effect of GS regression on correlation matrices can be just as problematic for analyses involving single groups of participants.

DISCUSSION

The main goal of the current paper was to examine several theoretically motivated predictions regarding the detrimental impact of GS regression on group comparisons of functional connectivity. We tested these predictions in our previously published resting-state data of ASD and TD participants relative to three other preprocessing models of interest, including our original ANATICOR approach and a novel alternative to GS regression that we refer to as GCOR (see also Saad et al., 2013). In summary, we have demonstrated the following points:

(1) GS regression does not simply re-center and/or re-scale a matrix of correlation values. It "warps"the values differentially in different voxel/ROI pairs as a function of the initial covariance matrix (see also Saad et al., 2012, 2013). This effect is not small. It reduced the Spearman rank correlations of matrices pre- and post-GS regression to approximately 0.7, sharing around 50% of the variance. This was not simply a function of removing unwanted global artifacts that influence BOLD fMRI. Results from two alternative methods, our ANATICOR approach that models physiological

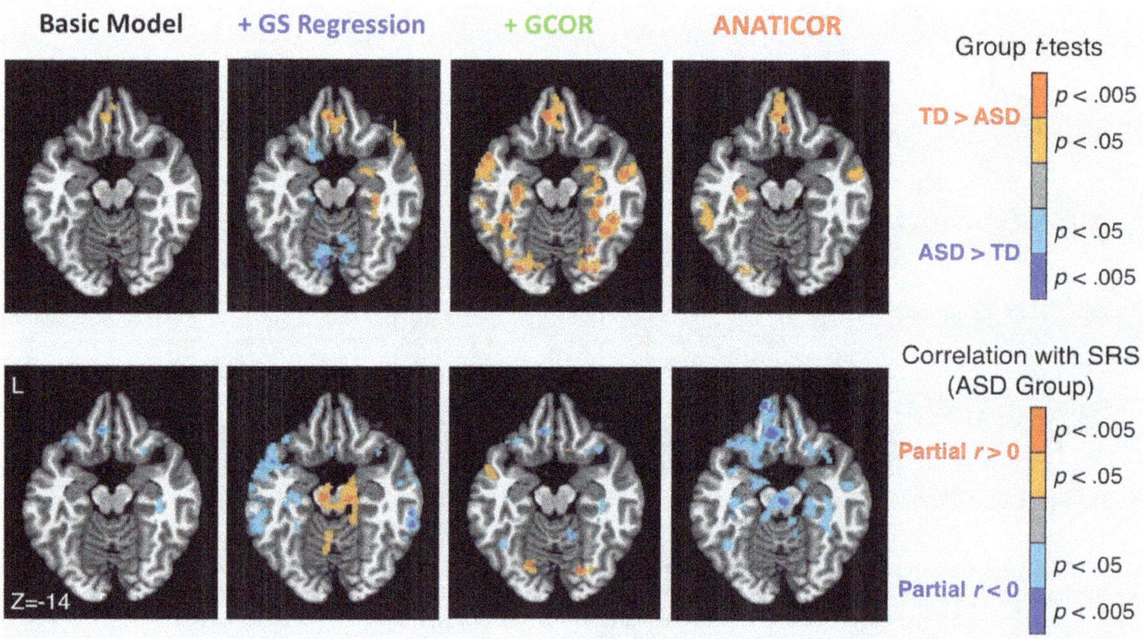

FIGURE 11 | Effect of preprocessing model on the agreement of group differences and ASD social symptom correlations using whole-brain connectedness. Whole-brain connectedness was compared between groups for each of the four preprocessing models (top row; see colorbar to right for scale and direction of effects). Whole-brain connectedness for the ASD participants was also correlated with SRS total score, partialling Age and IQ, for the four models (bottom row; see colorbar to the right for scale and direction of effects). While select locations overlapped between the two effects for the Basic and +GCOR models, the best correspondence was still obtained under the ANATICOR model. The two effects were robust individually under the +GS model, but they exhibited little spatial overlap with each other and only minor overlap with the effects under the other models (e.g., TD > ASD in the ventromedial prefrontal cortex). Only the +GS model exhibited prominent reversed effects (ASD > TD) for the group comparisons (see also **Figure 8**).

nuisance signals more explicitly and GCOR that partials the influence of the global level of correlation from the single-participant correlation values, were not altered comparably, with Spearman rank correlations of approximately 0.9 or higher (sharing better than 80% of the variance). The distortion of correlation values under GS regression was also well predicted by our prior mathematical analyses (correlations above 0.97 and 95% of variance accounted for), despite the fact that signals were not included from nuisance brain tissue compartments (white matter, ventricles, sinuses). Given that the distortion is a *systematic* function of the initial covariance matrix, results are expected to replicate well across labs and studies. In fact, the use of GS regression does increase the consistency of correlation estimates and correlation differences due to a reduction in brain-wide noise sources when such sources are otherwise unaccounted for (e.g., Fox et al., 2009; Keller et al., 2013). However this increased consistency is not a justification for the use of GS regression because it comes at the cost of rendering contrasts between groups with differing correlation structures uninterpretable, as illustrated in theory (Saad et al., 2012, 2013) and in practice here. Even single-group results will become distorted with GS regression (see bottom panels of **Figures 10, 11**).

(2) GS regression substantially increases the number of locations that demonstrate greater correlation for ASD relative to TD participants, both long-range and local. Indeed, under GS regression the average *t*-value observed across all regions sampled ($N = 1880$) was significantly different from zero, favoring the ASD group. Greater correlations for the ASD relative to the TD group were not prominently observed in any of the other preprocessing models. Furthermore, the two alternative preprocessing methods that address more global artifacts (ANATICOR, GCOR) produced qualitatively similar results to one another, with reasonable agreement about the direction of effects and regions involved as in another recent whole-brain study of functional connectivity in ASD that did not apply GS regression (e.g., Anderson et al., 2011b). The locations involved also agree well with task-based studies of evoked responses in ASD and TD participants that employ social and linguistic stimuli (e.g., Castelli et al., 2002; Just et al., 2004; Di Martino et al., 2009; Kaiser et al., 2010; Lombardo et al., 2010; Dinstein et al., 2011; Weisberg et al., 2012). In contrast, a recent whole-brain resting-state study of ASD that applied GS regression found a mixture of increased and decreased correlations relative to TD participants (Rudie et al., 2013). Indeed, the negative correlations present under GS regression for both groups led to separate effects in both directions for the positive versus the negative correlations. Given the results reported in the current paper, it is not clear whether the greater correlations observed for the ASD group in the Rudie et al. study are real or produced by GS regression.

(3) GS regression has a tendency to distort group comparisons most in locations that exhibit the strongest effects under other preprocessing models. ROIs that elicited the largest average seed-based correlation differences were the same ROIs for which the average correlation differences were most attenuated under GS regression (**Figure 6C**). When examining correlation differences among the 27 ROIs that yielded the largest effects in our prior study (Gotts et al., 2012), group differences were also mostly non-significant after GS regression (**Figure 10**). As discussed in the introduction, this occurs for a relatively simple mathematical reason: whole-brain connectedness is a direct function of the fit to the GS. The process of GS regression is to subtract this portion of variation from the results. This is not to say that all studies that employ GS regression will fail to find group differences similar to what we report here for ANATICOR or GCOR. Indeed, we already know from functional connectivity studies using a more restricted number of seed locations that a similar subset of results can be obtained when using GS regression (e.g., Kennedy and Courchesne, 2008; Ebisch et al., 2011; von dem Hagen et al., 2012; see Di Martino et al., 2013, for related discussion). However, we would expect such results to be larger in amplitude if an alternative such as GCOR were used, and we would also expect convergence toward the pattern of mixed increases and decreases if more seed locations are used.

(4) Locations exhibiting group differences and ASD social symptom correlations no longer overlap with one another after GS regression. Using the matrix of 27 ROIs from our previous study to assess the quantitative agreement of these two effects, the correlation was near zero after GS regression, whereas there was a significant level of agreement using the ANATICOR model ($r = -0.277$, $p < 0.03$) (**Figures 10, 11**).

Taken together, our results strongly argue against using GS regression when comparing correlation values between groups of participants. It is difficult to avoid the conclusion that nothing can be demonstrated unequivocally about either the location or direction of group differences when this form of "de-noising" is applied. Given the further alteration of the SRS correlations solely within the ASD group (**Figures 10, 11**), it is clear that the "warping" effects of GS regression on individual correlation matrices may also affect results obtained within single groups of participants (e.g., whole-brain parcellations of functional areas/networks that utilize correlation measures). It may therefore be prudent to re-examine such results with an alternative approach, perhaps with GCOR or preferably with de-noising approaches that avoid signals from the gray matter regions of interest (e.g., Jo et al., 2010; Anderson et al., 2011a).

IS THERE EVER A LEGITIMATE REASON TO APPLY GS REGRESSION?

While our conclusions here regarding GS regression are quite negative, we would like to emphasize that there are good reasons for examining—and perhaps removing—global fluctuations in fMRI time series. In many respects, the Basic preprocessing model produced highly similar matrices to those produced by ANATICOR and GCOR; the Spearman rank correlations are all above 0.9 for both the average matrices and those of individual participants. However, the group comparisons using the Basic model failed to yield robust results, and it is worth considering why this occurred. The effect of removing global sources of variation, either by modeling physiological variation directly (ANATICOR) or partialling out the influence of the global level of correlation (GCOR), was not primarily to modulate the average correlation values for the ASD and TD groups (see results related to Prediction 1). Rather, the larger impact appeared to be on the variation across participants for a given pair of ROIs (as in **Figure 4**, top panel). A relatively small number of participants have large global levels of correlation in both groups (**Figure 4**, bottom panel), which when comparing the two groups has the effect of making the standard deviations that contribute to the denominator of the *t*-values large and thus the *t*-values themselves become small and non-significant. Attenuating the variation in each group then has the effect of shifting all of the *t*-values to be more positive (**Figure 6A**). Indeed, this is one of the primary motivations for applying GS regression, and it demonstrates that if global artifacts in the data are not modeled and removed sufficiently, then one will be at risk of making Type II statistical errors.

One possible example of doing too little to remove global artifacts is provided in the recent study by Tyszka et al. (2013). These authors did an admirable job of assessing the impact of head motion on group differences, which is one source of global artifact in fMRI time series. They found mostly weak and non-significant group differences between ASD and TD participants, smaller on average than the influence of high versus low levels of head motion. This led them to conclude that resting-state correlations in ASD participants are largely typical. However, no aspect of the preprocessing in this study directly addressed global artifacts other than head motion, and GS regression was not applied. Physiological variation will not typically be well removed by the popular bandpass filtering step (Tyszka et al., 2013, removed independent components with more than 33% of spectral power above 0.1 Hz), since the problematic frequencies (~0.3 Hz for respiration cycles and ~0.9–1 Hz for cardiac cycles) have already been aliased to frequencies below the Nyquist frequency (0.25 Hz in Tyszka et al. for $TR = 2$ s). Slower fluctuations in the BOLD response that result from spontaneous breath withholding during fMRI scans, due to end-tidal CO_2 effects on BOLD measurements (Chang and Glover, 2009) and that are modeled by our RVT regressors (Birn et al., 2008), can have quite a large impact on resting-state correlations (>20–30% of total variance in some of our participants; see Supplementary Figure 1, Gotts et al., 2012). Since RVT regressors have most of their power (>90%) in frequencies below 0.1 Hz, bandpass filtering below 0.1 Hz will also fail to address this source of variation. Overall, one expects a preprocessing pipeline that does not address more global physiological artifacts to fail to find strong group differences, as shown in the supplement to our original paper (Gotts et al., 2012) and in the Basic model of the current paper (using regressors for motion, ventricles, and local white matter). In that sense, the results of Tyszka et al. (2013) are exactly in accord with our expectations. It would be quite useful to re-examine their results with a method such as GCOR to establish whether the *t*-values would shift to be more positive and significant as in our current study. Hardware artifacts, addressed by the local white matter regressor in all of the models in the current study (see Jo et al., 2010, 2013 for discussion), are another source of relatively global artifact that has received much less attention than merited. We agree with advocates of GS regression that removing the GS will be expected to attenuate all of these more global artifacts in the data, leading to stronger group differences, higher reliability of results, etc. This is the case for our current results relative to the Basic model. However, it will do so at the high cost of warping the matrices of interest, preventing any straightforward conclusions about group comparisons. Therefore, we cannot recommend its application, especially when cleaner alternative methods exist for removing global artifacts—including the distant-dependent effects of transient head motion documented by Power et al. (2012) and addressed recently in Jo et al. (2013).

GCOR AS AN ALTERNATIVE TO GS REGRESSION

The GCOR model yielded a pattern of group differences that largely replicated what we reported originally for ANATICOR. The strongest group differences were between limbic-related (ROIs 1–7) and non-limbic social brain regions (ROIs 8-27) (**Figures 8, 10, 11**). If anything, the group comparisons under GCOR were larger in magnitude. However, it failed to replicate the correlations with SRS score within the ASD group. This failure was not entirely unanticipated, since the approach explicitly alters the variation in individual correlation values around the mean (or median), which is the same as the primary measure used for the SRS correlations. Under the GCOR approach, there is no *a priori* way to correctly partition the global level of correlation into different sources, some of which should be removed (global artifacts such as head motion, physiological and hardware artifacts) and some of which should not (neurally generated global variation; e.g., Schölvinck et al., 2010). It is this issue that prevents us from enthusiastically endorsing it for general use as a covariate. However, its good performance for the group comparisons in the current study suggests that it may be useful for conducting group comparisons in seed-based correlation studies when physiological de-noising is not possible due to lack of cardiac and respiration measures. It is also useful as a diagnostic tool to assess the distribution of global correlation levels in different groups. With subsequent work on this and other forms of data standardization (e.g., Yan et al., 2013), a post-hoc correction that works well for both group comparisons and symptom correlations may eventually be discovered, preserving datasets that were acquired without independent physiological measures. However, any time that nuisance measures are taken from the data that they are intended to clean, the risk is high for collinearity with the grouping variable, necessarily leading to GS-regression-like effects to some degree (Saad et al., 2013). It will be essential to examine any such methods with both simulations and mathematical analyses for the biases that they can introduce into single- and multi-group analyses. For example, in the current GCOR method, it is critical to examine the issue of data centering and to verify that the distributions of the covariates in the two groups are substantially overlapping (see **Figure 4**). If covariate distributions are non-overlapping in the two groups and a single grand mean center for the covariate is used, GCOR will introduce distortions similar to those introduced by GS regression (Saad et al., 2013), although such distortions will likely fail to reach significance because the covariate is highly collinear with the grouping variable. If group-specific centering is chosen (as in the current study), then it is possible that the difference in average correlation between the two groups is based on an artifactual source of global variation rather than a real neural difference. The best current alternative is to collect independent measures of physiological variation, modeling their influences separately. Given the impact that these preprocessing choices can have on the results that one obtains, it is difficult to overstate the importance of collecting heart rate and respiratory waveforms at the time of data acquisition.

ARE STUDIES OF FUNCTIONAL CONNECTIVITY DOOMED BY ARTIFACTS?

One reaction to the data that we have presented is that the pattern of data one finds is strongly influenced by choice of preprocessing model. Without knowing which model is the correct one to use, how can we be confident in any of the results? Our reaction to the data is more optimistic than that. For three of the models examined (Basic, GCOR, and ANATICOR), the overall ROI-ROI structure of the correlation matrices and group comparisons was remarkably similar across models. One would not be led down a substantially different theoretical pathway by either of the two non-GS models that address global artifacts. Instead, our results highlight the importance of addressing *all* of the major classes of time-varying artifacts that MR methods research has identified for BOLD fMRI (i.e., head motion, physiological, and hardware). In principle, many preprocessing models - including ICA-based models, can do a sufficient job at addressing this family of artifacts. We view certain alternatives to standard regression-based data cleaning, such as multi-echo fMRI with ICA to sort BOLD from non-BOLD variation (Kundu et al., 2012), as extremely promising. Future studies comparing such alternatives with single-echo fMRI that is acquired along with independent physiological measures should help to clarify which data-cleaning approaches work the best.

ACKNOWLEDGMENTS

The authors would like to thank Lauren Kenworthy, John Strang, and Rafael Oliveras-Rentas for guidance and aid in ASD participant testing, and Kelly Barnes and Dale Stevens for useful discussions. This study was supported by the National Institute of Mental Health, NIH, Division of Intramural Research, and it was conducted under NIH Clinical Study Protocol 10-M-0027 (ClinicalTrials.gov ID: NCT01031407).

REFERENCES

Anderson, J. S., Druzgal, T. J., Lopez-Larson, M., Jeong, E.-K., Desai, K., and Yurgelun-Todd, D. (2011a). Network anticorrelations, global regression, and phase-shifted soft tissue correction. *Hum. Brain Mapp.* 32, 919–934. doi: 10.1002/hbm.21079

Anderson, J. S., Nielsen, J. A., Froehlich, A. L., DuBray, M. B., Druzgal, T. J., Cariello, A. N., et al. (2011b). Functional connectivity magnetic resonance imaging classification of autism. *Brain* 134, 3742–3754. doi: 10.1093/brain/awr263

Assaf, M., Jagannathan, K., Calhoun, V. D., Miller, L., Stevens, M. C., Sahl, R., et al. (2010). Abnormal functional connectivity of default mode sub-networks in autism spectrum disorder patients. *Neuroimage* 53, 247–256. doi: 10.1016/j.neuroimage.2010.05.067

Belmonte, M. K., Allen, G., Beckel-Mitchener, A., Boulanger, L. M., Carper, R. A., and Webb, S. J. (2004). Autism and abnormal development of brain connectivity. *J. Neurosci.* 24, 9228–9231. doi: 10.1523/JNEUROSCI.3340-04.2004

Birn, R. M., Diamond, J. B., Smith, M. A., and Bandettini, P. A. (2006). Separating respiratory-variation-related fluctuations from neuronal-activity-related fluctuations in fMRI. *Neuroimage* 31, 1536–1548. doi: 10.1016/j.neuroimage.2006.02.048

Birn, R. M., Smith, M. A., Jones, T. B., and Bandettini, P. A. (2008). The respiration response function: the temporal dynamics of fMRI signal fluctuations related to changes in respiration. *Neuroimage* 40, 644–654. doi: 10.1016/j.neuroimage.2007.11.059

Buckner, R. L., Sepulcre, J., Talukdar, T., Krienen, F. M., Liu, H., Hedden, T., et al. (2009). Cortical hubs revealed by intrinsic functional connectivity: mapping, assessment of stability, and relation to Alzheimer's disease. *J. Neurosci.* 29, 1860–1873. doi: 10.1523/JNEUROSCI.5062-08.2009

Castelli, F., Frith, C., Happe, F., and Frith, U. (2002). Autism, Asperger syndrome and brain mechanisms for the attribution of mental states to animated shapes. *Brain* 125, 1839–1849. doi: 10.1093/brain/awf189

Chang, C., Cunningham, J. P., and Glover, G. H. (2009). Influence of heart rate on the BOLD signal: The cardiac response function. *Neuroimage* 44, 857–869. doi: 10.1016/j.neuroimage.2008.09.029

Chang, C., and Glover, G. H. (2009). Relationship between respiration, end-tidal CO2, and BOLD signals in resting-state fMRI. *Neuroimage* 47, 1381–1393. doi: 10.1016/j.neuroimage.2009.04.048

Cole, M. W., Pathak, S., and Schneider, W. (2010). Identifying the brain's most globally connected regions. *Neuroimage* 49, 3132–3148. doi: 10.1016/j.neuroimage.2009.11.001

Constantino, J. N. (2002). *The Social Responsiveness Scale.* Los Angeles, CA: Western Psychological Services.

Cordes, D., Haughton, V., Carew, J. D., Arfanakis, K., and Maravilla, K. (2002). Hierarchical clustering to measure connectivity in fMRI resting-state data. *Magn. Reson. Imaging* 20, 305–317. doi: 10.1016/S0730-725X(02)00503-9

Cox, R. W. (1996). AFNI: Software for analysis and visualization of functional magnetic resonance neuroimages. *Comp. Biomed. Res.* 29, 162–173. doi: 10.1006/cbmr.1996.0014

Deen, B., and Pelphrey, K. (2012). Perspective: Brain scans need a rethink. *Nature* 491, S20. doi: 10.1038/491S20a

Di Martino, A., Ross, K., Uddin, L. Q., Sklar, A. B., Castellanos, F. X., and Milham, M. P. (2009). Functional brain correlates of social and nonsocial processes in autism spectrum disorders: an activation likelihood estimation meta-analysis. *Biol. Psychiatry* 65, 63–74. doi: 10.1016/j.biopsych.2008.09.022

Di Martino, A., Zuo, X. N., Kelly, C., Grzadzinski, R., Mennes, M., Schvarcz, A., et al. (2013). Shared and distinct intrinsic functional network centrality in autism and attention-deficit/hyperactivity disorder. *Biol. Psychiatry.* doi: 10.1016/j.biopsych.2013.02.011. [Epub ahead of print].

Dinstein, I., Pierce, K., Eyler, L., Solso, S., Malach, R., Behrmann, M., et al. (2011). Disrupted neural synchronization in toddlers with autism. *Neuron* 70, 1218–1225. doi: 10.1016/j.neuron.2011.04.018

Ebisch, S. J., Gallese, V., Willems, R. M., Mantini, D., Groen, W. B., Romani, G. L., et al. (2011). Altered intrinsic functional connectivity of anterior and posterior insula regions in high-functioning participants with autism spectrum disorder. *Hum. Brain Mapp.* 32, 1013–1028. doi: 10.1002/hbm.21085

Fischl, B., Salat, D. H., Busa, E., Albert, M., Dieterich, M., Haselgrove, C., et al. (2002). Whole brain segmentation: automated labeling of neuroanatomical structures in the human brain. *Neuron* 33, 341–355. doi: 10.1016/S0896-6273(02)00569-X

Fox, M. D., and Greicius, M. (2010). Clinical applications of resting state functional connectivity. *Front. Syst. Neurosci.* 4:19. doi: 10.3389/fnsys.2010.00019

Fox, M. D., and Raichle, M. E. (2007). Spontaneous fluctuations in brain activity observed with functional magnetic resonance imaging. *Nat. Rev. Neurosci.* 8, 700–711. doi: 10.1038/nrn2201

Fox, M. D., Zhang, D., Snyder, A. Z., and Raichle, M. E. (2009). The global signal and observed anticorrelated resting state brain networks. *J. Neurophysiol.* 101, 3270–3283. doi: 10.1152/jn.90777.2008

Fransson, P., Skiold, B., Horsch, S., Nordell, A., Blennow, M., Lagercrantz, H., et al. (2007). Resting-state networks in the infant brain. *Proc. Natl. Acad. Sci. U.S.A.* 104, 15531–15536. doi: 10.1073/pnas.0704380104

Glover, G. H., Li, T. Q., and Ress, D. (2000). Image-based method for retrospective correction of physiological motion effects in fMRI: RETROICOR. *Magn. Reson. Med.* 44, 162–167.

Gotts, S. J., Simmons, W. K., Milbury, L. A., Wallace, G. L., Cox, R. W., and Martin, A. (2012). Fractionation of social brain circuits in autism spectrum disorders. *Brain* 135, 2711–2725. doi: 10.1093/brain/aws160

Jiang, X., Bollich, A., Cox, P., Hyder, E., James, J., Gowani, S. A., et al. (2013). A quantitative link between face discrimination deficits and neuronal selectivity for faces in autism. *Neuroimage Clin.* 2, 320–331. doi: 10.1016/j.nicl.2013.02.002

Jo, H. J., Gotts, S. J., Reynolds, R. C., Bandettini, P. A., Martin, A., and Cox, R. W. (2013). Effective preprocessing procedures virtually eliminate distance-dependent motion artifacts in resting state FMRI. *J. Appl. Math.* 2013, 9. doi: 10.1155/2013/935154

Jo, H. J., Saad, Z. S., Simmons, W. K., Milbury, L. A., and Cox, R. W. (2010). Mapping sources of correlation in resting state FMRI, with artifact detection and removal. *Neuroimage* 52, 571–582. doi: 10.1016/j.neuroimage.2010.04.246

Jones, T. B., Bandettini, P. A., Kenworthy, L., Case, L. K., Milleville, S. C., Martin, A., et al. (2010). Sources of group differences in functional connectivity: an investigation applied to autism spectrum disorder. *Neuroimage* 49, 401–414. doi: 10.1016/j.neuroimage.2009.07.051

Just, M. A., Cherkassky, V. L., Keller, T. A., and Minshew, N. J. (2004). Cortical activation and synchronization during sentence comprehension in high-functioning autism: evidence of underconnectivity. *Brain* 127, 1811–1821. doi: 10.1093/brain/awh199

Kaiser, M. D., Hudac, C. M., Shultz, S., Lee, S. M., Cheung, C., Berken, A. M., et al. (2010). Neural signatures of autism. *Proc. Natl. Acad. Sci. U.S.A.* 107, 21223–21228. doi: 10.1073/pnas.1010412107

Keller, C. J., Bickel, S., Honey, C. J., Groppe, D. M., Entz, L., Craddock, R. C., et al. (2013). Neurophysiological investigation of spontaneous correlated and anticorrelated fluctuations of the BOLD signal. *J. Neurosci.* 33, 6333–6342. doi: 10.1523/JNEUROSCI.4837-12.2013

Kennedy, D. P., and Courchesne, E. (2008). Functional abnormalities of the default network during self- and other-reflection in autism. *Soc. Cogn. Affect. Neurosci.* 3, 177–190. doi: 10.1093/scan/nsn011

Khan, S., Gramfort, A., Shetty, N. R., Kitzbichler, M. G., Ganesan, S., Moran, J. M., et al. (2013). Local and long-range functional connectivity is reduced in concert in autism spectrum disorders. *Proc. Natl. Acad. Sci. U.S.A.* 110, 3107–3112. doi: 10.1073/pnas.1214533110

Kundu, P., Inati, S. J., Evans, J. W., Luh, W. M., and Bandettini, P. A. (2012). Differentiating BOLD and non-BOLD signals in fMRI time series using multi-echo EPI. *Neuroimage* 60, 1759–1770. doi: 10.1016/j.neuroimage.2011.12.028

Lainhart, J. E., Bigler, E. D., Bocian, M., Coon, H., Dinh, E., Dawson, G., et al. (2006). Head circumference and height in autism: a study by the Collaborative Program of Excellence in Autism. *Am. J. Med. Genet. A* 140, 2257–2274. doi: 10.1002/ajmg.a.31465

Le Couteur, A., Rutter, M., Lord, C., Rios, P., Robertson, S., Holdgrafer, M., et al. (1989). Autism diagnostic interview: a standardized investigator-based instrument. *J. Autism Dev. Disord.* 19, 363–387. doi: 10.1007/BF02212936

Lombardo, M. V., Chakrabarti, B., Bullmore, E. T., Sadek, S. A., Pasco, G., Wheelwright, S. J., et al. (2010). Atypical neural self-representation in autism. *Brain* 133, 611–624. doi: 10.1093/brain/awp306

Lord, C., Risi, S., Lambrecht, L., Cook, E. H. Jr., Leventhal, B. L., Dilavore, P. C., et al. (2000). The autism diagnostic observation schedule-generic: a standard measure of social and communication deficits associated with the spectrum of autism. *J. Autism Dev. Disord.* 30, 205–223. doi: 10.1023/A:1005592401947

Lord, C., Rutter, M., and Le Couteur, A. (1994). Autism Diagnostic Interview-Revised: a revised version of a diagnostic interview for caregivers of individuals with possible pervasive developmental disorders. *J. Autism Dev. Disord.* 24, 659–685. doi: 10.1007/BF02172145

Margulies, D. S., Vincent, J. L., Kelly, C., Lohmann, G., Uddin, L. Q., Biswal, B. B., et al. (2009). Precuneus shares intrinsic functional architecture in humans and monkeys. *Proc. Natl. Acad. Sci. U.S.A.* 106, 20069–20074.

Maris, E., and Oostenveld, R. (2007). Nonparametric statistical testing of EEG- and MEG-data. *J. Neurosci. Methods* 25, 2862–2874.

Monk, C. S., Peltier, S. J., Wiggins, J. L., Weng, S. J., Carrasco, M., Risi, S., et al. (2009). Abnormalities of intrinsic functional connectivity in autism spectrum disorders. *Neuroimage* 47, 764–772. doi: 10.1016/j.neuroimage.2009.04.069

Müller, R. A., Shih, P., Keehn, B., Deyoe, J. R., Leyden, K. M., and Shukla, D. K. (2011). Underconnected, but how? A survey of functional connectivity MRI studies in autism spectrum disorders. *Cereb. Cortex* 21, 2233–2243. doi: 10.1093/cercor/bhq296

Murphy, K., Birn, R. M., Handwerker, D. A., Jones, T. B., and Bandettini, P. A. (2009). The impact of global signal regression on resting state correlations: are anti-correlated networks introduced? *Neuroimage* 44, 893–905. doi: 10.1016/j.neuroimage.2008.09.036

Paakki, J. J., Rahko, J., Long, X., Moilanen, I., Tervonen, O., Nikkinen, J., et al. (2010). Alteration in regional homogeneity of resting-state brain activity in autism spectrum disorders. *Brain Res.* 1321, 169–179. doi: 10.1016/j.brainres.2009.12.081

Power, J. D., Barnes, K. A., Snyder, A. Z., Schlaggar, B. L., and Petersen, S. E. (2012). Spurious but systematic correlations in functional connectivity MRI networks arise from subject motion. *Neuroimage* 59, 2142–2154. doi: 10.1016/j.neuroimage.2011.10.018

Rudie, J. D., Brown, J. A., Beck-Pancer, D., Hernandez, L. M., Dennis, E. L., Thompson, P. M., et al. (2013). Altered functional and structural brain network organization in autism. *Neuroimage Clin.* 2, 79–94. doi: 10.1016/j.nicl.2012.11.006

Saad, Z. S., Gotts, S. J., Murphy, K., Chen, G., Jo, H. J., Martin, A., et al. (2012). Trouble at rest: how correlation patterns and group differences become distorted after global signal regression. *Brain Connect.* 2, 25–32. doi: 10.1089/brain.2012.0080

Saad, Z. S., Reynolds, R. C., Jo, H. J., Gotts, S. J., Chen, G., Martin, A., et al. (2013). Correcting brain-wide correlation differences in resting-state FMRI. *Brain Connect.* doi: 10.1089/brain.2013.0156. [Epub ahead of print].

Salomon, R., Bleich-Cohen, M., Hahamy-Dubossarsky, A., Dinstien, I., Weizman, R., Poyurovsky, M., et al. (2011). Global functional connectivity deficits in schizophrenia depend on behavioral state. *J. Neurosci.* 31, 12972–12981. doi: 10.1523/JNEUROSCI.2987-11.2011

Satterthwaite, T. D., Elliott, M. A., Gerraty, R. T., Ruparel, K., Loughead, J., Calkins, M. E., et al. (2013). An improved framework for confound regression and filtering for control of motion artifact in the preprocessing of resting-state functional connectivity data. *Neuroimage* 64, 240–256. doi: 10.1016/j.neuroimage.2012.08.052

Satterthwaite, T. D., Wolf, D. H., Loughead, J., Ruparel, K., Elliott, M. A., Hakonarson, H., et al. (2012). Impact of in-scanner head motion on multiple measures of functional connectivity: relevance for studies of neurodevelopment in youth. *Neuroimage* 60, 623–632. doi: 10.1016/j.neuroimage.2011.12.063

Schölvinck, M. L., Maier, A., Ye, F. Q., Duyn, J. H., and Leopold, D. A. (2010). Neural basis of global resting-state fMRI activity. *Proc. Natl. Acad. Sci. U.S.A.* 107, 10238–10243. doi: 10.1073/pnas.0913110107

Shmueli, K., Van Gelderen, P., De Zwart, J. A., Horovitz, S. G., Fukunaga, M., Jansma, J. M., et al. (2007). Low-frequency fluctuations in the cardiac rate as a source of variance in the resting-state fMRI BOLD signal. *Neuroimage* 38, 306–320. doi: 10.1016/j.neuroimage.2007.07.037

Shukla, D. K., Keehn, B., and Müller, R. A. (2010). Regional homogeneity of fMRI time series in autism spectrum disorders. *Neurosci. Lett.* 26, 46–51. doi: 10.1016/j.neulet.2010.03.080

Snyder, A. Z., and Raichle, M. E. (2012). A brief history of the resting state: the Washington University perspective. *Neuroimage* 62, 902–910. doi: 10.1016/j.neuroimage.2012.01.044

Talairach, J., and Tournoux, P. (1988). *Co-planar Stereotaxic Atlas of the Human Brain.* New York, NY: Thieme Medical Publishers.

Tyszka, J. M., Kennedy, D. P., Paul, L. K., and Adolphs, R. (2013). Largely typical patterns of resting-state functional connectivity in high-functioning adults with autism. *Cereb. Cortex.* doi: 10.1093/cercor/bht040. [Epub ahead of print].

Van Dijk, K. R., Sabuncu, M. R., and Buckner, R. L. (2012). The influence of head motion on intrinsic functional connectivity MRI. *Neuroimage* 59, 431–438. doi: 10.1016/j.neuroimage.2011.07.044

Vincent, J. L., Patel, G. H., Fox, M. D., Snyder, A. Z., Baker, J. T., Van Essen, D. C., et al. (2007). Intrinsic functional architecture in the anaesthetized monkey brain. *Nature* 447, 83–86. doi: 10.1038/nature05758

von dem Hagen, E. A., Stoyanova, R. S., Baron-Cohen, S., and Calder, A. J. (2012). Reduced functional connectivity within and between 'social' resting state networks in autism spectrum conditions. *Soc. Cogn. Affect. Neurosci.* doi: 10.1093/scan/nss053. [Epub ahead of print].

Weisberg, J., Milleville, S. C., Kenworthy, L., Wallace, G. L., Gotts, S. J., Beauchamp, M. S., et al. (2012). Social Perception in Autism Spectrum Disorders: impaired category selectivity for dynamic but not static images in ventral temporal cortex. *Cereb. Cortex.* doi: 10.1093/cercor/bhs276. [Epub ahead of print].

Weng, S. J., Wiggins, J. L., Peltier, S. J., Carrasco, M., Risi, S., Lord, C., et al. (2010). Alterations of resting state functional connectivity in the default network in adolescents with autism spectrum disorders. *Brain Res.* 1313, 202–214. doi: 10.1016/j.brainres.2009.11.057

Yan, C.-G., Cheung, B., Kelly, C., Colcombe, S., Craddock, R. C., Di Martino, A., et al. (2013). A comprehensive assessment of regional variation in the impact of head micromovements on functional connectomics. *Neuroimage* 76C, 183–201. doi: 10.1016/j.neuroimage.2013.03.004

Yan, C.-G., Craddock, R. C., Zuo, X.-N., Zang, Y.-F., and Milham, M. P. (2013). Standardizing the intrinsic brain: Towards robust measurement of inter-individual variation in 1000 functional connectomes. *Neuroimage* doi: 10.1016/j.neuroimage.2013.04.081. [Epub ahead of print].

Zang, Y., Jiang, T., Lu, Y., He, Y., and Tian, L. (2004). Regional homogeneity approach to fMRI data analysis. *Neuroimage* 22, 394–400. doi: 10.1016/j.neuroimage.2003.12.030

Altered neural connectivity in excitatory and inhibitory cortical circuits in autism

Basilis Zikopoulos * and Helen Barbas

Neural Systems Laboratory, Department of Health Sciences, Boston University, Boston, MA, USA

Edited by:
Diane Chugani, Wayne State University, USA

Reviewed by:
Jeffrey J. Hutsler, University of Nevada, Reno, USA
Cyndi Schumann, UC Davis MIND Institute, USA

****Correspondence:***
Basilis Zikopoulos, Neural Systems Laboratory, Department of Health Sciences, Boston University, 635 Commonwealth Avenue, Boston, MA 02215, USA
e-mail: zikopoul@bu.edu

Converging evidence from diverse studies suggests that atypical brain connectivity in autism affects in distinct ways short- and long-range cortical pathways, disrupting neural communication and the balance of excitation and inhibition. This hypothesis is based mostly on functional non-invasive studies that show atypical synchronization and connectivity patterns between cortical areas in children and adults with autism. Indirect methods to study the course and integrity of major brain pathways at low resolution show changes in fractional anisotropy (FA) or diffusivity of the white matter in autism. Findings in *post-mortem* brains of adults with autism provide evidence of changes in the fine structure of axons below prefrontal cortices, which communicate over short- or long-range pathways with other cortices and subcortical structures. Here we focus on evidence of cellular and axon features that likely underlie the changes in short- and long-range communication in autism. We review recent findings of changes in the shape, thickness, and volume of brain areas, cytoarchitecture, neuronal morphology, cellular elements, and structural and neurochemical features of individual axons in the white matter, where pathology is evident even in gross images. We relate cellular and molecular features to imaging and genetic studies that highlight a variety of polymorphisms and epigenetic factors that primarily affect neurite growth and synapse formation and function in autism. We report preliminary findings of changes in autism in the ratio of distinct types of inhibitory neurons in prefrontal cortex, known to shape network dynamics and the balance of excitation and inhibition. Finally we present a model that synthesizes diverse findings by relating them to developmental events, with a goal to identify common processes that perturb development in autism and affect neural communication, reflected in altered patterns of attention, social interactions, and language.

Keywords: prefrontal cortex (PFC), parvalbumin-positive interneurons, anterior cingulate cortex, ratio of excitation and inhibition, myelinated axons, GAP-43, white matter, short-range and long-distance pathways

INTRODUCTION—THE GENERAL HYPOTHESIS FOR DISRUPTED CONNECTIVITY IN ASD

The balance of excitation and inhibition is disrupted in autism spectrum disorders (ASD) with widespread repercussions on neural communication (Rubenstein and Merzenich, 2003; Amaral et al., 2008; Rubenstein, 2011). Connections are the conduit for neural communication, forming local or interareal circuits, which collectively construct large scale networks. In the primate brain, cortico-cortical, and cortico-subcortical pathways that travel through the white matter originate from excitatory neurons. The white matter pathways, which consist largely of axons of excitatory neurons, can be subdivided into short/medium- or long-range based on the distance they travel to connect with other neural structures. When these pathways reach their targets in the cortex or in subcortical structures they form excitatory synapses with local excitatory or inhibitory neurons, participating in local microcircuits within a column/minicolumn, or neighboring columns in the cortex, or within subcortical structures. Axons from inhibitory neurons in primates are largely confined within the gray matter and innervate nearby neurons found in the same or different layers within the same or neighboring columns.

This brief description of structural connectivity highlights multiple levels at the macro and micro scales that may be disrupted in varying degrees in ASD, affecting neural communication, and the balance of excitation and inhibition. Converging evidence from genetic, functional, and structural studies suggests that there are changes in excitatory and inhibitory neural communication in ASD and in the structure of the underlying cortical circuits or networks. At the microcircuit and synaptic level, numerous genetic studies have highlighted a large variety of polymorphisms and epigenetic factors that primarily affect neurite growth, synapse formation, and synaptic transmission of excitatory and inhibitory neurons (see Samaco et al., 2005; Hogart et al., 2007; Weiss et al., 2009; Gilman et al., 2011; Hallmayer et al., 2011; Hussman et al., 2011; Voineagu et al., 2011; Shulha et al., 2012; reviewed in Geschwind, 2011). At the level of the network, most imaging studies have also focused on affected brain systems by identifying abnormalities in the gray and white matter, primarily in frontal and temporal lobes, or in their major pathways (Belmonte et al., 2004a; Herbert, 2005; Casanova, 2007; Courchesne et al., 2007; Kumar et al., 2009; Schumann et al., 2010; Schipul et al., 2011; Just et al., 2012).

However, there is a paucity of data about specific changes in neural elements that form excitatory and inhibitory brain circuits and underlie mechanisms of imbalance in ASD. While in short supply, studies at the cellular level have described changes in the cytoarchitecture, density and neurochemical features of excitatory and inhibitory neurons in frontal and temporal areas in autism (Bauman and Kemper, 2005; Casanova, 2007; Amaral et al., 2008; Schmitz and Rezaie, 2008; Blatt and Fatemi, 2011; Penzes et al., 2011; Schumann and Nordahl, 2011; Srivastava et al., 2012). Only a few studies have employed a combination of high resolution methods to study the neural pathophysiology of autism, by identifying specific structural, neurochemical, and molecular changes of neuronal elements that may underlie atypical development of synaptic interactions within functional cortical networks (Weidenheim et al., 2001; Garbern et al., 2010; Zikopoulos and Barbas, 2010). The present review focuses on these structural aspects that likely tip the balance of excitation and inhibition at the level of circuits and networks in ASD.

Several cortical and subcortical areas including frontal and temporal cortices, the amygdala, and the cerebellum exhibit atypical functional and structural characteristics in ASD; it should be noted however, that pathology may also be present in other and as yet not studied brain regions. Frontal cortical pathways have received considerable attention because they consistently show functional disruption in ASD (Hill, 2004; Pickett and London, 2005; Wass, 2011; Just et al., 2012). For this reason, here we focus on three robustly interconnected prefrontal regions: anterior paracingulate and cingulate areas (referred thereafter as ACC) in the medial prefrontal cortex, orbitofrontal cortex (OFC) in the ventral and ventrolateral prefrontal cortex, and lateral prefrontal areas (LPFC). These areas have a key role in attention, social interactions, emotions, and executive control (Barbas, 2000a,b; Barbas et al., 2011), in processes that are severely affected in autism (Baron-Cohen, 1991; Ozonoff et al., 1991; Carper et al., 2002; Maestro et al., 2002; Sparks et al., 2002; Mundy, 2003; Hill, 2004; Girgis et al., 2007; Jiao et al., 2010). In some cases we include relevant findings in temporal or parietal cortices that are connected with the above prefrontal cortices.

The ACC, OFC, LPFC and their pathways are functionally disorganized in autism. There is evidence that at least some of these areas exhibit local over-connectivity and long-distance disconnection (Casanova et al., 2002b; Barnea-Goraly et al., 2004; Casanova, 2004; Herbert et al., 2004; Courchesne and Pierce, 2005; Herbert, 2005; Kana et al., 2006b; Girgis et al., 2007; Just et al., 2007; Pardini et al., 2009; Assaf et al., 2010; Hyde et al., 2010; Anagnostou and Taylor, 2011; Bernardi et al., 2011; Wass, 2011). Aberrant function of ACC in autism includes hyperactivity during response monitoring and social target detection (Thakkar et al., 2008; Dichter et al., 2009) and desynchronized activity during working memory tasks (Kana et al., 2006b), while LPFC shows lower activity in working memory tasks (Luna et al., 2002; Koshino et al., 2008; reviewed in Schipul et al., 2011). Activity in LPFC and OFC is correlated with intellectual level and predicts poor performance of individuals with autism in neuropsychological tasks (Loveland et al., 2008). In addition, in autism there is decreased functional connectivity between OFC, other areas that process emotions, reward, and social interactions, like the amygdala or insula, and language areas in the posterior superior temporal sulcus (Sabbagh, 2004; Bachevalier and Loveland, 2006; Hardan et al., 2006; Girgis et al., 2007; Abrams et al., 2013).

The goal of this article is to synthesize recent high resolution neuropathological findings at the cellular level of circuits and relate the observed changes to relevant gross anatomical, functional, genetic, or epidemiological data. The focus is on axons and neurons that form local or distant circuits. We highlight similarities and differences in the way local vs. long-distance circuits may be affected in ASD and propose refinements to the hypothesis of disrupted connectivity in ASD that may reconcile conflicting findings regarding the prevalence and significance of over-connectivity or under-connectivity in frontal and temporal networks. We additionally report preliminary findings of changes in the ratio of distinct types of inhibitory neurons in dorsolateral prefrontal area 9 of adults with ASD. This pilot study presents novel evidence that addresses the overarching hypothesis of disruption in the balance of excitation and inhibition in autism. Finally, by grounding findings within a developmental framework we propose potential common mechanisms that may underlie the disruption of neural communication and the imbalance of excitation and inhibition in ASD.

WHAT BRINGS ABOUT CHANGES IN STRUCTURAL CONNECTIVITY?

Structural connectivity can change by direct alterations in the physical connections between neurons, reflected in the numbers of synapses, and the biophysical attributes of individual synapses that affect synaptic efficacy. Significant structural changes likely affect functional connectivity, reflected in ASD as atypical synchronization and connectivity patterns of frontal or temporal areas in children and adults with autism, suggesting abnormal engagement and interactions of short-range and long-range excitatory pathways and local inhibitory circuits (Rubenstein and Merzenich, 2003). The study of structural connectivity at the synaptic level in humans is challenging, primarily due to limited tissue availability and variability in tissue preservation that may impede rigorous analyses. Despite these limitations there is considerable evidence for changes in neuronal elements in cortical areas that could affect synaptic function in ASD. Studies report changes in the structure of presynaptic and post-synaptic elements, pathways in the white and gray matter, and density and size of various neuronal and glial cell types, as elaborated below.

AXON PATHOLOGY IS AT THE CORE OF ATYPICAL CONNECTIVITY IN ASD

Imaging studies in children and adults with autism, show decreased functional connectivity between frontal and other areas and gross changes in the structural integrity of frontal gray and white matter (Barnea-Goraly et al., 2004; Kana et al., 2006a; Just et al., 2007; Keller et al., 2007; Minshew and Williams, 2007; Koshino et al., 2008; Thakkar et al., 2008; Pardini et al., 2009; Minshew and Keller, 2010). Typical findings in the white matter include lower fractional anisotropy (FA) and higher radial diffusivity in ASD groups than in controls, which may come about by a reduction of diffusion barriers between axons (reviewed in Muller et al., 2011). These findings suggest decreased axon diameter and/or decreased myelination that reduce axon volume, and may result in changes in the density of axons.

The relative position and size of axons in the white matter below the cortex can be used as an indicator of their termination in nearby or distant brain areas. The deep (inner or sagittal) white matter includes long-range excitatory pathways (Herbert et al., 2004; Hilgetag and Barbas, 2006; Petrides and Pandya, 2006, 2007; Schmahmann and Pandya, 2006; Sundaram et al., 2008), with thicker axons than found in the superficial white matter just below the cortex (Zikopoulos and Barbas, 2010; **Figure 1**). The superficial (outer or radiate) white matter is situated below cortical layer 6, and carries mostly thin excitatory fibers as axons branch to connect with nearby areas (**Figure 1**).

Based on the relationship of pathways within the white matter, functional imaging and physiological studies have shown that long-range cortico-cortical pathways that link frontal areas with

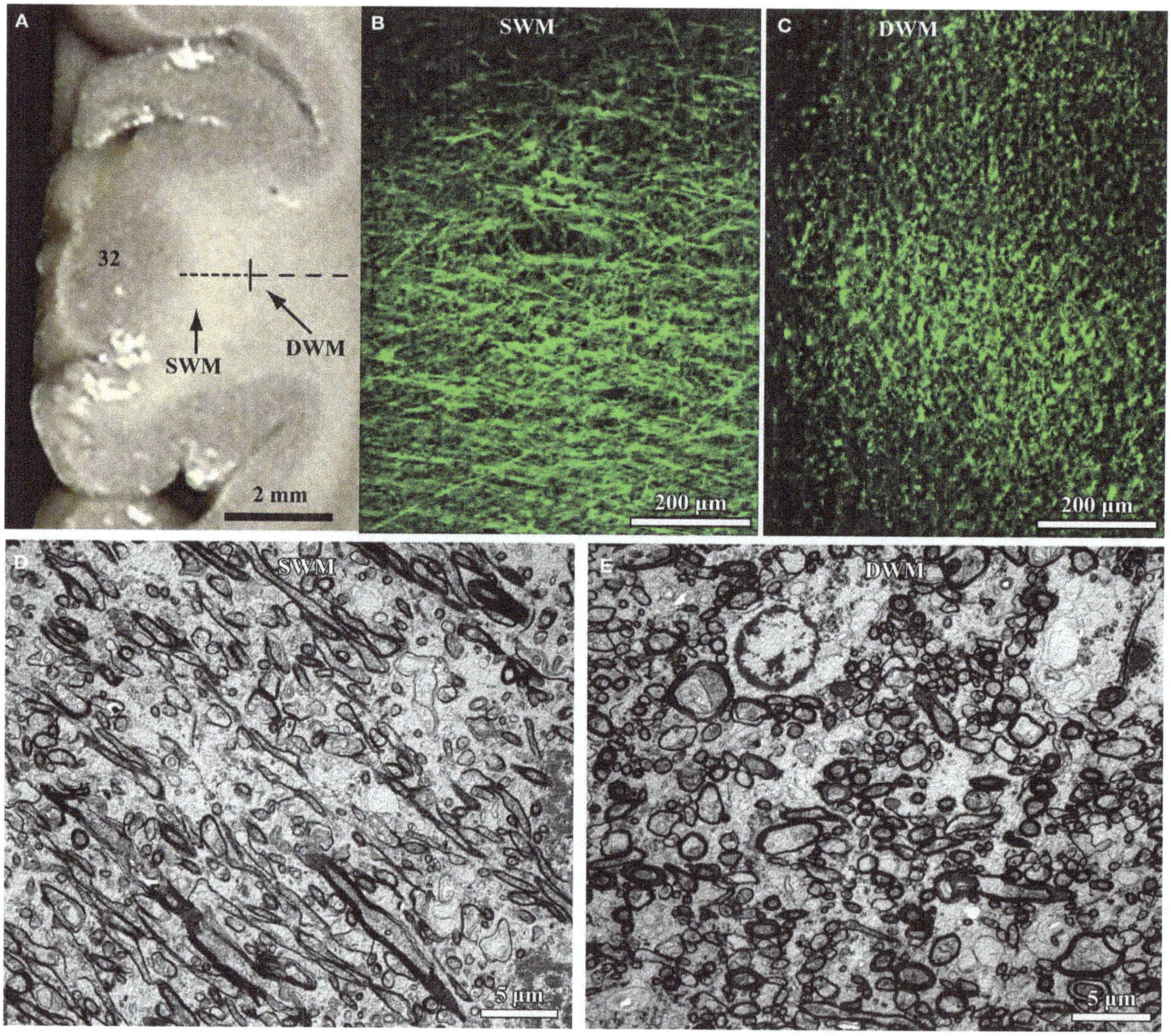

FIGURE 1 | High resolution segmentation of the white matter. (A) Coronal view of a representative ACC (A32) tissue slab. Dotted lines indicate gross (macroscopic) distinction of superficial (SWM) and deep (DWM) white matter, based on subsequent microscopic analysis. **(B,C)** Fluorescent photomicrographs of coronal sections from A32 white matter after labeling of axons with a neurofilament protein antibody (NFP-200; green). Light microscopic segmentation of superficial **(B)** and deep **(C)** white matter is based on the distinct orientation of axons at different depths from the gray matter. Axons in the superficial white matter travel mainly perpendicular to the surface of the cortex (**B**, axons appear mainly as thin lines), whereas in the deep white matter most axons travel parallel to the cortical surface (**C**, axons appear mainly as green dots). **(D,E)** EM photomicrographs show mostly elongated axon profiles in the superficial white matter **(D)** and mostly circular axon profiles in the deep white matter **(E)**. Adapted from Zikopoulos and Barbas (2010).

other cortices are weak and disorganized in autism. Specifically, there is reduced coherence and correlation in task-related activity of distant areas, which constitutes decreased functional connectivity (Just et al., 2004, 2007; Courchesne and Pierce, 2005). In addition, gross structural imaging studies have shown reduced size, FA, and diffusivity in deep white matter tracts, suggesting differential composition or compromised structural integrity of long-distance pathways in adults and children with autism (Alexander et al., 2007; Just et al., 2007; Frazier and Hardan, 2009; Casanova et al., 2011; Jou et al., 2011; Shukla et al., 2011a). In contrast, gross structural imaging studies have reported transient enlargement of the superficial white matter in the frontal cortex of children with autism (Belmonte et al., 2004a; Herbert et al., 2004; Herbert, 2005). Concomitantly, functional studies have shown aberrant or excessive activation and increased synchrony within frontal cortices, suggesting local overconnectivity in autism (Courchesne and Pierce, 2005; Kennedy et al., 2006).

Our recent work in adult human *post-mortem* brain tissue (Zikopoulos and Barbas, 2010) provides novel evidence for specific structural and molecular changes in individual prefrontal axons (**Figure 2**). In agreement with the long-range underconnectivity hypothesis, we found that below the anterior cingulate/paracingulate cortices (ACC) in the brains of adults with autism there are fewer large myelinated axons in the deep white matter, which link distant areas (Herbert et al., 2004; Hilgetag and Barbas, 2006; Petrides and Pandya, 2006, 2007; Schmahmann and Pandya, 2006; Sundaram et al., 2008). In sharp contrast, we found a higher density of thin myelinated axons in the superficial white matter below ACC, which was partially due to excessive branching of thin and medium-sized axons, which link nearby areas. In addition, axons below OFC had thinner myelin in ASD cases than in controls (**Figure 2**). The thinner myelin in OFC was not due to a reduction in the density of oligodendroglia in the white matter (Zikopoulos and Barbas, 2010).

The significance of these findings is twofold. First, the ACC has a key role in attentional control (Gehring and Knight, 2000; Paus, 2001; Ito et al., 2003; Johnston et al., 2007), and OFC in emotions (Barbas and Zikopoulos, 2006; Zikopoulos and Barbas, 2012), and both processes are seriously disrupted in autism (Gomot et al., 2006; Steele et al., 2007; Vlamings et al., 2008; Norbury et al., 2009; Markram and Markram, 2010; Bernardi et al., 2011). Second, in non-human primates, the ACC has the most widespread connections with other prefrontal cortices (Barbas et al., 1999). The OFC is distinguished for its multimodal input from every sensory modality through high-order sensory association and multimodal cortices (Barbas, 1993; Barbas and Zikopoulos, 2006). These findings suggest that changes in axons below ACC and OFC have widespread repercussions on prefrontal networks and beyond. That is why, even though axon features below lateral prefrontal cortices (LPFC) appear unaffected (Zikopoulos and Barbas, 2010), the altered white matter composition below ACC and OFC changes the relationship among prefrontal areas. The changes in the relationship of axons below prefrontal areas could affect LPFC function, because these regions are robustly interconnected in primates (Petrides and Pandya, 1988; Seltzer and Pandya, 1989; Barbas et al., 1999; Barbas, 2000a; Fullerton and Pandya, 2007; Schmahmann et al., 2007).

Two well-studied networks can be used to illustrate additional, and perhaps more specific, implications for the pathology of intrinsic or distant prefrontal circuits in ASD. First, studies of the ACC-LPFC intrinsic circuit in non-human primates show that ACC sends a robust feedback projection that targets primarily the superficial layers of LPFC (Medalla and Barbas, 2009, 2010, 2012). As is typical in cortico-cortical networks in primates, excitatory axons from ACC mainly target excitatory pyramidal neurons in LPFC. However, a smaller but significant proportion (~20%) of excitatory ACC axons form synapses with inhibitory neurons in the superficial layers of LPFC, where they innervate preferentially calbindin (CB) inhibitory neurons (Medalla and Barbas, 2009). Anatomic, physiologic, and computational studies have shown that CB inhibitory neurons innervate the distal dendrites of excitatory pyramidal neurons (Peters and Sethares, 1997) and modulate their activity, increasing the signal-to-noise ratio (Peters and Sethares, 1997; Gonzalez-Albo et al., 2001; Wang et al., 2004). These synaptic specializations suggest that ACC can enhance relevant signals and reduce noise in LPFC, to facilitate focusing attention on a task, and are especially useful during challenging cognitive tasks (Gehring and Knight, 2000; MacDonald et al., 2000; Paus, 2001; Schall, 2001; Ito et al., 2003; Badre and Wagner, 2004; Johnston et al., 2007; Tanji and Hoshi, 2008). The exuberance of thin, short-range axons found in adults with autism (Zikopoulos and Barbas, 2010) that link ACC with nearby areas, including LPFC, suggests a potential exaggeration of this mechanism that could underlie the difficulty of even high-functioning individuals with autism to shift attention. Distant regions that are likely affected are temporal lobe structures, including auditory or multimodal temporal cortices and the amygdala, which have strong bidirectional interactions with prefrontal cortices in non-human primates (e.g., Barbas and Mesulam, 1985; Barbas et al., 1999, 2005b; Ghashghaei and Barbas, 2002; Germuska et al., 2006; Ghashghaei et al., 2007; Medalla et al., 2007; Zikopoulos et al., 2008).

In spite of the small number of cases and heterogeneity on the ASD spectrum, changes in axons below ACC were present in all autistic cases studied, suggesting a fundamental autism phenotype in axons below some prefrontal areas (Zikopoulos and Barbas, 2010). The power and generalizability of these findings are high likely because the cases were well-matched and within a narrow age range (30–44 years), obviating differences in the developmental trajectory that can increase variability. Importantly, the findings are based on multiple independent methods to estimate the same or related variables. For example, axon size and branching were independently evaluated both at the confocal and electron microscopes, and additionally corroborated by independently labeling and estimating the proportion of axons that express axon growth factors, as elaborated below.

MOLECULAR MECHANISMS THAT REGULATE AXON GROWTH ARE AFFECTED IN AUTISM

In the study of adults with autism (Zikopoulos and Barbas, 2010), supernumerary branching, and density of thin axons below ACC are associated with increased expression of the Growth Associated Protein 43 (GAP-43; **Figure 2**). This intracellular protein is produced in the cell body and is quickly transported down the axon

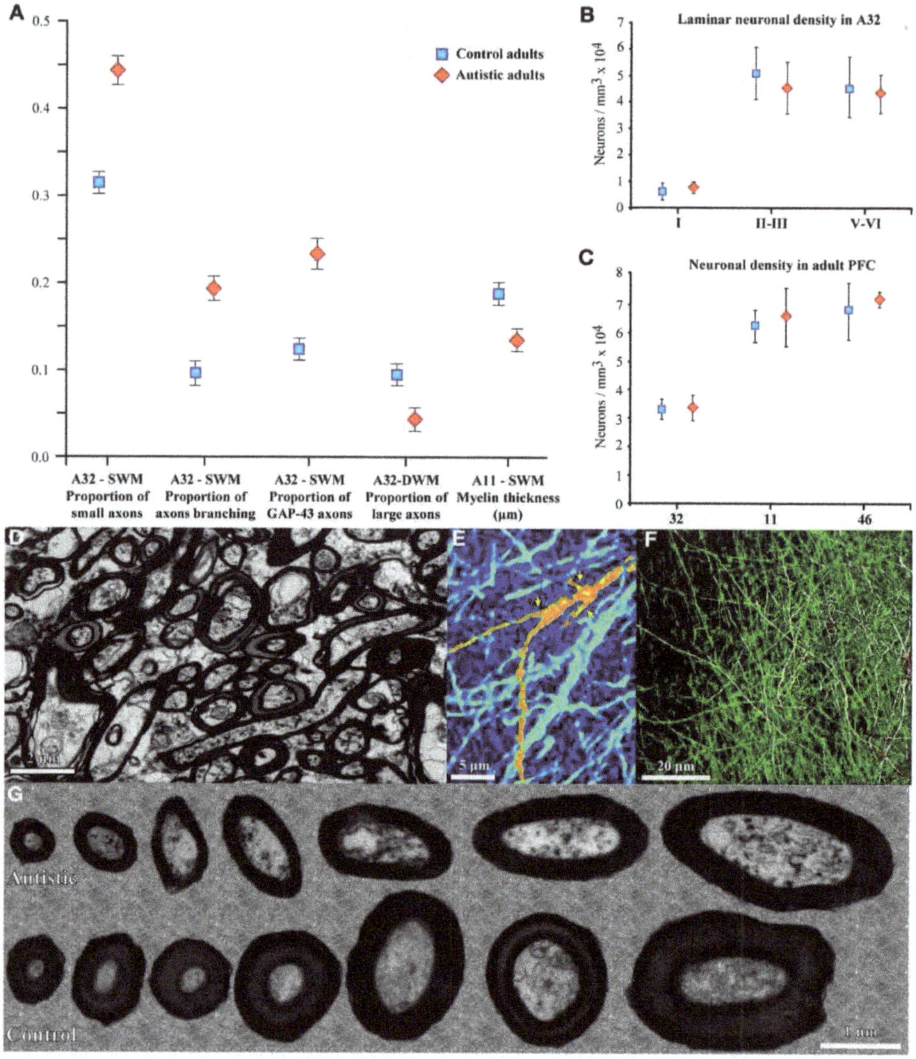

FIGURE 2 | Changes in myelinated axons below prefrontal cortices in adults with ASD. (A) In the superficial white matter (SWM) below ACC (area 32) the relative density of small (thin) axons (±SEM) is increased in the autistic cases, and more axons branch and express GAP-43. These data suggest increased local connectivity of ACC in ASD. In contrast, in the deep white matter (DWM) below ACC the relative density of large axons is reduced in ASD, suggesting weakening of long-range connectivity. Thinning of the myelin in axons of all sizes just below OFC (area 11) suggests weak local connections. **(B,C)** Laminar and overall neuronal density below ACC, OFC, and LPFC is similar in adults with ASD and controls and is not correlated with the changes in axons below PFC. **(D)** EM photomicrograph of axons in the superficial white matter below ACC of an adult with ASD. **(E)** Collapsed image (z-projection) from a three-dimensional confocal stack shows myelinated axons branching, labeled with NFP-200 (green). A branching axon is pseudo colored with orange/yellow hue for visualization (yellow arrowheads point to branches). **(F)** Image from a three-dimensional confocal stack with double immunofluorescence shows GAP-43 (red) in axons labeled with NFP-200 (green). Some myelinated axons contain GAP-43 in their axolemma, which is transported to axon terminals and branching points. Colocalization of the two antibodies is rendered white. **(G)** EM photomicrographs show differences in myelin thickness in OFC between control and autistic adults, apparent in all axon size groups.

to reach branching points, growth cones, and axon terminals (reviewed in Benowitz and Routtenberg, 1997). It is, therefore, most abundant in the superficial part of the white matter and in the gray matter, as axons branch to innervate their targets. GAP-43 also promotes neurotransmitter release, endocytosis and synaptic vesicle recycling (Denny, 2006). These actions are contingent upon phosphorylation of GAP-43 by protein kinase C, which induces local actin filament-membrane attachment. GAP-43 is expressed at high levels during late prenatal and early postnatal stages of axon growth, and is subsequently markedly reduced with the onset of myelination (Kapfhammer and Schwab, 1994; Benowitz and Routtenberg, 1997). In the adult brain GAP-43 is found in significant amounts only in some limbic areas, including the hippocampus and ACC, where it also promotes axon growth, and acts as a lateral stabilizer of actin filaments presynaptically, strengthening synapses to promote long-term potentiation, spatial memory formation, and learning (Maviel et al., 2004; Holahan et al., 2007; Holahan and Routtenberg,

2008). In addition, GAP-43 is found at focal sites after brain injury, where it promotes axon sprouting and regeneration (Neve et al., 1988; Benowitz and Routtenberg, 1997).

In autism, an increase in GAP-43 may persist in adulthood in response to reported inflammation (Vargas et al., 2005; Morgan et al., 2010), or due to axon damage. Interestingly, GAP-43 transcription is directly regulated by calcineurin and nuclear factor of activated T cells (Yoshida and Mishina, 2005; Nguyen et al., 2009), which are targets of immunosuppressants like rapamycin (Ho et al., 1996). Rapamycin inhibits the mTOR signaling pathway, and improves neurological dysfunction in animal models of tuberous sclerosis that are relevant for autism (Ehninger and Silva, 2011). Therefore, it seems plausible that GAP-43 and related signaling proteins may provide the link between neurological deficits and the extensive immune dysregulation in autism (Smith et al., 2007; Atladottir et al., 2009; Becker and Schultz, 2010; Patterson, 2011; Garbett et al., 2012; Hsiao et al., 2012; Malkova et al., 2012; Patterson, 2012).

A variety of external factors up-regulate GAP-43 expression, including estrogenic agents that disrupt endocrine function, such as bisphenol A, and immunosuppressive and psychiatric drugs used for a variety of common disorders, including psoriasis, asthma, rheumatoid arthritis, dry eye, depression, and anxiety (Wong et al., 1989; Jyonouchi et al., 2001; Granda et al., 2003; Croen et al., 2005, 2011; Ostensen et al., 2006; Sairanen et al., 2007; Brown, 2009; Nguyen et al., 2009). Several of these substances came into heavy use in the early 80s at a time when the prevalence of autism began to rise (Blaxill, 2004). The use of endocrine disruptors during pregnancy has been correlated with increased autism risk (Croen et al., 2011; Simpson et al., 2011; de Cock et al., 2012).

Information on the developmental trajectory of axon growth and relevant signaling pathways will help delineate a more detailed timeline for the development of autism pathology, narrow down the temporal window for the insult, and spur new research to identify affected signaling pathways and factors that may be targeted for therapeutic interventions. Importantly, epidemiologic studies are necessary to investigate the relationship between signaling pathways and possible cumulative effects of environmental agents, diet, and drugs on the uterine and postnatal environment that may perturb the expression of factors implicated in axon growth and guidance in autism.

DENDRITIC SPINE PATHOLOGY IN ASD

Structural evidence for the disturbance of neural communication in ASD is also apparent in the cortical gray matter, specifically on post-synaptic targets of cortical or subcortical afferents, the dendrites of excitatory pyramidal neurons. In dorsolateral prefrontal area 9, temporal area 21, and parietal area 7, there is increased dendritic spine density in layer II pyramidal neurons, and in neurons of layer V only in area 21, among those studied (Hutsler and Zhang, 2010). These differences were found in all major dendritic branches (apical, basilar, and oblique), and along the length of apical dendrites of pyramidal cells for several hundred micrometers from the cell body. Based on these results, ASD seems to be part of a small group of developmental disorders where there is no apparent loss of dendritic spines.

Since the majority of synapses on spines of pyramidal neurons are excitatory (e.g., Lowenstein and Somogyi, 1991; Peters et al., 1991; Ahmed et al., 1997; Somogyi et al., 1998; Alonso-Nanclares et al., 2004; Douglas and Martin, 2004; Anderson and Martin, 2009; Medalla and Barbas, 2009, 2010; Micheva et al., 2010), changes in spine density suggest an alteration in the density of excitatory synapses on dendritic segments within prefrontal, temporal, and parietal cortices in ASD. However, one cannot rule out possible changes in the density of inhibitory synapses onto cortical neurons, which also target dendritic spines and shafts in various ratios, depending on the pathway. Moreover, preliminary morphological analysis (Hutsler and Zhang, 2010; Avino et al., 2012) shows immature morphology and excessive fluctuation in the length and shape of spines in ASD cases, suggesting synaptic lability. The same morphological changes could affect dendritic cytosolic compartmentalization, dendritic computations, and ultimately neuronal processing (for a review see London and Hausser, 2005).

The findings on spine features are limited to studies by one group so far and do not offer explicit clues about the potential local or distant presynaptic origin of the connections affected, but are nevertheless informative about the overall pathology in ASD. Specifically, a consistent finding is increased layer II connectivity in ASD in association areas examined by (Hutsler and Zhang, 2010). Neurons in the superficial layers of the cortex are primarily involved in ipsilateral and contralateral cortico-cortical connections, and receive feedback projections from areas that have fewer layers or lower neuronal density, such as the ACC (Barbas and Rempel-Clower, 1997), and these pathways may be disproportionately affected in ASD. Layer II in LPFC receives strong input from the amygdala (Ghashghaei et al., 2007), most subcortical neuromodulatory systems (Berger et al., 1988; Lewis et al., 1988; Gaspar et al., 1989; Lewis and Morrison, 1989; Raghanti et al., 2008), and the ACC (Barbas et al., 1999; Medalla and Barbas, 2009, 2010). Another type of pathway that targets the superficial cortical layers, including layer II, originates from the widely projecting matrix neurons of the thalamus, which can effectively propagate and synchronize thalamocortical activity over large expansions of the cortex (Zikopoulos and Barbas, 2007; Jones, 2009). It is possible that within the frontal lobe, potential thalamocortical pathology in the upper layers may be restricted to lateral prefrontal areas, because at least the gross features of myelinated thalamocortical axons in the deep white matter below the ACC are not affected in ASD (Zikopoulos and Barbas, 2010). Further work is needed to determine if thalamocortical axons are more specifically affected as they branch to innervate different prefrontal cortices.

Further, based on the inside-out model of development of the cortex, layer II is the last layer to develop. The maturation period of layer II is protracted as connections are formed, in accord with the fact that long-distance cortico-cortical and callosal connections that these superficial layers participate in also develop late. It seems that changes in white matter axons, described in previous sections (Zikopoulos and Barbas, 2010), as well as changes in dendritic spines in the gray matter (Hutsler and Zhang, 2010), point toward late prenatal or early postnatal critical periods for the development of ASD neuropathology. This is also supported by the fact that callosal pathways, which also develop late, are severely compromised in ASD as well (Alexander et al., 2007; Just et al., 2007; Frazier and Hardan, 2009; Jou et al., 2010; Anderson et al., 2011b; Cantlon et al., 2011; Casanova et al., 2011; Fame et al., 2011; Schipul et al., 2011).

The finding of increased dendritic spine density in layer V pyramidal neurons only in temporal area 21 (Hutsler and Zhang, 2010) may be associated with atypical auditory or language processing and with deficits in social-emotional interactions in ASD. This idea is in accord with imaging studies (e.g., Just et al., 2004; Gomot et al., 2006; Bigler et al., 2007; Lee et al., 2007). Within the cortex, atypical activation patterns of layer V neurons in temporal areas may have an effect in feedback pathways to other cortical areas. Moreover, the amygdala, thalamus, and striatum are major subcortical targets of cortical layer V neurons, and structural as well as functional studies indicate that these subcortical structures and their circuits may be affected in autism (e.g., Bauman and Kemper, 1985; Tsatsanis et al., 2003; Schumann et al., 2004; Haznedar et al., 2006; Schumann and Amaral, 2006; Shukla et al., 2010; Tamura et al., 2010; Cheon et al., 2011; Di Martino et al., 2011; Langen et al., 2012).

NEURONAL AND GLIAL CELL DENSITIES AND MORPHOLOGY IN ASD

Several structural imaging studies have shown that there is abnormal acceleration of brain growth in ASD. The brains of young children with ASD are larger than those of typically developing controls, and although this enlargement is attributed mostly to increased white matter volume, there is also significant enlargement of gray matter, especially in frontal and temporal areas (reviewed in Courchesne et al., 2011a). The white matter or cortical enlargement appears to be transient and is not evident in adults with ASD (Herbert, 2005; Redcay and Courchesne, 2005). In agreement with these data, recent preliminary findings suggest that the increase in gray matter volume in children with ASD may, in some cases, be due to increased number of neurons, at least in some prefrontal cortices (Courchesne et al., 2011b). The authors of this study reported that children with ASD have, on average, 79% more neurons in dorsolateral prefrontal cortices (DLPFCs) and 29% more neurons in mesial prefrontal cortices (mesial: medial prefrontal cortices excluding cingulate areas). An earlier study also reported neuropathological thickening of the subependymal cell layer, multifocal subependymal nodular dysplasia, and heterotopias in some children and adults with ASD (Wegiel et al., 2010). These developmental changes may reflect multiregional cortical and subcortical dysregulation of neurogenesis, neuronal migration, and maturation in ASD.

In the brains of adults with autism there are no significant changes in the overall number or density of neurons (Zikopoulos and Barbas, 2010), or in the laminar density of neurons in medial areas 24, 32, orbital area 11, or dorsolateral areas 9 and 46. This evidence indicates that in autism the numbers of neurons in prefrontal cortices are comparable to controls in adulthood. Several other studies also report no differences in the numbers or density of neurons in other cortical areas, including ventrolateral language-related frontal areas 44 and 45 (Jacot-Descombes et al., 2012), area 23 in the posterior cingulate cortex (PCC) and area 37 in the fusiform gyrus (FFG; Oblak et al., 2011b, but see van Kooten et al., 2008), and in areas 3b, 4, 9, 10, 11, 17, 24, 43, and 44 (Casanova et al., 2002b, 2006) in children or adults with ASD. In line with this evidence, there appear to be no differences in cortical layering and thickness in prefrontal, temporal, and parietal areas of children and adults with ASD (Hutsler et al., 2007; Zikopoulos and Barbas, 2010). However, parts of areas 24 and 23 in the dorsal and posterior cingulate cortices display altered cytoarchitecture with irregularly distributed neurons, leading to irregular lamination and poor demarcation of layers IV and V in some ASD cases (Simms et al., 2009; Oblak et al., 2011b).

Detection of potential changes in the number or density of neurons in ASD additionally depends on the types of neurons analyzed. A recent study showed that children with autism consistently had a significantly higher ratio of von Economo neurons (VENs, also known as spindle neurons) to pyramidal neurons than control subjects in frontoinsular cortex (Santos et al., 2011). The authors of this study posit that higher numbers of VENs in autism may be related to alterations in migration, cortical lamination, and apoptosis, and may also underlie a heightened interoception, described in some clinical observations. It seems though that VEN numbers may be regionally specific and age-dependent, because there are no overall differences between autism and control brains in ACC area 24 in teenagers and young adults (Simms et al., 2009). However, among the autism cases, there were two subsets; 1/3 of the cases had significantly increased VEN density and the remaining 2/3 of the cases had reduced VEN density compared to controls.

Changes in the density of glia in the cortex in ASD appear to be type- and region-specific, as well. In a recent study, we did not find differences in the densities of oligodendrocytes, astrocytes, and microglia in the white matter below OFC (Zikopoulos and Barbas, 2010). However, findings suggest a role of glia in ASD pathology in the gray matter based on increased density of astrocytes in frontal cortices in ASD, although the results were not based on stereological analysis (Cao et al., 2012). Another intriguing finding pertains to a higher density of microglia in the gray matter of DLPFC, accompanied by increased activation of microglia in some ASD cases (Morgan et al., 2010). The same group recently showed that microglia are more frequently present near neurons in DLPFC leading to aberrantly close microglia–neuron association (Morgan et al., 2012). Interestingly, the density of activated microglia is additionally elevated in the gray matter of medial prefrontal, cingulate, orbitofrontal, and the gyral fusiform cortices in ASD (Pardo et al., 2005; Vargas et al., 2005; Suzuki et al., 2013). These findings indicate the potential for neuroinflammation and immune responses in some ASD cases that may be linked to higher levels of GAP-43 (Zikopoulos and Barbas, 2010).

Finally, a frequently observed change in the structure of cortical gray matter in children and adults with ASD is minicolumnopathy, defined by decreased columnar width, characterized by diminished and disrupted peripheral neuropil compartment (Casanova et al., 2002a,b, 2006; Buxhoeveden et al., 2006). More specifically, minicolumns in ASD appear to have less peripheral neuropil space and increased spacing among the constituent cells in several areas (3b, 4, 9, 10, 11, 17, 24, 43, 44).

Frontal area 44 seems to be the most affected, and the pathology is evident in children and adults with ASD. The increased number of minicolumns in autism may be accompanied or brought about by changes in the size of neurons, the number of cells per column, or their greater dispersion, resulting in no global difference in neuronal density. In line with this evidence, there are reports of decreased size of pyramidal neurons in layers III, V, VI in language related areas 44, 45 (Jacot-Descombes et al., 2012), in layers I-III and layers V-VI of cingulate area 24b and in cell packing density in layers V-VI of cingulate area 24c (Simms et al., 2009) in children and adults with ASD. In addition, areas 24 and 23 in the ACC and PCC display altered cytoarchitecture and increased density of neurons in the subcortical white matter (Simms et al., 2009; Oblak et al., 2011b). The latter is in agreement with observations of abnormal cell patterning at the cortical gray-white matter border of areas 9, 21, and 7 in ASD (Avino and Hutsler, 2010).

All these reported changes in neuron density and morphology, as well as laminar and columnar distribution, can affect both excitatory and inhibitory connections and circuits. In particular, the peripheral neuropil space surrounding the minicolumn is the conduit for inhibitory and excitatory local circuit projections (Peters and Sethares, 1996; Mountcastle, 1997, 1998; Casanova et al., 2003; Douglas and Martin, 2004) that may also be affected, further tipping the balance of excitation and inhibition in ASD, as elaborated below.

STRUCTURAL CHANGES IN CORTICAL INHIBITORY NEUROTRANSMISSION

CHANGES IN INHIBITORY NEUROTRANSMISSION IN ASD

Key evidence for irregular inhibition patterns in autism comes from functional data, suggesting decreased levels of synchronization during response inhibition tasks (Rubenstein and Merzenich, 2003; Yizhar et al., 2011). In addition, molecular studies of autistic individuals and relevant animal models have identified dysregulation of inhibitory biomarkers and mutations in genes associated with the development of cortical inhibitory neurons and their synaptic communication (Ma et al., 2005; Collins et al., 2006; Selby et al., 2007; Tabuchi et al., 2007; Yip et al., 2008; Fatemi et al., 2009a,b; Chao et al., 2010; Blatt and Fatemi, 2011; Gandal et al., 2012).

Importantly, a number of recent studies have consistently found changes in the levels of GABA receptors in frontal and temporal areas. The mean density of $GABA_A$ receptors and the density of benzodiazepine binding sites in all layers of area 24 are decreased in ASD (Oblak et al., 2009). Similar reduction is found in the superficial layers of areas 23 (PCC) and 37 (FFG). In the deep layers of the FFG there is also reduction in the number of benzodiazepine binding sites (Oblak et al., 2011a), found on inhibitory neurons (Murray and Wise, 2012). Interestingly, in the superficial layers of PCC and FFG the autism group appears to have higher binding affinity for ligands of the $GABA_A$ receptor. The authors suggest that the observed downregulation of receptors may be the result of increased GABA innervation and/or release. In addition, there are significant reductions in $GABA_B$ receptor density in the ACC, PCC and FFG in the brains of people with autism compared to matched controls (Oblak et al., 2010). These changes in the $GABA_B$ receptor subtype may contribute to the functional deficits in socio-emotional and cognitive processing, as well as identification of faces and facial expressions by individuals with ASD.

The reduction in GABA receptors and benzodiazepine binding in the cortex is a consistent deficit in autism, with similar findings in the hippocampus (Blatt et al., 2001; Guptill et al., 2007), suggesting widespread GABA receptor abnormalities in ASD. Based on recent findings (Fatemi et al., 2009b) of reduced levels of proteins in three of the $GABA_A$ receptor subunits in autism in multiple cortical regions, it is possible that a defect in one or more of the $GABA_A$ receptor subunits exists as well. Moreover, genetic studies found significant association and molecular interactions of specific GABA receptor subunit genes in autism (Ma et al., 2005). However, despite the evidence for widespread disruption of inhibitory neurotransmission in the cortex little is known about the state of the GABAergic interneurons themselves in the cortex in ASD (Lawrence et al., 2010; Oblak et al., 2011b), whose organization and function is highlighted below.

CIRCUIT BASIS FOR THE INITIATION OF INHIBITORY CONTROL

In the cortex, inhibitory control is primarily mediated through local GABAergic interneurons, which comprise a diverse group distinguished by morphology, the types of neurons and sites they synapse with, physiologic properties, and efficacy of inhibitory control (White, 1989; Kawaguchi and Kubota, 1997; Thomson and Deuchars, 1997; Somogyi et al., 1998; Gupta et al., 2000). Inhibitory neurons represent 20–30% of all neurons in the mammalian neocortex and in the frontal cortex of humans they make up ~21% of the neuronal population (Hornung and De Tribolet, 1994; Kalus and Senitz, 1996; Benes et al., 2001; Sherwood et al., 2010). In primates, inhibitory neurons can be classified by their expression of the calcium-binding proteins parvalbumin (PV), calbindin (CB), and calretinin (CR), which comprise largely non-overlapping neurochemical groups of inhibitory neurons in the cortex (Hendry et al., 1989; Defelipe, 1997). PV labels basket and chandelier inhibitory neurons (Defelipe et al., 1989b; Kawaguchi and Kubota, 1997), which are most prevalent in the middle layers of the cortex, where they form perisomatic synapses on pyramidal neurons, providing strong inhibition (Defelipe et al., 1989b; Shao and Burkhalter, 1999). CB labels several cortical morphologic types of inhibitory neurons, which are most densely distributed in cortical layers 2 and upper layer 3, and innervate distal dendrites of pyramidal neurons (Peters and Sethares, 1997), modulating their activity. CR inhibitory neurons are found mostly in the upper layers (I-IIIa) as well, where they innervate mostly other GABAergic neurons, at least in the upper layers (Gabbott et al., 1997; Meskenaite, 1997; Defelipe et al., 1999; Gonchar and Burkhalter, 1999). This regularity in the laminar distribution of PV, CB, and CR neurons is seen in frontal, temporal, and sensory association areas, which have been studied in primates (Defelipe et al., 1989a, 1990; Conde et al., 1994; Kondo et al., 1999; Dombrowski et al., 2001; Barbas et al., 2005b).

In the cortex there is also regularity in the laminar origin and termination of excitatory pathways, which can be predicted based on the structure of interconnected areas, as described by the structural model for connections (Barbas, 1986; Barbas and Rempel-Clower, 1997; Rempel-Clower and Barbas, 2000). Briefly, according to this model, limbic areas, which have fewer than 6 layers and lower cell density, send mainly feedback projections to eulaminate areas, which have 6 layers and higher cell density. These projections originate mainly from the deep layers and terminate mostly in the superficial layers. Projections in the opposite direction are feedforward, predominantly originate from the superficial layers of eulaminate areas and terminate in the middle/deep layers of limbic cortices. Connections between areas with similar architecture originate and terminate equally in all layers. Numerous studies, have consistently supported this model for ipsilateral and callosal connections among diverse cortices in non-human primates (Barbas, 1986; Barbas and Rempel-Clower, 1997; Barbas et al., 2005a,b; Medalla and Barbas, 2006; Medalla et al., 2007; Bunce and Barbas, 2011), and in other species (Grant and Hilgetag, 2005; Hilgetag and Grant, 2010).

Moreover, a series of studies in non-human primates has established that whereas excitatory prefrontal pathways innervate mostly excitatory neurons at the site of termination, they also innervate a smaller but significant (~10–30%) proportion of inhibitory neurons (Barbas et al., 2005b; Medalla et al., 2007; Medalla and Barbas, 2009, 2010; Anderson et al., 2011a; Bunce and Barbas, 2011; reviewed in Barbas and Zikopoulos, 2007). These findings provide the circuit basis for initiation of inhibitory control by prefrontal areas. Connections thus originate and terminate in distinct laminar microenvironments where the distribution of specific classes of inhibitory neurons also varies, providing the framework to examine the structural underpinnings for the imbalance in excitation and inhibition in autism, as elaborated in the preliminary experiments presented below.

DECREASED RATIO OF PV/CB INHIBITORY NEURONS IN DORSOLATERAL PREFRONTAL AREA 9 IN ASD

The balance of excitation and inhibition is affected in autism with detrimental effects on neural communication. Elements of inhibitory neurons are affected in autism, but the state of distinct neurochemical classes of inhibitory neurons in prefrontal cortex is unknown. Here we performed a preliminary study to examine the laminar distribution of cortical inhibitory neurons in ASD, using *post-mortem* adult human brain tissue from dorsolateral prefrontal area 9 ($n = 2$ autistic; $n = 2$ matched controls for age, sex, and hemisphere; **Figure 3**; **Table 1**). We compared the density of two non-overlapping, functionally distinct classes of local inhibitory interneurons, which, in primates, are also neurochemically distinct, based on their expression of the calcium-binding proteins calbindin (CB) or parvalbumin (PV).

There was a significant reduction of PV neurons in the autistic brains, in both cases [(density: cells/mm^3 ± standard deviation) control, PV: 3747 ± 786; CB: 3747 ± 337; ASD, PV: 2390 ± 564; CB: 3693 ± 511; $p = 0.01$; **Figure 4**]. The ratio of PV/CB inhibitory neurons thus decreased by approximately a third in ASD (to 0.65), potentially affecting inhibitory efficacy and overall network dynamics. In typical controls the ratio is close to 1, as is also found in non-human primates (Gabbott and Bacon, 1996; Dombrowski et al., 2001).

PV inhibitory neurons are most prevalent in the middle cortical layers, and provide strong perisomatic inhibition of excitatory neurons (Defelipe et al., 1989b; Kawaguchi and Kubota, 1997; Shao and Burkhalter, 1999). Reduction in PV inhibitory neurons in area 9 may help explain abnormally high columnar activation and desynchronization of oscillatory activity in autism (reviewed in Defelipe, 1999). Our findings are in accord with evidence of compromised inhibitory neurotransmission in autism, reflected by reduced gamma band power of auditory responses in children and adolescents with autism (Wilson et al., 2007), and absence of stimulus-driven synchronization effects on sensory perception (Tommerdahl et al., 2008). These findings suggest atypical coordination of local excitatory-inhibitory cortical activity. Our preliminary findings are also in line with a recent report, showing that in the fusiform face area (FFA) there is less synchrony between alpha and gamma waves, when subjects with autism look at faces, when compared to controls (Khan et al., 2013). Because both of these brain rhythms depend on local inhibition driven primarily by PV neurons (Chow et al., 1998; White et al., 2000; Whittington et al., 2000, 2011; Borgers and Kopell, 2003; Buzsaki and Draguhn, 2004), reduction in phase-amplitude coupling between slow alpha and fast gamma rhythms suggests compromised inhibitory neurotransmission.

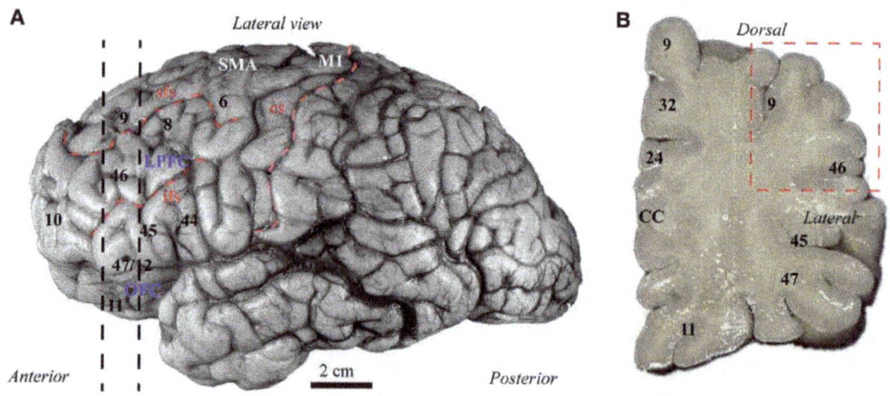

FIGURE 3 | Map of human frontal areas. (A) Lateral view of the human brain shows the dorsolateral prefrontal area 9 and its relationship with other frontal areas. Dotted lines indicate the coronal level used for analysis. **(B)** One centimeter thick slab of frontal cortex shows the region sampled in the dorsolateral prefrontal cortex (red dotted-line square). See Appendix for abbreviations.

Table 1 | Clinical characteristics of post-mortem cases studied.

Case number	Control-4786	Control-4981	Autism-4541	Autism-6677
Age at death (years)	36	42	44	30
Sex	Male	Male	Male	Male
Post-mortem interval (hours)	20	18	31	16
Primary cause of death	Myocardial infarction	Myocardial infarction	Acute myocardial infarction	Congestive heart failure
Hemisphere	Right	Right	Right	Right
AUTISM DIAGNOSTIC INTERVIEW–REVISED (ADI-R) SCORES FOR AUTISTIC CASES				
(A) Qualitative impairments in reciprocal social interactions (cutoff: 10)			26	26
(B) Qualitative abnormalities in communication (Verbal; cutoff: 8)			18	22
(C) Qualitative abnormalities in communication (Non-verbal; cutoff: 7)			13	#
(D) Restricted, repeated, and stereotyped patterns of behavior (cutoff: 3)			6	12
(E) Abnormality of development evident at or before 36 months (cutoff: 1)			5	5

 # Scores were not obtained/not applicable due to lack of communication skills. All donors in the autism group had difficulties with communication, social behaviors, and atypical interests, consistent with a diagnosis of autism, and the ADI-R scores met and exceeded cutoffs for autism in each of these areas.

On the other hand, we found no differences in the density of CB inhibitory neurons in area 9, which are most numerous in the superficial cortical layers, and have modulatory effects (e.g., Peters and Sethares, 1997; Gonzalez-Albo et al., 2001). CB neurons in LPFC have a role in gain modulation during attentional processes, and among inhibitory classes, they are targeted preferentially by ACC pathways (Medalla and Barbas, 2009).

Previous findings of changes in the white matter suggest that pathways linking ACC with nearby prefrontal areas are excessively dense in autism (Zikopoulos and Barbas, 2010). These findings are consistent with functional studies showing that ACC in autism is hyperactive, especially during response monitoring (Thakkar et al., 2008). This could lead to over activation of CB inhibitory neurons in area 9. This circuit mechanism suggests heightened ability to focus attention, which, on one hand, can be advantageous for complex problem solving. On the other hand, excessive strength in the pathway from ACC to LPFC may also disrupt the ability to shift attention flexibly, and may contribute to the rigid and repetitive behavior seen in autism. In line with this hypothesis, the reported increase in the density of dendritic spines on layer II pyramidal neurons of dorsolateral area 9 (Hutsler and Zhang, 2010), may reflect a plasticity change that spines can undergo (Nimchinsky et al., 2002), perhaps to accommodate the excess fiber input of feedback pathways from ACC in ASD.

A potential change in the ratio of the functionally distinct classes of inhibitory neurons in lateral area 9 in autism can have an impact on the activity of other areas both locally and in widespread distributed circuits, affecting neural dynamics of communication in the cortex. In accordance with our preliminary data, a reduction in PV inhibitory neurons, which mediate perisomatic inhibition of pyramidal excitatory neurons, may diminish strong inhibition in prefrontal areas, leading to over excitation and desynchronization of neuronal activity over large brain networks. This outcome could offer clues on the high prevalence of epilepsy in autism (about 30%) (reviewed in Levisohn, 2007; Hughes, 2008), and has profound implications for LPFC function, like working memory, as reported for autism (Luna et al., 2002; Steele et al., 2007). The ability of LPFC to dynamically adjust the attentional gain in these processes relies heavily on the activity of local PV inhibitory neurons, which underlie shifts in cortical rhythms during cognitive tasks (Abbott and Chance, 2005; Borgers et al., 2008), a process that is also necessary to shift attention flexibly.

To date, DLPFC is the only cortical area in which changes in the ratio of inhibitory neurons in ASD have been reported, since Oblak et al. (2011b) found no differences in parvalbumin, or calbindin interneurons in areas in the posterior cingulate and FFG. It should be noted however, that given the extensive physiological evidence for atypical inhibitory activity patterns in ASD more cortical areas need to be examined. If supported with data from more cases, our findings will have important implications for the pathology in autism. In addition, studies in a variety of animals and humans have established that CB neurons develop earlier than PV neurons (Alcantara et al., 1993; Yan et al., 1997; Letinic and Kostovic, 1998; Hof et al., 1999), and the selective reduction of PV neurons in area 9 in autism suggests the likely timing of the pathology. The status of axons below prefrontal areas also point to changes that have their root in development, as discussed below in the context of a model that relates pathological findings to developmental events.

A MODEL FOR THE DEVELOPMENT OF DISRUPTED FRONTAL NETWORKS IN ASD

LOCAL OVERCONNECTIVITY, LONG-DISTANCE DISCONNECTION, OR BOTH? IT DEPENDS ON THE AREA

Findings from a variety of functional and structural imaging studies suggest that the breakdown in neural communication in autism involves local overconnectivity and long-distance

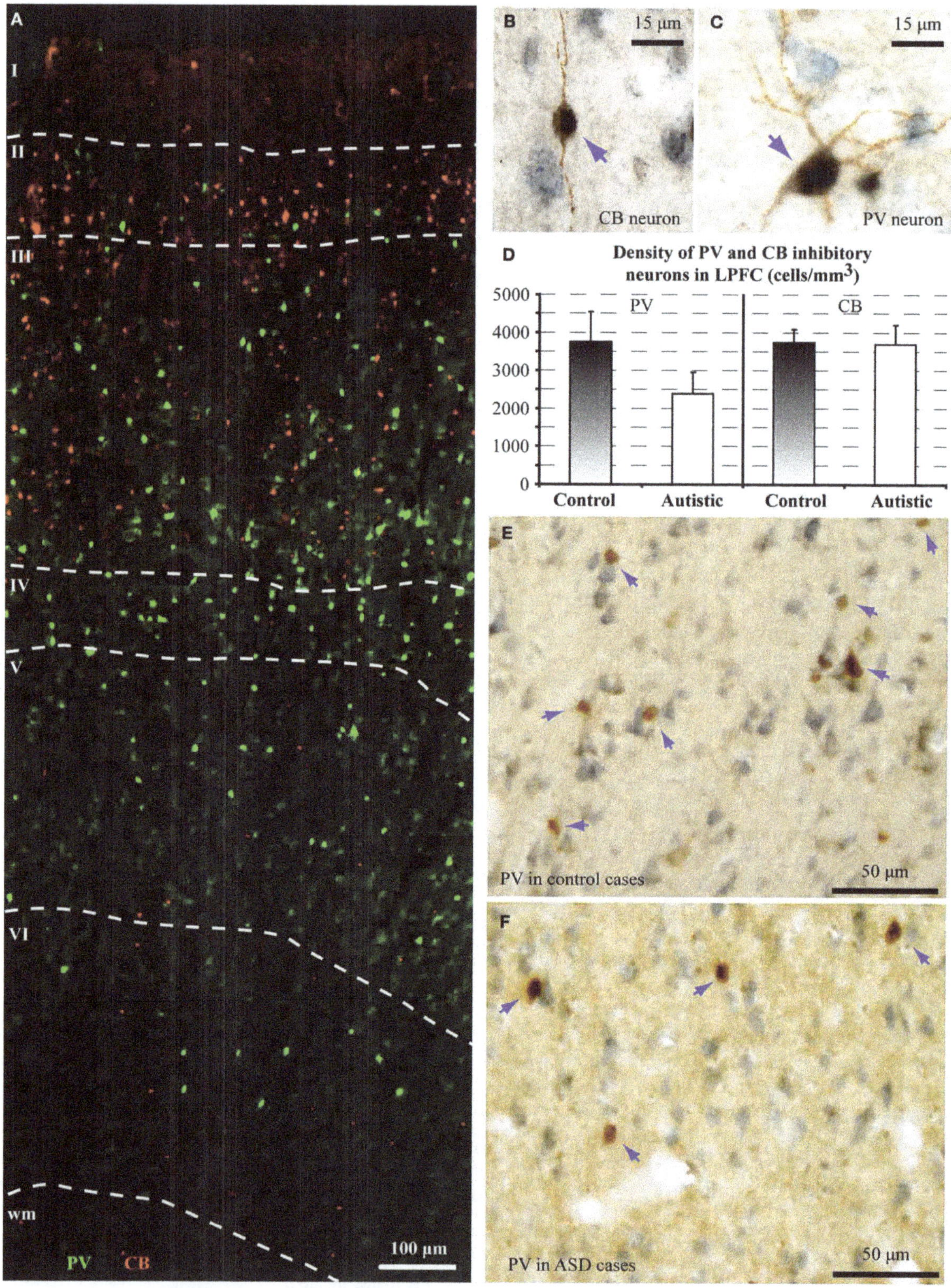

FIGURE 4 | There is a decrease in the ratio of parvalbumin (PV) to calbindin (CB) inhibitory neurons in area 9 of the human brain in autism. (A) Fluorescent photomicrograph shows the preferential laminar distribution of CB (red) in the superficial layers and PV (green) in the middle-deep layers of the human dorsolateral prefrontal cortex. **(B,C)** High magnification photographs of CB and PV neurons in the human dorsolateral prefrontal cortex (indicated by blue arrows). **(D)** Preliminary results show lower density of PV neurons in autistic cases (cells/mm^3 ± standard deviation). **(E,F)** Low magnification photographs of PV neurons in the dorsolateral prefrontal cortex (indicated by blue arrows) of control and ASD adults.

disconnection, especially in pathways that include the frontal lobe (Herbert et al., 2003; Belmonte et al., 2004b; Carper and Courchesne, 2005; Courchesne and Pierce, 2005; Kennedy et al., 2006; Thakkar et al., 2008). There is general agreement that long-distance connections are weak in autism, but some studies suggest that local connections are also weak, or at least not excessive (e.g., Sundaram et al., 2008; Shukla et al., 2011a,b). The disparity in findings on first blush may be attributed to methodological issues inherent in the limited resolution of MRI and DTI, specific methodological and data analysis choices (reviewed in Muller et al., 2011), or poor contrast of the gray-white matter boundary in autism that renders automatic segmentation ambiguous (Bailey et al., 1998; Avino and Hutsler, 2010).

The most likely scenario, however, is that connectivity is affected differentially in distinct cortical regions in autism (**Figure 5**). This hypothesis is consistent with findings that suggest weak local connectivity in some sensory areas or the face region (Sundaram et al., 2008; Shukla et al., 2011a,b; Khan et al., 2013), contrasted with excessive connectivity between some prefrontal cortices in autism (Herbert et al., 2003; Kennedy et al., 2006; Thakkar et al., 2008; Zikopoulos and Barbas, 2010). We found evidence suggesting overconnectivity by the ACC, no change in lateral prefrontal, and weak connectivity in OFC in autism. These findings are based on high resolution methods to view individual axons at the level of the system and to zero in at axon segments at the electron microscope in *post-mortem* brain tissue (Zikopoulos and Barbas, 2010). The high resolution methods employed make it possible to differentiate not only the gray-white matter border, but also to separate the superficial from the deep white matter based on axon orientation. In coronal sections, axons that course in the superficial white matter appear as elongated rods of variable size and direction. In contrast, axons that dive down to the deep white matter en route to distant areas appear as small circular, doughnut-like, structures, because they travel parallel to the cortical surface (**Figure 1**).

Precise segmentation of the superficial white matter revealed an excess number of medium and thin axons and more branching just below the ACC in the brains of adults with autism (Zikopoulos and Barbas, 2010). The affected superficial white matter links nearby areas. We found no such changes in axons below lateral areas 9, 46, or orbital area 11. But just below area 11 the myelin was thinner in the brains of autistic people than in controls, consistent with decreased functional anisotropy (FA) in some frontal areas (Sundaram et al., 2008). The above findings demonstrate that the connectivity status in autism varies depending on cortical region.

The changes in axons below the ACC are of special interest for several reasons. To begin with, in non-human primates the ACC has the most widespread connections with neighboring prefrontal cortices (Barbas et al., 1999). The ACC may exercise its critical role in allocating attention through its normally extensive influence on the rest of the prefrontal cortex. Further, in non-human primates, excitatory pathways from the ACC innervate not only excitatory neurons in LPFC, but also a smaller but significant proportion of inhibitory neurons. Importantly, pathways from ACC form large and efficient synapses with inhibitory neurons in LPFC, and innervate preferentially the neurochemical class of inhibitory neurons labeled for calbindin (Medalla and Barbas, 2009, 2010), which are suited to reduce neural noise and enhance signal (Constantinidis et al., 2002; Wang et al., 2004). The exuberance of axons that connect the ACC with LPFC over short or medium distances may help explain why people with autism focus on a stimulus and have difficulty in orienting to other stimuli in the environment when needed. The problems in shifting

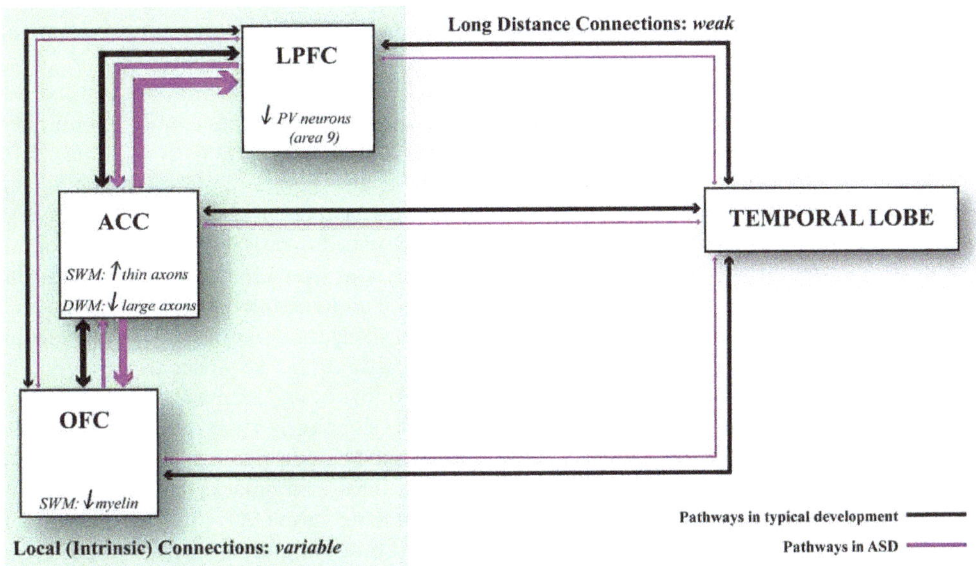

FIGURE 5 | Relationship of axonal features to developmental events. Changes in axons and inhibitory neurotransmission affect network dynamics in ASD. ACC exhibits local overconnectivity in ASD, which combined with changes in the ratio of inhibitory neurons in LPFC can tip the balance of excitation and inhibition. OFC exhibits weak local connectivity in ASD due to thinning of the myelin, which may affect conduction velocity. Overall, prefrontal areas exhibit weakening in their long-distance connections. This connectivity pattern is supported by structural and functional data. Black lines indicate typical connectivity and purple lines indicate connectivity in ASD. The thickness of the line indicates the strength of a connection.

attention are universal among people with autism, who are otherwise heterogeneous with regard to language acquisition, or the presence or absence of mental retardation or epilepsy (Zikopoulos and Barbas, 2010).

On the other hand, there is general agreement that pathways that travel over long distances are weak in autism, based on a variety of physiological and structural data (Courchesne and Pierce, 2005; Lepagnol-Bestel et al., 2008; Zikopoulos and Barbas, 2010; Muller et al., 2011; Schipul et al., 2011; Just et al., 2012), including findings at the level of single axons (Zikopoulos and Barbas, 2010). This consistent finding in autism likely contributes to the incongruence of cortical rhythms that engage distant cortices in autism (Thatcher et al., 2009; Lai et al., 2010; Khan et al., 2013). The physiological changes within large scale networks may help explain why people with autism have difficulty in shifting attention from one stimulus to another as the situation demands. In non-human primates, long-distance pathways are sparse in comparison with short-range pathways, which account for about 80% of connections (Barbas, 1988; Hilgetag et al., 2000; Hilgetag and Grant, 2000; Hilgetag and Kaiser, 2004; Barbas et al., 2005a). Nevertheless, long-distance pathways have considerable influence on the cortex. The prefrontal cortex, in particular, relies on sparse long-distance pathways for sensory input. Long-distance pathways also include interhemispheric connections, which have a critical role for synthesizing information across the commissures for a large variety of cognitive tasks, including language. In non-human primates, connections across the two hemispheres are less dense than connections within one hemisphere but involve just as many areas as the ipsilateral, at least for the prefrontal cortex (Barbas et al., 2005a). Contralateral pathways are also severely compromised in autism (Alexander et al., 2007; Just et al., 2007; Frazier and Hardan, 2009; Jou et al., 2010; Anderson et al., 2011b; Cantlon et al., 2011; Casanova et al., 2011; Fame et al., 2011; Schipul et al., 2011). In view of their functional significance and lower density, even small changes in long-range connections in autism likely have devastating effects on function.

In conclusion, areas are affected in varied ways in their connections in autism (**Figure 5**). In the superficial white matter below ACC, there is exuberance of short- or medium-range axons that link areas over short or medium distances. The white matter below lateral areas 9 and 46 shows no differences in axon density. On the other hand, in the superficial white matter below orbitofrontal area 11 the myelin is thinner, suggesting weak local connectivity. In the deep white matter below ACC there is a paucity of large axons that connect it with distant sensory and association areas. Pathology in ACC, which has a key role in attention, suggests that it may be the epicenter for abnormalities elsewhere, resulting in deficits in attention—excessive focusing on one stimulus or thought, and inability to disengage and attend to other stimuli flexibly. The deficits in ACC are consistent with the universal problems in attention in people with autism regardless of the severity of symptoms.

A TESTABLE BIOLOGICAL MODEL RELATES STRUCTURAL AXON FEATURES IN AUTISM TO DEVELOPMENT

Why are thin and medium axons in excess just below the ACC, large axons in short supply in long-distance pathways, and myelin is insufficient in orbital area 11? Are these disparate findings independent or related? Autism is a disorder with its roots in development and to begin to sort out what may go awry with connections it is necessary to consider the development of affected areas (**Figure 5**). Let us first consider the ACC, which appears to have more than its share of deficiencies in autism. In non-human primates the ACC develops early in ontogeny (Rakic, 2002). When migrating neurons take their position in the cortex they extend axons that branch to connect with other areas. Several proteins expressed in development are critical for axon growth and guidance. One of these proteins is GAP-43, which is expressed at high levels in all areas during development (Milosevic et al., 1995; Kanazir et al., 1996; Oishi et al., 1998). In adult brains GAP-43 is expressed in significant levels only in some areas, albeit less than in development, and the ACC is one such region. The continued presence of GAP-43 into normal adulthood may help explain the numerous pathways that connect the ACC with neighboring areas, as seen in normal non-human primates (Barbas et al., 1999).

In contrast to the early migration of neurons in ACC, myelination begins much later, and is nearly as late as the last myelinating lateral prefrontal areas (Flechsig, 1901; Von Bonin, 1950; Yakovlev and Lecours, 1967; Hasegawa et al., 1992). Why are two developmental processes so much separated in time in the ACC? It turns out that GAP-43 and myelin proteins inhibit each other and consequently there is an inverse relationship between GAP-43 expression and myelination (Kapfhammer and Schwab, 1994; Benowitz and Routtenberg, 1997). Axons first elongate and then myelinate. The onset and duration of myelination varies among cortical areas, starting prenatally, gradually increasing postnatally, and continuing throughout childhood in most prefrontal cortices (Flechsig, 1901; Von Bonin, 1950; Yakovlev and Lecours, 1967; Benes, 1989; Paus et al., 1999, 2001; Levitt, 2003; Suzuki et al., 2003). The differences in development and myelination among areas may help explain why areas are not equally affected in autism.

In the brains of adults with autism just below ACC, GAP-43 is expressed in more than double the number of axons than in normal controls (Zikopoulos and Barbas, 2010). If expression of GAP-43 is also higher in children with autism that would help explain the exuberant branching of axons below ACC in adults. We used data from development and our findings from *post-mortem* brains from adults with autism to construct a biological model (Zikopoulos and Barbas, 2010). The model shows in broad terms the likely fate of axons and their branching and myelination based strictly on the sequence of developmental events in non-human primates and humans. A high level of GAP-43 in ACC, which develops early (Rakic, 2002), promotes axon growth and branching. The selective increase in medium and thin axons in the superficial white matter below the ACC is explained by the exposure of axons to GAP-43, which is highest at the growing end of axons, mediating branching as axons enter or leave the white matter to link nearby areas. This pattern is expected to increase the density of medium and thin axons. The model shows that myelination should not be affected, because the ACC myelinates very late (Flechsig, 1901; Von Bonin, 1950; Yakovlev and Lecours, 1967), when GAP-43 level drops relative to its expression early in development.

Development takes a different temporal course in OFC, where there is no excessive branching of axons but the myelin is thinner in the brains of autistic adults (Zikopoulos and Barbas, 2010). In OFC, neurons normally migrate to the cortex later than in ACC, but myelinate earlier, effectively shortening the interval between neuronal migration and axonal myelination. Based on these developmental events, the model predicts that a small increase in GAP-43 in OFC in development can affect myelination but not axon branching, as seen in the brains of adults with autism (Zikopoulos and Barbas, 2010). In lateral prefrontal areas 9 and 46, neurogenesis and migration are completed much later (Rakic, 2002), when levels of GAP-43 are comparatively low, which helps explain why neither axon branching nor myelination are affected in adults with autism (Zikopoulos and Barbas, 2010).

The predictions of our biological model, which is testable, are bolstered by recent genetic studies that have associated single nucleotide polymorphisms in the GAP-43 gene with autism (Allen-Brady et al., 2009), and identified its extended chromosomal region as an autism risk locus (Trikalinos et al., 2006; Szatmari et al., 2007). In addition, studies in mice have shown that wide changes in the levels of GAP-43 can lead to autistic-like behaviors, including learning disability and stereotypical behaviors (Routtenberg et al., 2000; Zaccaria et al., 2010).

Atypical GAP-43 levels in autism may, therefore, help explain the exuberance of short-range pathways below ACC, which leads to intrinsic overconnectivity in the frontal lobe (Courchesne and Pierce, 2005). Importantly, based on the late onset and completion of the development of connections between distant cortices, high levels of GAP-43 in ACC may also help explain the weakened long-distance connections that course in the deep white matter below ACC. Reduction in strength of long-distance pathways that course through the deep white matter in autism may be secondary to the excessive short-range connections, which develop first, reach their targets fast, and occupy sites that normally would be available to the sparser long-distance pathways (Zikopoulos and Barbas, 2010). Pathways that reach the ACC from a long distance thus may be at a competitive disadvantage, not only because they develop late, but also because their axons must continue to elongate to reach and form synapses in the prefrontal cortex.

In conclusion, using the distinct findings in ACC, orbitofrontal and lateral prefrontal areas and their relationship to developmental events, including neuronal migration, axonal branching in the presence of GAP-43, and myelination, a biological model can help explain the varied effects within the frontal lobe. The findings suggest overconnectivity of the ACC with nearby areas, long-distance disconnection, weakening of nearby connections of the OFC, and sparing of axonal structure in lateral prefrontal areas 9 and 46. However, even though none of the changes seen in axons below ACC or orbitofrontal area 11 were evident below prefrontal areas 9 and 46, the interlinkage of these areas suggests that they do not remain unscathed. Indeed, the relationship of axon types was seriously altered among prefrontal areas, suggesting widespread repercussions beyond the immediate areas affected.

In line with the above findings, the increased density of spines of the late-developing neurons in the superficial layers of lateral prefrontal areas may help accommodate excessive feedback from ACC in autism. Moreover, lateral prefrontal areas appear to have reduced PV/CB ratio, due to fewer PV inhibitory neurons, which also develop later than CB neurons in animals and humans. Future studies with more cases are needed to investigate if the ratio of distinct inhibitory neurons is altered in autism and may help explain the changes seen in GABA receptors. Combined, these findings provide converging information about the developmental timeline of ASD, pointing to a critical perinatal period for the emergence of axon pathology and neural communication deficits in autism.

MATERIALS AND METHODS

TISSUE PREPARATION

Post-mortem prefrontal brain tissue was obtained from the Harvard Brain Tissue Resource Center through the Autism Tissue Program from two autistic male adults and two typically developed, age-matched, male controls, ages 30–44 years. The selection of cases used was based on tissue availability of cases with closely matched characteristics, including *post-mortem* interval (**Table 1**), and period of storage of tissue in formalin (mean $\pm$ standard deviation $= 137 \pm 37$ months), which minimized variability of tissue immunolabeling and shrinkage. The study was approved by the Institutional Review Board of Boston University. The diagnosis of autism was based on the Autism Diagnostic Interview-Revised (ADI-R) in both cases (**Table 1**). Clinical characteristics are summarized in **Table 1**. We excised small blocks ($\sim 2 \times 3$ cm) of matched frontal coronal tissue slabs (~ 1 cm thick), containing gray and white matter from DLPFC area 9 (**Figure 3**) based on the human brain atlas from the Autism Tissue Portal (www.atpportal.org) and (Von Economo, 2009, re-issued), and additional cytoarchitectonic studies of human prefrontal cortex (Selemon et al., 1998; Stark et al., 2004; Miguel-Hidalgo et al., 2006). We matched all samples to minimize variability and maximize statistical power. To ensure adequate preservation of the tissue the blocks were stored at −20°C in anti-freeze solution (30% ethylene glycol, 30% glycerol, 0.05% azide in PB). The blocks were rinsed in 0.1 M PB and cut coronally in series of adjacent sections (50 μm) on a vibratome (Pelco, series 1000).

IMMUNOHISTOCHEMISTRY

We used standard immunohistochemical procedures to label inhibitory neurons, as described (e.g., Barbas et al., 2005b; Zikopoulos and Barbas, 2006, 2007). Briefly, free-floating sections (50 μm thick) were treated with 1% H_2O_2 aqueous solution to suppress endogenous peroxidase activity, followed by 0.05 M glycine in 0.01 M phosphate buffered saline (PBS), pH: 7.4, to reduce cross-linking of lipids due to fixation. Tissue was placed in blocking solution of 0.3% Triton-X, 5% bovine serum albumin (BSA), 5% normal goat serum (NGS) in PBS, and then incubated in mouse monoclonal antibody (0.3% Triton-X in PBS) against CB, or PV, (1:2000, Swant). The sections were then incubated with a secondary biotinylated anti-mouse antibody (1:200 in PBS with 0.1% Triton-X; Vector), followed by avidin-biotin-peroxidase solution (Vector ABC Elite kit). We visualized positive neurons by the peroxidase-catalyzed polymerization of 0.05% 3,3-diaminobenzidine tetrahydrochloride (DAB; Zymed Laboratories) in 0.01% H_2O_2 buffer solution (pH, 7.5). After binding of the primary antibodies some sections were rinsed in

PBS, incubated for 4 h with goat anti-mouse secondary antibodies conjugated with the fluorescent probes Alexa Fluor 488 (green) or 568 (red; 1:100; Invitrogen) and rinsed with PBS. To test for non-specific labeling we performed control experiments with sections adjacent to the experimental, omitting the primary antibodies, and incubating with secondary antisera. A small number of CB+ neurons in the cortex are pyramidal, but their labeling is minimized by using a monoclonal antibody (Gonzalez-Albo et al., 2001; and personal observations). In addition, we can morphologically identify these neurons, since they are larger and have spiny dendrites as opposed to smooth, small bipolar inhibitory CB neurons.

STEREOLOGICAL ANALYSIS—LIGHT AND CONFOCAL MICROSCOPY

We estimated the laminar density of labeled PV and CB inhibitory neurons as well as total neuronal density in tissue blocks of similar size and volume of DLPFC area 9 using the stereological method of the optical fractionator (Gundersen, 1986; Howard and Reed, 1998) and specific software (StereoInvestigator; Microbrightfield) under the microscope at high magnification (×400), as we have described (e.g., Dombrowski et al., 2001; Zikopoulos and Barbas, 2006, 2010). For microscopic analyses we used a minimum of three sections from one series of coronal sections (50 μm thick) from each case. To estimate the number of neurons we first measured the thickness of each section, and used StereoInvestigator to set a guard zone at the bottom and top of each section to correct for objects plucked during sectioning; the disector thickness was thus smaller than the thickness of the section (Gundersen, 1986; West et al., 1991; Howard and Reed, 1998). The sampling fraction was 1/50 of the total volume of the area examined. The use of uniform random sampling ensured that every part of the area examined had the same chance of being included in the sample. The estimated numbers of neurons and the volumes of the corresponding layers (estimated with the Cavalieri method) were divided to assess relative density of label. In all experiments we stained one series of sections for Nissl (thionin) to place cytoarchitectonic borders. The section surface, the cytoarchitectonic borders of areas of interest, and layers, were outlined with the aid of a commercial computerized microscope system and motorized stage at a magnification ×400.

It should be noted here that the densities we report are relative, not absolute, since we did not apply a correction factor to account for inevitable tissue shrinkage during prolonged fixation and immunohistochemical processing. Variability due to tissue shrinkage was likely minimal because the period of storage of tissue in fixative was comparable across cases, and brain sections were simultaneously processed, using a standardized protocol, under identical conditions. This resulted in comparable shrinkage of tissue due to processing, mounting, and air drying, which was minimal in the X and Y dimensions (~2%) and within expected levels in the Z dimension (~65%), as reported previously (Dombrowski et al., 2001). Matching of normal and autistic brain sections and simultaneous processing under identical conditions, minimized experimental variability and made it possible to use a small number of brains, as each brain yields a large amount of data. This is particularly critical with the use of a rare and valuable resource of human brain tissue.

STATISTICAL ANALYSIS

We gathered data blind to condition and cortical region. Random codes for cases and images were broken after completion of each part of the study, as described (Zikopoulos and Barbas, 2010). In all cases data collection was performed by at least two investigators. Values obtained from the two independent measures were highly correlated (Pearson $R = 0.97$, $p = 0.001$). Data distributions for continuous variables were not significantly different from normal as determined by the Kolmogorov–Smirnov test, and thus allowed the use of parametric statistics. Data were evaluated with Statistica (StatSoft, Tulsa, OK), through a two-tailed *t*-test. For all analyses *p*-values <0.05 were taken as statistically significant.

AUTHOR CONTRIBUTIONS

Basilis Zikopoulos and Helen Barbas designed the experiments. Basilis Zikopoulos performed and analyzed the experiments. Basilis Zikopoulos and Helen Barbas prepared the manuscript.

ACKNOWLEDGMENTS

We thank Dr. Nenad Bogdanovic for useful comments on the manuscript, Marcia Feinberg for assistance with electron microscopy, and Mary Louise Fowler for assistance with cell counts. This work was supported by grants from: Autism Speaks; CELEST, the Center of Excellence for Learning in Education, Science, and Technology (a National Science Foundation Science of Learning Center, grant SBE-0354378) and the National Institutes of Health (National Institute of Mental Health RO1MH057414, and the National Institute of Neurological Disorders and Stroke, R01NS024760). We gratefully acknowledge the families of the donors and the following brain banks that make *post-mortem* research possible: The Autism Tissue Program (ATP; Dr. Jane Pickett, Director), The Eunice Kennedy Shriver NICHD Brain and Tissue Bank at the University of Maryland, Baltimore, MD, USA (Dr. Ronald Zielke, Director), and the Harvard Brain and Tissue Resource Center (HBTRC; Dr. Francine Benes, Director).

REFERENCES

Abbott, L. F., and Chance, F. S. (2005). Drivers and modulators from push-pull and balanced synaptic input. *Prog. Brain Res.* 149, 147–155. doi: 10.1016/S0079-6123(05)49011-1

Abrams, D. A., Lynch, C. J., Cheng, K. M., Phillips, J., Supekar, K., Ryali, S., et al. (2013). Underconnectivity between voice-selective cortex and reward circuitry in children with autism. *Proc. Natl. Acad. Sci. U.S.A.* 110, 12060–12065. doi: 10.1073/pnas.1302982110

Ahmed, B., Anderson, J. C., Martin, K. A., and Nelson, J. C. (1997). Map of the synapses onto layer 4 basket cells of the primary visual cortex of the cat. *J. Comp. Neurol.* 380, 230–242. doi: 10.1002/(SICI)1096-9861(19970407)380:2<230::AID-CNE6>3.0.Co;2-4

Alcantara, S., Ferrer, I., and Soriano, E. (1993). Postnatal development of parvalbumin and calbindin D28K immunoreactivities in the cerebral cortex of the rat. *Anat. Embryol.* 188, 63–73. doi: 10.1007/BF00191452

Alexander, A. L., Lee, J. E., Lazar, M., Boudos, R., Dubray, M. B., Oakes, T. R., et al. (2007). Diffusion tensor imaging of the corpus callosum in Autism. *Neuroimage* 34, 61–73. doi: 10.1016/j.neuroimage.2006.08.032

Allen-Brady, K., Miller, J., Matsunami, N., Stevens, J., Block, H., Farley, M., et al. (2009). A high-density SNP genome-wide linkage scan in a large autism extended pedigree.

Mol. Psychiatry 14, 590–600. doi: 10.1038/mp.2008.14
Alonso-Nanclares, L., White, E. L., Elston, G. N., and Defelipe, J. (2004). Synaptology of the proximal segment of pyramidal cell basal dendrites. *Eur. J. Neurosci.* 19, 771–776. doi: 10.1111/j.0953-816X.2003.03166.x
Amaral, D. G., Schumann, C. M., and Nordahl, C. W. (2008). Neuroanatomy of autism. *Trends Neurosci.* 31, 137–145. doi: 10.1016/j.tins.2007.12.005
Anagnostou, E., and Taylor, M. (2011). Review of neuroimaging in autism spectrum disorders: what we have learned and where we go from here. *Mol. Autism* 2:4. doi: 10.1186/2040-2392-2-4
Anderson, J. C., Kennedy, H., and Martin, K. A. C. (2011a). Pathways of attention: synaptic relationships of frontal eye field to V4, lateral intraparietal cortex, and area 46 in macaque monkey. *J. Neurosci.* 31, 10872–10881. doi: 10.1523/JNEUROSCI.0622-11.2011
Anderson, J. S., Druzgal, T. J., Froehlich, A., Dubray, M. B., Lange, N., Alexander, A. L., et al. (2011b). Decreased interhemispheric functional connectivity in autism. *Cereb. Cortex* 21, 1134–1146. doi: 10.1093/Cercor/bhq190
Anderson, J. C., and Martin, K. A. (2009). The synaptic connections between cortical areas V1 and V2 in macaque monkey. *J. Neurosci.* 29, 11283–11293. doi: 10.1523/JNEUROSCI.5757-08.2009
Assaf, M., Jagannathan, K., Calhoun, V. D., Miller, L., Stevens, M. C., Sahl, R., et al. (2010). Abnormal functional connectivity of default mode sub-networks in autism spectrum disorder patients. *Neuroimage* 53, 247–256. doi: 10.1016/j.neuroimage.2010.05.067
Atladottir, H. O., Pedersen, M. G., Thorsen, P., Mortensen, P. B., Deleuran, B., Eaton, W. W., et al. (2009). Association of family history of autoimmune diseases and autism spectrum disorders. *Pediatrics* 124, 687–694. doi: 10.1542/peds.2008-2445
Avino, T. A., and Hutsler, J. J. (2010). Abnormal cell patterning at the cortical gray-white matter boundary in autism spectrum disorders. *Brain Res.* 1360, 138–146. doi: 10.1016/j.brainres.2010.08.091
Avino, T. A., Wojcik, C., Mann, A., and Hutsler, J. J. (2012). "Morphological analysis of dendritic spines on cortical pyramidal cells in ASD," in *2012 International Meeting for Autism Research* (Toronto, ON).
Bachevalier, J., and Loveland, K. A. (2006). The orbitofrontal-amygdala circuit and self-regulation of social-emotional behavior in autism. *Neurosci. Biobehav. Rev.* 30, 97–117. doi: 10.1016/j.neubiorev.2005.07.002
Badre, D., and Wagner, A. D. (2004). Selection, integration, and conflict monitoring; assessing the nature and generality of prefrontal cognitive control mechanisms. *Neuron* 41, 473–487. doi: 10.1016/S0896-6273(03)00851-1
Bailey, A., Luthert, P., Dean, A., Harding, B., Janota, I., Montgomery, M., et al. (1998). A clinicopathological study of autism. *Brain* 121(Pt 5), 889–905. doi: 10.1093/brain/121.5.889
Barbas, H. (1986). Pattern in the laminar origin of corticocortical connections. *J. Comp. Neurol.* 252, 415–422. doi: 10.1002/cne.902520310
Barbas, H. (1988). Cortical projections to orbitofrontal limbic cortices in the rhesus monkey. *Neurosci. Abstr.* 14, 922.
Barbas, H. (1993). Organization of cortical afferent input to orbitofrontal areas in the rhesus monkey. *Neuroscience* 56, 841–864. doi: 10.1016/0306-4522(93)90132-Y
Barbas, H. (2000a). Complementary role of prefrontal cortical regions in cognition, memory and emotion in primates. *Adv. Neurol.* 84, 87–110.
Barbas, H. (2000b). Connections underlying the synthesis of cognition, memory, and emotion in primate prefrontal cortices. *Brain Res. Bull.* 52, 319–330. doi: 10.1016/S0361-9230(99)00245-2
Barbas, H., and Mesulam, M. M. (1985). Cortical afferent input to the principalis region of the rhesus monkey. *Neuroscience* 15, 619–637. doi: 10.1016/0306-4522(85)90064-8
Barbas, H., and Rempel-Clower, N. (1997). Cortical structure predicts the pattern of corticocortical connections. *Cereb. Cortex* 7, 635–646. doi: 10.1093/cercor/7.7.635
Barbas, H., and Zikopoulos, B. (2006). "Sequential and parallel circuits for emotional processing in primate orbitofrontal cortex," in *The Orbitofrontal Cortex*, eds Z. David and R. Scott (Oxford: Oxford University Press), 57–91.
Barbas, H., and Zikopoulos, B. (2007). The prefrontal cortex and flexible behavior. *Neuroscientist* 13, 532–545. doi: 10.1177/1073858407301369
Barbas, H., Ghashghaei, H., Dombrowski, S. M., and Rempel-Clower, N. L. (1999). Medial prefrontal cortices are unified by common connections with superior temporal cortices and distinguished by input from memory-related areas in the rhesus monkey. *J. Comp. Neurol.* 410, 343–367. doi: 10.1002/(SICI)1096-9861(19990802)410:3<343::AID-CNE1>3.0.CO;2-1
Barbas, H., Hilgetag, C. C., Saha, S., Dermon, C. R., and Suski, J. L. (2005a). Parallel organization of contralateral and ipsilateral prefrontal cortical projections in the rhesus monkey. *BMC Neurosci.* 6:32. doi: 10.1186/1471-2202-6-32
Barbas, H., Medalla, M., Alade, O., Suski, J., Zikopoulos, B., and Lera, P. (2005b). Relationship of prefrontal connections to inhibitory systems in superior temporal areas in the rhesus monkey. *Cereb. Cortex* 15, 1356–1370. doi: 10.1093/cercor/bhi018
Barbas, H., Zikopoulos, B., and Timbie, C. (2011). Sensory pathways and emotional context for action in primate prefrontal cortex. *Biol. Psychiatry* 69, 1133–1139. doi: 10.1016/j.biopsych.2010.08.008
Barnea-Goraly, N., Kwon, H., Menon, V., Eliez, S., Lotspeich, L., and Reiss, A. L. (2004). White matter structure in autism: preliminary evidence from diffusion tensor imaging. *Biol. Psychiatry* 55, 323–326. doi: 10.1016/j.biopsych.2003.10.022
Baron-Cohen, S. (1991). The development of a theory of mind in autism: deviance and delay? *Psychiatr. Clin. North Am.* 14, 33–51.
Bauman, M. L., and Kemper, T. L. (2005). Neuroanatomic observations of the brain in autism: a review and future directions. *Int. J. Dev. Neurosci.* 23, 183–187. doi: 10.1016/j.ijdevneu.2004.09.006
Bauman, M., and Kemper, T. L. (1985). Histoanatomic observations of the brain in early infantile autism. *Neurology* 35, 866–874. doi: 10.1212/WNL.35.6.866
Becker, K. G., and Schultz, S. T. (2010). Similarities in features of autism and asthma and a possible link to acetaminophen use. *Med. Hypotheses* 74, 7–11. doi: 10.1016/j.mehy.2009.08.033
Belmonte, M. K., Allen, G., Beckel-Mitchener, A., Boulanger, L. M., Carper, R. A., and Webb, S. J. (2004a). Autism and abnormal development of brain connectivity. *J. Neurosci.* 24, 9228–9231. doi: 10.1523/JNEUROSCI.3340-04.2004
Belmonte, M. K., Cook, E. H., Anderson, G. M., Rubenstein, J. L. R., Greenough, W. T., Beckel-Mitchener, A., et al. (2004b). Autism as a disorder of neural information processing: directions for research and targets for therapy. *Mol. Psychiatry* 9, 646–663.
Benes, F. M. (1989). Myelination of cortical-hippocampal relays during late adolescence. *Schizophr. Bull.* 15, 585–593. doi: 10.1093/schbul/15.4.585
Benes, F. M., Vincent, S. L., and Todtenkopf, M. (2001). The density of pyramidal and nonpyramidal neurons in anterior cingulate cortex of schizophrenic and bipolar subjects. *Biol. Psychiatry* 50, 395–406. doi: 10.1016/S0006-3223(01)01084-8
Benowitz, L. I., and Routtenberg, A. (1997). GAP-43: an intrinsic determinant of neuronal development and plasticity. *Trends Neurosci.* 20, 84–91. doi: 10.1016/S0166-2236(96)10072-2
Berger, B., Trottier, S., Verney, C., Gaspar, P., and Alvarez, C. (1988). Regional and laminar distribution of the dopamine and serotonin innervation in the macaque cerebral cortex: a radioautographic study. *J. Comp. Neurol.* 273, 99–119. doi: 10.1002/cne.902730109
Bernardi, S., Anagnostou, E., Shen, J., Kolevzon, A., Buxbaum, J. D., Hollander, E., et al. (2011). *In vivo* (1)H-magnetic resonance spectroscopy study of the attentional networks in autism. *Brain Res.* 1380, 198–205. doi: 10.1016/j.brainres.2010.12.057
Bigler, E. D., Mortensen, S., Neeley, E. S., Ozonoff, S., Krasny, L., Johnson, M., et al. (2007). Superior temporal gyrus, language function, and autism. *Dev. Neuropsychol.* 31, 217–238. doi: 10.1080/87565640701190841
Blatt, G. J., and Fatemi, S. H. (2011). Alterations in GABAergic biomarkers in the autism brain. *Anat. Rec.* 294, 1646–1652. doi: 10.1002/ar.21252
Blatt, G. J., Fitzgerald, C. M., Guptill, J. T., Booker, A. B., Kemper, T. L., and Bauman, M. L. (2001). Density and distribution of hippocampal neurotransmitter receptors in autism: an autoradiographic study. *J. Autism Dev. Disord.* 31, 537–543. doi: 10.1023/A:1013238809666
Blaxill, M. F. (2004). What's going on? The question of time trends in autism. *Public Health Rep.* 119, 536–551. doi: 10.1016/j.phr.2004.09.003
Borgers, C., and Kopell, N. (2003). Synchronization in networks of excitatory and inhibitory neurons with sparse, random connectivity.

Neural Comput. 15, 509–538. doi: 10.1162/089976603321192059
Borgers, C., Epstein, S., and Kopell, N. J. (2008). Gamma oscillations mediate stimulus competition and attentional selection in a cortical network model. *Proc. Natl. Acad. Sci. U.S.A.* 105, 18023–18028. doi: 10.1073/pnas.0809511105
Brown, J. S. Jr. (2009). Effects of bisphenol-A and other endocrine disruptors compared with abnormalities of schizophrenia: an endocrine-disruption theory of schizophrenia. *Schizophr. Bull.* 35, 256–278. doi: 10.1093/schbul/sbm147
Bunce, J. G., and Barbas, H. (2011). Prefrontal pathways target excitatory and inhibitory systems in memory-related medial temporal cortices. *Neuroimage* 55, 1461–1474. doi: 10.1016/j.neuroimage.2011.01.064
Buxhoeveden, D. P., Semendeferi, K., Buckwalter, J., Schenker, N., Switzer, R., and Courchesne, E. (2006). Reduced minicolumns in the frontal cortex of patients with autism. *Neuropathol. Appl. Neurobiol.* 32, 483–491. doi: 10.1111/j.1365-2990.2006.00745.x
Buzsaki, G., and Draguhn, A. (2004). Neuronal oscillations in cortical networks. *Science* 304, 1926–1929. doi: 10.1126/science.1099745
Cantlon, J. F., Davis, S. W., Libertus, M. E., Kahane, J., Brannon, E. M., and Pelphrey, K. A. (2011). Inter-parietal white matter development predicts numerical performance in young children. *Learn. Individ. Differ.* 21, 672–680. doi: 10.1016/j.lindif.2011.09.003
Cao, F., Yin, A., Wen, G., Sheikh, A. M., Tauqeer, Z., Malik, M., et al. (2012). Alteration of astrocytes and Wnt/beta-catenin signaling in the frontal cortex of autistic subjects. *J. Neuroinflammation* 9, 223. doi: 10.1186/1742-2094-9-223
Carper, R. A., and Courchesne, E. (2005). Localized enlargement of the frontal cortex in early autism. *Biol. Psychiatry* 57, 126–133. doi: 10.1016/j.biopsych.2004.11.005
Carper, R. A., Moses, P., Tigue, Z. D., and Courchesne, E. (2002). Cerebral lobes in autism: early hyperplasia and abnormal age effects. *Neuroimage* 16, 1038–1051. doi: 10.1006/nimg.2002.1099
Casanova, M. F. (2004). White matter volume increase and minicolumns in autism. *Ann. Neurol.* 56, 453. doi: 10.1002/ana.20196
Casanova, M. F. (2007). The neuropathology of autism. *Brain Pathol.* 17, 422–433. doi: 10.1111/j.1750-3639.2007.00100.x
Casanova, M. F., Buxhoeveden, D. P., and Brown, C. (2002a). Clinical and macroscopic correlates of minicolumnar pathology in autism. *J. Child Neurol.* 17, 692–695. doi: 10.1177/088307380201700908
Casanova, M. F., Buxhoeveden, D. P., Switala, A. E., and Roy, E. (2002b). Minicolumnar pathology in autism. *Neurology* 58, 428–432. doi: 10.1212/WNL.58.3.428
Casanova, M. F., Buxhoeveden, D., and Gomez, J. (2003). Disruption in the inhibitory architecture of the cell minicolumn: implications for autism. *Neuroscientist* 9, 496–507. doi: 10.1177/1073858403253552
Casanova, M. F., El Baz, A., Elnakib, A., Switala, A. E., Williams, E. L., Williams, D. L., et al. (2011). Quantitative analysis of the shape of the corpus callosum in patients with autism and comparison individuals. *Autism* 15, 223–238. doi: 10.1177/1362361310386506
Casanova, M. F., van Kooten, I. A., Switala, A. E., van Engeland, H., Heinsen, H., Steinbusch, H. W., et al. (2006). Minicolumnar abnormalities in autism. *Acta Neuropathol.* 112, 287–303. doi: 10.1007/s00401-006-0085-5
Chao, H. T., Chen, H., Samaco, R. C., Xue, M., Chahrour, M., Yoo, J., et al. (2010). Dysfunction in GABA signalling mediates autism-like stereotypies and Rett syndrome phenotypes. *Nature* 468, 263–269. doi: 10.1038/nature09582
Cheon, K. A., Kim, Y. S., Oh, S. H., Park, S. Y., Yoon, H. W., Herrington, J., et al. (2011). Involvement of the anterior thalamic radiation in boys with high functioning autism spectrum disorders: a Diffusion Tensor Imaging study. *Brain Res.* 1417, 77–86. doi: 10.1016/j.brainres.2011.08.020
Chow, C. C., White, J. A., Ritt, J., and Kopell, N. (1998). Frequency control in synchronized networks of inhibitory neurons. *J. Comput. Neurosci.* 5, 407–420. doi: 10.1023/A:1008889328787
Collins, A. L., Ma, D., Whitehead, P. L., Martin, E. R., Wright, H. H., Abramson, R. K., et al. (2006). Investigation of autism and GABA receptor subunit genes in multiple ethnic groups. *Neurogenetics* 7, 167–174. doi: 10.1007/s10048-006-0045-1
Conde, F., Lund, J. S., Jacobowitz, D. M., Baimbridge, K. G., and Lewis, D. A. (1994). Local circuit neurons immunoreactive for calretinin, calbindin D- 28k or parvalbumin in monkey prefrontal cortex: distribution and morphology. *J. Comp. Neurol.* 341, 95–116. doi: 10.1002/cne.903410109
Constantinidis, C., Williams, G. V., and Goldman-Rakic, P. S. (2002). A role for inhibition in shaping the temporal flow of information in prefrontal cortex. *Nat. Neurosci.* 5, 175–180. doi: 10.1038/nn799
Courchesne, E., and Pierce, K. (2005). Why the frontal cortex in autism might be talking only to itself: local over-connectivity but long-distance disconnection. *Curr. Opin. Neurobiol.* 15, 225–230. doi: 10.1016/j.conb.2005.03.001
Courchesne, E., Campbell, K., and Solso, S. (2011a). Brain growth across the life span in autism: age-specific changes in anatomical pathology. *Brain Res.* 1380, 138–145.
Courchesne, E., Mouton, P. R., Calhoun, M. E., Semendeferi, K., Ahrens-Barbeau, C., Hallet, M. J., et al. (2011b). Neuron number and size in prefrontal cortex of children with autism. *JAMA* 306, 2001–2010. doi: 10.1001/jama.2011.1638
Courchesne, E., Pierce, K., Schumann, C. M., Redcay, E., Buckwalter, J. A., Kennedy, D. P., et al. (2007). Mapping early brain development in autism. *Neuron* 56, 399–413. doi: 10.1016/j.neuron.2007.10.016
Croen, L. A., Grether, J. K., Yoshida, C. K., Odouli, R., and Hendrick, V. (2011). Antidepressant use during pregnancy and childhood autism spectrum disorders. *Arch. Gen. Psychiatry.* 68, 1104–1112. doi: 10.1001/archgenpsychiatry.2011.73
Croen, L. A., Grether, J. K., Yoshida, C. K., Odouli, R., and Van de, W. J. (2005). Maternal autoimmune diseases, asthma and allergies, and childhood autism spectrum disorders: a case-control study. *Arch. Pediatr. Adolesc. Med.* 159, 151–157. doi: 10.1001/archpedi.159.2.151
de Cock, M., Maas, Y. G., and van de Bor, M. (2012). Does perinatal exposure to endocrine disruptors induce autism spectrum and attention deficit hyperactivity disorders? Review. *Acta Paediatr.* 101, 811–818. doi: 10.1111/j.1651-2227.2012.02693.x
Defelipe, J. (1997). Types of neurons, synaptic connections and chemical characteristics of cells immunoreactive for calbindin-D28K, parvalbumin and calretinin in the neocortex. *J. Chem. Neuroanat.* 14, 1–19. doi: 10.1016/S0891-0618(97)10013-8
Defelipe, J. (1999). Chandelier cells and epilepsy. *Brain* 122(Pt 10), 1807–1822. doi: 10.1093/brain/122.10.1807
Defelipe, J., Gonzalez-Albo, M. C., Del Rio, M. R., and Elston, G. N. (1999). Distribution and patterns of connectivity of interneurons containing calbindin, calretinin, and parvalbumin in visual areas of the occipital and temporal lobes of the macaque monkey. *J. Comp. Neurol.* 412, 515–526. doi: 10.1002/(SICI)1096-9861(19990927)412:3<515::AID-CNE10>3.0.CO;2-1
Defelipe, J., Hendry, S. H., and Jones, E. G. (1989a). Synapses of double bouquet cells in monkey cerebral cortex visualized by calbindin immunoreactivity. *Brain Res.* 503, 49–54. doi: 10.1016/0006-8993(89)91702-2
Defelipe, J., Hendry, S. H., and Jones, E. G. (1989b). Visualization of chandelier cell axons by parvalbumin immunoreactivity in monkey cerebral cortex. *Proc. Natl. Acad. Sci. U.S.A.* 86, 2093–2097. doi: 10.1073/pnas.86.6.2093
Defelipe, J., Hendry, S. H., Hashikawa, T., Molinari, M., and Jones, E. G. (1990). A microcolumnar structure of monkey cerebral cortex revealed by immunocytochemical studies of double bouquet cell axons. *Neuroscience* 37, 655–673. doi: 10.1016/0306-4522(90)90097-N
Denny, J. B. (2006). Molecular mechanisms, biological actions, and neuropharmacology of the growth-associated protein GAP-43. *Curr. Neuropharmacol.* 4, 293–304. doi: 10.2174/157015906778520782
Di Martino, A., Kelly, C., Grzadzinski, R., Zuo, X. N., Mennes, M., Mairena, M. A., et al. (2011). Aberrant striatal functional connectivity in children with autism. *Biol. Psychiatry* 69, 847–856. doi: 10.1016/j.biopsych.2010.10.029
Dichter, G. S., Felder, J. N., and Bodfish, J. W. (2009). Autism is characterized by dorsal anterior cingulate hyperactivation during social target detection. *Soc. Cogn. Affect. Neurosci.* 4, 215–226. doi: 10.1093/scan/nsp017
Dombrowski, S. M., Hilgetag, C. C., and Barbas, H. (2001). Quantitative architecture distinguishes prefrontal cortical systems in the rhesus monkey. *Cereb. Cortex* 11, 975–988. doi: 10.1093/cercor/11.10.975
Douglas, R. J., and Martin, K. A. (2004). Neuronal circuits of the neocortex. *Annu. Rev. Neurosci.* 27, 419–451. doi: 10.1146/annurev.neuro.27.070203.144152
Ehninger, D., and Silva, A. J. (2011). Rapamycin for treating Tuberous

sclerosis and Autism spectrum disorders. *Trends Mol. Med.* 17, 78–87. doi: 10.1016/j.molmed.2010.10.002

Fame, R. M., MacDonald, J. L., and Macklis, J. D. (2011). Development specification, and diversity of callosal projection neurons. *Trends Neurosci.* 34, 41–50. doi: 10.1016/j.tins.2010.10.002

Fatemi, S. H., Folsom, T. D., Reutiman, T. J., and Thuras, P. D. (2009a). Expression of GABA(B) receptors is altered in brains of subjects with autism. *Cerebellum* 8, 64–69. doi: 10.1007/s12311-008-0075-3

Fatemi, S. H., Reutiman, T. J., Folsom, T. D., and Thuras, P. D. (2009b). GABA(A) receptor downregulation in brains of subjects with autism. *J. Autism Dev. Disord.* 39, 223–230. doi: 10.1007/s10803-008-0646-7

Flechsig, P. (1901). Developmental (myelogenetic) localisation of the cerebral cortex in the human subject. *Lancet* 158, 1027–1029. doi: 10.1016/S0140-6736(01)01429-5

Frazier, T. W., and Hardan, A. Y. (2009). A meta-analysis of the corpus callosum in autism. *Biol. Psychiatry* 66, 935–941. doi: 10.1016/j.biopsych.2009.07.022

Fullerton, B. C., and Pandya, D. N. (2007). Architectonic analysis of the auditory-related areas of the superior temporal region in human brain. *J. Comp. Neurol.* 504, 470–498. doi: 10.1002/cne.21432

Gabbott, P. L. A., Jays, P. R. L., and Bacon, S. J. (1997). Calretinin neurons in human medial prefrontal cortex (areas 24a,b,c, 32', and 25). *J. Comp. Neurol.* 381, 389–410. doi: 10.1002/(SICI)1096-9861(19970519)381:4<389::AID-CNE1>3.0.CO;2-Z

Gabbott, P. L., and Bacon, S. J. (1996). Local circuit neurons in the medial prefrontal cortex (areas 24a,b,c, 25 and 32) in the monkey: II. Quantitative areal and laminar distributions. *J. Comp. Neurol.* 364, 609–636. doi: 10.1002/(SICI)1096-9861 (19960122)364:4<609::AID-CNE2>3.0.CO;2-7

Gandal, M. J., Sisti, J., Klook, K., Ortinski, P. I., Leitman, V., Liang, Y., et al. (2012). GABAB-mediated rescue of altered excitatory-inhibitory balance, gamma synchrony and behavioral deficits following constitutive NMDAR-hypofunction. *Transl. Psychiatry* 2:e142. doi: 10.1038/tp.2012.69

Garbern, J. Y., Neumann, M., Trojanowski, J. Q., Lee, V. M., Feldman, G., Norris, J. W., et al. (2010). A mutation affecting the sodium/proton exchanger, SLC9A6, causes mental retardation with tau deposition. *Brain* 133, 1391–1402. doi: 10.1093/brain/awq071

Garbett, K. A., Hsiao, E. Y., Kalman, S., Patterson, P. H., and Mirnics, K. (2012). Effects of maternal immune activation on gene expression patterns in the fetal brain. *Transl. Psychiatry* 2:e98. doi: 10.1038/tp.2012.24

Gaspar, P., Berger, B., Febvret, A., Vigny, A., and Henry, J. P. (1989). Catecholamine innervation of the human cerebral cortex as revealed by comparative immunohistochemistry of tyrosine hydroxylase and dopamine-beta-hydroxylase. *J. Comp. Neurol.* 279, 249–271. doi: 10.1002/cne.902790208

Gehring, W. J., and Knight, R. T. (2000). Prefrontal-cingulate interactions in action monitoring. *Nat. Neurosci.* 3, 516–520. doi: 10.1038/74899

Germuska, M., Saha, S., Fiala, J. C., and Barbas, H. (2006). Synaptic distinction of laminar specific prefrontal-temporal pathways in primates. *Cereb. Cortex* 16, 865–875. doi: 10.1093/cercor/bhj030

Geschwind, D. H. (2011). Genetics of autism spectrum disorders. *Trends Cogn. Sci.* 15, 409–416. doi: 10.1016/j.tics.2011.07.003

Ghashghaei, H. T., and Barbas, H. (2002). Pathways for emotions: interactions of prefrontal and anterior temporal pathways in the amygdala of the rhesus monkey. *Neuroscience* 115, 1261–1279. doi: 10.1016/S0306-4522(02)00446-3

Ghashghaei, H. T., Hilgetag, C. C., and Barbas, H. (2007). Sequence of information processing for emotions based on the anatomic dialogue between prefrontal cortex and amygdala. *Neuroimage* 34, 905–923. doi: 10.1016/j.neuroimage.2006.09.046

Gilman, S. R., Iossifov, I., Levy, D., Ronemus, M., Wigler, M., and Vitkup, D. (2011). Rare de novo variants associated with autism implicate a large functional network of genes involved in formation and function of synapses. *Neuron* 70, 898–907. doi: 10.1016/j.neuron.2011.05.021

Girgis, R. R., Minshew, N. J., Melhem, N. M., Nutche, J. J., Keshavan, M. S., and Hardan, A. Y. (2007). Volumetric alterations of the orbitofrontal cortex in autism. *Prog. NeuroPsychopharmacol. Biol. Psychiatry* 31, 41–45. doi: 10.1016/j.pnpbp.2006.06.007

Gomot, M., Bernard, F. A., Davis, M. H., Belmonte, M. K., Ashwin, C., Bullmore, E. T., et al. (2006). Change detection in children with autism: an auditory event-related fMRI study. *Neuroimage* 29, 475–484. doi: 10.1016/j.neuroimage.2005.07.027

Gonchar, Y., and Burkhalter, A. (1999). Connectivity of GABAergic calretinin-immunoreactive neurons in rat primary visual cortex. *Cereb. Cortex* 9, 683–696. doi: 10.1093/cercor/9.7.683

Gonzalez-Albo, M. C., Elston, G. N., and Defelipe, J. (2001). The human temporal cortex: characterization of neurons expressing nitric oxide synthase, neuropeptides and calcium-binding proteins, and their glutamate receptor subunit profiles. *Cereb. Cortex* 11, 1170–1181. doi: 10.1093/cercor/11.12.1170

Granda, B., Tabernero, A., Tello, V., and Medina, J. M. (2003). Oleic acid induces GAP-43 expression through a protein kinase C-mediated mechanism that is independent of NGF but synergistic with NT-3 and NT-4/5. *Brain Res.* 988, 1–8. doi: 10.1016/S0006-8993(03)03253-0

Grant, S., and Hilgetag, C. C. (2005). Graded classes of cortical connections: quantitative analyses of laminar projections to motion areas of cat extrastriate cortex. *Eur. J. Neurosci.* 22, 681–696. doi: 10.1111/j.1460-9568.2005.04232.x

Gundersen, H. J. (1986). Stereology of arbitrary particles. A review of unbiased number and size estimators and the presentation of some new ones, in memory of William R. Thompson. *J. Microsc.* 143(Pt 1), 3–45. doi: 10.1111/j.1365-2818.1986.tb02764.x

Gupta, A., Wang, Y., and Markram, H. (2000). Organizing principles for a diversity of GABAergic interneurons and synapses in the neocortex. *Science* 287, 273–278. doi: 10.1126/science.287.5451.273

Guptill, J. T., Booker, A. B., Gibbs, T. T., Kemper, T. L., Bauman, M. L., and Blatt, G. J. (2007). [3H]-flunitrazepam-labeled benzodiazepine binding sites in the hippocampal formation in autism: a multiple concentration autoradiographic study. *J. Autism Dev. Disord.* 37, 911–920. doi: 10.1007/s10803-006-0226-7

Hallmayer, J., Cleveland, S., Torres, A., Phillips, J., Cohen, B., Torigoe, T., et al. (2011). Genetic heritability and shared environmental factors among twin pairs with autism. *Arch. Gen. Psychiatry* 68, 1095–1102. doi: 10.1001/archgenpsychiatry.2011.76

Hardan, A. Y., Girgis, R. R., Lacerda, A. L. T., Yorbik, O., Kilpatiick, M., Keshavan, M. S., et al. (2006). Magnetic resonance imaging study of the orbitofrontal cortex in autism. *J. Child Neurol.* 21, 866–871. doi: 10.1177/08830738060210100701

Hasegawa, M., Houdou, S., Mito, T., Takashima, S., Asanuma, K., and Ohno, T. (1992). Development of myelination in the human fetal and infant cerebrum: a myelin basic protein immunohistochemical study. *Brain Dev.* 14, 1–6. doi: 10.1016/S0387-7604(12)80271-3

Haznedar, M. M., Buchsbaum, M. S., Licalzi, E. M., Cartwright, C., and Hollander, E. (2006). Volumetric analysis and three-dimensional glucose metabolic mapping of the striatum and thalamus in patients with autism spectrum disorders. *Am. J. Psychiatry* 163, 1252–1263. doi: 10.1176/appi.ajp.163.7.1252

Hendry, S. H. C., Jones, E. G., Emson, P. C., Lawson, D. E. M., Heizmann, C. W., and Streit, P. (1989). Two classes of cortical GABA neurons defined by differential calcium binding protein immunoreactivities. *Exp. Brain Res.* 76, 467–472. doi: 10.1007/BF00247904

Herbert, M. R. (2005). Large brains in autism: the challenge of pervasive abnormality. *Neuroscientist* 11, 417–440. doi: 10.1177/0091270005278866

Herbert, M. R., Ziegler, D. A., Deutsch, C. K., O'Brien, L. M., Lange, N., Bakardjiev, A., et al. (2003). Dissociations of cerebral cortex, subcortical and cerebral white matter volumes in autistic boys. *Brain* 126, 1182–1192. doi: 10.1093/brain/awg110

Herbert, M. R., Ziegler, D. A., Makris, N., Filipek, P. A., Kemper, T. L., Normandin, J. J., et al. (2004). Localization of white matter volume increase in autism and developmental language disorder. *Ann. Neurol.* 55, 530–540. doi: 10.1002/ana.20032

Hilgetag, C. C., and Barbas, H. (2006). Role of mechanical factors in the morphology of the primate cerebral cortex. *PLoS Comput. Biol.* 2:e22. doi: 10.1371/journal.pcbi.0020022

Hilgetag, C. C., and Grant, S. (2000). Uniformity, specificity and variability of corticocortical connectivity. *Philos. Trans. R. Soc. Lond. B Biol. Sci.* 355, 7–20. doi: 10.1098/rstb.2000.0546

Hilgetag, C. C., and Grant, S. (2010). Cytoarchitectural differences are a key determinant of laminar projection origins in the visual cortex. *Neuroimage* 51, 1006–1017. doi: 10.1016/j.neuroimage.2010.03.006

Hilgetag, C. C., and Kaiser, M. (2004). Clustered organization of cortical connectivity. *Neuroinformatics* 2, 353–360. doi: 10.1385/NI:2:3:353

Hilgetag, C. C., Burns, G. A., O'Neill, M. A., Scannell, J. W., and Young, M. P. (2000). Anatomical connectivity defines the organization of clusters of cortical areas in the macaque monkey and the cat. *Philos. Trans. R. Soc. Lond. B Biol. Sci.* 355, 91–110. doi: 10.1098/rstb.2000.0551

Hill, E. L. (2004). Executive dysfunction in autism. *Trends Cogn. Sci.* 8, 26–32. doi: 10.1016/j.tics.2003.11.003

Ho, S., Clipstone, N., Timmermann, L., Northrop, J., Graef, I., Fiorentino, D., et al. (1996). The mechanism of action of cyclosporin A and FK506. *Clin. Immunol. Immunopathol.* 80, S40–S45. doi: 10.1006/clin.1996.0140

Hof, P. R., Glezer, I. I., Conde, F., Flagg, R. A., Rubin, M. B., Nimchinsky, E. A., et al. (1999). Cellular distribution of the calcium-binding proteins parvalbumin, calbindin, and calretinin in the neocortex of mammals: phylogenetic and developmental patterns. *J. Chem. Neuroanat.* 16, 77–116. doi: 10.1016/S0891-0618(98)00065-9

Hogart, A., Nagarajan, R. P., Patzel, K. A., Yasui, D. H., and Lasalle, J. M. (2007). 15q11-13 GABAA receptor genes are normally biallelically expressed in brain yet are subject to epigenetic dysregulation in autism-spectrum disorders. *Hum. Mol. Genet.* 16, 691–703. doi: 10.1093/hmg/ddm014

Holahan, M. R., Honegger, K. S., Tabatadze, N., and Routtenberg, A. (2007). GAP-43 gene expression regulates information storage. *Learn. Mem.* 14, 407–415. doi: 10.1101/lm.581907

Holahan, M., and Routtenberg, A. (2008). The protein kinase C phosphorylation site on GAP-43 differentially regulates information storage. *Hippocampus* 18, 1099–1102. doi: 10.1002/hipo.20486

Hornung, J. P., and De Tribolet, N. (1994). Distribution of GABA-containing neurons in human frontal cortex: a quantitative immunocytochemical study. *Anat. Embryol. (Berl.)* 189, 139–145. doi: 10.1007/BF00185772

Howard, C. V., and Reed, M. G. (1998). *Unbiased Stereology, Three-dimensional Measurement in Microscopy.* Oxford: BIOS Scientific Publishers Limited.

Hsiao, E. Y., McBride, S. W., Chow, J., Mazmanian, S. K., and Patterson, P. H. (2012). Modeling an autism risk factor in mice leads to permanent immune dysregulation. *Proc. Natl. Acad. Sci. U.S.A.* 109, 12776–12781. doi: 10.1073/pnas.1202556109

Hughes, J. R. (2008). A review of recent reports on autism: 1000 studies published in 2007. *Epilepsy Behav.* 13, 425–437. doi: 10.1016/j.yebeh.2008.06.015

Hussman, J. P., Chung, R., Griswold, A., Jaworski, J., Salyakina, D., Ma, D., et al. (2011). A noise-reduction GWAS analysis implicates altered regulation of neurite outgrowth and guidance in autism. *Mol. Autism* 2:1. doi: 10.1186/2040-2392-2-1

Hutsler, J. J., and Zhang, H. (2010). Increased dendritic spine densities on cortical projection neurons in autism spectrum disorders. *Brain Res.* 1309, 83–94. doi: 10.1016/j.brainres.2009.09.120

Hutsler, J. J., Love, T., and Zhang, H. (2007). Histological and magnetic resonance imaging assessment of cortical layering and thickness in autism spectrum disorders. *Biol. Psychiatry* 61, 449–457. doi: 10.1016/j.biopsych.2006.01.015

Hyde, K. L., Samson, F., Evans, A. C., and Mottron, L. (2010). Neuroanatomical differences in brain areas implicated in perceptual and other core features of autism revealed by cortical thickness analysis and voxel-based morphometry. *Hum. Brain Mapp.* 31, 556–566.

Ito, S., Stuphorn, V., Brown, J. W., and Schall, J. D. (2003). Performance monitoring by the anterior cingulate cortex during saccade countermanding. *Science* 302, 120–122. doi: 10.1126/science.1087847

Jacot-Descombes, S., Uppal, N., Wicinski, B., Santos, M., Schmeidler, J., Giannakopoulos, P., et al. (2012). Decreased pyramidal neuron size in Brodmann areas 44 and 45 in patients with autism. *Acta Neuropathol.* 124, 67–79. doi: 10.1007/s00401-012-0976-6

Jiao, Y., Chen, R., Ke, X. Y., Chu, K. K., Lu, Z. H., and Herskovits, E. H. (2010). Predictive models of autism spectrum disorder based on brain regional cortical thickness. *Neuroimage* 50, 589–599. doi: 10.1016/j.neuroimage.2009.12.047

Johnston, K., Levin, H. M., Koval, M. J., and Everling, S. (2007). Top-down control-signal dynamics in anterior cingulate and prefrontal cortex neurons following task switching. *Neuron* 53, 453–462. doi: 10.1016/j.neuron.2006.12.023

Jones, E. G. (2009). Synchrony in the interconnected circuitry of the thalamus and cerebral cortex. *Ann. N.Y. Acad. Sci.* 1157, 10–23. doi: 10.1111/j.1749-6632.2009.04534.x

Jou, R. J., Mateljevic, N., Kaiser, M. D., Sugrue, D. R., Volkmar, F. R., and Pelphrey, K. A. (2011). Structural neural phenotype of autism: preliminary evidence from a diffusion tensor imaging study using tract-based spatial statistics. *Am. J. Neuroradiol.* 32, 1607–1613. doi: 10.3174/ajnr.A2558

Jou, R. J., Minshew, N. J., Keshavan, M. S., and Hardan, A. Y. (2010). Cortical gyrification in autistic and asperger disorders: a preliminary magnetic resonance imaging study. *J. Child Neurol.* 25, 1462–1467. doi: 10.1177/0883073810368311

Just, M. A., Cherkassky, V. L., Keller, T. A., and Minshew, N. J. (2004). Cortical activation and synchronization during sentence comprehension in high-functioning autism: evidence of underconnectivity. *Brain* 127, 1811–1821. doi: 10.1093/brain/awh199

Just, M. A., Cherkassky, V. L., Keller, T. A., Kana, R. K., and Minshew, N. J. (2007). Functional and anatomical cortical underconnectivity in autism: evidence from an fMRI study of an executive function task and corpus callosum morphometry. *Cereb. Cortex* 17, 951–961. doi: 10.1093/cercor/bhl006

Just, M. A., Keller, T. A., Malave, V. L., Kana, R. K., and Varma, S. (2012). Autism as a neural systems disorder: a theory of frontal-posterior underconnectivity. *Neurosci. Biobehav. Rev.* 36, 1292–1313. doi: 10.1016/j.neubiorev.2012.02.007

Jyonouchi, H., Sun, S., and Le, H. (2001). Proinflammatory and regulatory cytokine production associated with innate and adaptive immune responses in children with autism spectrum disorders and developmental regression. *J. Neuroimmunol.* 120, 170–179. doi: 10.1016/S0165-5728(01)00421-0

Kalus, P., and Senitz, D. (1996). Parvalbumin in the human anterior cingulate cortex: morphological heterogeneity of inhibitory interneurons. *Brain Res.* 729, 45–54. doi: 10.1016/0006-8993(96)00415-5

Kana, R. K., Keller, T. A., Cherkassky, V. L., Minshew, N. J., and Just, M. A. (2006a). Sentence comprehension in autism: thinking in pictures with decreased functional connectivity. *Brain* 129, 2484–2493. doi: 10.1093/brain/awl164

Kana, R. K., Keller, T. A., Minshew, N. J., and Just, M. A. (2006b). Inhibitory control in high-functioning autism: decreased activation and underconnectivity in inhibition networks. *Biol. Psychiatry* 62, 198–206. doi: 10.1016/j.biopsych.2006.08.004

Kanazir, S., Ruzdijic, S., Vukosavic, S., Ivkovic, S., Milosevic, A., Zecevic, N., et al. (1996). GAP-43 mRNA expression in early development of human nervous system. *Brain Res. Mol. Brain Res.* 38, 145–155. doi: 10.1016/0169-328X(96)00008-3

Kapfhammer, J. P., and Schwab, M. E. (1994). Inverse patterns of myelination and GAP-43 expression in the adult CNS: neurite growth inhibitors as regulators of neuronal plasticity? *J. Comp. Neurol.* 340, 194–206. doi: 10.1002/cne.903400206

Kawaguchi, Y., and Kubota, Y. (1997). GABAergic cell subtypes and their synaptic connections in rat frontal cortex. *Cereb. Cortex* 7, 476–486. doi: 10.1093/cercor/7.6.476

Keller, T. A., Kana, R. K., and Just, M. A. (2007). A developmental study of the structural integrity of white matter in autism. *Neuroreport* 18, 23–27. doi: 10.1097/01.wnr.0000239965.21685.99

Kennedy, D. P., Redcay, E., and Courchesne, E. (2006). Failing to deactivate: resting functional abnormalities in autism. *Proc. Natl. Acad. Sci. U.S.A.* 103, 8275–8280. doi: 10.1073/pnas.0600674103

Khan, S., Gramfort, A., Shetty, N. R., Kitzbichler, M. G., Ganesan, S., Moran, J. M., et al. (2013). Local and long-range functional connectivity is reduced in concert in autism spectrum disorders. *Proc. Natl. Acad. Sci. U.S.A.* 110, 3107–3112. doi: 10.1073/pnas.1214533110

Kondo, H., Tanaka, K., Hashikawa, T., and Jones, E. G. (1999). Neurochemical gradients along monkey sensory cortical pathways: calbindin-immunoreactive pyramidal neurons in layers II and III. *Eur. J. Neurosci.* 11, 4197–4203. doi: 10.1046/j.1460-9568.1999.00844.x

Koshino, H., Kana, R. K., Keller, T. A., Cherkassky, V. L., Minshew, N. J., and Just, M. A. (2008). fMRI investigation of working memory for faces in autism: visual coding and underconnectivity with frontal areas. *Cereb. Cortex* 18, 289–300. doi: 10.1093/cercor/bhm054

Kumar, A., Sundaram, S. K., Sivaswamy, L., Behen, M. E., Makki, M. I., Ager, J., et al. (2009). Alterations in frontal lobe tracts and corpus callosum in young children with autism spectrum disorder. *Cereb. Cortex* 20, 2103–2113. doi: 10.1093/cercor/bhp278

Lai, M. C., Lombardo, M. V., Chakrabarti, B., Sadek, S. A., Pasco, G., Wheelwright, S. J., et al. (2010). A shift to randomness of brain oscillations in people with autism. *Biol. Psychiatry* 68, 1092–1099. doi: 10.1016/j.biopsych.2010.06.027

Langen, M., Leemans, A., Johnston, P., Ecker, C., Daly, E., Murphy, C. M., et al. (2012). Fronto-striatal circuitry and inhibitory control in autism: findings from diffusion tensor imaging tractography. *Cortex* 48, 183–193. doi: 10.1016/j.cortex.2011.05.018

Lawrence, Y. A., Kemper, T. L., Bauman, M. L., and Blatt, G. J. (2010). Parvalbumin-, calbindin-, and calretinin-immunoreactive hippocampal interneuron density in autism. *Acta Neurol. Scand.* 121, 99–108. doi: 10.1111/j.1600-0404.2009.01234.x

Lee, J. E., Bigler, E. D., Alexander, A. L., Lazar, M., Dubray, M. B., Chung, M. K., et al. (2007). Diffusion tensor imaging of white matter in the superior temporal gyrus and temporal stem in autism. *Neurosci. Lett.* 424, 127–132. doi: 10.1016/j.neulet.2007.07.042

Lepagnol-Bestel, A. M., Maussion, G., Boda, B., Cardona, A., Iwayama, Y., Delezoide, A. L., et al. (2008). SLC25A12 expression is associated with neurite outgrowth and is upregulated in the prefrontal cortex of autistic subjects. *Mol. Psychiatry* 13, 385–397. doi: 10.1038/sj.mp.4002120

Letinic, K., and Kostovic, I. (1998). Postnatal development of calcium-binding proteins calbindin and parvalbumin in human visual cortex. *Cereb. Cortex* 8, 660–669. doi: 10.1093/cercor/8.7.660

Levisohn, P. M. (2007). The autism-epilepsy connection. *Epilepsia* 48(Suppl. 9), 33–35. doi: 10.1111/j.1528-1167.2007.01399.x

Levitt, P. (2003). Structural and functional maturation of the developing primate brain. *J. Pediatr.* 143, S35–S45. doi: 10.1067/S0022-3476(03)00400-1

Lewis, D. A., and Morrison, J. H. (1989). Noradrenergic innervation of monkey prefrontal cortex: a dopamine-á-hydoxylase immunohistochemical study. *J. Comp. Neurol.* 282, 317–330. doi: 10.1002/cne.902820302

Lewis, D. A., Foote, S. L., Goldstein, M., and Morrison, J. H. (1988). The dopaminergic innervation of monkey prefrontal cortex: a tyrosine hydroxylase immunohistochemical study. *Brain Res.* 449, 225–243. doi: 10.1016/0006-8993(88)91040-2

London, M., and Hausser, M. (2005). Dendritic computation. *Annu. Rev. Neurosci.* 28, 503–532. doi: 10.1146/annurev.neuro.28.061604.135703

Loveland, K. A., Bachevalier, J., Pearson, D. A., and Lane, D. M. (2008). Fronto-limbic functioning in children and adolescents with and without autism. *Neuropsychologia* 46, 49–62. doi: 10.1016/j.neuropsychologia.2007.08.017

Lowenstein, P. R., and Somogyi, P. (1991). Synaptic organization of cortico-cortical connections from the primary visual cortex to the posteromedial lateral suprasylvian visual area in the cat. *J. Comp. Neurol.* 310, 253–266. doi: 10.1002/cne.903100209

Luna, B., Minshew, N. J., Garver, K. E., Lazar, N. A., Thulborn, K. R., Eddy, W. F., et al. (2002). Neocortical system abnormalities in autism: an fMRI study of spatial working memory. *Neurology* 59, 834–840. doi: 10.1212/WNL.59.6.834

Ma, D. Q., Whitehead, P. L., Menold, M. M., Martin, E. R., Ashley-Koch, A. E., Mei, H., et al. (2005). Identification of significant association and gene-gene interaction of GABA receptor subunit genes in autism. *Am. J. Hum. Genet.* 77, 377–388. doi: 10.1086/433195

MacDonald, A. W. III., Cohen, J. D., Stenger, V. A., and Carter, C. S. (2000). Dissociating the role of the dorsolateral prefrontal and anterior cingulate cortex in cognitive control. *Science* 288, 1835–1838. doi: 10.1126/science.288.5472.1835

Maestro, S., Muratori, F., Cavallaro, M. C., Pei, F., Stern, D., Golse, B., et al. (2002). Attentional skills during the first 6 months of age in autism spectrum disorder. *J. Am. Acad. Child Adolesc. Psychiatry* 41, 1239–1245. doi: 10.1097/00004583-200210000-00014

Malkova, N. V., Yu, C. Z., Hsiao, E. Y., Moore, M. J., and Patterson, P. H. (2012). Maternal immune activation yields offspring displaying mouse versions of the three core symptoms of autism. *Brain Behav. Immun.* 26, 607–616. doi: 10.1016/j.bbi.2012.01.011

Markram, K. M., and Markram, H. (2010). The intense world theory - a unifying theory of the neurobiology of autism. *Front. Hum. Neurosci.* 4:224. doi: 10.3389/fnhum.2010.00224

Maviel, T., Durkin, T. P., Menzaghi, F., and Bontempi, B. (2004). Sites of neocortical reorganization critical for remote spatial memory. *Science* 305, 96–99. doi: 10.1126/science.1098180

Medalla, M., and Barbas, H. (2006). Diversity of laminar connections linking periarcuate and lateral intraparietal areas depends on cortical structure. *Eur. J. Neurosci.* 23, 161–179. doi: 10.1111/j.1460-9568.2005.04522.x

Medalla, M., and Barbas, H. (2009). Synapses with inhibitory neurons differentiate anterior cingulate from dorsolateral prefrontal pathways associated with cognitive control. *Neuron* 61, 609–620. doi: 10.1016/j.neuron.2009.01.006

Medalla, M., and Barbas, H. (2010). Anterior cingulate synapses in prefrontal areas 10 and 46 suggest differential influence in cognitive control. *J. Neurosci.* 30, 16068–16081. doi: 10.1523/JNEUROSCI.1773-10.2010

Medalla, M., and Barbas, H. (2012). The anterior cingulate cortex may enhance inhibition of lateral prefrontal cortex via m2 cholinergic receptors at dual synaptic sites. *J. Neurosci.* 32, 15611–15625. doi: 10.1523/JNEUROSCI.2339-12.2012

Medalla, M., Lera, P., Feinberg, M., and Barbas, H. (2007). Specificity in inhibitory systems associated with prefrontal pathways to temporal cortex in primates. *Cereb. Cortex* 17(Suppl. 1), i136-i150. doi: 10.1093/cercor/bhm068

Meskenaite, V. (1997). Calretinin-immunoreactive local circuit neurons in area 17 of the cynomolgus monkey, *Macaca fascicularis*. *J. Comp. Neurol.* 379, 113–132. doi: 10.1002/(SICI)1096-9861(19970303)379:1<113::AID-CNE8>3.0.CO;2-7

Micheva, K. D., Busse, B., Weiler, N. C., O'Rourke, N., and Smith, S. J. (2010). Single-synapse analysis of a diverse synapse population: proteomic imaging methods and markers. *Neuron* 68, 639–653. doi: 10.1016/j.neuron.2010.09.024

Miguel-Hidalgo, J. J., Overholser, J. C., Meltzer, H. Y., Stockmeier, C. A., and Rajkowska, G. (2006). Reduced glial and neuronal packing density in the orbitofrontal cortex in alcohol dependence and its relationship with suicide and duration of alcohol dependence. *Aging Clin. Exp. Res.* 30, 1845–1855. doi: 10.1111/j.1530-0277.2006.00221.x

Milosevic, A., Kanazir, S., and Zecevic, N. (1995). Immunocytochemical localization of growth-associated protein GAP-43 in early human development. *Brain Res. Dev. Brain Res.* 84, 282–286. doi: 10.1016/0165-3806(94)00187-5

Minshew, N. J., and Keller, T. A. (2010). The nature of brain dysfunction in autism: functional brain imaging studies. *Curr. Opin. Neurol.* 23, 124–130. doi: 10.1097/WCO.0b013e32833782d4

Minshew, N. J., and Williams, D. L. (2007). The new neurobiology of autism: cortex, connectivity, and neuronal organization. *Arch. Neurol.* 64, 945–950. doi: 10.1001/archneur.64.7.945

Morgan, J. T., Chana, G., Abramson, I., Semendeferi, K., Courchesne, E., and Everall, I. P. (2012). Abnormal microglial-neuronal spatial organization in the dorsolateral prefrontal cortex in autism. *Brain Res.* 1456, 72–81. doi: 10.1016/j.brainres.2012.03.036

Morgan, J. T., Chana, G., Pardo, C. A., Achim, C., Semendeferi, K., Buckwalter, J., et al. (2010). Microglial activation and increased microglial density observed in the dorsolateral prefrontal cortex in autism. *Biol. Psychiatry* 68, 368–376. doi: 10.1016/j.biopsych.2010.05.024

Mountcastle, V. (1998). "The columnar organization of the neocortex," in *Perceptual Neuroscience: The Cerebral Cortex*, ed V. Mountcastle (Cambridge: Harvard University Press), 165–203.

Mountcastle, V. B. (1997). The columnar organization of the neocortex. *Brain* 120(Pt 4), 701–722. doi: 10.1093/brain/120.4.701

Muller, R. A., Shih, P., Keehn, B., Deyoe, J. R., Leyden, K. M., and Shukla, D. K. (2011). Underconnected, but how? A survey of functional connectivity MRI studies in autism spectrum disorders. *Cereb. Cortex* 21, 2233–2243. doi: 10.1093/cercor/bhq296

Mundy, P. (2003). Annotation: the neural basis of social impairments in autism: the role of the dorsal medial-frontal cortex and anterior cingulate system. *J. Child Psychol. Psychiatry* 44, 793–809. doi: 10.1111/1469-7610.00165

Murray, E. A., and Wise, S. P. (2012). Why is there a special issue on perirhinal cortex in a journal called hippocampus? The perirhinal cortex in historical perspective. *Hippocampus* 22, 1941–1951. doi: 10.1002/hipo.22055

Neve, R. L., Finch, E. A., Bird, E. D., and Benowitz, L. I. (1988). Growth-associated protein GAP-43 is expressed selectively in associative regions of the adult human brain. *Proc. Natl. Acad. Sci. U.S.A.* 85, 3638–3642. doi: 10.1073/pnas.85.10.3638

Nguyen, T., Lindner, R., Tedeschi, A., Forsberg, K., Green, A., Wuttke, A., et al. (2009). NFAT-3 is a transcriptional repressor of the growth-associated protein 43 during neuronal maturation. *J. Biol. Chem.* 284, 18816–18823. doi: 10.1074/jbc.M109.015719

Nimchinsky, E. A., Sabatini, B. L., and Svoboda, K. (2002). Structure and function of dendritic spines. *Annu. Rev. Physiol.* 64, 313–353. doi: 10.1146/annurev.physiol.64.081501.160008

Norbury, C. F., Brock, J., Cragg, L., Einav, S., Griffiths, H., and Nation, K. (2009). Eye-movement patterns are associated with communicative competence in autistic spectrum disorders. *J. Child Psychol. Psychiatry* 50, 834–842. doi: 10.1111/j.1469-7610.2009.02073.x

Oblak, A. L., Gibbs, T. T., and Blatt, G. J. (2010). Decreased GABA(B) receptors in the cingulate cortex and fusiform gyrus in autism. *J. Neurochem.* 114, 1414–1423.

Oblak, A. L., Gibbs, T. T., and Blatt, G. J. (2011a). Reduced GABAA receptors and benzodiazepine binding sites in the posterior cingulate cortex and fusiform gyrus in autism. *Brain Res.* 1380, 218–228. doi: 10.1016/j.brainres.2010.09.021

Oblak, A. L., Rosene, D. L., Kemper, T. L., Bauman, M. L., and Blatt, G. J. (2011b). Altered posterior cingulate cortical cyctoarchitecture, but normal density of neurons and interneurons in the posterior cingulate cortex and fusiform gyrus in autism. *Autism Res.* 4, 200–211. doi: 10.1002/aur.188

Oblak, A., Gibbs, T. T., and Blatt, G. J. (2009). Decreased GABAA receptors and benzodiazepine binding sites in the anterior cingulate cortex in autism. *Autism Res.* 2, 205–219. doi: 10.1002/aur.88

Oishi, T., Higo, N., Umino, Y., Matsuda, K., and Hayashi, M. (1998). Development of GAP-43 mRNA in the macaque cerebral cortex. *Brain Res. Dev. Brain Res.* 109, 87–97. doi: 10.1016/S0165-3806(98)00067-4

Ostensen, M., Khamashta, M., Lockshin, M., Parke, A., Brucato, A., Carp, H., et al. (2006). Anti-inflammatory and immunosuppressive drugs and reproduction. *Arthritis Res.Ther.* 8, 209. doi: 10.1186/ar1957

Ozonoff, S., Pennington, B. F., and Rogers, S. J. (1991). Executive function deficits in high-functioning autistic individuals: relationship to theory of mind. *J. Child Psychol. Psychiatry* 32, 1081–1105. doi: 10.1111/j.1469-7610.1991.tb00351.x

Pardini, M., Garaci, F. G., Bonzano, L., Roccatagliata, L., Palmieri, M. G., Pompili, E., et al. (2009). White matter reduced streamline coherence in young men with autism and mental retardation. *Eur. J. Neurol.* 16, 1185–1190. doi: 10.1111/j.1468-1331.2009.02699.x

Pardo, C. A., Vargas, D. L., and Zimmerman, A. W. (2005). Immunity, neuroglia and neuroinflammation in autism. *Int. Rev. Psychiatry* 17, 485–495. doi: 10.1080/02646830500381930

Patterson, P. H. (2011). Maternal infection and immune involvement in autism. *Trends Mol. Med.* 17, 389–394. doi: 10.1016/j.molmed.2011.03.001

Patterson, P. H. (2012). Maternal infection and autism. *Brain Behav. Immun.* 26, 393. doi: 10.1016/j.bbi.2011.09.008

Paus, T. (2001). Primate anterior cingulate cortex: where motor control, drive and cognition interface. *Nat. Rev. Neurosci.* 2, 417–424. doi: 10.1038/35077500

Paus, T., Collins, D. L., Evans, A. C., Leonard, G., Pike, B., and Zijdenbos, A. (2001). Maturation of white matter in the human brain: a review of magnetic resonance studies. *Brain Res. Bull.* 54, 255–266. doi: 10.1016/S0361-9230(00)00434-2

Paus, T., Zijdenbos, A., Worsley, K., Collins, D. L., Blumenthal, J., Giedd, J. N., et al. (1999). Structural maturation of neural pathways in children and adolescents: *in vivo* study. *Science* 283, 1908–1911. doi: 10.1126/science.283.5409.1908

Penzes, P., Cahill, M. E., Jones, K. A., Vanleeuwen, J. E., and Woolfrey, K. M. (2011). Dendritic spine pathology in neuropsychiatric disorders. *Nat. Neurosci.* 14, 285–293. doi: 10.1038/nn.2741

Peters, A., and Sethares, C. (1996). Myelinated axons and the pyramidal cell modules in monkey primary visual cortex. *J. Comp. Neurol.* 365, 232–255. doi: 10.1002/(SICI)1096-9861(19960205)365: 2< 232::AID-CNE3>3.0.CO;2-6

Peters, A., and Sethares, C. (1997). The organization of double bouquet cells in monkey striate cortex. *J. Neurocytol.* 26, 779–797. doi: 10.1023/A:1018518515982

Peters, A., Palay, S. L., and Webster, H. D. (1991). *The Fine Structure of the Nervous System. Neurons and Their Supporting Cells.* New York, NY: Oxford University Press.

Petrides, M., and Pandya, D. N. (1988). Association fiber pathways to the frontal cortex from the superior temporal region in the rhesus monkey. *J. Comp. Neurol.* 273, 52–66. doi: 10.1002/cne.902730106

Petrides, M., and Pandya, D. N. (2006). Efferent association pathways originating in the caudal prefrontal cortex in the macaque monkey. *J.Comp Neurol.* 498, 227–251. doi: 10.1002/cne.21048

Petrides, M., and Pandya, D. N. (2007). Efferent association pathways from the rostral prefrontal cortex in the macaque monkey. *J. Neurosci.* 27, 11573–11586. doi: 10.1523/JNEUROSCI.2419-07.2007

Pickett, J., and London, E. (2005). The neuropathology of autism: a review. *J. Neuropathol. Exp. Neurol.* 64, 925–935. doi: 10.1097/01.jnen.0000186921.42592.6c

Raghanti, M. A., Stimpson, C. D., Marcinkiewicz, J. L., Erwin, J. M., Hof, P. R., and Sherwood, C. C. (2008). Differences in cortical serotonergic innervation among humans, chimpanzees, and macaque monkeys: a comparative study. *Cereb. Cortex* 18, 584–597. doi: 10.1093/cercor/bhm089

Rakic, P. (2002). Neurogenesis in adult primate neocortex: an evaluation of the evidence. *Nat. Rev. Neurosci.* 3, 65–71. doi: 10.1038/nrn700

Redcay, E., and Courchesne, E. (2005). When is the brain enlarged in autism? A meta-analysis of all brain size reports. *Biol. Psychiatry* 58, 1–9. doi: 10.1016/j.biopsych.2005.03.026

Rempel-Clower, N. L., and Barbas, H. (2000). The laminar pattern of connections between prefrontal and anterior temporal cortices in the rhesus monkey is related to cortical structure and function. *Cereb. Cortex* 10, 851–865. doi: 10.1093/cercor/10.9.851

Routtenberg, A., Cantallops, I., Zaffuto, S., Serrano, P., and Namgung, U. (2000). Enhanced learning after genetic overexpression of a brain growth protein. *Proc. Natl. Acad. Sci. U.S.A.* 97, 7657–7662. doi: 10.1073/pnas.97.13.7657

Rubenstein, J. L. R. (2011). Development of the cerebral cortex: implications for neurodevelopmental disorders. *J. Child Psychol. Psychiatry* 52, 339–355. doi: 10.1111/j.1469-7610.2010.02307.x

Rubenstein, J. L., and Merzenich, M. M. (2003). Model of autism: increased ratio of excitation/inhibition in key neural systems. *Genes Brain Behav.* 2, 255–267. doi: 10.1034/j.1601-183X.2003.00037.x

Sabbagh, M. A. (2004). Understanding orbitofrontal contributions to theory-of-mind reasoning: implications for autism. *Brain Cogn.* 55, 209–219. doi: 10.1016/j.bandc.2003.04.002

Sairanen, M., O'Leary, O. F., Knuuttila, J. E., and Castren, E. (2007). Chronic antidepressant treatment selectively increases expression of plasticity-related proteins in the hippocampus and medial prefrontal cortex of the rat. *Neuroscience* 144, 368–374. doi: 10.1016/j.neuroscience.2006.08.069

Samaco, R. C., Hogart, A., and Lasalle, J. M. (2005). Epigenetic overlap in autism-spectrum neurodevelopmental disorders: MECP2 deficiency causes reduced expression of UBE3A and GABRB3. *Hum. Mol. Genet.* 14, 483–492. doi: 10.1093/hmg/ddi045

Santos, M., Uppal, N., Butti, C., Wicinski, B., Schmeidler, J., Giannakopoulos, P., et al. (2011). Von Economo neurons in autism: a stereologic study of the frontoinsular cortex in children. *Brain Res.* 1380, 206–217. doi: 10.1016/j.brainres.2010.08.067

Schall, J. D. (2001). Neural basis of deciding, choosing and acting. *Nat. Rev. Neurosci.* 2, 33–42. doi: 10.1038/35049054

Schipul, S., Keller, T., and Just, M. A. (2011). Inter-regional brain communication and its disturbance in autism. *Front. Syst. Neurosci.* 5:10. doi: 10.3389/fnsys.2011.00010

Schmahmann, J. D., and Pandya, D. N. (2006). *Fiber Pathways of the Brain.* New York, NY: Oxford University Press Inc. doi: 10.1093/acprof:oso/9780195104233.001.0001

Schmahmann, J. D., Pandya, D. N., Wang, R., Dai, G., D'Arceuil, H. E., De Crespigny, A. J., et al. (2007). Association fibre pathways of the brain: parallel observations from diffusion spectrum imaging and autoradiography. *Brain* 130, 630–653. doi: 10.1093/brain/awl359

Schmitz, C., and Rezaie, P. (2008). The neuropathology of autism: where do we stand? *Neuropathol. Appl. Neurobiol.* 34, 4–11.

Schumann, C. M., and Amaral, D. G. (2006). Stereological analysis of amygdala neuron number in autism. *J. Neurosci.* 26, 7674–7679. doi: 10.1523/JNEUROSCI.1285-06.2006

Schumann, C. M., and Nordahl, C. W. (2011). Bridging the gap between MRI and postmortem research in autism. *Brain Res.* 1380, 175–186. doi: 10:1016/j.brainres.2010.09.061

Schumann, C. M., Bloss, C. S., Barnes, C. C., Wideman, G. M., Carper, R. A., Akshoomoff, N., et al. (2010). Longitudinal magnetic resonance imaging study of cortical development through early childhood in autism. *J. Neurosci.* 30, 4419–4427. doi: 10.1523/JNEUROSCI.5714-09.2010

Schumann, C. M., Hamstra, J., Goodlin-Jones, B. L., Lotspeich, L. J., Kwon, H., Buonocore, M. H., et al. (2004). The amygdala is enlarged in children but not adolescents with autism; the hippocampus is enlarged at all ages. *J. Neurosci.* 24, 6392–6401. doi: 10.1523/JNEUROSCI.1297-04.2004

Selby, L., Zhang, C., and Sun, Q. Q. (2007). Major defects in neocortical GABAergic inhibitory circuits in mice lacking the fragile X mental retardation protein. *Neurosci. Lett.* 412, 227–232. doi: 10.1016/j.neulet.2006.11.062

Selemon, L. D., Rajkowska, G., and Goldman-Rakic, P. S. (1998). Elevated neuronal density in prefrontal area 46 in brains from schizophrenic patients: application of a three-dimensional, stereologic counting method. *J. Comp. Neurol.* 392, 402–412. doi: 10.1002/(SICI)1096-9861(19980316)392:3<402::AID-CNE9>3.0.CO;2-5

Seltzer, B., and Pandya, D. N. (1989). Frontal lobe connections of the superior temporal sulcus in the rhesus monkey. *J. Comp. Neurol.* 281, 97–113. doi: 10.1002/cne.902810108

Shao, Z., and Burkhalter, A. (1999). Role of GABAB receptor-mediated inhibition in reciprocal interareal pathways of rat visual cortex. *J. Neurophysiol.* 81, 1014–1024.

Sherwood, C. C., Raghanti, M. A., Stimpson, C. D., Spocter, M. A., Uddin, M., Boddy, A. M., et al. (2010). Inhibitory interneurons of the human prefrontal cortex display conserved evolution of the phenotype and related genes. *Proc. Biol. Sci.* 277, 1011–1020. doi: 10.1098/rspb.2009.1831

Shukla, D. K., Keehn, B., Lincoln, A. J., and Muller, R. A. (2010). White matter compromise of callosal and subcortical fiber tracts in children with autism spectrum disorder: a diffusion tensor imaging study. *J. Am. Acad. Child Adolesc. Psychiatry* 49, 1269–1278, 1278 e1261-1262.

Shukla, D. K., Keehn, B., and Muller, R. A. (2011a). Tract-specific analyses of diffusion tensor imaging show widespread white matter compromise in autism spectrum disorder. *J. Child Psychol. Psychiatry* 52, 286–295. doi: 10.1111/j.1469-7610.2010.02342.x

Shukla, D. K., Keehn, B., Smylie, D. M., and Muller, R. A. (2011b). Microstructural abnormalities of short-distance white matter tracts in autism spectrum disorder. *Neuropsychologia* 49, 1378–1382. doi: 10.1016/j.neuropsychologia.2011.02.022

Shulha, H. P., Cheung, I., Whittle, C., Wang, J., Virgil, D., Lin, C. L., et al. (2012). Epigenetic signatures of autism: trimethylated H3K4 landscapes in prefrontal neurons. *Arch. Gen. Psychiatry* 69, 314–324. doi: 10.1001/archgenpsychiatry.2011.151

Simms, M. L., Kemper, T. L., Timbie, C. M., Bauman, M. L., and Blatt, G. J. (2009). The anterior cingulate cortex in autism: heterogeneity of qualitative and quantitative cytoarchitectonic features suggests possible subgroups. *Acta Neuropathol.* 118, 673–684. doi: 10.1007/s00401-009-0568-2

Simpson, K. L., Weaver, K. J., de Villers-Sidani, E., Lu, J. Y., Cai, Z., Pang, Y., et al. (2011). Perinatal antidepressant exposure alters cortical network function in rodents. *Proc. Natl. Acad. Sci. U.S.A.* 108, 18465–18470. doi: 10.1073/pnas.1109353108

Smith, S. E., Li, J., Garbett, K., Mirnics, K., and Patterson, P. H. (2007). Maternal immune activation alters fetal brain development through interleukin-6. *J. Neurosci.* 27, 10695–10702. doi: 10.1523/JNEUROSCI.2178-07.2007

Somogyi, P., Tamas, G., Lujan, R., and Buhl, E. H. (1998). Salient features of synaptic organisation in the cerebral cortex. *Brain Res. Brain Res. Rev.* 26, 113–135. doi: 10.1016/S0165-0173(97)00061-1

Sparks, B. F., Friedman, S. D., Shaw, D. W., Aylward, E. H., Echelard, D., Artru, A. A., et al. (2002). Brain structural abnormalities in young children with autism spectrum disorder. *Neurology* 59, 184–192. doi: 10.1212/WNL.59.2.184

Srivastava, D. P., Woolfrey, K. M., Jones, K. A., Anderson, C. T., Smith, K. R., Russell, T. A., et al. (2012). An autism-associated variant of Epac2 reveals a role for Ras/Epac2 signaling in controlling basal dendrite maintenance in mice. *PLoS Biol.* 10:e1001350. doi: 10.1371/journal.pbio.1001350

Stark, A. K., Uylings, H. B., Sanz-Arigita, E., and Pakkenberg, B. (2004). Glial cell loss in the anterior cingulate cortex, a subregion of the prefrontal cortex, in subjects with schizophrenia. *Am. J. Psychiatry* 161, 882–888. doi: 10.1176/appi.ajp.161.5.882

Steele, S. D., Minshew, N. J., Luna, B., and Sweeney, J. A. (2007). Spatial working memory deficits in autism. *J. Autism Dev. Disord.* 37, 605–612. doi: 10.1007/s10803-006-0202-2

Sundaram, S. K., Kumar, A., Makki, M. I., Behen, M. E., Chugani, H. T., and Chugani, D. C. (2008). Diffusion tensor imaging of frontal lobe in autism spectrum disorder. *Cereb. Cortex* 18, 2659–2665. doi: 10.1093/cercor/bhn031

Suzuki, K., Sugihara, G., Ouchi, Y., Nakamura, K., Futatsubashi, M., Takebayashi, K., et al. (2013). Microglial activation in young adults with autism spectrum disorder. *JAMA Psychiatry* 70, 49–58. doi: 10.1001/jamapsychiatry.2013.272

Suzuki, Y., Matsuzawa, H., Kwee, I. L., and Nakada, T. (2003). Absolute eigenvalue diffusion tensor analysis for human brain maturation. *NMR Biomed.* 16, 257–260. doi: 10.1002/nbm.848

Szatmari, P., Paterson, A. D., Zwaigenbaum, L., Roberts, W., Brian, J., Liu, X. Q., et al. (2007). Mapping autism risk loci using genetic linkage and chromosomal rearrangements. *Nat. Genet.* 39, 319–328. doi: 10.1038/ng1985

Tabuchi, K., Blundell, J., Etherton, M. R., Hammer, R. E., Liu, X., Powell, C. M., et al. (2007). A neuroligin-3 mutation implicated in autism increases inhibitory synaptic transmission in mice. *Science* 318, 71–76. doi: 10.1126/science.1146221

Tamura, R., Kitamura, H., Endo, T., Hasegawa, N., and Someya, T. (2010). Reduced thalamic volume observed across different subgroups of autism spectrum disorders. *Psychiatry Res.* 184, 186–188. doi: 10.1016/j.pscychresns.2010.07.001

Tanji, J., and Hoshi, E. (2008). Role of the lateral prefrontal cortex in executive behavioral control. *Physiol. Rev.* 88, 37–57. doi: 10.1152/physrev.00014.2007

Thakkar, K. N., Polli, F. E., Joseph, R. M., Tuch, D. S., Hadjikhani, N., Barton, J. J., et al. (2008). Response monitoring, repetitive behaviour and anterior cingulate abnormalities in autism spectrum disorders (ASD). *Brain* 131, 2464–2478. doi: 10.1093/brain/awn099

Thatcher, R. W., North, D. M., Neubrander, J., Biver, C. J., Cutler, S., and Defina, P. (2009). Autism and EEG phase reset: deficient GABA mediated inhibition in thalamo-cortical circuits. *Dev. Neuropsychol.* 34, 780–800. doi: 10.1080/87565640903265178

Thomson, A. M., and Deuchars, J. (1997). Synaptic interactions in neocortical local circuits: dual intracellular recordings *in vitro*. *Cereb. Cortex* 7, 510–522. doi: 10.1093/cercor/7.6.510

Tommerdahl, M., Tannan, V., Holden, J. K., and Baranek, G. T. (2008). Absence of stimulus-driven synchronization effects on sensory perception in autism: evidence for local underconnectivity? *Behav. Brain Funct.* 4, 19. doi: 10.1186/1744-9081-4-19

Trikalinos, T. A., Karvouni, A., Zintzaras, E., Ylisaukko-Oja, T., Peltonen, L., Jarvela, I., et al. (2006). A heterogeneity-based genome search meta-analysis for autism-spectrum disorders. *Mol. Psychiatry* 11, 29–36. doi: 10.1038/sj.mp.4001750

Tsatsanis, K. D., Rourke, B. P., Klin, A., Volkmar, F. R., Cicchetti, D., and Schultz, R. T. (2003). Reduced thalamic volume in high-functioning individuals with autism. *Biol. Psychiatry* 53, 121–129. doi: 10.1016/S0006-3223(02)01530-5

van Kooten, I. A., Palmen, S. J., von Cappeln, P., Steinbusch, H. W., Korr, H., Heinsen, H., et al. (2008). Neurons in the fusiform gyrus are fewer and smaller in autism. *Brain* 131, 987–999. doi: 10.1093/brain/awn033

Vargas, D. L., Nascimbene, C., Krishnan, C., Zimmerman, A. W., and Pardo, C. A. (2005). Neuroglial activation and neuroinflammation in the brain of patients with autism. *Ann. Neurol.* 57, 67–81. doi: 10.1002/ana.20315

Vlamings, P. H. J. M., Jonkman, L. M., Hoeksma, M. R., van Engeland, H., and Kemner, C. (2008). Reduced error monitoring in children with autism spectrum disorder: an ERP study. *Eur. J. Neurosci.* 28, 399–406. doi: 10.1111/j.1460-9568.2008.06336.x

Voineagu, I., Wang, X. C., Johnston, P., Lowe, J. K., Tian, Y., Horvath, S., et al. (2011). Transcriptomic analysis of autistic brain reveals convergent molecular pathology. *Nature* 474, 380–384. doi: 10.1038/nature10110

Von Bonin, G. (1950). *Essay on the Cerebral Cortex.* Springfield, IL: Thomas, C.C.

Von Economo, C. (2009). *Cellular structure of the human cerebral cortex.* Basel: Karger.

Wang, X. J., Tegner, J., Constantinidis, C., and Goldman-Rakic, P. S. (2004). Division of labor among distinct subtypes of inhibitory neurons in a cortical microcircuit of working memory. *Proc. Natl. Acad.*

Sci. U.S.A. 101, 1368–1373. doi: 10.1073/pnas.0305337101

Wass, S. (2011). Distortions and disconnections: disrupted brain connectivity in autism. *Brain Cogn.* 75, 18–28. doi: 10.1016/j.bandc.2010.10.005

Wegiel, J., Kuchna, I., Nowicki, K., Imaki, H., Marchi, E., Ma, S. Y., et al. (2010). The neuropathology of autism: defects of neurogenesis and neuronal migration, and dysplastic changes. *Acta Neuropathol.* 119, 755–770. doi: 10.1007/s00401-010-0655-4

Weidenheim, K. M., Goodman, L., Dickson, D. W., Gillberg, C., Rastam, M., and Rapin, I. (2001). Etiology and pathophysiology of autistic behavior: clues from two cases with an unusual variant of neuroaxonal dystrophy. *J. Child Neurol.* 16, 809–819. doi: 10.1177/08830738010160110601

Weiss, L. A., Arking, D. E., Daly, M. J., Chakravarti, A., Brune, C. W., West, K., et al. (2009). A genome-wide linkage and association scan reveals novel loci for autism. *Nature* 461, 802–808. doi: 10.1038/nature08490

West, M. J., Slomianka, L., and Gundersen, H. J. G. (1991). Unbiased stereological estimation of the total number of neurons in the subdivisions of the rat hippocampus using the optical fractionator. *Anat. Rec.* 231, 482–497. doi: 10.1002/ar.1092310411

White, E. L. (1989). *Cortical Circuits. Synaptic Organization of the Cerebral Cortex. Structure, Function and Theory.* Boston, MA: Birkhäuser. doi: 10.1007/978-1-4684-8721-3

White, J. A., Banks, M. I., Pearce, R. A., and Kopell, N. J. (2000). Networks of interneurons with fast and slow gamma-aminobutyric acid type A (GABAA) kinetics provide substrate for mixed gamma-theta rhythm. *Proc. Natl. Acad. Sci. U.S.A.* 97, 8128–8133. doi: 10.1073/pnas.100124097

Whittington, M. A., Cunningham, M. O., Lebeau, F. E., Racca, C., and Traub, R. D. (2011). Multiple origins of the cortical gamma rhythm. *Dev. Neurobiol.* 71, 92–106. doi: 10.1002/dneu.20814

Whittington, M. A., Traub, R. D., Kopell, N., Ermentrout, B., and Buhl, E. H. (2000). Inhibition-based rhythms: experimental and mathematical observations on network dynamics. *Int. J. Psychophysiol.* 38, 315–336. doi: 10.1016/S0167-8760(00)00173-2

Wilson, T. W., Rojas, D. C., Reite, M. L., Teale, P. D., and Rogers, S. J. (2007). Children and adolescents with autism exhibit reduced MEG steady-state gamma responses. *Biol. Psychiatry* 62, 192–197. doi: 10.1016/j.biopsych.2006.07.002

Wong, K. L., Murakami, K., and Routtenberg, A. (1989). Dietary cis-fatty acids that increase protein F1 phosphorylation enhance spatial memory. *Brain Res.* 505, 302–305. doi: 10.1016/0006-8993(89)91456-X

Yakovlev, P. I., and Lecours, A. R. (1967). "The myelogenetic cycles of regional maturation of the brain," in *Regional Development of the Brain in Early Life*, ed A. Minowski (Oxford and Edinburgh: Blackwell Scientific Publications), 3–70.

Yan, X. X., Cao, Q. L., Luo, X. G., and Garey, L. J. (1997). Prenatal development of calbindin D-28K in human visual cortex. *Cereb. Cortex* 7, 57–62. doi: 10.1093/cercor/7.1.57

Yip, J., Soghomonian, J. J., and Blatt, G. J. (2008). Increased GAD67 mRNA expression in cerebellar interneurons in autism: implications for Purkinje cell dysfunction. *J. Neurosci. Res.* 86, 525–530. doi: 10.1002/jnr.21520

Yizhar, O., Fenno, L. E., Prigge, M., Schneider, F., Davidson, T. J., O'Shea, D. J., et al. (2011). Neocortical excitation/inhibition balance in information processing and social dysfunction. *Nature* 477, 171–178. doi: 10.1038/nature10360

Yoshida, T., and Mishina, M. (2005). Distinct roles of calcineurin-nuclear factor of activated T-cells and protein kinase A-cAMP response element-binding protein signaling in presynaptic differentiation. *J. Neurosci.* 25, 3067–3079. doi: 10.1523/JNEUROSCI.3738-04.2005

Zaccaria, K. J., Lagace, D. C., Eisch, A. J., and McCasland, J. S. (2010). Resistance to change and vulnerability to stress: autistic-like features of GAP43-deficient mice. *Genes Brain Behav.* 9, 985–996. doi: 10.1111/j.1601-183X.2010.00638.x

Zikopoulos, B., and Barbas, H. (2006). Prefrontal projections to the thalamic reticular nucleus form a unique circuit for attentional mechanisms. *J. Neurosci.* 26, 7348–7361. doi: 10.1523/JNEUROSCI.5511-05.2006

Zikopoulos, B., and Barbas, H. (2007). Parallel driving and modulatory pathways link the prefrontal cortex and thalamus. *PLoS ONE* 2:e848. doi: 10.1371/journal.pone.0000848

Zikopoulos, B., and Barbas, H. (2010). Changes in prefrontal axons may disrupt the network in autism. *J. Neurosci.* 30, 14595–14609. doi: 10.1523/JNEUROSCI.2257-10.2010

Zikopoulos, B., and Barbas, H. (2012). Pathways for emotions and attention converge on the thalamic reticular nucleus in primates. *J. Neurosci.* 32, 5338–5350. doi: 10.1523/JNEUROSCI.4793-11.2012

Zikopoulos, B., Hoistad, M., and Barbas, H. (2008). "Differential projections and synaptic interactions of posterior orbitofrontal and anterior cingulate cortices with the amygdala," in *Program No.35.5.2008 Neuroscience 2008 Abstracts,* Vol. 34. (Washington, DC: Society for Neuroscience [Online]).

12

Functional connectivity in the first year of life in infants at-risk for autism: a preliminary near-infrared spectroscopy study

Brandon Keehn[1,2], Jennifer B. Wagner[3], Helen Tager-Flusberg[4] and Charles A. Nelson[1,2]*

[1] *Laboratories of Cognitive Neuroscience, Division of Developmental Medicine, Boston Children's Hospital, Boston, MA, USA*
[2] *Harvard Medical School, Boston, MA, USA*
[3] *Department of Psychology, The College of Staten Island, The City University of New York, Staten Island, NY, USA*
[4] *Department of Psychology, Boston University, Boston, MA, USA*

Edited by:
Lucina Q. Uddin, Stanford University, USA

Reviewed by:
Jeff Anderson, University of Utah, USA
Ilan Dinstein, Ben Gurion University of the Negev, Israel

****Correspondence:***
Charles A. Nelson, Laboratories of Cognitive Neuroscience, Division of Developmental Medicine, Boston Children's Hospital, 1 Autumn Street, 6th Floor, Boston, 02115 MA, USA
e-mail: charles.nelson@childrens.harvard.edu

Background: Autism spectrum disorder (ASD) has been called a "developmental disconnection syndrome," however the majority of the research examining connectivity in ASD has been conducted exclusively with older children and adults. Yet, prior ASD research suggests that perturbations in neurodevelopmental trajectories begin as early as the first year of life. Prospective longitudinal studies of infants at risk for ASD may provide a window into the emergence of these aberrant patterns of connectivity. The current study employed functional connectivity near-infrared spectroscopy (NIRS) in order to examine the development of intra- and inter-hemispheric functional connectivity in high- and low-risk infants across the first year of life.

Methods: NIRS data were collected from 27 infants at high risk for autism (HRA) and 37 low-risk comparison (LRC) infants who contributed a total of 116 data sets at 3-, 6-, 9-, and 12-months. At each time point, HRA and LRC groups were matched on age, sex, head circumference, and Mullen Scales of Early Learning scores. Regions of interest (ROI) were selected from anterior and posterior locations of each hemisphere. The average time course for each ROI was calculated and correlations for each ROI pair were computed. Differences in functional connectivity were examined in a cross-sectional manner.

Results: At 3-months, HRA infants showed increased overall functional connectivity compared to LRC infants. This was the result of increased connectivity for intra- and inter-hemispheric ROI pairs. No significant differences were found between HRA and LRC infants at 6- and 9-months. However, by 12-months, HRA infants showed decreased connectivity relative to LRC infants.

Conclusions: Our preliminary results suggest that atypical functional connectivity may exist within the first year of life in HRA infants, providing support to the growing body of evidence that aberrant patterns of connectivity may be a potential endophenotype for ASD.

Keywords: autism, functional connectivity, near-infrared spectroscopy, endophenotype, infancy

INTRODUCTION

Autism spectrum disorder (ASD) is considered by many to be a "developmental disconnection syndrome" (Geschwind and Levitt, 2007), reflecting a shift in perspective from conceptualizing ASD as a disorder of region-specific dysfunction toward one associated with atypical neural circuitry (Belmonte et al., 2004; Muller, 2007; Wass, 2010). Despite being termed a developmental disconnection syndrome, the majority of the research examining anatomical and functional connectivity in ASD has focused on school-aged children, adolescents, and adults, with a small minority of imaging studies examining changes in connectivity across time. However, in ASD, perturbations in neurodevelopmental trajectories begin as early as the first year of life (e.g., Redcay and Courchesne, 2005), indicating that important neuropathological processes are operating in infancy if not earlier.

Prospective longitudinal studies of infants at high-risk for ASD (HRA; because they have an older sibling diagnosed with ASD) provide a window into the earliest manifestations of these aberrant patterns of neurofunctional and structural connectivity. Moreover, studies investigating siblings of individuals diagnosed with ASD also have potential to shed light on possible endophenotypes. Endophenotypes reflect characteristic behavioral or neurobiological features that are present in both affected individuals and their first-degree family members (Gottesman and Gould, 2003), and may lead to a more straightforward decomposition of complex genetic disorders, such as ASD. Both children with ASD and their siblings atypically evidence reductions in white matter connectivity (Barnea-Goraly et al., 2010). More recently, altered developmental trajectories of anatomical connectivity in high-risk infants later diagnosed with ASD were found (Wolff et al., 2012), indicating that atypical connectivity may represent an endophenotype or potential biomarker for ASD.

Much of the ASD anatomical and functional connectivity literature focusing on older individuals supports the underconnectivity theory of ASD originally put forward by Just et al. (2004, 2012). Findings from diffusion tensor imaging (DTI) studies, an imaging modality used to measure microstructural properties of white matter, have generally reported indices of reduced anatomical connectivity in school-aged children, adolescents, and adults with ASD (see Travers et al., 2012, for review). However, in contrast to DTI studies of older individuals with ASD, work with children with ASD as young as one-year-old has shown increased fractional anisotropy (FA) as compared to typically developing (TD) children (Ben Bashat et al., 2007; Weinstein et al., 2011). These results may be indicative of accelerated white matter development in ASD (although see Walker et al., 2012, for discussion of the difficulties interpreting DTI indices), and provide evidence that patterns of over- and under-connectivity may differ as a function of development.

Prior studies investigating connectivity using functional connectivity MRI (fcMRI), an analytical approach used to investigate inter-regional signal cross-correlations that reflect distributed functional networks, have reported both over- and under-connectivity in older individuals with ASD (which may be dependent on specific methodological decisions; see Muller et al., 2011). In the only study to examine functional connectivity in toddlers and younger children with ASD, Dinstein et al. (2011) reported reduced inter-hemispheric connectivity similar to findings from older individuals diagnosed with ASD. In typically developing infants, fcMRI analyses have shown that functional networks exist in neonates and mature gradually across the first years of life (see Smyser et al., 2011, for review). However, to date, no study has examined the development of functional brain networks in the first year of life in ASD.

Recently, functional connectivity has been investigated using near-infrared spectroscopy (fcNIRS) in typically developing infants (Homae et al., 2010, 2011; White et al., 2012) and adults (Mesquita et al., 2010; Zhang et al., 2010; Duan et al., 2012; Sasai et al., 2012). Near-infrared spectroscopy (NIRS) is a relatively new, non-invasive method used to measure concentrations of oxy- (oxy-Hb) and deoxy-hemoglobin (deoxy-Hb) in the cortex, and therefore provides an indirect measure of neuronal activity (similar to functional magnetic resonance imaging; fMRI) (see Gervain et al., 2011, for review). Unlike fMRI, NIRS does not require rigid head stabilization or that the infant be asleep (to avoid motion), making it a more suitable tool to study infant brain development. Furthermore, simultaneous NIRS-fcMRI studies have demonstrated that both methods produce similar functional networks (Duan et al., 2012; Sasai et al., 2012). The current study employed NIRS to examine functional connectivity in the first year of life in infants at high- and low-risk for ASD as they passively listened to linguistic stimuli (Gervain et al., 2008).

Although a failure of neurotypical development of functional brain networks is thought to characterize ASD, only a handful of studies have investigated early differences in connectivity. The current study addresses this gap in the literature by examining functional connectivity in infants at risk for autism as early as 3-months of age. Additionally, while our study is cross-sectional in nature, by investigating infants at risk for ASD we are able to examine *changes* in connectivity across the first year of life (before a reliable diagnosis of ASD can be made), and therefore provide insight into how atypical network organization may emerge in ASD. To our knowledge, this is the first study to examine functional connectivity in infants at risk for ASD. Specifically, the current study employed fcNIRS in order to examine the development of intra- and inter-hemispheric functional connectivity in high- and low-risk comparison (LRC) infants across the first year of life in order to determine if atypical connectivity represents an endophenotype in ASD.

MATERIALS AND METHODS

PARTICIPANTS

A total of 76 infants ($n = 33$ HRA; $n = 43$ LRC) completed visits at 3-, 6-, 9-, and/or 12-months of age. All infants had a minimum gestational age of 36 weeks, no history of prenatal or postnatal medical or neurological problems, and no known genetic disorders (e.g., fragile-X, tuberous sclerosis). Low-risk infants had a typically developing older sibling and no family history of autism or other neurodevelopmental disorders; infants at high-risk for ASD were defined by having at least one older full sibling with a diagnosis of Autistic disorder, Aspergers disorder, or Pervasive Developmental Disorder–Not Otherwise Specified. Community diagnosis of the older sibling with ASD was confirmed using the Social Communication Questionnaire (SCQ; Rutter et al., 2003). At 6- and 12-month visits, infants were administered the Mullen Scales of Early Learning (MSEL; Mullen, 1995) in order to obtain a measure of developmental functioning. Independent-samples t-tests and Fisher's Exact tests confirmed that, at 3-, 6-, 9-, and 12-month visits, HRA and LRC infants that contributed usable NIRS data did not differ significantly with regard to age, sex, head circumference, and at 6- and 12-months, did not differ on MSEL Early Learning Composite score (ELCS) (all $p > 0.1$) (see **Table 1**). Total attrition rates for the current study (26%) were similar to previous infant NIRS studies (~40%; see Lloyd-Fox et al., 2010, for review). At each visit time point, infants were excluded if they were unable to tolerate the NIRS hat, did not complete at least 14 blocks of the task, or did not have at least one usable channel in any region of interest (see **Table 2** for more information). The final sample included a total of 64 infants ($n = 27$ HRA; $n = 37$ LRC) who contributed 116 data sets. Informed consent was obtained from all caregivers in accordance with the Boston Children's Hospital and Boston University Institutional Review Boards.

STIMULI

Stimuli consisted of trisyllabic sequences presented in either an ABB (e.g., "ba-lo-lo") or ABC (e.g., "ba-lo-ti") artificial grammar (see Gervain et al., 2008, for further details). Trisyllabic sequences were grouped into blocks of 10 sounds

Table 1 | Participant infomation.

	HRA				LRC			
	3 months (*n* = 17)	**6 months (*n* = 12)**	**9 months (*n* = 8)**	**12 months (*n* = 6)**	**3 months (*n* = 13)**	**6 months (*n* = 18)**	**9 months (*n* = 21)**	**12 months (*n* = 21)**
Age [days]	106 (11) 91–121	217 (15) 193–242	296 (17) 272–329	396 (13) 382–416	110 (12) 94–135	207 (17) 186–241	297 (17) 276–336	388 (13) 364–422
Sex [males; females]	10; 7	5; 7	3; 5	2; 4	7; 6	8; 10	10; 11	11; 10
MSEL ELCS	n/a	91 (8) 79–110	n/a	105 (24) 81–138	n/a	93 (9) 74–113	n/a	103 (12) 77–116
Blocks completed	27 (3) 17–28	26 (4) 15–28	27 (2) 24–28	27 (2) 23–28	27 (3) 19–28	28 (2) 19–28	27 (2) 22–28	27 (3) 18–28
HC	0.38 (0.80) −0.9–1.8	0.78 (0.69) 0–2.3	1.0 (0.85) −0.1–2.7	1.1 (1.0) −0.5–2.3	0.58 (1.3) −1.2–3.2	0.99 (1.3) −0.6–3.4	0.99 (1.3) −1.8–3.4	0.84 (1.2) −1.3–3.2

Mean (SD); Range. Early Learning Composite Score (ELCS); Head circumference z-score (HC).

Table 2 | Attrition rates for entire sample of infants.

	HRA				LRC				Total
	3 months	**6 months**	**9 months**	**12 months**	**3 months**	**6 months**	**9 months**	**12 months**	
Included	17 (94%)	12 (67%)	8 (62%)	6 (43%)	13 (100%)	18 (78%)	21 (78%)	21 (68%)	116 (74%)
Excluded: refused cap; fussed-out	0 (0%)	0 (0%)	1 (8%)	0 (0%)	0 (0%)	0 (0%)	1 (4%)	1 (3%)	3 (2%)
Excluded: <14 blocks administered	1 (6%)	4 (22%)	2 (15%)	5 (36%)	0 (0%)	1 (4%)	1 (4%)	2 (6%)	16 (10%)
Excluded: no usable channels in ROI	0 (0%)	2 (11%)	2 (15%)	3 (21%)	0 (0%)	4 (17%)	4 (15%)	7 (23%)	22 (14%)

with a random inter-trial interval of 500–1500 ms. Each block lasted ~16 s and was separated by a silent pause of varying duration (15 s minimum). In general, the examiner initiated subsequent blocks after the 15 s silent pause that followed each block; however, in instances in which the infant became upset the experimenter would initiate the subsequent block only after the infant was no longer fussy. Up to 28 blocks were presented in one of two semi-randomized sequences.

PROCEDURE

Data were acquired in a dimly lit electrically- and acoustically-shielded room. Infants were seated on their caregivers' lap. During the visit, infants completed three tasks in the following order: (1) a NIRS experiment examining facial identity and emotion processing, (2) an upright-inverted face eye-tracking paradigm, and (3) the task reported here, a NIRS language processing paradigm. For this task, each block was initiated by an examiner who monitored the infant's movement. Blocks were presented until a total of 28 were completed or until the infant no longer tolerated the task. Infants were also presented with a continuous video of different moving shapes. If infants became uninterested in the video or upset, an experimenter used silent toys and bubbles in an attempt to keep the infant calm and still. Infants who became fussy were permitted to nurse, feed from a bottle, or to eat in order to expose them to as many blocks as possible. While these techniques have the potential to introduce motion artifacts, prior electrophysiological studies (a methodology more susceptible to motion artifacts than NIRS) have demonstrated sufficient amounts of artifact-free data can be acquired under similar circumstances. A subset of infants fell asleep during the course of the experiment; in these cases, the experiment proceeded as described above as most infant fcNIRS studies have been completed during natural sleep. Given the nature of the study visit (which required awake infants to attend to visual stimuli prior to the current experiment) and infant experimental research in general, infant state varied across the task (i.e., including awake and attending to visual information, eating or nursing, and/or asleep). Because connectivity measures are dependent on levels of wakefulness and arousal (e.g., awake vs. asleep; see Heine et al., 2012, for review) as well as task-related activation (e.g., Arfanakis et al., 2000), we examined whether groups differed with respect to the frequency of attentive, feeding, and sleeping states across the task. Based on notes taken from each visit, infant state was coded according to three broadly defined categories: (1) visual attention: infant watched video, bubbles, and/or silent toys, (2) feeding: infant nursed, fed from a bottle, or ate, and (3) sleep: infant fell asleep. Relative to the total number of blocks completed, infants were coded as whether they spent 0%, <50%, or ≥50%

of their time in each state. Distributions of visual attention, feeding, and sleeping between groups were compared at each age using chi-squared tests (see **Figure 1**). Groups only differed significantly in the distribution of sleep at 3-months, $X^2(2, n = 30) = 6.3$, $p < 0.05$, with a greater percentage of HRA infants sleeping relative to LRC infants. Furthermore, to confirm that variability of NIRS signal did not differ between groups, the root mean square (RMS) of the average ROI time courses was calculated (Larson-Prior et al., 2009). RMS did not differ between groups for any ROI at any time point with the exception of the left anterior ROI at 6-months, $t_{(28)} = 2.1$, $p < 0.05$, where the LRC group had significantly larger RMS compared to the HRA group.

NEAR-INFRARED SPECTROSCOPY (NIRS)

Acquisition and processing

A 24-channel Hitachi ETG-4000 NIRS system was used to measure levels of oxy- and deoxy-hemoglobin (oxy-Hb and deoxy-Hb). Two wavelengths of light (695 and 830 nm) were used to detect hemodynamic responses with a sampling rate of 10 Hz. The NIRS probes were arranged in two 3 × 3 chevron arrays, each with five incident and four detecting fibers with 3 cm spacing. Each pair of emitting-detecting fibers defines a single channel. Probes were attached to a soft hat designed for infants (see **Figure 2**). NIRS probe sets were upgraded over the course of our longitudinal study. There was no significant difference between groups for the number of data sets collected with each probe set at 3-, 9-, or 12-months ($p > 0.4$); at 6-months, groups did differ on the distribution of data collected with old (HRA $n = 9$; LRC $n = 22$) vs. new (HRA $n = 5$; LRC $n = 0$) probes ($p < 0.05$). However, at the ages at which significant group differences emerged (i.e., 3- and 12-months), there were no significant main effects of probe type (new, old) or interactions between probe and group ($p > 0.3$) for overall mean connectivity.

Analyses were conducted on NIRS data that were acquired continuously 5 s prior to the onset of the first block until 10 s after the end of the final block. Average time series duration was approximately 15 min and did not differ between HRA and LRC groups at any age ($ps > 0.3$). Based on light intensity detection through each channel, relative concentrations of oxy-Hb and deoxy-Hb were calculated for the absorbance

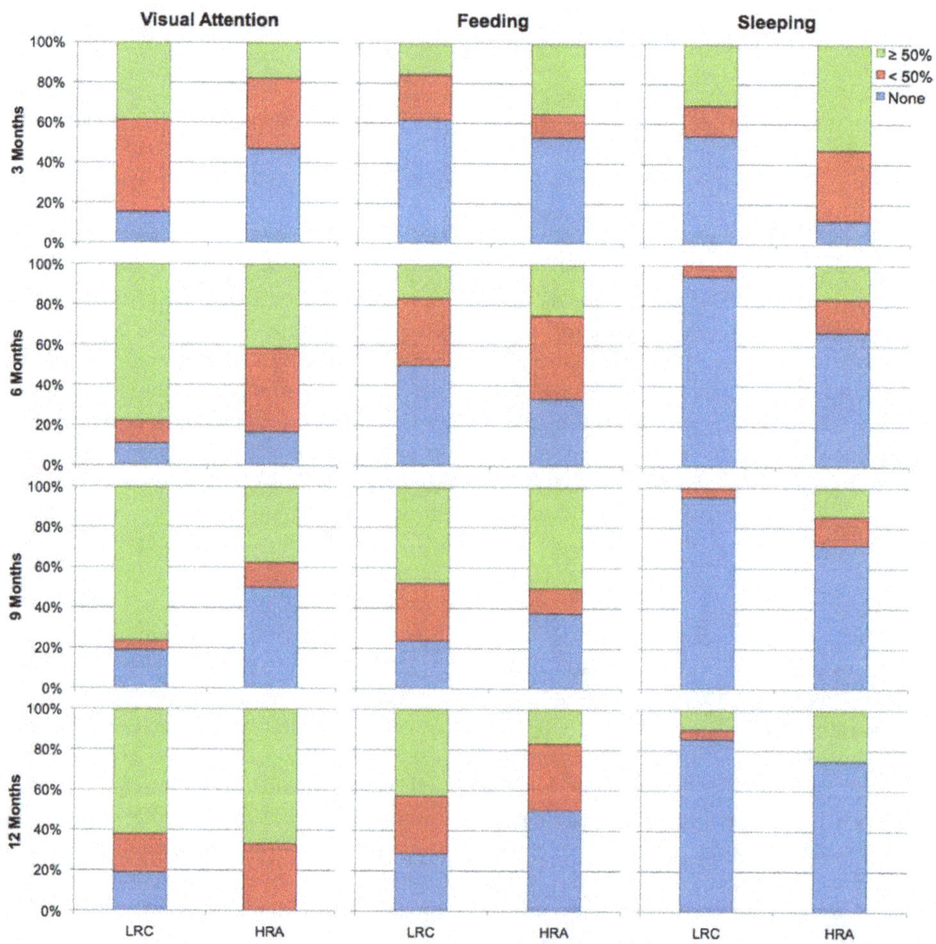

FIGURE 1 | Coded behavioral data for time spent attending to visual stimuli, feeding, and sleeping for LRC and HRA groups at 3-, 6-, 9-, and 12-months.

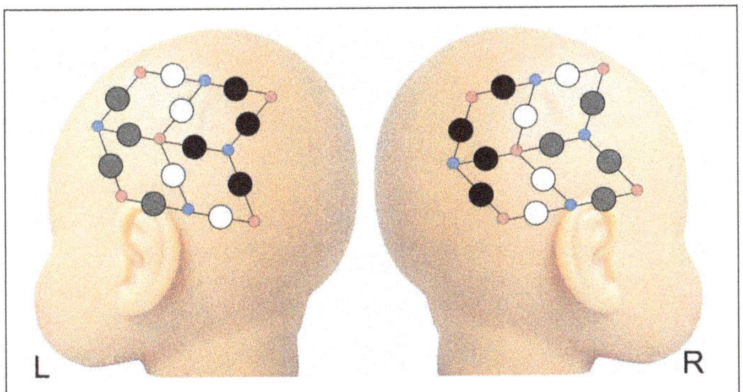

FIGURE 2 | Four regions of interest (ROI) selected from anterior and posterior recording sites on each hemisphere. Gray circles represent channels included in anterior ROIs; black circles are channels included in posterior ROIs. Probes not included in ROIs are depicted in white. Smaller red and blue circles represent infrared emitters and detectors, respectively.

of each wavelength using the modified Beer-Lambert law. Data were then band-pass filtered ($0.008 < f < 0.08$) and the linear trend was removed. Next, given the impact of head motion on functional connectivity measured using fcMRI (Power et al., 2012; Van Dijk et al., 2012), a series of quality control procedures were conducted to insure that only artifact-free data were included in the functional connectivity analysis. First, individual time points were censored if the raw signal exceeded 4.95 (indicating saturation signals) or if total-Hb change exceeded 0.3 mM*mm within a two sample time window. Next, for each channel, the RMS of the first temporal derivative was calculated for the oxy-Hb signal; channels were excluded if the RMS exceeded a threshold of 0.25 or if more than 50% of time points exceeded saturation threshold.

Functional connectivity analysis

Similar to previous studies investigating functional connectivity in infants using NIRS (Homae et al., 2010, 2011), we chose to focus on oxy-Hb, as the oxy-Hb signal has a higher signal-to-noise ratio than deoxy-Hb (Tong and Frederick, 2010) and overlaps to a greater degree with functional networks defined by the fMRI BOLD signal (Duan et al., 2012). Four regions of interest (ROI) were selected from anterior and posterior locations for each hemisphere (LA, left anterior; LP, left posterior; RA, right anterior; RP, right posterior) (see **Figure 2**). The average time course for each ROI was calculated from signals from usable channels within each ROI. Because findings of over- and under-connectivity in ASD-related studies may be associated with specific methodological choices (Muller et al., 2011), we chose to examine the data using two separate pipelines–with and without task regression. For the task-regression pipeline (referred to below as intrinsic connectivity), task-related signal fluctuations were removed in order to examine intrinsic cortical connectivity. Task regressors for both ABB and ABC conditions were included in a general linear model to remove hemodynamic responses associated with auditory stimuli. Next, correlations between the residual time courses for each ROI pair (for all 6 ROI pairs) were computed. For the non-task-regressed pipeline (referred to below as co-activation connectivity), task related activation was not removed. Instead, correlations between mean time courses for each ROI pair were computed. For both pipelines, ROI pair correlations were transformed using Fisher's r to z' transformation. Next, mean z' scores were created for all (all 6 ROI pairs), inter-hemispheric (LA-RA, LA-RP, LP-RA, LP-RP; which includes both homo- and hetero-topic connections), and intra-hemispheric (LA-LP, RA-RP) ROI pairs. Finally, differences in functional connectivity were examined in a cross-sectional manner at 3-, 6-, 9-, and 12-months. Z-transformed data were entered into a series of independent-samples t-tests to assess between-group differences in connectivity at each time point. A secondary bootstrap analysis (10,000 iterations) was used to confirm t-test results. Shapiro–Wilk test of normality confirmed the data for each group met the normality assumption for tests that showed between-group differences. All statistical analyses were performed using SPSS, version 18.0.0.

RESULTS

Intrinsic and co-activation connectivity z-scores for all ROI pairs for both HRA and LRC groups at 3-, 6-, 9-, and 12-months are shown in **Figure 3**. At 3-months, differences between HRA and LRC infants for intrinsic connectivity were present only for the LA-RP ROI pair, $t_{(28)} = -2.3$, $p < 0.05$. More robust group differences emerged for co-activation connectivity as HRA infants showed marginally increased overall functional connectivity, $t_{(28)} = -2.0$, $p = 0.054$. This was mainly due to increased connectivity for intra-hemispheric ROI pairs, $t_{(28)} = -2.3$, $p < 0.05$. Analysis of individual ROI pairs revealed significantly increased connectivity between LA-RP, $t_{(28)} = -2.5$, $p < 0.05$, and marginally increased connectivity between LA-LP, $t_{(28)} = -1.8$, $p < 0.1$, in HRA as compared to LRC infants. Results for both intrinsic and co-activation t-tests at 3-months were confirmed by a bootstrap analysis (10,000 iterations).

There were no significant differences between any average z' score or individual ROI pair for either intrinsic or co-activation analysis at 6- or 9-months (all $p > 0.4$). However, by 12-months, LRC infants showed increased intrinsic connectivity relative to HRA infants. Specifically, LRC infants had increased intra-hemispheric connectivity relative to HRA infants, $t_{(20.7)} = 2.3$, $p < 0.05$, which was primarily due to significantly increased connectivity of the LA-LP ROI pair, $t_{(25)} = 2.7$, $p < 0.05$. Increases in global connectivity did not reach significance; however, as can be seen in **Figure 4**, differences in connectivity across the first year of life shift from marginally increased connectivity for HRA infants at 3-months to increased connectivity for LRC infants by 12-months. Findings for co-activation connectivity were identical to intrinsic connectivity results; relative to the LRC group, the HRA group showed decreased connectivity for intra-hemispheric connections, $t_{(22.2)} = 2.5$, $p < 0.05$, which was driven by significantly decreased LA-LP connectivity, $t_{(25)} = 2.7$, $p < 0.05$. Results for both intrinsic and co-activation t-tests at 12-months were confirmed by a bootstrap analysis (10,000 iterations) with the exception of mean intra-hemispheric connectivity, which was marginally increased in LRC infants for co-activation analysis, $t_{(25)} = 1.6$, $p < 0.1$,

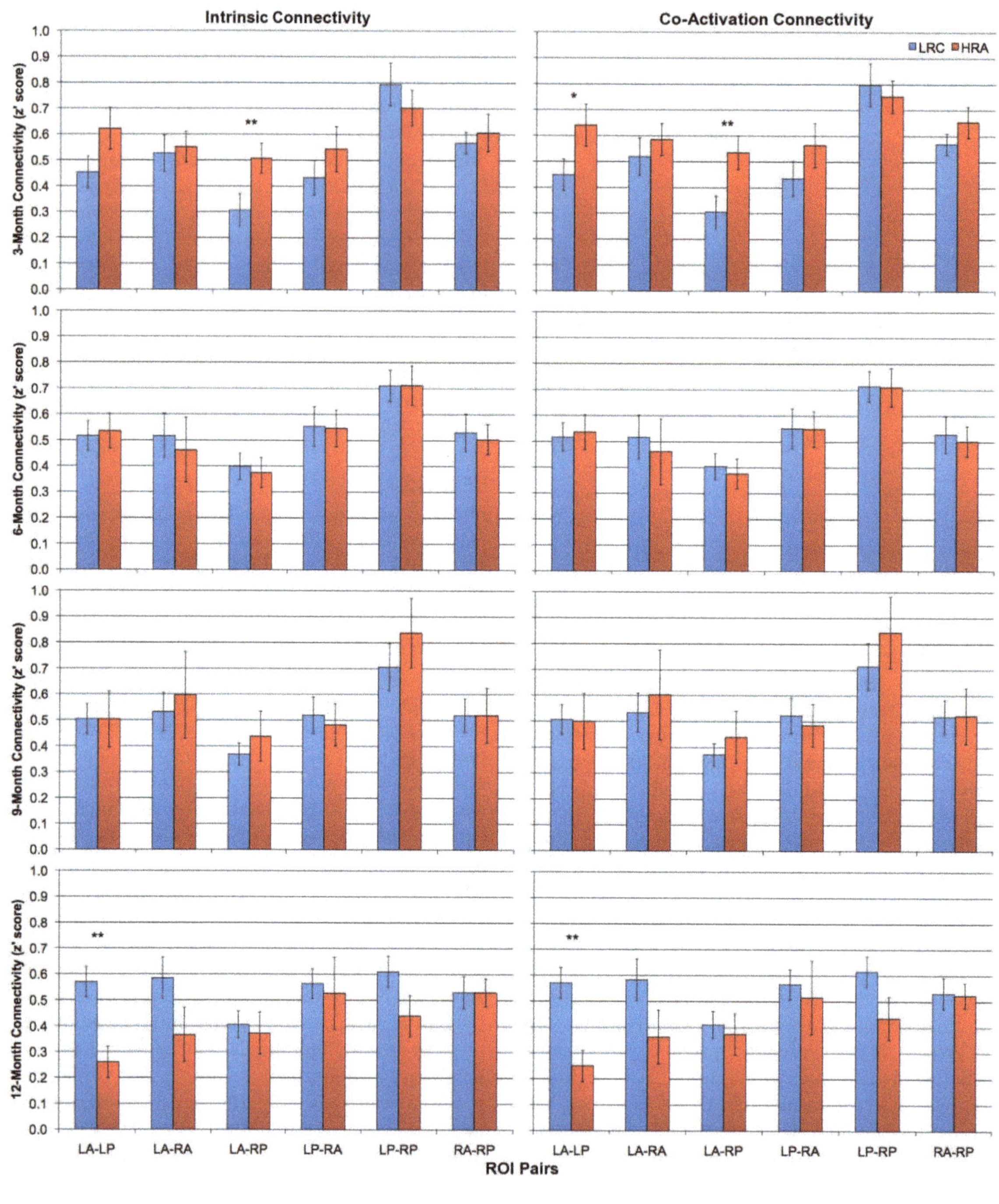

FIGURE 3 | Intrinsic (left column) and co-activation (right column) connectivity for HRA and LRC groups at 3-, 6-, 9-, and 12-months for all six ROI pairs. Error bars represent one standard error of the mean. *$p < 0.1$, **$p < 0.05$.

and no longer significant for intrinsic analysis, $t_{(25)} = 1.5$, $p > 0.1$.

DISCUSSION

The current study is the first to use NIRS to examine functional connectivity in infants at-risk for developing ASD. Our preliminary findings suggest that divergent patterns of functional connectivity emerge across the first year of life. Whereas LRC infants showed a pattern of increasing functional connectivity from 3- to 12-months, HRA infants exhibited a pattern of *decreasing* connectivity. These contrasting patterns resulted in increased connectivity at 3-months in HRA compared to LRC infants and, by 12-months, decreased connectivity in HRA compared to LRC infants.

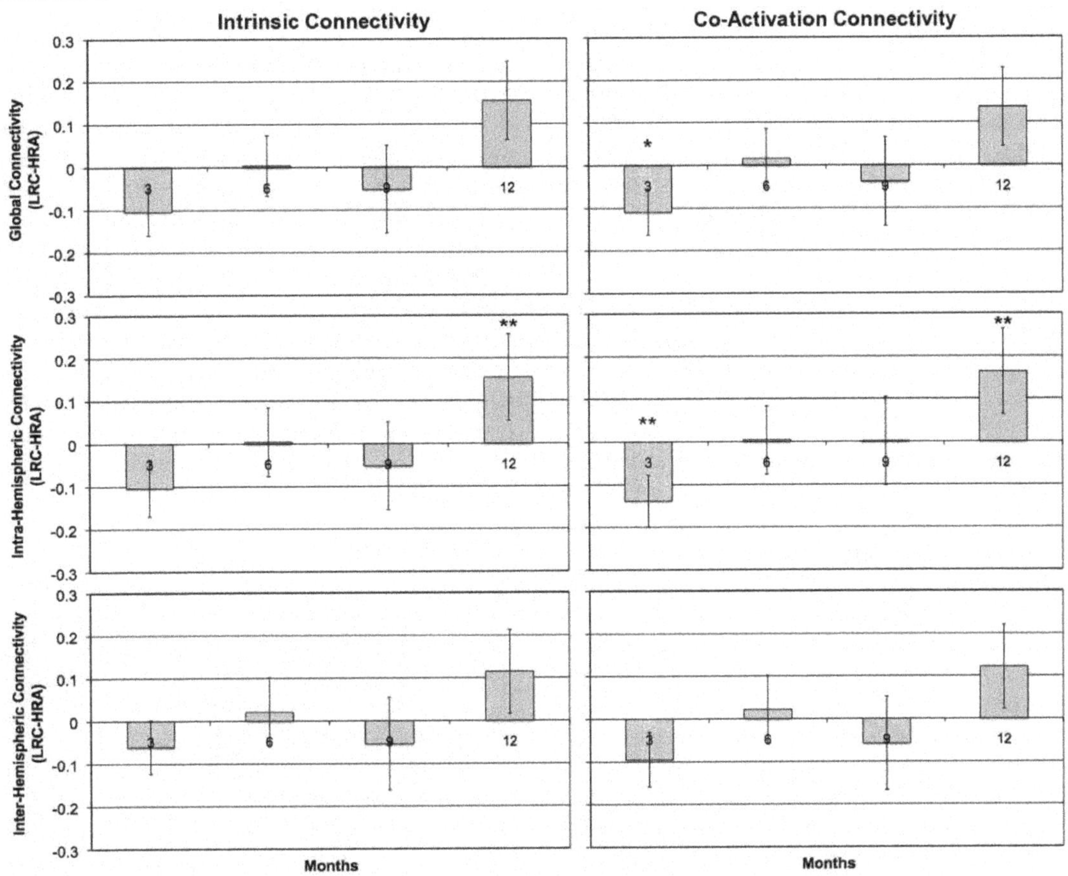

FIGURE 4 | Group differences in mean *z*′-scores for global connectivity and intra- and inter-hemispheric connectivity measures at 3-, 6-, 9-, and 12-months for task-regressed, intrinsic functional (left column) and co-activation (right column) connectivity pipelines. Positive scores reflect LRC > HRA; negative scores reflect HRA > LRC for connectivity measures. Error bars represent one standard error of the mean. *$p < 0.1$, **$p < 0.05$.

Differences in functional connectivity at 3-months suggest that prenatal or early postnatal differences in brain connectivity exist in infants at-risk for ASD. A comparison to the findings of Wolff et al. (2012), which previously reported early connectivity differences in at-risk infants, is difficult because the study did not include a neurotypical comparison group. However, findings from other DTI studies suggest elevated indices of white matter connectivity and, perhaps, accelerated white matter growth (Ben Bashat et al., 2007; Weinstein et al., 2011), which is followed by reduced FA in school-aged children, adolescents, and adults with ASD (Travers et al., 2012). Our findings of increased functional connectivity at 3-months is in agreement with the idea that, early in development, individuals with (or at-risk for) ASD may potentially have diffusely increased connectivity.

However, similar to Dinstein et al. (2011) fcMRI study of toddlers with ASD, our preliminary 12-month results show reduced connectivity of both anterior and posterior inter-hemispheric connections (albeit not significantly so). Further, our results show that, at 12-months, HRA infants have reduced intra-hemispheric connectivity (both co-activation and intrinsic) for the left hemisphere compared to LRC infants. These results, in conjunction with weaker inter-hemisphere connectivity of inferior frontal and superior temporal gyri reported by Dinstein et al. (2011), suggest that early atypical development of the language-processing network may exist in infants and toddlers at risk for or diagnosed with ASD. Although we are currently unable to determine whether differences in connectivity at 3- and 12-months were driven by infants that will later go on to meet diagnostic criteria for ASD, the results add to a growing body of evidence suggesting that atypical connectivity may be an potential endophenotype for ASD (e.g., Barnea-Goraly et al., 2010).

Previous functional connectivity studies in neurotypical adults have shown state (e.g., awake vs. asleep) may alter degree of network connectivity (see Heine et al., 2012, for review). Although state-dependent deviations in connectivity may be network-specific and vary according to level of wakefulness [e.g., descent to sleep (Larson-Prior et al., 2009) vs. deep sleep (Horovitz et al., 2009)], reduced levels of awareness are generally associated with decreased levels of connectivity. In the current study, NIRS data were acquired during different levels of wakefulness and arousal. Differences in the distribution of visual attention, feeding, and sleeping were similar for HRA and LRC infants except at

3-months where a larger proportion of at-risk infants slept during the task compared to the LRC infants. Assuming similar properties of connectivity dynamics exist in the infant brain (which remains undetermined as no study to date has examined differences in functional connectivity in sleep-wake states in infants), we would assume that high-risk infants would show reduced connectivity relative to LRC infants based on state alone. However, our results show that infants at-risk have increased connectivity relative to low-risk infants despite spending a larger portion of the assessment sleeping.

Although infants at risk for ASD have been shown to have similar brain volume measurements at 6-months compared to LRC infants (Hazlett et al., 2012; Shen et al., 2013), ASD is associated with accelerated brain growth over the first years of life (Redcay and Courchesne, 2005; Shen et al., 2013). Lewis and Elman (2008) hypothesized that early overgrowth results in atypical patterns of connectivity, specifically reduced long-distance connectivity, and demonstrated that developmental differences in connectivity emerged at between 12 and 24 simulated months using a neural network model. Further, Lewis et al. (2009) have shown that larger brains are associated with reduced long distance connectivity (potentially due to increased conduction delays and cellular costs associated with long-distance connections), and that corpus callosum size in individuals with ASD is inversely related to intracranial volume (i.e., larger brain, smaller corpus callosum) (Lewis et al., 2012). Although the current study did not find any between-group differences in head circumference, future studies may wish to examine the relations between trajectories of brain size or head circumference and the emergence of group differences in patterns of anatomical and functional connectivity.

Lastly, the current study employed task-regressed, intrinsic and non-task-regressed, co-activation analyses as task regression in fcMRI studies may result in different patterns of over- and under-connectivity in ASD (Jones et al., 2010; Muller et al., 2011). Although general patterns of over- and under-connectivity were consistent for both methods across 3-, 6-, 9-, and 12-month time points, group differences (specifically, increased connectivity in the HRA group) were more robust for co-activation analyses at 3-month of age.

LIMITATIONS

There are several limitations to the current study. First, our sample sizes, especially for the 9- and 12-month time points, are small and therefore the current results should be viewed as preliminary and interpreted with caution. Furthermore, small sample sizes restricted current analyses to a cross-sectional examination of the data. Future studies with larger sample sizes will employ longitudinal statistical analyses to examine developmental trajectories of functional connectivity across the first year of life. Second, measurement of oxy- and deoxy-Hb responses requires transmission of light through scalp, skull, cerebral spinal fluid, and meninges; however, scalp-brain distance increases across development and is significantly shorter in the left compared to right hemisphere (Beauchamp et al., 2011). Additionally, the presence of hair (which increases throughout development) can result in the attenuation of light and result in unreliable measurements. It is unclear how these developmental changes differentially impact low- and high-risk infants (although see Shen et al., 2013, for example of differences in cerebral spinal fluid); nevertheless, future studies may wish to address these potentially confounding issues. Third, although levels of wakefulness and arousal varied within each infant's visit, the distribution of infant state rarely varied across group. Nevertheless, the current results should be interpreted with caution as subtle variations in infant state could have potentially impacted our group comparisons. Additionally, while we took steps to remove time points and channels corrupted by movement artifacts, head motion was not measured in the current study and therefore we are unable to determine whether group differences in motion artifacts were present. Lastly, ROIs in the current study included large areas of lateral frontal and posterior cortex and are therefore unlikely to sample homogeneous cortical areas. As a result, our current measure has limited spatial resolution, which is likely to introduce variability within our connectivity measures.

CONCLUSIONS

Distributed functional brain networks arise from the complex interaction of genes, environmental factors, and experience-dependent processes. Our findings suggest that, in infants with a family history of ASD, there are early differences in brain connectivity and an atypical developmental trajectory of functional connectivity compared to LRC infants. Because the majority of our current sample of infants have yet to reach 36 months of age, we do not have data regarding diagnostic outcome. Therefore, our current analysis has only examined whether *risk* for autism is associated with differences in connectivity (i.e., an endophenotype), rather than whether infants that are later diagnosed with ASD exhibit unique patterns of connectivity in the first year of life. In conjunction with previous findings (e.g., Barnea-Goraly et al., 2010), the current results suggest that atypical network connectivity may represent a putative endophenotype in ASD. Although our findings are in accord with other functional and structural connectivity studies of high-risk infants and toddlers with ASD (Dinstein et al., 2011; Wolff et al., 2012), our results should be interpreted with caution given the small sample sizes. Ongoing data collection will provide a larger sample for more sophisticated longitudinal analyses, as well as the ability to examine whether differences in connectivity exist between high-risk infants that do and do not go on to develop ASD.

ACKNOWLEDGMENTS

We are extremely grateful to the families for their invaluable contribution to the Infant Sibling Project. We would also like to acknowledge the Infant Sibling Project staff—Tara Augenstein, Leah Casner, Kristin Concannon, Kerri Downing, Sharon Fox, Nina Leezenbaum, Vanessa Loukas, Rhiannon Luyster, Stephanie Marshall, Anne Seery, Meagan Thompson, Vanessa Vogel-Farley, and Anne-Marie Zuluaga—for their assistance in data acquisition. Supported by NIH R01-DC010290 to Helen Tager-Flusberg and Charles A. Nelson and The Simons Foundation (137186) to Charles A. Nelson. Jennifer B. Wagner was supported by a NARSAD Young Investigator Abrams Award (17708). Brandon Keehn was supported by an Autism Speaks Translational Postdoctoral Fellowship (7629).

REFERENCES

Arfanakis, K., Cordes, D., Haughton, V. M., Moritz, C. H., Quigley, M. A., and Meyerand, M. E. (2000). Combining independent component analysis and correlation analysis to probe interregional connectivity in fMRI task activation datasets. *Magn. Reson. Imaging* 18, 921–930. doi: 10.1016/S0730-725X(00)00190-9

Barnea-Goraly, N., Lotspeich, L. J., and Reiss, A. L. (2010). Similar white matter aberrations in children with autism and their unaffected siblings: a diffusion tensor imaging study using tract-based spatial statistics. *Arch. Gen. Psychiatry* 67, 1052–1060. doi: 10.1001/archgenpsychiatry.2010.123

Beauchamp, M. S., Beurlot, M. R., Fava, E., Nath, A. R., Parikh, N. A., Saad, Z. S., et al. (2011). The developmental trajectory of brain-scalp distance from birth through childhood: implications for functional neuroimaging. *PLoS ONE* 6: e24981. doi: 10.1371/journal.pone.0024981

Belmonte, M. K., Allen, G., Beckel-Mitchener, A., Boulanger, L. M., Carper, R. A., and Webb, S. J. (2004). Autism and abnormal development of brain connectivity. *J. Neurosci.* 24, 9228–9231. doi: 10.1523/JNEUROSCI.3340-04.2004

Ben Bashat, D., Kronfeld-Duenias, V., Zachor, D. A., Ekstein, P. M., Hendler, T., Tarrasch, R., et al. (2007). Accelerated maturation of white matter in young children with autism: a high b value DWI study. *Neuroimage* 37, 40–47. doi: 10.1016/j.neuroimage.2007.04.060

Dinstein, I., Pierce, K., Eyler, L., Solso, S., Malach, R., Behrmann, M., et al. (2011). Disrupted neural synchronization in toddlers with autism. *Neuron* 70, 1218–1225. doi: 10.1016/j.neuron.2011.04.018

Duan, L., Zhang, Y. J., and Zhu, C. Z. (2012). Quantitative comparison of resting-state functional connectivity derived from fNIRS and fMRI: a simultaneous recording study. *Neuroimage* 60, 2008–2018. doi: 10.1016/j.neuroimage.2012.02.014

Gervain, J., Macagno, F., Cogoi, S., Pena, M., and Mehler, J. (2008). The neonate brain detects speech structure. *Proc. Natl. Acad. Sci. U.S.A.* 105, 14222–14227. doi: 10.1073/pnas.0806530105

Gervain, J., Mehler, J., Werker, J. F., Nelson, C. A., Csibra, G., Lloyd-Fox, S., et al. (2011). Near-infrared spectroscopy: a report from the McDonnell infant methodology consortium. *Dev. Cogn. Neurosci* 1, 22–46. doi: 10.1016/j.dcn.2010.07.004

Geschwind, D. H., and Levitt, P. (2007). Autism spectrum disorders: developmental disconnection syndromes. *Curr. Opin. Neurobiol.* 17, 103–111. doi: 10.1016/j.conb.2007.01.009

Gottesman, I. I., and Gould, T. D. (2003). The endophenotype concept in psychiatry: etymology and strategic intentions. *Am. J. Psychiatry* 160, 636–645. doi: 10.1176/appi.ajp.160.4.636

Hazlett, H. C., Gu, H., McKinstry, R. C., Shaw, D. W., Botteron, K. N., Dager, S. R., et al. (2012). Brain volume findings in 6-month-old infants at high familial risk for autism. *Am. J. Psychiatry* 169, 601–608. doi: 10.1176/appi.ajp.2012.11091425

Heine, L., Soddu, A., Gomez, F., Vanhaudenhuyse, A., Tshibanda, L., Thonnard, M., et al. (2012). Resting state networks and consciousness: alterations of multiple resting state network connectivity in physiological, pharmacological, and pathological consciousness States. *Front. Psychol.* 3:295. doi: 10.3389/fpsyg.2012.00295

Homae, F., Watanabe, H., Nakano, T., and Taga, G. (2011). Large-scale brain networks underlying language acquisition in early infancy. *Front. Psychol.* 2:93. doi: 10.3389/fpsyg.2011.00093

Homae, F., Watanabe, H., Otobe, T., Nakano, T., Go, T., Konishi, Y., et al. (2010). Development of global cortical networks in early infancy. *J. Neurosci.* 30:4877–4882. doi: 10.1523/JNEUROSCI.5618-09.2010

Horovitz, S. G., Braun, A. R., Carr, W. S., Picchioni, D., Balkin, T. J., Fukunaga, M., et al. (2009). Decoupling of the brain's default mode network during deep sleep. *Proc. Natl. Acad. Sci. U.S.A.* 106, 11376–11381. doi: 10.1073/pnas.0901435106

Jones, T. B., Bandettini, P. A., Kenworthy, L., Case, L. K., Milleville, S. C., Martin, A., et al. (2010). Sources of group differences in functional connectivity: an investigation applied to autism spectrum disorder. *Neuroimage* 49, 401–414. doi: 10.1016/j.neuroimage.2009.07.051

Just, M. A., Cherkassky, V. L., Keller, T. A., and Minshew, N. J. (2004). Cortical activation and synchronization during sentence comprehension in high-functioning autism: evidence of underconnectivity. *Brain* 127, 1811–1821. doi: 10.1093/brain/awh199

Just, M. A., Keller, T. A., Malave, V. L., Kana, R. K., and Varma, S. (2012). Autism as a neural systems disorder: a theory of frontal-posterior underconnectivity. *Neurosci. Biobehav. Rev.* 36, 1292–1313. doi: 10.1016/j.neubiorev.2012.02.007

Larson-Prior, L. J., Zempel, J. M., Nolan, T. S., Prior, F. W., Snyder, A. Z., and Raichle, M. E. (2009). Cortical network functional connectivity in the descent to sleep. *Proc. Natl. Acad. Sci. U.S.A.* 106, 4489–4494. doi: 10.1073/pnas.0900924106

Lewis, J. D., and Elman, J. L. (2008). Growth-related neural reorganization and the autism phenotype: a test of the hypothesis that altered brain growth leads to altered connectivity. *Dev. Sci.* 11, 135–155. doi: 10.1111/j.1467-7687.2007.00634.x

Lewis, J. D., Theilmann, R. J., Fonov, V., Bellec, P., Lincoln, A., Evans, A. C., et al. (2012). Callosal fiber length and interhemispheric connectivity in adults with autism: brain overgrowth and underconnectivity. *Hum. Brain Mapp.* 34, 1685–1695. doi: 10.1002/hbm.22018

Lewis, J. D., Theilmann, R. J., Sereno, M. I., and Townsend, J. (2009). The relation between connection length and degree of connectivity in young adults: a DTI analysis. *Cereb. Cortex* 19, 554–562. doi: 10.1093/cercor/bhn105

Lloyd-Fox, S., Blasi, A., and Elwell, C. E. (2010). Illuminating the developing brain: the past, present and future of functional near infrared spectroscopy. *Neurosci. Biobehav. Rev.* 34, 269–284. doi: 10.1016/j.neubiorev.2009.07.008

Mesquita, R. C., Franceschini, M. A., and Boas, D. A. (2010). Resting state functional connectivity of the whole head with near-infrared spectroscopy. *Biomed. Opt. Express* 1, 324–336. doi: 10.1364/BOE.1.000324

Mullen, E. M. (1995). *Mullen Scales of Early Learning.* Circle Pines, MN: American Guidance Service, Inc.

Muller, R. A. (2007). The study of autism as a distributed disorder. *Ment. Retard. Dev. Disabil. Res. Rev.* 13, 85–95. doi: 10.1002/mrdd.20141

Muller, R. A., Shih, P., Keehn, B., Deyoe, J. R., Leyden, K. M., and Shukla, D. K. (2011). Underconnected, but how? A survey of functional connectivity MRI studies in autism spectrum disorders. *Cereb. Cortex* 21, 2233–2243. doi: 10.1093/cercor/bhq296

Power, J. D., Barnes, K. A., Snyder, A. Z., Schlaggar, B. L., and Petersen, S. E. (2012). Spurious but systematic correlations in functional connectivity MRI networks arise from subject motion. *Neuroimage* 59, 2142–2154. doi: 10.1016/j.neuroimage.2011.10.018

Redcay, E., and Courchesne, E. (2005). When is the brain enlarged in autism? A meta-analysis of all brain size reports. *Biol. Psychiatry* 58, 1–9. doi: 10.1016/j.biopsych.2005.03.026

Rutter, M., Bailey, A., and Lord, C. (2003). *Social Communication Questionnaire.* Los Angeles, CA: Western Psychological Services.

Sasai, S., Homae, F., Watanabe, H., Sasaki, A. T., Tanabe, H. C., Sadato, N., et al. (2012). A NIRS-fMRI study of resting state network. *Neuroimage* 63, 179–193. doi: 10.1016/j.neuroimage.2012.06.011

Shen, M. D., Nordahl, C. W., Young, G. S., Wootton-Gorges, S. L., Lee, A., Liston, S. E., et al. (2013). Early brain enlargement and elevated extra-axial fluid in infants who develop autism spectrum disorder. *Brain.* doi: 10.1093/brain/awt166. [Epub ahead of print].

Smyser, C. D., Snyder, A. Z., and Neil, J. J. (2011). Functional connectivity MRI in infants: exploration of the functional organization of the developing brain. *Neuroimage* 56, 1437–1452. doi: 10.1016/j.neuroimage.2011.02.073

Tong, Y., and Frederick, B. D. (2010). Time lag dependent multimodal processing of concurrent fMRI and near-infrared spectroscopy (NIRS) data suggests a global circulatory origin for low-frequency oscillation signals in human brain. *Neuroimage* 53, 553–564. doi: 10.1016/j.neuroimage.2010.06.049

Travers, B. G., Adluru, N., Ennis, C., Tromp Do, P. M., Destiche, D., Doran, S., et al. (2012). Diffusion tensor imaging in autism spectrum disorder: a review. *Autism Res.* 5, 289–313. doi: 10.1002/aur.1243

Van Dijk, K. R., Sabuncu, M. R., and Buckner, R. L. (2012). The influence of head motion on intrinsic functional connectivity MRI. *Neuroimage* 59, 431–438. doi: 10.1016/j.neuroimage.2011.07.044

Walker, L., Gozzi, M., Lenroot, R., Thurm, A., Behseta, B., Swedo,

S., et al. (2012). Diffusion tensor imaging in young children with autism: biological effects and potential confounds. *Biol. Psychiatry* 72, 1043–1051. doi: 10.1016/j.biopsych.2012.08.001

Wass, S. (2010). Distortions and disconnections: disrupted brain connectivity in autism. *Brain Cogn.* 75, 18–28. doi: 10.1016/j.bandc.2010.10.005

Weinstein, M., Ben-Sira, L., Levy, Y., Zachor, D. A., Ben Itzhak, E., Artzi, M., et al. (2011). Abnormal white matter integrity in young children with autism. *Hum. Brain Mapp.* 32, 534–543. doi: 10.1002/hbm.21042

White, B. R., Liao, S. M., Ferradal, S. L., Inder, T. E., and Culver, J. P. (2012). Bedside optical imaging of occipital resting-state functional connectivity in neonates. *Neuroimage* 59, 2529–2538. doi: 10.1016/j.neuroimage.2011.08.094

Wolff, J. J., Gu, H., Gerig, G., Elison, J. T., Styner, M., Gouttard, S., et al. (2012). Differences in white matter fiber tract development present from 6 to 24 months in infants with autism. *Am. J. Psychiatry* 169, 589–600.

Zhang, Y. J., Lu, C. M., Biswal, B. B., Zang, Y. F., Peng, D. L., and Zhu, C. Z. (2010). Detecting resting-state functional connectivity in the language system using functional near-infrared spectroscopy. *J. Biomed. Opt.* 15, 047003. doi: 10.1117/1.3462973

13

Atypical modulation of distant functional connectivity by cognitive state in children with Autism Spectrum Disorders

Xiaozhen You[1]*, Megan Norr[1], Eric Murphy[1], Emily S. Kuschner[2], Elgiz Bal[2], William D. Gaillard[2], Lauren Kenworthy[2] and Chandan J. Vaidya[1,2]*

[1] *Department of Psychology, Georgetown University, Washington, DC, USA*
[2] *Children's Research Institute, Children's National Medical Center, Washington DC, USA*

Edited by:
Ralph-Axel Müller, San Diego State University, USA

Reviewed by:
Christopher Monk, University Hospitals Bristol NHS Foundation Trust, UK
Brandon Keehn, Children's Hospital Boston, USA

*Correspondence:
Xiaozhen You and Chandan J. Vaidya, Department of Psychology, Georgetown University, 306 White-Gravenor, Washington, DC 20057, USA
e-mail: xy34@georgetown.edu; cjv2@georgetown.edu

We examined whether modulation of functional connectivity by cognitive state differed between pre-adolescent children with Autism Spectrum Disorders (ASD) and age and IQ-matched control children. Children underwent functional magnetic resonance imaging (fMRI) during two states, a resting state followed by a sustained attention task. A voxel-wise method was used to characterize functional connectivity at two levels, local (within a voxel's 14 mm neighborhood) and distant (outside of the voxel's 14 mm neighborhood to the rest of the brain) and regions exhibiting Group × State interaction were identified for both types of connectivity maps. Distant functional connectivity of regions in the left frontal lobe (dorsolateral [BA 11, 10]; supplementary motor area extending into dorsal anterior cingulate [BA 32/8]; and premotor [BA 6, 8, 9]), right parietal lobe (paracentral lobule [BA 6]; angular gyrus [BA 39/40]), and left posterior middle temporal cortex (BA 19/39) showed a Group × State interaction such that relative to the resting state, connectivity reduced (i.e., became focal) in control children but increased (i.e., became diffuse) in ASD children during the task state. Higher state-related increase in distant connectivity of left frontal and right angular gyrus predicted worse inattention in ASD children. Two graph theory measures (global efficiency and modularity) were also sensitive to Group × State differences, with the magnitude of state-related change predicting inattention in the ASD children. Our results indicate that as ASD children transition from an unconstrained to a sustained attentional state, functional connectivity of frontal and parietal regions with the rest of the brain becomes more widespread in a manner that may be maladaptive as it was associated with attention problems in everyday life.

Keywords: fMRI, intrinsic, spontaneous, task, ASD

INTRODUCTION

Disturbed functional connectivity across distant regions is posited to mediate functional impairment in Autism Spectrum Disorders (ASD). Functional impairment in ASD comprises symptoms of ASD (e.g., difficulty with social interaction and communication, repetitive and restricted behaviors and interests) as well as problems with executive function, the goal-directed regulation of attention, actions and thoughts (Hill, 2004; Kenworthy et al., 2005, 2008). While executive dysfunction is not part of ASD diagnosis, it is associated with symptom presentation (e.g., Lopez et al., 2005; Kenworthy et al., 2009; Yerys et al., 2009a) and decreased independence and poor outcomes in adulthood [see review Hume et al. (2009)]. An emerging theoretical view of ASD is that frontal-posterior temporal synchronization of blood-oxygen level dependent (BOLD) signal is reduced in ASD subjects while they are engaged in social/communicative or executive functions (Just et al., 2012). Such "underconnectivity" has also been observed in spontaneous low-frequency BOLD fluctuations while subjects are not engaged in a directed task, a state of unconstrained cognition that is referred to as "resting" (Cherkassky et al., 2006; Kennedy and Courchesne, 2008; Assaf et al., 2010; Weng et al., 2010; Wiggins et al., 2011; Gotts et al., 2012; Von dem Hagen et al., 2012). In addition to evidence supporting under-connectivity in ASD, greater than normal functional connectivity ("overconnectivity") has also been noted, either across cortical regions or between subcortical and cortical regions, during task-evoked (Noonan et al., 2009; Shih et al., 2011; Lai et al., 2012) as well as resting (Monk et al., 2009; Di Martino et al., 2011) states. Cognitive conditions that yield abnormally weaker or stronger functional connectivity in ASD are currently not well understood (Müller et al., 2011).

Functional connectivity may be atypical in ASD not only with respect to overall strength but also in its modulation by cognitive state. Studies of healthy adults show that the topology of functional network organization is remarkably similar during task-evoked and resting states. Networks delineated from spontaneous BOLD fluctuations while subjects rest (termed intrinsic connectivity networks) conform to activation patterns observed during visual, auditory, sensorimotor, executive, and self/internally-oriented tasks (Smith et al., 2009) and predict individual differences in task-evoked activation and associated performance (Fox et al., 2006; Mennes et al., 2010;

Gordon et al., 2012c). Further, intrinsic connectivity networks are preserved during sleep (Fukunaga et al., 2006) and light anesthesia (Vincent et al., 2007; Greicius et al., 2008), suggesting that they do not depend upon conscious cognition. While their topology is preserved across states, their strength differs in several ways: First, intrinsic connectivity was stronger, within networks and in anticorrelation across networks, during awake than non-conscious states [see review Heine et al. (2012)]. Second, within-subjects' comparison showed that functional connectivity became stronger from resting to a task-evoked state selectively, in regions activated during the task such as auditory (Arfanakis et al., 2000), visual (Arfanakis et al., 2000; Hampson et al., 2004; Nir et al., 2006), or motor (Arfanakis et al., 2000; Jiang et al., 2004). Third, functional connectivity decreased across some networks during task performance relative to a resting state (Fransson, 2006; Gordon et al., 2012b), suggesting that specific networks became more segregated when subjects were in a cognitive state constrained by a task. Fourth, the extent to which functional connectivity changed from resting to task states, particularly across networks, varied across individuals based upon dopamine neurotransmitter function and traits of distractibility and impulsivity (Gordon et al., 2012b). Together, these findings support the notion that functional connectivity is dynamic, and its modulation by cognitive state is associated with individual variability in attentional function. Whether state-related changes in functional connectivity are atypical in ASD and whether they predict attentional function is unknown.

The goal of the present study was to examine whether changes in functional connectivity, from a resting to a sustained attention state differ between ASD and typically developing (control) 9–13 year-old children. We focused on this narrow age range later in childhood in order to minimize developmental differences and maximize chances of acquiring two motion-free back-to-back fMRI runs from each child. We measured the strength of functional connectivity using a voxel-wise method that distinguished local connectivity, defined as within a voxel's 14 mm neighborhood, and distant connectivity, defined as connectivity of a voxel to the rest of the brain, outside of its 14 mm neighborhood. Such a voxel-wise data-driven method allows testing predictions without regard to a priori functional divisions, an approach that distinguishes the present study from past functional connectivity studies of ASD. For distant connectivity, we predicted a Group × State interaction such that control but not ASD children would modulate connectivity in response to the sustained attention state. As adult findings reviewed above showed that connectivity of selective networks became stronger during a task relative to a resting state, we reasoned that in control children, such a change suggestive of focal connectivity networks (i.e., task-relevant connections get stronger while task-irrelevant connections get weaker) ought to be expressed as a net reduction in our estimate of distant connectivity, which considers all voxels in the brain. In contrast, in light of the many underconnectivity findings in ASD during both task-evoked and resting states reviewed above, we expected overall weaker distant connectivity and little change from resting to task states. Further, we also explored whether whole-brain metrics of connectivity using two graph theory measures, global efficiency and modularity, would be sensitive to Group × State interaction. Global efficiency, measured by path length and reflecting network integration, characterizes the average "speed" of information transfer between any pair of nodes (Latora and Marchiori, 2001; Achard and Bullmore, 2007), and was lower in ASD subjects in a resting state magnetoencephalography study (Tsiaras et al., 2011). Modularity, on the other hand, reflects network segregation, through defining how well an entire network is organized into modules of densely interconnected nodes (Newman, 2006), and was higher in ASD subjects in a resting state electroencephalography study (Barttfeld et al., 2011). For regions (and graph theory metrics) showing the predicted interaction, we examined whether the state-related change in functional connectivity was related to attention problems measured by the inattention score of the ADHD Rating Scale (DuPaul et al., 1998). We focused upon attention, rather than hyperactivity/impulsivity or ASD symptoms, as it is most closely related to sustained attention, the task-state examined here. Due to the lack of past work on local connectivity changes by state in healthy or ASD adults or children, we tested for the same Group × State interaction but made no predictions.

METHODS

SUBJECTS

Thirty-one children aged 9–13 years, 15 with a diagnosis of ASD (3 left handed and 12 right handed) and 16 control children (all right handed), matched for age, IQ, and gender (see **Table 1**), participated in the study after complying with consenting guidelines of the Georgetown University and Children's National Medical

Table 1 | Demographic characteristics (Mean and standard deviation in parenthesis).

	ASD	Control
N	15	16
Gender (females) ($\chi^2 = 1.06$, $p = 0.30$)	3	7
Age (in years) ($p = 0.96$)	11.2 (1.4)	11.2 (1.3)
Full scale IQ ($p = 0.26$)	118.7 (11.5)	123.0 (9.2)
Performance IQ ($p = 0.17$)	112.7 (12.9)	118.5 (9.8)
Verbal IQ ($p = 0.44$)	120.4 (11.3)	123.5 (11.0)
ADHD Rating scale inattentive raw score (0–25) ($p < 0.0001$)	13.9 (6.2)	4.1 (3.5)
ADHD Rating scale hyperactive/impulsive raw score (0–25) ($p < 0.001$)	8.6 (5.5)	2.4 (3.0)
ADOS Communication total (1–7)	3.0 (1.8)	–
ADOS Social interaction total (2–13)	7.5 (3.1)	–
ADOS Stereotypical behaviors and restricted interests total (0–5)	1.8 (1.7)	–
ADI-R Total verbal score (7–24)	16.0 (4.8)	–
ADI-R Total social interaction score (11–28)	19.9 (5.5)	–
ADI-R Restrictive interests and repetitive behaviors score (3–7)	4.9 (1.3)	–

center Institutional Review Boards. This sample was retained after applying criteria for head motion, from a total sample of 24 ASD and 26 control children. ASD children were recruited through the Center for ASD at Children's National Medical Center. Control children were recruited from the Washington DC area community through advertisements at public venues and pediatrician offices.

ASD case classification followed diagnosis by a trained and experienced clinician based on the DSM-IV-TR criteria (American Psychiatric Association, 2000) and was confirmed with the Autism Diagnostic Interview—Revised (ADI-R) (Lord et al., 1994) and the Autism Diagnostic Observation Schedule—Generic (ADOS-G) (Lord et al., 2000) following the criteria established by the NICHD/NIDCD Collaborative Programs for Excellence in Autism (Lainhart et al., 2006). These criteria require that the child meet ADI-R cutoff for autism in the social domain and at least one other domain (communication and/or repetitive behaviors and restricted interests), and meet ADOS cutoff (autism or ASD) for the combined social and communication score. One ASD subject met criteria for an ASD diagnosis on the ADI and ADOS, and by clinical diagnosis two years prior to this study, but on re-evaluation showed significant improvement on the ADOS.

Exclusion criteria included: (1) Full-Scale IQ below 80 as measured by the Wechsler Intelligence Scale for Children (WISC-IV) or Wechsler Abbreviated Scale of Intelligence (WASI) (Wechsler, 1999); (2) Other neurological diagnosis(e.g., epilepsy) based on parent report; (3) Psychiatric diagnosis based on Child and Adolescent Symptom Inventory—4R (Lavigne et al., 2009) for control children; and (4) Contraindications for MRI such as metallic implants or pregnancy. We used the WISC-IV General Ability Index (GAI) as a measure of Full Scale IQ. The GAI provides a comparable approximation of overall intellectual ability as represented by the WISC-IV Full-Scale IQ score, yet is less sensitive to the influence of working memory and processing speed (Prifitera et al., 1998; Weiss et al., 1999; Saklofske et al., 2004). For participants with WASI scores, we used the Tellegen and Briggs (1967) formula to convert WASI subtest scores into WISC-IV Index scores. In addition, we collected the ADHD Rating Scale: Home Version from parents (DuPaul et al., 1998). Five children in the ASD group were on stimulants that were withheld for at least 24 h before scanning; in addition one child with ASD was on non-stimulant and anti-anxiety medications that could not be withdrawn. All remaining children were not medicated.

IMAGING PROTOCOL

Echo-planar images were acquired on a Siemens Trio 3T with parameters: 3 mm isotropic resolution (3.0 × 3.0 × 2.5 mm), $TR = 2000$ ms, $TE = 30$ ms, flip angle $= 90°$, FOV $= 192 \times 192$ mm. Each child underwent two functional runs, a resting state run for 5:14 min in which children were asked to rest with eyes open and stay awake, followed by a task run during which children performed a sustained attention task modified from Zink et al. (2003). Children were instructed to focus on the center of the screen and press a button with their right hand for a triangle (target stimuli) among serially presented squares, circles, and rectangles, and to ignore anything else that may come up elsewhere on the screen. Each stimulus was presented for 750 ms within a 2000 ms interstimulus interval. Targets appeared on 25% of the trials and the remaining trials were non-targets, requiring no motor response. Of these non-target trials, 25% were presented with the central stimuli only and on the remaining trials, a distracter, a small flickering shape was flashed in the periphery in one of the four corners of the display. On half of these distracter trials, the flickering shape was an open circle, whereas on the remaining half of the distracter trials, the shape was variable (e.g., star, diamond) and colorful. Therefore, the breakdown of the types of trials was 25% target, 25% non-target without distracter, 25% non-target with familiar distracter, and 25% non-target with novel distracter. The task consisted of 168 total trials presented in an event-related design with appropriate jitter determined by Optseq2 (http://surfer.nmr.mgh.harvard.edu/optseq/) and lasted 5:46 min. Trial types are not pertinent to the present results as they were regressed out from the connectivity analysis, and therefore, the only difference in connectivity between the resting and task runs was driven by the attentional state of the subject, unconstrained in the resting run and sustained in the task run. Structural images were also acquired for each subject, with a high resolution sagittal T1-weighted structural scan using a 3D MPRAGE sequence with a scan time of 8:05 min and the following parameters: $TR = 2530$ ms, $TE = 3.5$ ms, 256 × 256-mm FOV, 176-mm slab with 1-mm-thick slices, and a 7° flip angle. Head motion was minimized by foam cushions padding the space between the subject's head and the headcoil.

IMAGE PREPROCESSING

Images were processed in SPM8 (Wellcome Department of Cognitive Neurology, London, UK) using MATLAB (Version 7.1 Mathworks, Inc., Sherborn, MA) for both rest and task runs. The first four time points were excluded to allow for signal stabilization. Images were corrected for slice timing and translational and rotational motion by realigning to the first image of the session with INRIAlign (Freire et al., 2002). Images were then normalized to the SPM8 EPI template and resliced to 4 mm for computational efficiency, low pass filtered to exclude frequencies higher than 0.08 Hz, followed by spatial smoothing with 4 mm FWHM. Contributions of motion and physiological noise to the time course of each voxel were removed by including the six motion parameters, signal from ventricle and white matter regions of interest with their respective first temporal derivatives, as regressors of no interest (Wise et al., 2004; Birn et al., 2006; Van Dijk et al., 2010). Further, constant offsets and linear trends were also removed. For the task run, an additional regressor of task conditions was included as being of no interest in order to prevent inflation of functional connectivity estimates by activation differences associated with task conditions (e.g., distracter present vs. absent trials; motor response vs. no motor response). If task conditions are not regressed out, even regions with no moment-to-moment correlations would appear functionally connected because subjects were responding to task conditions over the course of trials [see Jones et al. (2010) for discussion of this point]. Thus, this preprocessing step made the resting and task data comparable, differing only in the subjects' cognitive state [following Gordon et al. (2012a,b)]. The observed pattern of results did not change when task conditions were not regressed out (See Supplementary Materials).

To further restrict the effect of motion on functional connectivity estimates, volumes with greater than 0.5 mm framewise displacement (FD) or temporal derivative of timecourses-root mean square variance over voxel (DVARS) greater than.5% of the whole brain mode value were excluded (as recommended by Power et al. (2012). This "scrubbing" procedure retained 120 timepoints (4 min) for each child for further analysis. For retained volumes, mean FD did not differ between control (Rest: $M = 0.158$ mm, $SD = 0.061$ mm; Task: $M = 0.167$ mm, $SD = 0.090$ mm) and ASD (Rest: $M = 0.171$ mm, $SD = 0.071$ mm; Task: $M = 0.151$ mm, $SD = 0.069$ mm) children during rest ($p = 0.58$) or task ($p = 0.57$); further main effect of state ($p = 0.63$) and the group × state interaction was not significant ($p = 0.16$) indicating that head micromovements did not depend on state. Further, the effects of any residual micromovements were removed by including Mean FD as a regressor in the second-level group analysis [following Satterthwaite et al. (2012)].

LOCAL AND DISTANT CONNECTIVITY STRENGTH

Following Sepulcre et al. (2010), the resulting smoothed images were used to map the local and distant functional connectivity. The time course of each voxel within a whole-brain mask excluding the cerebellum was correlated to every other voxel's time course, resulting in an $n \times n$ correlation matrix, where n is the dimension of the whole-brain mask ($n = 33839$). The correlation calculation is based on Pearson correlation coefficients (r) and thresholded at $p = 0.001$ FDR corrected at the individual level, to exclude less reliable pairwise connections [following Buckner et al. (2009)], resulting in a r threshold range of 0.32–0.34 across individuals, after retaining only positive correlations. For each subject, a resting and task functional connectivity map was computed by averaging the r-to-Z Fisher transformed correlation values, for each voxel to voxels inside (for local connectivity map) and outside (for distant connectivity map) of a 14 mm radius. A 14 mm radius was chosen following Sepulcre et al. (2010) as they observed stable estimates of local connectivity for neighborhood radius values greater than 10 mm and no significant effect on distant connectivity estimates for radius more than 10–14 mm. For discussion of the effects of neighborhood threshold, mask, smoothing kernels and r threshold see Buckner et al. (2009) and Sepulcre et al. (2010). We used connectivity degree weighted by strength (taking both the count of how many links connected to one voxel and their connectivity strength into account– see formulae in Supplementary Materials) as our connectivity estimate rather than connectivity degree alone as used by Sepulcre et al. (2010).

In order to identify regions where group differences in connectivity depended on cognitive state, we tested for Group (ASD, Control) X State (rest, task) interaction in second-level analysis. Subject-specific local and distant functional connectivity maps were entered into separate ANOVA models in SPM8 with Group and State as categorical variables and age and Mean FD as covariates of no interest. This analysis was thresholded at $p < 0.05$ corrected for multiple comparisons based on Monte Carlo simulation (Ward, 2000), which established the correction threshold at height $p < 0.001$, $k = 5$ voxels (for voxel size of 64 mm^3). For clusters that survived the threshold, functional connectivity values were extracted using MarsBaR toolbox (Brett et al., 2002) from both resting and task runs and graphed to identify the nature of Group and State differences. Further, in regions showing Group × State interaction, we examined whether the magnitude of state-related functional connectivity change was related to inattention. For this analysis, a difference score was computed by subtracting the functional connectivity values from the Resting and Task runs and these difference scores were correlated with the inattention scores from the ADHD Rating Scale, separately for ASD and control children.

To visualize the change in distant functional connectivity patterns from resting to task states, we conducted a seed-based connectivity analysis using regions showing Group × Task interaction as seeds. For each subject at each state, the average timecourse of each significant seed cluster was extracted using MarsBaR and correlated with the timecourse of all other voxels in the brain; r values were converted to Z using Fisher's transformation. During the correlation calculation, we also regressed out signals of no interest, including timecourses from ventricle, white matter and six motion parameters with their respective first temporal derivatives. Then an averaged group map for each state was generated and visualized (at a range of thresholds 0.1–0.4) on the cortical surface using the population-average, landmark- and surface-based (PALS) surface and plotted using Caret software (Van Essen, 2005). These results are depicted in **Figures 1–4**. This analysis allowed us to see the nature of change in the pattern of distant connectivity across states.

GLOBAL GRAPH THEORY MEASURES

We calculated two measures of network topology on a voxel-level graph, global efficiency and modularity, using the brain connectivity toolbox created by Sporns and colleagues (https://sites.google.com/site/bctnet/measures/list); the images were downsampled to 6 mm voxel size for computational efficiency [see Rubinov and Sporns (2010) and formulae in Supplementary Materials]. These graph measures were calculated by generating the undirected binary whole brain graph (excluding cerebellum as mentioned before), through thresholding the 9736 × 9736 correlation matrix (each 6 mm^3 voxel to every other voxel) with the same FDR-corrected r threshold used for calculating local and distant connectivity. We also examined the effect of lower r thresholds (0.2, 0.1 respectively) on the two graph measures (see Supplementary Materials) to show that our findings were not biased by more stringent r threshold selection. For each subject, global efficiency and modularity were calculated for both the resting and task runs and entered into separate ANOVA models in R (http://cran.r-project.org) with Group and State as categorical variables with age and mean FD as covariates of no interest similar to the local/distant connectivity analysis above. Similarly, we also examined whether the magnitude of state-related change in global efficiency and modularity (Task—Resting difference) correlated with the inattention score of the ADHD Rating Scale, separately in the two groups.

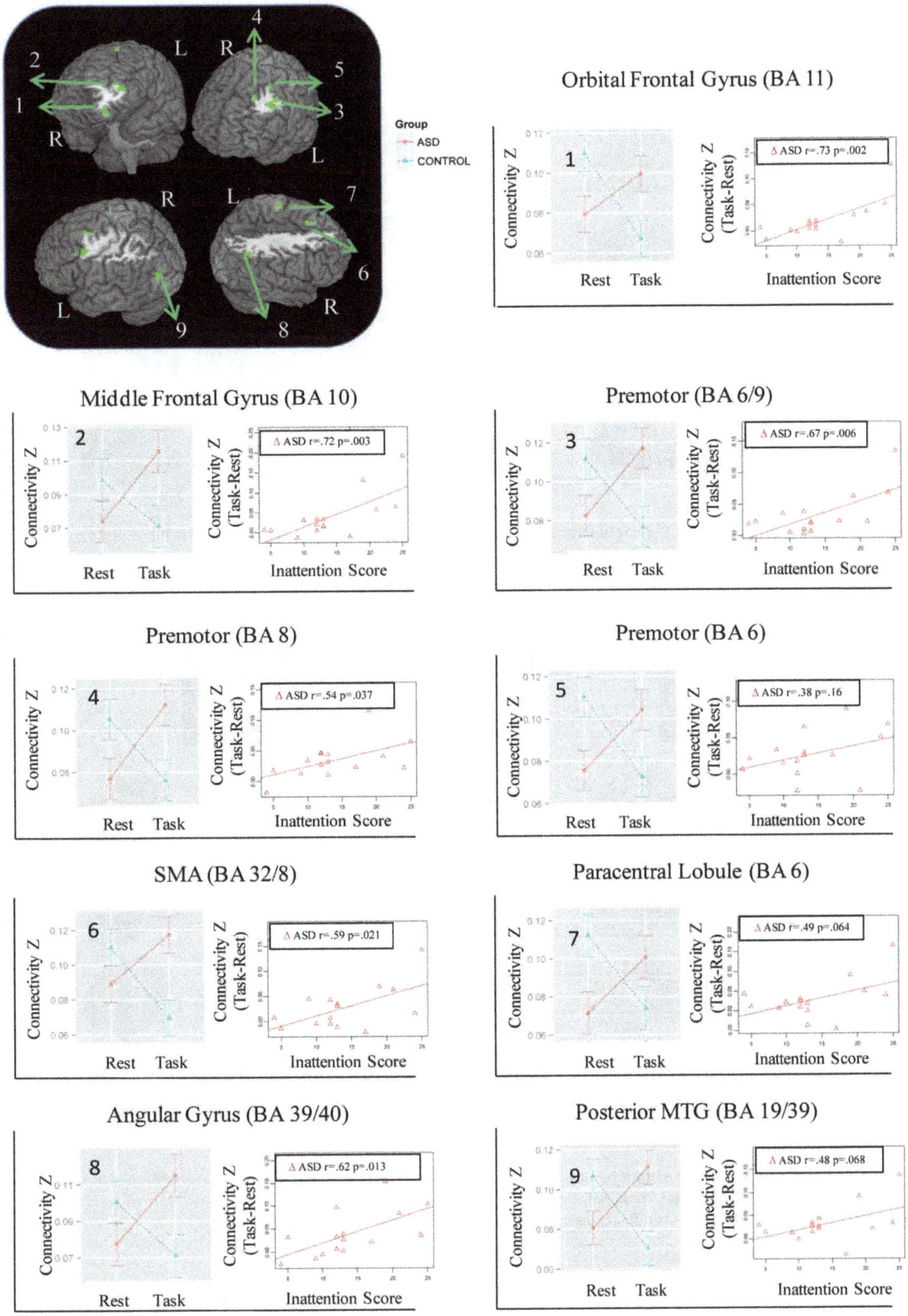

FIGURE 1 | Regions showing Group × State interaction for distant connectivity. Each region is identified with a number on the brain image in the top left corner. The corresponding graphs showing the interaction and correlation with inattention scores in the ASD group are identified with the same number.

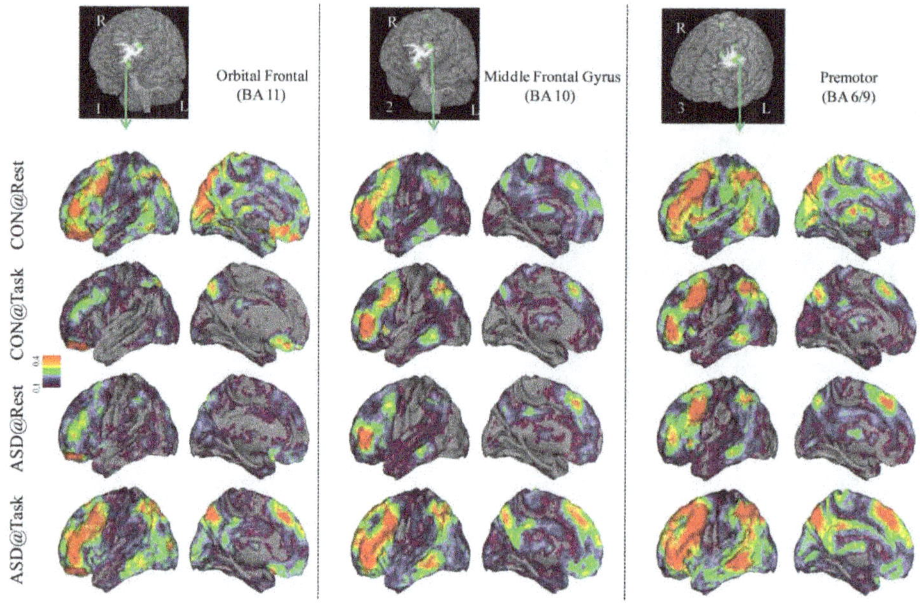

FIGURE 2 | Seed-based connectivity maps of distant functional connectivity patterns in resting and task states, for three clusters showing Group × Task interaction: left orbital frontal gyrus (BA 11) (left panel), left middle frontal gyrus (BA 10) (middle panel) and left premotor (BA 6/9) (right panel). Region numbers 1–3 on the left corner in the brain image correspond to the region number in **Figure 1**.

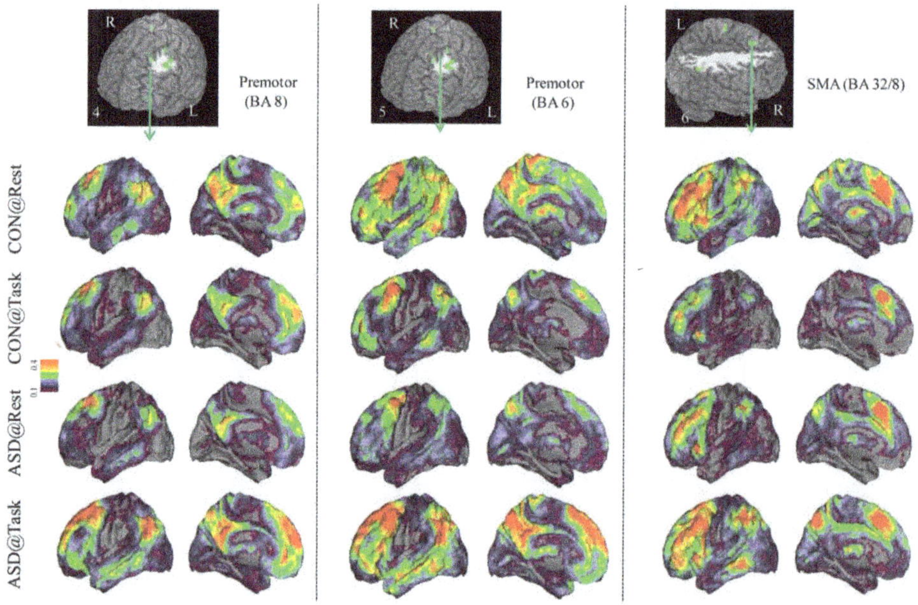

FIGURE 3 | Seed-based connectivity maps of distant functional connectivity patterns in resting and task states, for three clusters showing Group × Task interaction: left premotor (BA 8) (left panel), left premotor (BA 6) (middle panel) and SMA (BA 32/8) (right panel). Region numbers 4–6 on the left corner in the brain image correspond to the region number in **Figure 1**.

RESULTS

BEHAVIOR

For the task run, groups did not differ in target hits [ASD: $M = 96.2\%$, $SD = 8.0\%$; Controls: $M = 100\%$, $SD = 0\%$, $t_{(14)} = 1.9$, $p = 0.08$] and false alarms [ASD: $M = 0.08\%$, $SD = 0.3\%$; Controls: $M = 0.2\%$, $SD = 0.5\%$, $t_{(25.7)} = 1$, $p = 0.33$]. However, target response was slower in ASD than control children [ASD: $M = 602.1$ ms, $SD = 77.6$ ms; Controls: $M = 513.2$ ms, $SD = 70.6$ ms, $t_{(28.3)} = 3.3$, $p = 0.002$]. Mean ADHD Rating scores for Inattention [$t_{(21.7)} = 5.4$, $p < 0.0001$] and Hyperactivity-impulsivity [$t_{(21.4)} = 3.9$, $p < 0.001$] were higher in ASD than control

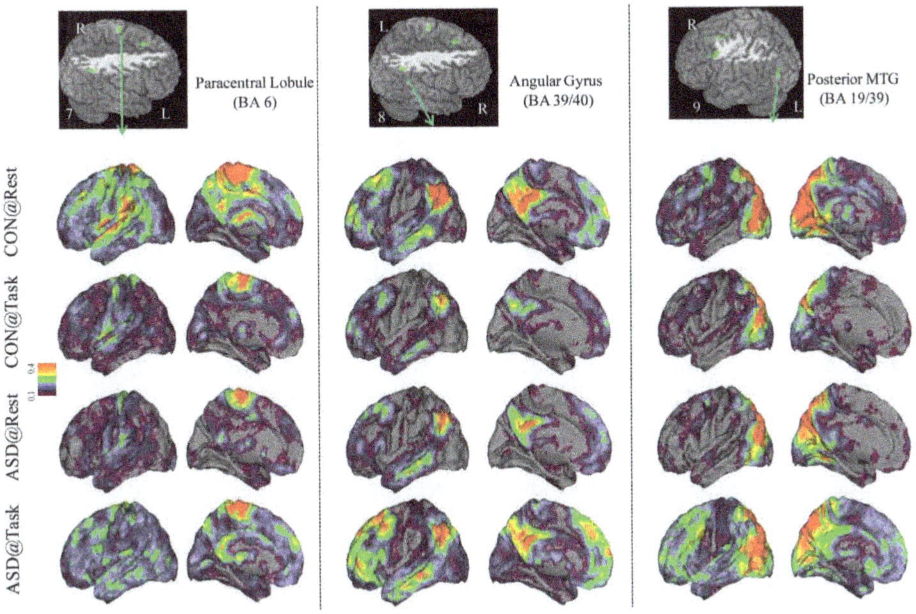

FIGURE 4 | Seed-based connectivity maps to understand distant functional connectivity patterns in resting and task states, for three clusters showing Group × Task interaction: paracentral Lobule (BA 6) (left panel), right Angular Gyrus (BA 39/40) (middle panel) and Posterior MTG (BA 19/39) (right panel). Region numbers 7–9 on the left corner in the brain image correspond to the region number in **Figure 1**.

children, indicating worse attentional function in ASD (see **Table 1**).

LOCAL AND DISTANT FUNCTIONAL CONNECTIVITY

While no regions showed a significant Group × State interaction for local connectivity, left frontal, right parietal, and left posterior temporal cortices showed the interaction in distant connectivity (**Figure 1**). In left frontal cortex, there were six clusters, a medial one including dorsal anterior cingulate extending into Supplementary Motor Area (SMA) (BA 32/8), and five lateral ones including dorsolateral prefrontal (middle frontal gyrus, BA 10; orbital gyrus, BA 11), and three in premotor cortex (BA 8, 6, 6/9). In right parietal cortex, there were two clusters, a dorsomedial one in paracentral lobule (BA 6) and an inferior lateral one near angular gyrus (BA 39/40). The final posterior cluster was in left posterior middle temporal gyrus (BA 19/39). As can be seen in graphs in **Figure 1** (cluster information in **Table 2**), in each of these regions, distant connectivity estimates were reduced in control children but increased in ASD children from resting to task state (See Table S1 for summary of mean, standard deviation and *p*-values in Supplementary Materials). Upon repeating the same analysis without regressing out trial conditions from the task run, similar Group × State interaction regions were found as above but with three exceptions—the paracentral lobule and BA 6 clusters did not survive the corrected threshold and the BA 6/9 cluster became larger (19 voxel vs. 16 voxel) (see Table S2 for summary of mean, standard deviation and p values in Supplementary Materials).

Seed-based connectivity maps for each of these regions showed that the connectivity map was more focal (i.e., smaller areas in the red-yellow intensity range) during the task relative to the resting run, for the control group. In contrast, for the ASD group, the connectivity map was more diffuse (i.e., larger areas in the red-orange intensity range) during the task relative to the resting run (See **Figures 2–4**); Figures showing difference maps (t-test $p < 0.005$, 5 voxels) comparing groups at each state (**Figures S1–S3**) and states for each group (**Figures S4–S6**) are in Supplementary Materials.

Table 2 | Regions showing Group (ASD, Control) × State (Resting, Sustained attention task) interaction for distant functional connectivity.

	Region	MNI coordinates			Cluster size (mm^3)	Peak Z-score
		x	y	z		
Left	Orbital frontal gyrus (BA 11)	−18	44	−22	320	3.72
Left	Middle frontal gyrus (BA 10)	−42	48	6	384	3.82
Left	Premotor (BA 6/9)	−42	12	38	1024	3.70
Left	Premotor (BA 8)	−26	20	50	512	4.26
Left	Premotor (BA 6)	−38	4	58	384	4.36
Medial	SMA (BA 32/8)	−2	24	46	384	3.57
Medial	Paracentral lobule (BA 6)	−2	−20	70	320	3.34
Right	Angular gyrus (BA 39/40)	50	−60	38	320	4.66
Left	Posterior MTG (BA 19/39)	−46	−80	18	512	3.87

GLOBAL GRAPH THEORY MEASURES

Group × State interaction was observed in global efficiency [$F_{(1,\ 29)} = 7.78$, $p = .009$]; *post-hoc* t-tests showed that global efficiency decreased from resting to the task run in control children [$t_{(15)} = 2.72, p = 0.016$] but did not change significantly in ASD children [$t_{(14)} = 0.96, p = 0.36$] (See bar graph in **Figure 5**). Further, the groups did not differ significantly in global efficiency during the resting [$t_{(22.\ 7)} = 1.3$, $p = 0.21$] or task [$t_{(26.\ 7)} = 1.22, p = 0.23$] runs.

Modularity also showed a Group × State interaction [$F_{(1,\ 29)} = 9.45$, $p = 0.005$]; *post-hoc* t-tests showed that modularity decreased in ASD children [$t_{(14)} = 2.62$, $p = 0.02$] but did not change significantly in control children [$t_{(15)} = 1.5, p = 0.15$] (See bar graph in **Figure 5**). Further, ASD children had higher modularity than controls [$t_{(23.5)} = 2.31, p = 0.03$] during the resting run, but the groups did not differ during the task run [$t_{(28.8)} = 0.85, p = 0.40$]. These observed patterns did not change when task conditions were not regressed out (See Table S3).

CORRELATION OF STATE-RELATED CHANGE IN DISTANT CONNECTIVITY WITH INATTENTION SCORES

The magnitude of increase in distant connectivity from resting to the task state in clusters showing Group × State interaction correlated positively with the inattention scores in ASD children, indicating that those with greater attention problems in everyday life showed a stronger increase in distant connectivity from resting to the task run (see scatterplots in **Figure 1**). Specifically, correlation was significant in dorsolateral prefrontal (BA 11: $r = 0.73$, $p = 0.002$; BA 10: $r = 0.72$, $p = 0.003$), premotor (BA 8: $r = 0.54, p = 0.037$; BA 6/9: $r = 0.67, p = 0.006$), supplementary motor (BA 32/8: $r = 0.59$, $p = 0.021$), and in right angular gyrus (BA 39/40: $r = 0.62$, $p = 0.013$). In the remaining three clusters, premotor (BA 6, $r = 0.38$, $p = 0.16$), paracentral lobule ($r = 0.49$, $p = 0.064$), and middle temporal ($r = 0.48, p = 0.068$), the correlation did not reach significance. The amount of task-related increase of global efficiency ($r = 0.53$, $p = 0.044$) and decrease of modularity ($r = -0.67$, $p = 0.007$) in ASD children also correlated with inattention scores (see scatterplots in **Figure 5**). Correlations were not significant in control children ($ps > 0.077$), for either regions showing Group × State interaction or graph theory measures.

DISCUSSION

We used a voxel-wise method to characterize local and distant functional connectivity in two cognitive states, resting and sustained attention, in pre-adolescent children with ASD and control children. Results showed that state-related changes in distant functional connectivity differed between groups in prefrontal, premotor, parietal, and posterior temporal cortical regions known to be associated with cognitive control and spatial attention. In these regions, distant connectivity, defined by the weighted strength of each voxel's temporal correlation with all voxels in the brain outside of its local neighborhood, increased in ASD children but reduced in control children, during sustained attention relative to a preceding resting state. Seed-based maps further confirmed that as hypothesized, reduced distant connectivity in control children reflected a more focal network topology during task than during the resting state. In contrast, contrary to our hypothesis, ASD children showed increased distant connectivity, reflected in a more diffuse network topology, during task than during the resting state. The magnitude of state-related increase in distant connectivity of prefrontal, premotor, and lateral parietal regions correlated positively with ASD children's inattention as measured by parent report on the ADHD Rating Scale. The resting versus task state comparison represents a distinction between attention that is unconstrained relative to

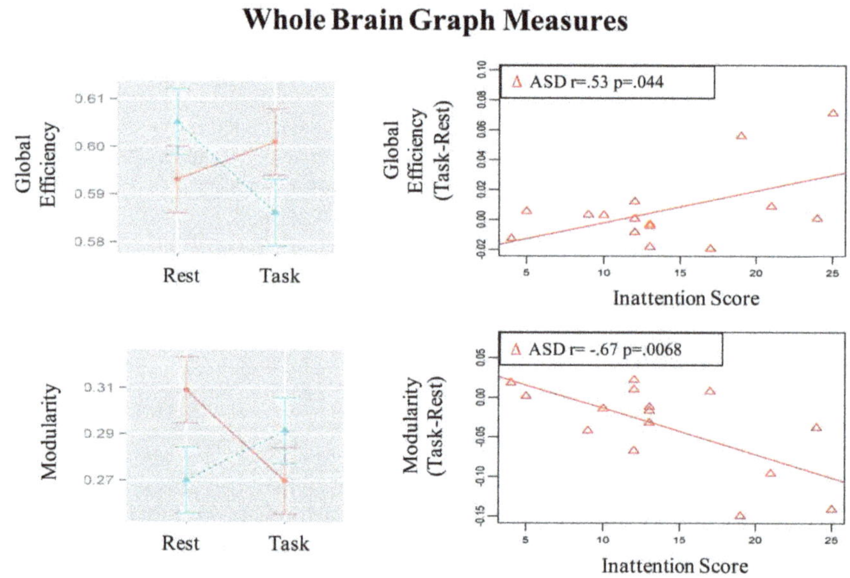

FIGURE 5 | Graphs depicting Group x State interaction for graph theory measures and correlation of the magnitude of state-related change (Task-Rest) with inattention scores in the ASD group.

that which is constrained by task-goals (e.g., monitoring for a target shape), respectively. As ASD children transition between the unconstrained state to a sustained attention demand, functional connectivity of frontal and parietal regions becomes more widespread, a property that may be maladaptive as it predicted greater attention problems in everyday life.

Some methodological considerations are important to note for interpreting the observed results. First, distant connectivity maps represent moderately high positive correlations (~0.33) between voxels. Further, global signal regression was not performed and therefore, positive/negative correlation value distributions were not altered during preprocessing (Murphy et al., 2009). Thus, interpretation of the observed results is limited to state-related changes in positive functional connectivity. Second, head motion was addressed using "scrubbing" procedures recommended by Power et al. (2012), resulting in retaining 4 min of data in each run for each child. While longer durations are desirable, 4 min is adequate to yield reliable connectivity estimates (Van Dijk et al., 2010). Residual motion was further addressed by using mean FD as a regressor in second-level analysis. As the number of volumes removed and mean FD did not differ between groups, the observed results cannot be attributed to differences in head motion. Third, the sustained attention task included manipulation of distracting information. As our primary aim was to examine effects of cognitive state, task conditions were regressed out, in order to ensure that group differences in connectivity were not driven by differential response to distraction. Importantly, repeating the analysis without regressing out task conditions resulted in a similar pattern of state-related group differences (Table S2), suggesting that the observed group differences were not driven by manipulation of task conditions. Fourth, scan order was fixed, with the resting state run acquired immediately before the task run. Order was not counterbalanced because pre-task and post-task resting state is not identical as task-related functional connectivity persists into the subsequent resting state, suggestive of a cognitive aftereffect (Gordon et al., 2012a). Fifth, our sample sizes of 15/16 children per group are relatively small due to our design requiring two back-to-back fMRI runs satisfying strict motion criteria from the same child. Nonetheless, it is important to note that the small samples limit the generalizability of the observed results.

Distant but not local functional connectivity was sensitive to group differences in modulation by cognitive state. Efficient cortical processing is posited to reflect the balance of connectivity within local regions supported by U-fibers, and across disparate regions supported by long-range white matter tracts (Mesulam, 1998; Schmahmann et al., 2008). While both types of connectivity are present throughout cortex, regions differ in their dominant (e.g. local or distant) connectivity properties. Local hierarchical connections are more representative of sensory cortical areas whereas association cortices such as prefrontal, parietal, lateral temporal, and limbic/paralimbic, have more long-range distributed connections (Felleman and Van Essen, 1991; Mesulam, 1998). In a study with healthy adults, Sepulcre et al. (2010) showed that the local/distant processing topology was paralleled in voxel-wise functional connectivity of low-frequency BOLD signals such that visual and somatosensory cortices showed higher local connectivity whereas association cortices showed higher distant connectivity. Further, while performing a semantic classification task, local and distant connectivity patterns of regions relevant to that task changed relative to a resting state. Here, we found that any state-related changes in local connectivity did not differ between ASD and control children, at least at a threshold that corrected for multiple comparisons. The size of the local neighborhood, 14 mm sphere, was selected based upon Sepulcre et al.'s (2010) recommendation as being optimal for distinguishing regional topography. While that recommendation is based upon adult brain size, it applies to children of the ages examined here as normalization of pediatric brain images to adult stereotactic space has been validated in children as young as 7 years (Burgund et al., 2002; Kang et al., 2003). Lack of significant group differences in state-related modulation of local connectivity suggests that local processing as reflected in voxel-wise BOLD temporal correlations is typical in ASD, at least in the context of transitioning to a relatively easy sustained attention task state.

Distant connectivity was modulated atypically in ASD children during sustained attention relative to a resting state, specifically in regions associated with attentional function. These regions included left dorsolateral prefrontal cortex (BA 10, 11), dorsal anterior cingulate extending to SMA (BA 32/8), and lateral premotor regions (BA 6, 8, 6/9), which are often engaged during tasks requiring cognitive control (Bunge et al., 2002; Vaidya et al., 2005). In addition, there were two parietal clusters, in right paracentral lobule, perhaps associated with motor responses and right inferior parietal cortex associated with spatial attention (Shulman et al., 2010). Finally, there was a cluster in left posterior middle temporal cortex (BA 19/39), a region that children sometimes engage during cognitive control tasks (Rubia et al., 1999; Durston et al., 2003; Vaidya et al., 2005). In all these regions, distant connectivity during sustained attention reduced in control children but increased in ASD children, relative to a resting state. Seed-based connectivity of each of these regions disambiguated the rest-to-task connectivity changes by showing that control children had a focal or less extensive pattern of anterior-posterior connectivity networks during the task relative to resting state. In contrast, ASD children showed the opposite pattern, diffuse or more extensive connectivity networks during the task relative to resting state, suggestive of a lack of selective engagement of task-relevant networks. Such a failure ought to lead to worse performance, which was evident in slower target detection speed in ASD children, while maintaining high accuracy. Further, the extent of increased distant connectivity from rest-to-task states in cognitive control (e.g., prefrontal, medial frontal, premotor) and spatial attention (e.g., lateral parietal) regions was associated with attention problems in everyday behavior as ASD children with larger increases in connectivity had worse inattention scores on the ADHD Rating Scale. Diffuse network engagement during an attentionally demanding state in ASD children may relate to the putative imbalance of inhibitory to excitatory connections associated with glutamatergic (Bejjani et al., 2012) and/or GABAergic dysfuntion (Rojas et al., 2013). If indeed so, then our results suggest that the inhibitory/excitatory milieu of the brain in ASD is modulated by cognitive state in a manner that differs from typical development. Whatever the physiological basis, it appears that in transitioning from a resting to sustained attention state, ASD children exhibited indiscriminate cortical network engagement, which may underlie their functional impairment in the domain of attention.

Group differences in state-related distant connectivity changes were apparent in two graph theory metrics, modularity and global efficiency, which quantify properties of global network organization (Rubinov and Sporns, 2010). Modularity describes the extent to which a network is organized into densely connected modules that are segregated from each other and global efficiency describes the average number of connections to be crossed to go from each voxel to every other voxel in the brain. In control children, global efficiency reduced during sustained attention compared to a resting state; this reduction reflects increased path length, which is consistent with a less extensive network observed during task relative to the resting state. This metric did not show significant difference across states in ASD children. ASD children's modularity reduced during task relative to the resting state, a pattern suggesting increased noise between modules (Bullmore and Sporns, 2009; Rubinov and Sporns, 2010), which is consistent with the observation of a more extensively connected network in ASD children during task than resting state. Even though state-related change was significant only for modularity in ASD children, their amount of change in both graph theory measures predicted inattention scores. Further, comparison of the groups during the resting state showed results that were consistent with past studies using scalp-based imaging measures showing higher modularity [electroencephalography (Barttfeld et al., 2011; Boersma et al., 2013)] in ASD compared to control subjects. While lower global efficiency [magnetoencephalography (Tsiaras et al., 2011)] has been reported in ASD children, it did not differ significantly between groups in the present study. These findings add to the growing volume of studies showing that graph theory metrics are sensitive to inter-individual differences [e.g., age, neurological, and psychiatric disorder (Bullmore and Sporns, 2009)] as well as intra-individual differences [e.g., learning (Bassett et al., 2011), working memory performance (Stevens et al., 2012), IQ (Van den Heuvel et al., 2009)]. Establishing the sensitivity of such whole-brain network metrics to subject factors or cognitive state is an important step in assessing their potential for serving as biomarkers for psychiatric and developmental disorders.

The present findings contribute to developing theories of functional connectivity in ASD in four novel ways. First, they extend the notion that functional connectivity is abnormal in ASD to include transitions across cognitive states. Studies examining functional connectivity during task states that are highly demanding of attention (e.g., theory of mind, working memory, face processing) show reduced connectivity of task-selective networks comprising distant frontal-posterior regions in ASD (Just et al., 2012; Khan et al., 2013). It is plausible that a failure of task-selective engagement such as that suggested by more extensive voxel-wise distant connectivity networks observed here is paralleled in reduced functional connectivity of specific networks or regions. We are unable to effectively test this prediction within the present data because procedures for addressing head motion required excluding volumes with high head motion, making for sparse sampling of individual trial-types.

Second, our findings highlight that examination of highly comorbid deficits in ASD such as attentional function may be insightful about pathophysiology of ASD. Attentional dysfunction is a common comorbid condition in ASD, with over 40% of ASD children estimated to also meet criteria for attention deficit hyperactivity disorder (ADHD) (Leyfer et al., 2006; Yerys et al., 2009b; Sikora et al., 2012). We cannot formally diagnose ADHD in the present sample based solely on parental report on the ADHD Rating scale. However, average scores for inattention and hyperactivity/impulsivity were higher in ASD than control children and 6 of the 15 ASD children had clinically elevated scores for either Inattention or Hyperactivity/impulsivity, consistent with past reports (Yerys et al., 2009b; Rosenthal et al., 2013; Smithson et al., 2013). Attentional and executive dysfunction are common targets for intervention in ASD as they are associated with worse adaptive functioning (Gilotty et al., 2002; Sikora et al., 2012) and outcome in adulthood [see review Hume et al. (2009)]. To the extent that some level of attentional dysfunction always accompanies ASD, it is important to characterize the underlying neural signatures, especially if they prove to be unique to ASD. Thus, it would be important to conduct a similar study in children with ADHD to specify the extent to which our results reflect a general or disorder-specific correlate of transitioning between attentional states.

Third, our graph theory findings contribute to the growing body of studies of large-scale network structure of the brain by showing that modularity and global efficiency were sensitive to ASD and to manipulation of cognitive state. Demonstrating such sensitivity contributes to the potential of such connectivity metrics to serve as biomarkers for psychiatric and developmental disorders. Fourth, the present results highlight the importance of considering cognitive state in current theories of functional connectivity in ASD. It is likely that neither under- nor over-connectivity may characterize ASD in absolute terms but that the nature of alteration may depend upon the specific cognitive state. Mixed findings across task-evoked functional connectivity studies may reflect nuanced differences in the subjects cognitive state induced not just by experimental demands but also the individual's experience of the task as high/low arousing, easy/hard, boring/enjoyable. Furthermore, specific networks may be more susceptible to cognitive state differences than others. As this area of investigation evolves, consideration of task demands, networks, and individual subject characteristics ought to be productive in resolving the status of connectivity abnormality in ASD.

ACKNOWLEDGMENTS

We thank Evan Gordon for helpful discussion of methods. This work was funded by MH084961 from NIMH to Chandan J. Vaidya, and supported by the Intellectual and Developmental Disabilities Research Center, Children's National Medical Center Grant [HD040677-07].

SUPPLEMENTARY MATERIAL

The Supplementary Material for this article can be found online at: http://www.frontiersin.org/Human_Neuroscience/10.3389/fnhum.2013.00482/abstract

FIGURE S1 | Group differences in seed-based connectivity maps in resting and task states, for three clusters showing Group × Task interaction: left orbital frontal gyrus (BA 11) (left panel), left middle frontal gyrus (BA 10) (middle panel) and left premotor (BA 6/9) (right panel). Region numbers 1–3 on the left corner in the brain image correspond to the region number in **Figure 1**.

FIGURE S2 | Group differences in seed-based connectivity maps in resting and task states, for three clusters showing Group × Task interaction: left premotor (BA 8) (left panel), left premotor (BA 6) (middle panel) and SMA (BA 32/8) (right panel). Region numbers 4–6 on the left corner in the brain image correspond to the region number in **Figure 1**.

FIGURE S3 | Group differences in seed-based connectivity maps in resting and task states, for three clusters showing Group × Task interaction: Paracentral Lobule (BA 6) (left panel), right Angular Gyrus (BA 39/40) (middle panel) and Posterior MTG (BA 19/39) (right panel). Region numbers 7–9 on the left corner in the brain image correspond to the region number in **Figure 1**.

FIGURE S4 | State differences in seed-based connectivity maps within each group, for three clusters showing Group × Task interaction: left orbital frontal gyrus (BA 11) (left panel), left middle frontal gyrus (BA 10) (middle panel) and left premotor (BA 6/9) (right panel). Region numbers 1–3 on the left corner in the brain image correspond to the region number in **Figure 1**.

FIGURE S5 | State differences in seed-based connectivity maps within each group, for three clusters showing Group × Task interaction: left premotor (BA 8) (left panel), left premotor (BA 6) (middle panel) and SMA (BA 32/8) (right panel). Region numbers 4–6 on the left corner in the brain image correspond to the region number in **Figure 1**.

FIGURE S6 | State differences in seed-based connectivity maps within each group, for three clusters showing Group × Task interaction: Paracentral Lobule (BA 6) (left panel), right Angular Gyrus (BA 39/40) (middle panel) and Posterior MTG (BA 19/39) (right panel). Region numbers 7–9 on the left corner in the brain image correspond to the region number in **Figure 1**.

REFERENCES

Achard, S., and Bullmore, E. (2007). Efficiency and cost of economical brain functional networks. *PLoS Comput. Biol.* 3:e17. doi: 10.1371/journal.pcbi.0030017

American Psychiatric Association. (2000). *Diagnostic and statistical manual of mental disorders (4th ed., text rev.).*

Arfanakis, K., Cordes, D., Haughton, V. M., Moritz, C. H., Quigley, M. A., and Meyerand, M. E. (2000). Combining independent component analysis and correlation analysis to probe interregional connectivity in fMRI task activation datasets. *Magn. Reson. Imaging* 18, 921–930. doi: 10.1016/S0730-725X(00)00190-9

Assaf, M., Jagannathan, K., Calhoun, V. D., Miller, L., Stevens, M. C., Sahl, R., et al. (2010). Abnormal functional connectivity of default mode sub-networks in autism spectrum disorder patients. *Neuroimage* 53, 247–256. doi: 10.1016/j.neuroimage.2010.05.067

Barttfeld, P., Wicker, B., Cukier, S., Navarta, S., Lew, S., and Sigman, M. (2011). A big-world network in ASD: dynamical connectivity analysis reflects a deficit in long-range connections and an excess of short-range connections. *Neuropsychologia* 49, 254–263. doi: 10.1016/j.neuropsychologia.2010.11.024

Bassett, D. S., Wymbs, N. F., Porter, M. A., Mucha, P. J., Carlson, J. M., and Grafton, S. T. (2011). Dynamic reconfiguration of human brain networks during learning. *Proc. Natl. Acad. Sci. U.S.A.* 108, 7641–7646. doi: 10.1073/pnas.1018985108

Bejjani, A., O'Neill, J., Kim, J. A., Frew, A. J., Yee, V. W., Ly, R., et al. (2012). Elevated glutamatergic compounds in pregenual anterior cingulate in pediatric autism spectrum disorder demonstrated by 1H MRS and 1H MRSI. *PLoS ONE* 7:e38786. doi: 10.1371/journal.pone.0038786

Birn, R. M., Diamond, J. B., Smith, M. A., and Bandettini, P. A. (2006). Separating respiratory-variation-related fluctuations from neuronal-activity-related fluctuations in fMRI. *Neuroimage* 31, 1536–1548. doi: 10.1016/j.neuroimage.2006.02.048

Boersma, M., Kemner, C., de Reus, M. A., Collin, G., Snijders, T. M., Hofman, D., et al. (2013). Disrupted functional brain networks in autistic toddlers. *Brain Connect.* 3, 41–49. doi: 10.1089/brain.2012.0127

Brett, M., Anton, J., Valabregue, R., and Pioline, J. (2002). "Region of interest analysis using an SPM toolbox," in *Presented at the 8th International Conferance on Functional Mapping of the Human Brain* (Sendai) [abstract].

Buckner, R. L., Sepulcre, J., Talukdar, T., Krienen, F. M., Liu, H., Hedden, T., et al. (2009). cortical hubs revealed by intrinsic functional connectivity: mapping, assessment of stability, and relation to Alzheimer's Disease. *J. Neurosci.* 29, 1860–1873. doi: 10.1523/JNEUROSCI.5062-08.2009

Bullmore, E., and Sporns, O. (2009). Complex brain networks: graph theoretical analysis of structural and functional systems. *Nat. Rev. Neurosci.* 10, 186–198. doi: 10.1038/nrn2575

Bunge, S. A., Dudukovic, N. M., Thomason, M. E., Vaidya, C. J., and Gabrieli, J. D. E. (2002). Immature frontal lobe contributions to cognitive control in children: evidence from fMRI. *Neuron* 33, 301–311. doi: 10.1016/S0896-6273(01)00583-9

Burgund, E. D., Kang, H. C., Kelly, J. E., Buckner, R. L., Snyder, A. Z., Petersen, S. E., et al. (2002). The feasibility of a common stereotactic space for children and adults in fMRI studies of development. *Neuroimage* 17, 184–200. doi: 10.1006/nimg.2002.1174

Cherkassky, V. L., Kana, R. K., Keller, T. A., and Just, M. A. (2006). Functional connectivity in a baseline resting-state network in autism. *Neuroreport* 17, 1687–1690. doi: 10.1097/01.wnr.0000239956.45448.4c

Di Martino, A., Kelly, C., Grzadzinski, R., Zuo, X.-N., Mennes, M., Mairena, M. A., et al. (2011). Aberrant striatal functional connectivity in children with autism. *Biol. Psychiatry* 69, 847–856. doi: 10.1016/j.biopsych.2010.10.029

DuPaul, G. J., Power, T. J., Anastopoulos, A. D., and Reid, R. (1998). *ADHD Rating Scale-IV: Checklists, Norms, and Clinical Interpretation.* (New York, NY: Guilford Press).

Durston, S., Tottenham, N. T., Thomas, K. M., Davidson, M. C., Eigsti, I.-M., Yang, Y., et al. (2003). Differential patterns of striatal activation in young children with and without ADHD. *Biol. Psychiatry* 53, 871–878. doi: 10.1016/S0006-3223(02)01904-2

Felleman, D. J., and Van Essen, D. C. (1991). Distributed hierarchical processing in the primate cerebral cortex. *Cereb. Cortex* 1, 1–47. doi: 10.1093/cercor/1.1.1

Fox, M. D., Snyder, A. Z., Zacks, J. M., and Raichle, M. E. (2006). Coherent spontaneous activity accounts for trial-to-trial variability in human evoked brain responses. *Nat. Neurosci.* 9, 23–25. doi: 10.1038/nn1616

Fransson, P. (2006). How default is the default mode of brain function? Further evidence from intrinsic BOLD signal fluctuations. *Neuropsychologia* 44, 2836–2845. doi: 10.1016/j.neuropsychologia.2006.06.017

Freire, L., Roche, A., and Mangin, J.-F. (2002). What is the best similarity measure for motion correction in fMRI time series. *IEEE Trans. Med. Imaging* 21, 470–484. doi: 10.1109/TMI.2002.1009383

Fukunaga, M., Horovitz, S. G., van Gelderen, P., de Zwart, J. A., Jansma, J. M., Ikonomidou, V. N., et al. (2006). Large-amplitude, spatially correlated fluctuations in BOLD fMRI signals during extended rest and early sleep stages. *Magn. Reson. Imaging* 24, 979–992. doi: 10.1016/j.mri.2006.04.018

Gilotty, L., Kenworthy, L., Sirian, L., Black, D. O., and Wagner, A. E. (2002). Adaptive skills and executive function in autism spectrum disorders. *Child Neuropsychol.* 8, 241–248. doi: 10.1076/chin.8.4.241.13504

Gordon, E. M., Breeden, A. L., Bean, S. E., and Vaidya, C. J. (2012a). Working memory-related changes in functional connectivity persist beyond task disengagement. *Hum. Brain Mapp.* doi: 10.1002/hbm.22230. [Epub ahead of print].

Gordon, E. M., Stollstorff, M., Devaney, J. M., Bean, S., and Vaidya, C. J. (2012b). Effect of dopamine transporter genotype on intrinsic functional connectivity depends on cognitive state. *Cereb. Cortex* 22, 2182–2196. doi: 10.1093/cercor/bhr305

Gordon, E. M., Stollstorff, M., and Vaidya, C. J. (2012c). Using spatial multiple regression to identify intrinsic connectivity networks involved in working memory performance. *Hum. Brain Mapp.* 33, 1536–1552. doi: 10.1002/hbm.21306

Gotts, S. J., Simmons, W. K., Milbury, L. A., Wallace, G. L., Cox, R. W., and Martin, A. (2012). Fractionation of social brain circuits in autism spectrum disorders. *Brain* 135, 2711–2725. doi: 10.1093/brain/aws160

Greicius, M. D., Kiviniemi, V., Tervonen, O., Vainionpää, V., Alahuhta, S., Reiss, A. L., et al. (2008). Persistent default-mode network connectivity during light sedation. *Hum. Brain Mapp.* 29, 839–847. doi: 10.1002/hbm.20537

Hampson, M., Olson, I. R., Leung, H.-C., Skudlarski, P., and Gore, J. C. (2004). Changes in functional connectivity of human MT/V5 with visual motion input. *Neuroreport* 15, 1315–1319. doi: 10.1097/01.wnr.0000129997.95055.15

Heine, L., Soddu, A., Gómez, F., Vanhaudenhuyse, A., Tshibanda, L., Thonnard, M., et al. (2012). Resting state networks and consciousness: alterations of multiple resting state network connectivity in physiological, pharmacological, and pathological consciousness States. *Front. Psychol.* 3:295. doi: 10.3389/fpsyg.2012.00295

Hill, E. L. (2004). Executive dysfunction in autism. *Trends Cogn. Sci.* 8, 26–32. doi: 10.1016/j.tics.2003.11.003

Hume, K., Loftin, R., and Lantz, J. (2009). Increasing independence in autism spectrum disorders: a review of three focused interventions. *J. Autism Dev. Disord.* 39, 1329–1338. doi: 10.1007/s10803-009-0751-2

Jiang, T., He, Y., Zang, Y., and Weng, X. (2004). Modulation of functional connectivity during the resting state and the motor task. *Hum. Brain Mapp.* 22, 63–71. doi: 10.1002/hbm.20012

Jones, T. B., Bandettini, P. A., Kenworthy, L., Case, L. K., Milleville, S. C., Martin, A., et al. (2010). Sources of group differences in functional connectivity: an investigation applied to autism spectrum disorder. *Neuroimage* 49, 401–414. doi: 10.1016/j.neuroimage.2009.07.051

Just, M. A., Keller, T. A., Malave, V. L., Kana, R. K., and Varma, S. (2012). Autism as a neural systems disorder: a theory of frontal-posterior underconnectivity. *Neurosci. Biobehav. Rev.* 36, 1292–1313. doi: 10.1016/j.neubiorev.2012.02.007

Kang, H. C., Burgund, E. D., Lugar, H. M., Petersen, S. E., and Schlaggar, B. L. (2003). Comparison of functional activation foci in children and adults using a common stereotactic space. *Neuroimage* 19, 16–28. doi: 10.1016/S1053-8119(03)00038-7

Kennedy, D. P., and Courchesne, E. (2008). The intrinsic functional organization of the brain is altered in autism. *Neuroimage* 39, 1877–1885. doi: 10.1016/j.neuroimage.2007.10.052

Kenworthy, L., Black, D. O., Harrison, B., Della Rosa, A., and Wallace, G. L. (2009). Are executive control functions related to autism symptoms in high-functioning children. *Child Neuropsychol.* 15, 425–440. doi: 10.1080/09297040802646983

Kenworthy, L., Yerys, B. E., Anthony, L. G., and Wallace, G. L. (2008). Understanding executive control in autism spectrum disorders in the lab and in the real world. *Neuropsychol. Rev.* 18, 320–338. doi: 10.1007/s11065-008-9077-7

Kenworthy, L. E., Black, D. O., Wallace, G. L., Ahluvalia, T., Wagner, A. E., and Sirian, L. M. (2005). Disorganization: the forgotten executive dysfunction in high-functioning autism (HFA) spectrum disorders. *Dev. Neuropsychol.* 28, 809–827. doi: 10.1207/s15326942dn2803_4

Khan, S., Gramfort, A., Shetty, N. R., Kitzbichler, M. G., Ganesan, S., Moran, J. M., et al. (2013). Local and long-range functional connectivity is reduced in concert in autism spectrum disorders. *Proc. Natl. Acad. Sci. U.S.A.* 110, 3107–3112. doi: 10.1073/pnas.1214533110

Lai, G., Pantazatos, S. P., Schneider, H., and Hirsch, J. (2012). Neural systems for speech and song in autism. *Brain* 135, 961–975. doi: 10.1093/brain/awr335

Lainhart, J. E., Bigler, E. D., Bocian, M., Coon, H., Dinh, E., Dawson, G., et al. (2006). Head circumference and height in autism: a study by the collaborative program of excellence in autism. *Am. J. Med. Genet. A* 140, 2257–2274. doi: 10.1002/ajmg.a.31465

Latora, V., and Marchiori, M. (2001). Efficient behavior of small-world networks. *Phys. Rev. Lett.* 87, 198701. doi: 10.1103/PhysRevLett.87.198701

Lavigne, J. V., Cromley, T., Sprafkin, J., and Gadow, K. D. (2009). The child and adolescent symptom inventory-progress monitor: a brief diagnostic and statistical manual of mental disorders, 4th edition-referenced parent-report scale for children and adolescents. *J. Child Adolesc. Psychopharmacol.* 19, 241–252. doi: 10.1089/cap.2008.052

Leyfer, O. T., Folstein, S. E., Bacalman, S., Davis, N. O., Dinh, E., Morgan, J., et al. (2006). Comorbid psychiatric disorders in children with autism: interview development and rates of disorders. *J. Autism Dev. Disord.* 36, 849–861. doi: 10.1007/s10803-006-0123-0

Lopez, B. R., Lincoln, A. J., Ozonoff, S., and Lai, Z. (2005). Examining the relationship between executive functions and restricted, repetitive symptoms of Autistic Disorder. *J. Autism Dev. Disord.* 35, 445–460. doi: 10.1007/s10803-005-5035-x

Lord, C., Risi, S., Lambrecht, L., Cook, E. H., Leventhal, B. L., DiLavore, P. C., et al. (2000). The autism diagnostic observation schedule-generic: a standard measure of social and communication deficits associated with the spectrum of autism. *J. Autism Dev. Disord.* 30, 205–223. doi: 10.1023/A:1005592401947

Lord, C., Rutter, M., and Le Couteur, A. (1994). Autism diagnostic interview-revised: a revised version of a diagnostic interview for caregivers of individuals with possible pervasive developmental disorders. *J. Autism Dev. Disord.* 24, 659–685. doi: 10.1007/BF02172145

Mennes, M., Kelly, C., Zuo, X.-N., Di Martino, A., Biswal, B., Castellanos, F. X., et al. (2010). Inter-individual differences in resting state functional connectivity predict task-induced BOLD activity. *Neuroimage* 50, 1690–1701. doi: 10.1016/j.neuroimage.2010.01.002

Mesulam, M. M. (1998). From sensation to cognition. *Brain* 121(Pt 6), 1013–1052. doi: 10.1093/brain/121.6.1013

Monk, C. S., Peltier, S. J., Wiggins, J. L., Weng, S.-J., Carrasco, M., Risi, S., et al. (2009). Abnormalities of intrinsic functional connectivity in autism spectrum disorders. *Neuroimage* 47, 764–772. doi: 10.1016/j.neuroimage.2009.04.069

Müller, R.-A., Shih, P., Keehn, B., Deyoe, J. R., Leyden, K. M., and Shukla, D. K. (2011). Underconnected, but how. A survey of functional connectivity MRI studies in autism spectrum disorders. *Cereb. Cortex* 21, 2233–2243. doi: 10.1093/cercor/bhq296

Murphy, K., Birn, R. M., Handwerker, D. A., Jones, T. B., and Bandettini, P. A. (2009). The impact of global signal regression on resting state correlations: are anti-correlated networks introduced. *Neuroimage* 44, 893–905. doi: 10.1016/j.neuroimage.2008.09.036

Newman, M. E. J. (2006). Modularity and community structure in networks. *Proc. Natl. Acad. Sci. U.S.A.* 103, 8577–8582. doi: 10.1073/pnas.0601602103

Nir, Y., Hasson, U., Levy, I., Yeshurun, Y., and Malach, R. (2006). Widespread functional connectivity and fMRI fluctuations in human visual cortex in the absence of visual stimulation. *Neuroimage* 30, 1313–1324. doi: 10.1016/j.neuroimage.2005.11.018

Noonan, S. K., Haist, F., and Müller, R.-A. (2009). Aberrant functional connectivity in autism: evidence from low-frequency BOLD signal fluctuations. *Brain Res.* 1262, 48–63. doi: 10.1016/j.brainres.2008.12.076

Power, J. D., Barnes, K. A., Snyder, A. Z., Schlaggar, B. L., and Petersen, S. E. (2012). Spurious but systematic correlations in functional connectivity MRI networks arise from subject motion. *Neuroimage* 59, 2142–2154. doi: 10.1016/j.neuroimage.2011.10.018

Prifitera, A., Weiss, L. G., and Saklofske, D. H. (1998). "The WISC–III in context," in *WISC–III Clinical Use and Interpretation: Scientist-Practitioner Perspectives*, eds A. Prifitera and D. H. Saklofske (NewYork, NY: Academic Press), 1–38. doi: 10.1016/B978-012564930-8/50002-4

Rojas, D. C., Singel, D., Steinmetz, S., Hepburn, S., and Brown, M. S. (2013). Decreased left perisylvian GABA concentration in children with autism and unaffected siblings. *Neuroimage.* doi: 10.1016/j.neuroimage.2013.01.045. [Epub ahead of print].

Rosenthal, M., Wallace, G. L., Lawson, R., Wills, M. C., Dixon, E., Yerys, B. E., et al. (2013). Impairments in real-world executive function increase from childhood to adolescence in autism spectrum disorders. *Neuropsychology* 27, 13–18. doi: 10.1037/a0031299

Rubia, K., Overmeyer, S., Taylor, E., Brammer, M., Williams, S. C., Simmons, A., et al. (1999). Hypofrontality in attention deficit hyperactivity disorder during higher-order motor control: a study with functional MRI. *Am. J. Psychiatry* 156, 891–896.

Rubinov, M., and Sporns, O. (2010). Complex network measures of brain connectivity: uses and interpretations. *Neuroimage* 52, 1059–1069. doi: 10.1016/j.neuroimage.2009.10.003

Saklofske, D. H., Prifitera, A., Weiss, L. G., Rolfhus, E., and Zhu, J. (2004). "Clinical Interpretation of the WISC-IV FSIQ and GAI," in *WISC-IV Clinical Use and Interpretation: Scientist-Practitioner Perspectives*, (New York, NY: Academic Press), 36–71.

Satterthwaite, T. D., Wolf, D. H., Loughead, J., Ruparel, K., Elliott, M. A., Hakonarson, H., et al. (2012). Impact of in-scanner head motion on multiple measures of functional connectivity: relevance for studies of neurodevelopment in youth. *Neuroimage* 60, 623–632. doi: 10.1016/j.neuroimage.2011.12.063

Schmahmann, J. D., Smith, E. E., Eichler, F. S., and Filley, C. M. (2008). Cerebral white matter: neuroanatomy, clinical neurology, and neurobehavioral correlates. *Ann. N.Y. Acad. Sci.* 1142, 266–309. doi: 10.1196/annals.1444.017

Sepulcre, J., Liu, H., Talukdar, T., Martincorena, I., Yeo, B. T. T., and Buckner, R. L. (2010). The organization of local and distant functional connectivity in the human brain. *PLoS Comput. Biol.* 6:e1000808. doi: 10.1371/journal.pcbi.1000808

Shih, P., Keehn, B., Oram, J. K., Leyden, K. M., Keown, C. L., and Müller, R.-A. (2011). Functional differentiation of posterior superior temporal sulcus in autism: a functional connectivity magnetic resonance imaging study. *Biol. Psychiatry* 70, 270–277. doi: 10.1016/j.biopsych.2011.03.040

Shulman, G. L., Pope, D. L. W., Astafiev, S. V., McAvoy, M. P., Snyder, A. Z., and Corbetta, M. (2010). Right hemisphere dominance during spatial selective attention and target detection occurs outside the dorsal frontoparietal network. *J. Neurosci.* 30, 3640–3651. doi: 10.1523/JNEUROSCI.4085-09.2010

Sikora, D. M., Vora, P., Coury, D. L., and Rosenberg, D. (2012). Attention-deficit/hyperactivity disorder symptoms, adaptive functioning, and quality of life in children with autism spectrum disorder. *Pediatrics* 130(Suppl. 2), S91–S97. doi: 10.1542/peds.2012-0900G

Smith, S. M., Fox, P. T., Miller, K. L., Glahn, D. C., Fox, P. M., Mackay, C. E., et al. (2009). Correspondence of the brain's functional architecture during activation and rest. *Proc. Natl. Acad. Sci. U.S.A* 106, 13040–13045. doi: 10.1073/pnas.0905267106

Smithson, P. E., Kenworthy, L., Wills, M. C., Jarrett, M., Atmore, K., and Yerys, B. E. (2013). Real world executive control impairments in preschoolers with autism spectrum disorders. *J. Autism Dev. Disord.* doi: 10.1007/s10803-012-1747-x. [Epub ahead of print].

Stevens, A. A., Tappon, S. C., Garg, A., and Fair, D. A. (2012). Functional brain network modularity captures inter- and intra-individual variation in working memory capacity. *PLoS ONE* 7:e30468. doi: 10.1371/journal.pone.0030468

Tellegen, A., and Briggs, P. F. (1967). Old wine in new skins: grouping Wechsler subtests into new scales. *J. Consult. Psychol.* 31, 499–506. doi: 10.1037/h0024963

Tsiaras, V., Simos, P. G., Rezaie, R., Sheth, B. R., Garyfallidis, E., Castillo, E. M., et al. (2011). Extracting biomarkers of autism from MEG resting-state functional connectivity networks. *Comput. Biol. Med.* 41, 1166–1177. doi: 10.1016/j.compbiomed.2011.04.004

Vaidya, C. J., Bunge, S. A., Dudukovic, N. M., Zalecki, C. A., Elliott, G. R., and Gabrieli, J. D. E. (2005). Altered neural substrates of cognitive control in childhood ADHD: evidence from functional magnetic resonance imaging. *Am. J. Psychiatry* 162, 1605–1613. doi: 10.1176/appi.ajp.162.9.1605

Van den Heuvel, M. P., Stam, C. J., Kahn, R. S., and Hulshoff Pol, H. E. (2009). Efficiency of functional brain networks and intellectual performance. *J. Neurosci.* 29, 7619–7624. doi: 10.1523/JNEUROSCI.1443-09.2009

Van Dijk, K. R. A., Hedden, T., Venkataraman, A., Evans, K. C., Lazar, S. W., and Buckner, R. L. (2010). Intrinsic functional connectivity as a tool for human connectomics: theory, properties, and optimization. *J. Neurophysiol.* 103, 297–321. doi: 10.1152/jn.00783.2009

Van Essen, D. C. (2005). A population-average, landmark- and surface-based (PALS) atlas of human cerebral cortex. *Neuroimage* 28, 635–662. doi: 10.1016/j.neuroimage.2005.06.058

Vincent, J. L., Patel, G. H., Fox, M. D., Snyder, A. Z., Baker, J. T., Van Essen, D. C., et al. (2007). Intrinsic functional architecture in the anaesthetized monkey brain. *Nature* 447, 83–86. doi: 10.1038/nature05758

Von dem Hagen, E. A. H., Stoyanova, R. S., Baron-Cohen, S., and Calder, A. J. (2012). *Reduced Functional Connectivity within and Between "social" Resting State Networks in Autism Spectrum Conditions. Social Cognitive and Affective Neuroscience.* Available online at: http://www.ncbi.nlm.nih.gov/pubmed/22563003 (Accessed: 16, July, 2012).

Ward, B. D. (2000). *Simultaneous Inference for fMRI Data. Biophysics Research Institute,Medical College of Wisconsin.* Available online at: http://afni.nimh.nih.gov/pub/dist/doc/manual/AlphaSim.pdf.

Wechsler, D. (1999). *Manual for the Wechsler Abbreviated Intelligence Scale (WASI).* San Antonio, TX: The Psychological Corporation.

Weiss, L. G., Saklofske, D. H., Prifitera, A., Chen, H.-Y., and Hildebrand, D. (1999). The calculation of the WISC-Ill general ability index using Canadian norms. *Can. J. Sch. Psychol.* 14, 1–10. doi: 10.1177/082957359901400202

Weng, S.-J., Wiggins, J. L., Peltier, S. J., Carrasco, M., Risi, S., Lord, C., et al. (2010). Alterations of resting state functional connectivity in the default network in adolescents with autism spectrum disorders. *Brain Res.* 1313, 202–214. doi: 10.1016/j.brainres.2009.11.057

Wiggins, J. L., Peltier, S. J., Ashinoff, S., Weng, S.-J., Carrasco, M., Welsh, R. C., et al. (2011). Using a self-organizing map algorithm to detect age-related changes in functional connectivity during rest in autism spectrum disorders. *Brain Res.* 1380, 187–197. doi: 10.1016/j.brainres.2010.10.102

Wise, R. G., Ide, K., Poulin, M. J., and Tracey, I. (2004). Resting fluctuations in arterial carbon dioxide induce significant low frequency variations in BOLD signal. *Neuroimage* 21, 1652–1664. doi: 10.1016/j.neuroimage.2003.11.025

Yerys, B. E., Wallace, G. L., Harrison, B., Celano, M. J., Giedd, J. N., and Kenworthy, L. E. (2009a). Set-shifting in children with autism spectrum disorders: reversal shifting deficits on the Intradimensional/Extradimensional Shift Test correlate with repetitive behaviors. *Autism* 13, 523–538.

Yerys, B. E., Wallace, G. L., Sokoloff, J. L., Shook, D. A., James, J. D., and Kenworthy, L. (2009b). Attention deficit/hyperactivity disorder symptoms moderate cognition and behavior in children with autism spectrum disorders. *Autism Res.* 2, 322–333.

Zink, C. F., Pagnoni, G., Martin, M. E., Dhamala, M., and Berns, G. S. (2003). Human striatal response to salient nonrewarding stimuli. *J. Neurosci.* 23, 8092–8097.

14

Resting state fMRI reveals a default mode dissociation between retrosplenial and medial prefrontal subnetworks in ASD despite motion scrubbing

Tuomo Starck[1,2]*, Juha Nikkinen[1], Jukka Rahko[3], Jukka Remes[1,4], Tuula Hurtig[3], Helena Haapsamo[3], Katja Jussila[3], Sanna Kuusikko-Gauffin[3], Marja-Leena Mattila[3], Eira Jansson-Verkasalo[5], David L. Pauls[6], Hanna Ebeling[3], Irma Moilanen[3], Osmo Tervonen[1,2] and Vesa J. Kiviniemi[1,2]

[1] Department of Diagnostic Radiology, Oulu University Hospital, Oulu, Finland
[2] Department of Diagnostic Radiology, Oulu University, Oulu, Finland
[3] Department of Child Psychiatry, Institute of Clinical Medicine, Oulu University Hospital and Oulu University, Oulu, Finland
[4] Department of Electrical and Information Engineering, Oulu University, Oulu, Finland
[5] Department of Behavioral Sciences and Philosophy, Logopedics, University of Turku, Turku, Finland
[6] Psychiatric and Neurodevelopmental Genetics Unit, Harvard Medical School, Boston, MA, USA

Edited by:
Lucina Q. Uddin, Stanford University, USA

Reviewed by:
Scott Peltier, University of Michigan, USA
Charles J. Lynch, Georgetown University, USA

***Correspondence:**
Tuomo Starck, Department of Diagnostic Radiology, Oulu University Hospital, PO Box 50, Kajaanintie, Oulu, 90029 OYS, Finland
e-mail: tuomo.starck@ppshp.fi

In resting state functional magnetic resonance imaging (fMRI) studies of autism spectrum disorders (ASDs) decreased frontal-posterior functional connectivity is a persistent finding. However, the picture of the default mode network (DMN) hypoconnectivity remains incomplete. In addition, the functional connectivity analyses have been shown to be susceptible even to subtle motion. DMN hypoconnectivity in ASD has been specifically called for re-evaluation with stringent motion correction, which we aimed to conduct by so-called scrubbing. A rich set of default mode subnetworks can be obtained with high dimensional group independent component analysis (ICA) which can potentially provide more detailed view of the connectivity alterations. We compared the DMN connectivity in high-functioning adolescents with ASDs to typically developing controls using ICA dual-regression with decompositions from typical to high dimensionality. Dual-regression analysis within DMN subnetworks did not reveal alterations but connectivity between anterior and posterior DMN subnetworks was decreased in ASD. The results were very similar with and without motion scrubbing thus indicating the efficacy of the conventional motion correction methods combined with ICA dual-regression. Specific dissociation between DMN subnetworks was revealed on high ICA dimensionality, where networks centered at the medial prefrontal cortex and retrosplenial cortex showed weakened coupling in adolescents with ASDs compared to typically developing control participants. Generally the results speak for disruption in the anterior-posterior DMN interplay on the network level whereas local functional connectivity in DMN seems relatively unaltered.

Keywords: autism, resting state, fMRI, ICA, default mode, motion

INTRODUCTION

In autism spectrum disorders (ASDs) the functional connectivity (FC) research with resting state functional magnetic resonance imaging (fMRI) has shown aberrant FC (Cherkassky et al., 2006; Kennedy and Courchesne, 2008; Monk et al., 2009; Assaf et al., 2010; Weng et al., 2010; Wiggins et al., 2012). The evidence for disrupted connectivity in ASD was seen in 1988 by positron emission tomography (Horwitz et al., 1988). Of the several resting state networks (RSNs), the Default mode network (DMN) can be readily designated as the most prominent with its cognitive associations in, such as self-referential processing and envisioning of the past and the future (Andreasen et al., 1995). DMN has recently gained interest as a functional entity due to a study (Anderson et al., 2011) where several DMN regions were found to be most informative for classifying individuals with autism and typically developing (TD) control subjects. In resting state fMRI, the majority of the findings have shown decreased DMN FC especially in frontal-posterior pairs in ASD (Schipul et al., 2011), thereby supporting the theory of frontal-posterior underconnectivity in autism (Just et al., 2004, 2007). While the underconnectivity is a typical finding in ASD it is important to bear in mind the developmental aspect of the disorder as which has recently been explored (Lynch et al., 2013; Washington et al., 2013).

It has lately been established that the resting state DMN constitutes of subsystems that manifest themselves in various ways, depending on the analysis method. Spatial ICA and spatial group ICA have been shown to work well in the DMN region-of-interest definition for FC analysis (Marrelec and Fransson, 2011). Temporal-concatenation based spatial group ICA (Calhoun et al., 2001) is known to split some components along increasing ICA dimensionality (i.e., model order) and the major DMN splitting into default mode subnetworks (DM-SN) already occurs at very low dimensionalities (Abou-Elseoud et al., 2010). Division of the DMN into anterior and posterior has been demonstrated (Calhoun et al., 2008; Uddin et al., 2009), but DMN dynamics are more complex than this (Buckner et al., 2008). With ICA, a ventral-dorsal splitting of the posterior DMN has been demonstrated in several publications around the typical ICA decomposition dimensionality of 20–30 components (Damoiseaux et al., 2008; Kim et al., 2009). However, different DMN parcellations with ICA in three subnetworks have also been presented (Jafri et al., 2008; Assaf et al., 2010). Using methods other than ICA, DMN has been shown to fractionate in several ways (Buckner et al., 2008; Uddin et al., 2009; Andrews-Hanna et al., 2010; Leech et al., 2011) and the posteromedial cortex has been shown to present heterogeneous FC (Margulies et al., 2009; Dastjerdi et al., 2011).

The versatile DMN manifestation combinations suggest that it has a very dynamic constellation that is insufficiently depicted with static maps. However, in an attempt to delineate this complex spatiotemporal connectivity it could be useful to study the DMN appearance at varying ICA decomposition levels. High dimensional group ICA of around 70–100 components has been increasingly studied for resting state fMRI data (Malinen et al., 2007; Kiviniemi et al., 2009; Ystad et al., 2010; Abou Elseoud et al., 2011) and the highly parcellated components obtained have been shown to be in good correspondence with the parcellation of fMRI activation data (Smith et al., 2009). On the other hand, ICA has been demonstrated not to suffer from the usage of such high model order but instead from the use of too low model order, for single subject analysis (Esposito and Goebel, 2011) and for group analysis (Allen et al., 2012). Moreover, there are indications that the source separation between physiological noise sources and RSNs is better at higher dimensionality (Beall and Lowe, 2010; Starck et al., 2010).

Recently a serious concern has emerged about motion induced spurious signal changes contaminating the FC analysis. Some long-distance correlations in the brain have been shown to decrease due to subject motion and the elimination of timepoints indicated with excess motion by "scrubbing" has been proposed as a solution (Power et al., 2012). In a DMN seed correlation analysis with a large sample size, a small group-wise difference in motion has been shown to alter the FC results between the anterior and posterior brain regions (Van Dijk et al., 2012). Also in an ICA combined with dual-regression analysis motion has been found to impact the DMN estimates although differently between two studies (Mowinckel et al., 2012; Satterthwaite et al., 2012). Altogether the motion issue has led to speculations (Deen and Pelphrey, 2012) about the validity of the frontal-posterior hypoconnectivity theory in ASD as children and adolescents with ASDs have a tendency to move more than TD subjects during fMRI scanning.

In this study we aimed to map the resting state DMN connectivity in adolescents with ASDs by ICA using dimensionalities within the usual range and high dimensionality. The rationale behind the deployment of a multi-dimensional data-driven approach is to investigate different functional hierarchies that represent heterogeneity of the DMN connectivity. We investigated FC within and between default mode subnetworks (DM-SNs) with a specific interest in the ICA manifestation of the reported anterior-posterior hypoconnectivity (Schipul et al., 2011). Additionally, we carried out the motion scrubbing procedure as motion has been suspected to undermine the hypoconnectivity theory in ASD. The results were compared to analysis without scrubbing.

METHODS

PARTICIPANTS AND fMRI DATA

Thirty high-functioning adolescents with ASDs were gathered from a community-based study conducted between 2000 and 2003 (Mattila et al., 2007, 2011, 2012) and from a clinic-based study conducted in 2003 (Kuusikko et al., 2009; Mattila et al., 2009; Weiss et al., 2009). Further information about the screening and diagnostic process can be found from these earlier publications. Thirty age and gender-matched TD controls were recruited from mainstream schools in Oulu (Jansson-Verkasalo et al., 2005; Kuusikko et al., 2008). All participants and their parents gave written informed consent, and the study was approved by the Ethical Committee of the University Hospital of Oulu, Finland.

After the screening process the DSM-IV-TR criteria (APA, 2000) were used to construct the consensus ASD diagnoses based on the information gathered. The information for diagnostic examination in the clinic-based study consisted of the Autism Diagnostic Interview-Revised (ADI-R; Lord et al., 1995), Autism Diagnostic Observation Schedule—module 3 (ADOS; Lord et al., 2000), Wechsler Intelligence Scale for Children—Third revision (WISC-III; Wechsler, 1991) and medical records of Oulu University Hospital. In the community-based study the gathered information consisted additionally of school-day observations and teacher interviews for some of the individuals. The ADI-R and ADOS were not used to make diagnostic classifications in this study. Instead, these instruments were used to obtain structured information from parents and for semi-structured observation of a child. The physicians and a Master of Education graduate who participated in the diagnostic process had been trained in the use of the ADI-R and ADOS for research purposes, but inter-rater reliabilities had not been established. The full-scale IQ was greater than 75 for the participants with ASDs. The ASD individuals with Tourette's disorder or hyperkinesia were excluded based on interviews using the Schedule for Affective Disorders and Schizophrenia for School-Age Children (K-SADS-PL) (Kaufman et al., 1997) following DSM-IV-TR criteria. In addition, the subjects with ASDs included in the neuroimaging were not allowed to have any medications. Psychometric information to be used in the present study was gathered in 2003, 4 years before the MRI, with the Social Responsiveness Scale (SRS) (Constantino, 2002).

TD control participants were screened using the Autism Spectrum Screening Questionnaire (ASSQ) (Ehlers et al., 1999) to exclude those with clinically significant ASD symptoms. Other psychiatric disorders were screened using the K-SADS-PL. The IQ of the controls was not measured, however, all control participants attended mainstream elementary schools and in Finland the majority of mainstream schools' students in each class have normal range IQ and only few children with intellectual disabilities may be integrated into a mainstream class with the help of a personal assistant.

Imaging was carried out during 2007 using a GE 1.5 T HDX scanner equipped with an 8-channel head coil employing parallel imaging with an acceleration factor of 2. During the resting state scan the participants were asked to lie still, stay relaxed and awake and look at a white cross on the middle of a dark-gray screen. Within the MRI session the resting state was scanned before any task-fMRI scans. BOLD fMRI scanning of 7.5 min consisted of 253 whole brain volumes of which the first three were discarded due to T1 equilibrium effects. Parameters of the GR-EPI scanning employing parallel imaging were TR 1.8 s, TE 40 ms, flip angle 90°, FOV 256 mm, 64 × 64 in-plane matrix, 4 × 4 × 4 mm voxel size, 28 oblique axial slices with a 0.4 mm gap and interleaved acquisition order. Structural data were acquired using a T1-weighted 3D FSPGR sequence with 1 mm oblique axial slices, FOV 24.0 × 24.0 cm with a 256 × 256 matrix.

The study population was reduced during the imaging phase due to the following issues: one participant with ASD refused to undergo imaging in the MRI scanner room and the dataset of one participant with ASD was lost. One control participant had teeth braces and due to the resulting imaging artifacts the scanning was aborted. Two control participants were discarded due to suprathreshold ASSQ scores >7. There remained 28 high-functioning adolescents with ASDs and 27 TD individuals for the current study before exclusion of participants with too much motion during the resting state scan.

After omitting the datasets with excess motion the final sample consisted of 24 participants with ASDs (18 ♂, 6 ♀, age 14.9 ± 1.4, three left-handed) and 26 TD participants (19 ♂,7 ♀; age 14.8 ± 1.7; two left-handed). In the ASD group there were 17 participants diagnosed with Asperger syndrome and 7 with autism. Mean FSIQ was 107.3 ± 16.9 in the ASD group. The average SRS psychometric measures ($n = 21$, not available for all participants with ASD) were the following for the ASD group: SRS total 83.4, SRS subscales: awareness 10.1, Cognition 15.6, Communication 27.7, Motivation 12.9 and Mannerism 15.2.

DATA PRE-PROCESSING

Raw time-series were subjected to a stringent motion control procedure known as scrubbing (Power et al., 2012), using the fsl_motion_outliers-tool in FSL 5.0. The threshold value for time-point exclusion based on a framewise displacement metric was set to 0.20 mm, a proposed best practice threshold by Power et al. (2012). One time-point following the time-point with motion threshold exceeding was always removed from the time-series, a decision based on measured motion effects on global BOLD time-series (Satterthwaite et al., 2013). Actual removal of time-points was carried out for fully pre-processed time-series that were not low-pass filtered. High-motion subjects (4 ASD, 1 TD) with less than 4 min of data remaining after scrubbing were excluded from the analysis according to criteria by Satterthwaite et al. (2013). For the remaining sample the percentage of average scrubbed time-points was 13.5% for the ASD and 11.4% for the TD group.

The first actual pre-processing step was the spike removal from the time-series with the AFNI 3dDespike tool using default threshold settings. All other pre-processing was carried out using functions embedded into the MELODIC version 3.05 tool in the FSL 4.0 software package. Head motion was corrected using multi-resolution rigid body co-registration of volumes (MCFLIRT) (Jenkinson et al., 2002); the middle volume was the reference. Subsequently, slice timing correction and brain extraction was carried out for fMRI data with MELODIC pre-processing, brain extraction for structural data was performed separately using BET (Smith, 2002). Temporal high-pass filtering (cut-off frequency 0.01 Hz), Gaussian temporal low-pass filtering (half width at half maximum 2.8 s), and spatial filtering with a Gaussian kernel (5 mm FWHM) were performed. Every fMRI dataset was intensity normalized by a single scaling factor (grand mean scaling). Multi-resolution affine co-registration (Jenkinson and Smith, 2001) was used to co-register fMRI volumes with 6°-of-freedom to structural scans of corresponding subjects, and structural images were co-registered with 12°-of-freedom to the MNI standard structural space template with a resampling resolution of 4 mm.

FUNCTIONAL CONNECTIVITY ANALYSIS

Group ICA in temporal concatenation mode using the MELODIC ICA version 3.05 (Beckmann and Smith, 2004) was conducted for a range of dimensionalities: typical (20 and 30), and very high (100). Stopping criteria for the iterative algorithm was set to be fairly stringent 0.0000001 in order to produce more robust decomposition especially on the high dimensionality. The DM-SN selection procedure utilized spatial correlation between unitary DMN from low dimensionality ICA and target components. The ICA dimensionality producing a single DMN component was manually searched.

The dim = 100 decomposition was subjected to ICA repeatability analysis with ICASSO (Himberg et al., 2004). In this check it was ascertained that the analysis would be carried out for DM-SNs closely resembling the ICASSO cluster centroid components. On the dim = 100 ICASSO was performed 100 times as done previously (Kiviniemi et al., 2009) and with similar algorithm settings as those of the above single MELODIC runs. The ICASSO centroid decomposition could not be used in the following dual-regression since it resulted in spuriously similar time-series (cc ~0.98) for different components, probably due to violation of the linear independence assumption in the general linear model algorithm.

The resulting decompositions from single MELODIC runs including all motion and physiological noise components were used as a spatial a priori for the Dual Regression—FSL tool (Filippini et al., 2009) version 0.5, which provides subject-level spatial maps and time-courses of the components. The procedure involves first using the obtained group ICA spatial maps in a linear model fit against the individual fMRI data sets (spatial regression) resulting in time-courses specific for each independent component in each subject. Secondly, using variance normalized time-courses, subject-specific spatial maps are calculated voxel-by-voxel (temporal regression). Unlike the datasets that were used for ICA computation, the dataset fed to the dual-regression were generated in an otherwise similar manner but without low-pass filtering. Dual-regression analysis was performed for both motion scrubbed and full time-series.

In addition to the above within network FC with dual-regression, the between networks FC was studied using subject-level network time-courses provided by the first regression step in dual-regression. For the between network FC the zero-lag correlation coefficient was computed between the DM-SN time-series in Matlab 7.3 (http://www.mathworks.com). Correlation coefficients were Z-transformed before statistical testing.

STATISTICAL TESTING

In the dual-regression procedure the group-level statistical inference was carried out with a non-parametric test using FSL Randomise (Nichols and Holmes, 2002). The number of permutations was set to 5000. Threshold-free cluster enhancement (TFCE) (Smith and Nichols, 2009) was used to control for multiple comparison correction on each component separately with corrected probability of 0.05 determined as the significance threshold.

In statistical testing of the between network FC, the correlations between DM-SNs were hypothesized to be decreased in ASD. Testing was carried out with FSL Randomise with 10,000 permutations and multiple comparison correction with significance threshold of $p = 0.05$ determined over all DM-SN pairs separately on each ICA dimensionality.

In all of the above statistical tests the demeaned absolute and relative gross motion estimates from MCFLIRT were set as covariates of no interest. Absolute (referenced to middle time-point) and relative (compared to previous time-point) estimates are root-mean-square values of translational and rotational movements.

All FC measures that were found to be significant in the above group comparison were a subject of further covariance testing within the ASD group. Specifically, we tested the covariance of age in order to investigate the developmental aspect of the disorder. Also, covariance of the psychometric SRS measures with FC measures was tested.

RESULTS

MOTION DIFFERENCES

The group averages and group differences of root-mean-square motion estimates computed by FSL MCFLIRT (Jenkinson et al., 2002) were as follows:

- relative motion of 0.059 mm for TD and 0.061 mm for ASD ($p = 0.37$).
- absolute motion of 0.24 mm for TD and 0.37 mm for ASD ($p = 0.03$).

DM-SN SELECTION

The unitary DMN component to be used in the selection procedure was found with ICA dim = 8 (**Figure 1**).

- DM-SNs revealed from dim = 20 were clearly distinguishable as anterior (DMN-A) and posterior (DMN-P) weighted compartments.
- ICA decomposition at dim = 30 revealed three DM-SNs principally similar to those of the previous study (Damoiseaux et al., 2008) and they correlated about equally with the single DMN reference. As a general outline, the ICA-based DMN fractionation on this typical ICA dimensionality (dim = 30) is represented by the following division:
    - o DMN-A covering mainly the medial prefrontal cortex (MPFC)
    - o dorsal (DMN-D) with the main nodes in the central-posterior precuneus and in the PCC
    - o ventral (DMN-V) centered at the retrosplenial cortex.
- DM-SN selection at 100 components yielded five components of which DMN-D had the highest correlation to the reference DMN. The spatial distribution of the DM-SNs was more confined compared to the lower dimensional ICA results.
    - o DMN-A covering mainly the MPFC, more ventrally than at dim = 20/30
    - o DMN-D centered at the central-posterior precuneus and the PCC
    - o DMN-V centered at the retrosplenial cortex
    - o Right (DMN-R) covering mainly the right parietal lobule
    - o Left (DMN-L) covering the left parietal lobule.

ICASSO reliability estimates of the dim = 100 decomposition showed that the DM-SNs were reasonably robust. DM-SNs had high cluster quality indexes between 0.85 and 0.95 except DMN-R had a quality index of 0.70, which is still sufficiently repeatable. Decomposition from a single ICA run, which was used in the actual statistical analysis, showed good correspondence in the selected DM-SNs to the ICASSO centroid components. Spatial correlation coefficients of the DM-SNs were between 0.91 and 0.96 except for DMN-L, which was slightly lower at 0.80. Overall, these measures guaranteed the robustness of the DM-SNs used in the analysis.

FUNCTIONAL CONNECTIVITY WITHIN DM-SNs

In FC analysis with normal ICA / dual-regression procedure, neither significant nor even near-significant group differences were detected on any model order for the DM-SNs. In this regard the result was similar for analyses with and without scrubbing.

FUNCTIONAL CONNECTIVITY BETWEEN DM-SNs

ASD participants showed significantly lower temporal correlation between the anterior DM-SN and varying posterior DM-SNs on every tested ICA dimensionality (**Figure 2**, **Table 1**). Firstly, antero-posterior hypoconnectivity in ASD was found on dim = 20 between the two DM-SNs. On dim = 30 the hypoconnectivity was dispersed between two pairs: there was a significant difference in the DMN-A—DMN-D connection, plus a near significant difference in the DMN-A—DMN-V connection. Finally the details of the antero-posterior hypoconnectivity in ASD were specified with dim = 100 where the DMN-A—DMN-V connection turned out to be the only distinct group difference. The finding on dim = 100 also remained statistically significant ($p < 0.05$) after multiple comparison correction also over the three ICA dimensionalities.

Age was not found to significantly covary with the above findings of decreased antero-posterior DMN connectivity in the ASD

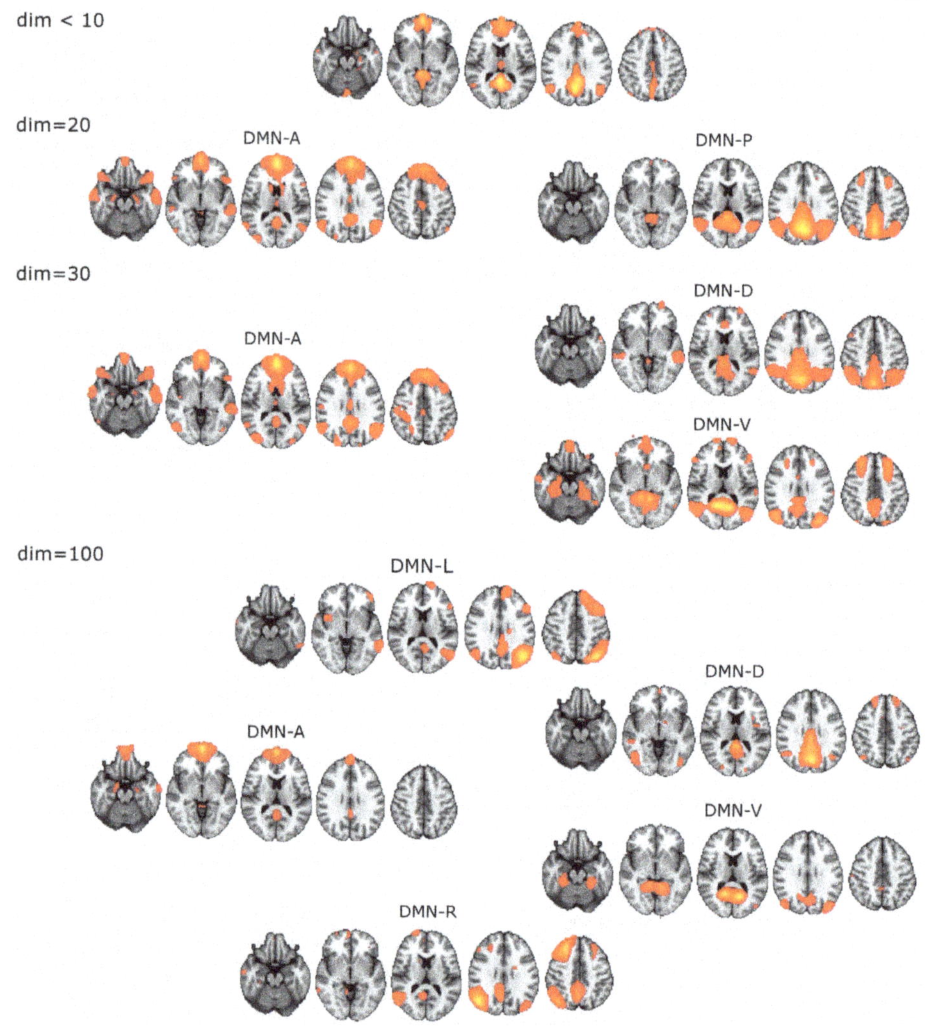

FIGURE 1 | Illustration of the DMN division into distinct DM-SNs presented across the studied ICA dimensionalities of 20, 30, and 100. First at dim = 20 the original low model order single DMN is split into anterior and posterior SNs and then the posterior SN is further split into dorsal and ventral components. At high dim = 100 clearly lateralized DMNs appear.

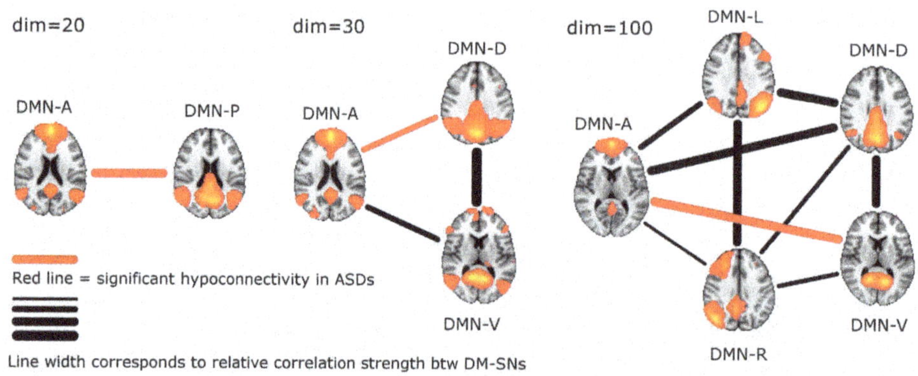

FIGURE 2 | The lines between DM-SNs illustrate the tested connections on varying ICA dimensionalities between the participants with ASDs and TDs. The red line denotes statistically significant hypoconnectivity in ASD between the nodes and the line width denotes the connection strength in the TD group (see **Table 1**).

Table 1 | The results of temporal correlation coefficients (Fisher Z-transformed) between DM-SNs with and without motion scrubbing.

ICA dim	20	30	30	30	100	100	100	100	100	100	100	100	100	100
DM-SN 1	A	A	A	D	A	A	D	A	A	D	D	V	V	L
DM-SN 2	P	D	V	V	D	V	V	L	R	L	R	L	R	R
WITH MOTION SCRUBBING														
TD mean cc	0.52	0.48	0.46	0.62	0.55	0.46	0.50	0.56	0.41	0.50	0.41	0.28	0.42	0.52
ASD mean cc	0.38	0.35	0.35	0.61	0.52	0.33	0.42	0.55	0.32	0.42	0.44	0.17	0.36	0.52
t-score	2.36	2.27	1.96	−0.38	0.12	2.81	1.10	0.46	1.20	0.85	−0.69	1.91	0.78	−0.23
p (corr.)	0.01	0.04	0.08	–	0.96	0.03	0.63	0.89	0.57	0.75	–	0.22	0.78	–
WITHOUT MOTION SCRUBBING														
TD mean cc	0.49	0.46	0.47	0.61	0.53	0.46	0.50	0.55	0.39	0.51	0.43	0.27	0.42	0.53
ASD mean cc	0.36	0.33	0.37	0.60	0.53	0.33	0.42	0.53	0.31	0.43	0.44	0.18	0.35	0.53
t-score	2.51	2.27	1.82	−0.33	−0.04	2.54	0.92	0.70	1.0	0.83	−0.67	1.77	0.87	−0.05
p (corr.)	0.009	0.04	0.10	–	–	0.06	0.70	0.82	0.68	0.74	–	0.28	0.74	–

Statistically significant differences between the ASD and TD groups are denoted with a gray cell background. Abbreviations of the DM-SNs: A, Anterior; P, Posterior; D, Dorsal; V, Ventral; L, Left; R, Right.

group. The relationship between connectivity and age was positive but the *p*-value close to one. Similarly, no signicant covariance between the antero-posterior FC measures with SRS total score or any of the SRS subscale scores was found. The relationship with the SRS total was slightly negative but the *p*-value was almost one.

Gross motion estimates were not found to reach statistical significance (results not shown) in co-variance with DM-SN correlations on any ICA dimensionality, with or without the scrubbing procedure. However, on dim = 100 the DMN-D—DMN-R correlation coefficient strength was near-significantly positively co-varying with motion estimates.

THE EFFECT OF MOTION SCRUBBING

The effect of motion scrubbing compared to full time-series analysis was studied for the FC between DM-SNs that were found to differ between the groups in the above analyses. The scrubbing procedure yielded somewhat greater group differences in some of the DMN antero-posterior connections, but decreases in others (**Table 1**). On average, the *t*-scores changed by 0.13 units while the maximum change was 0.27 units. The most influential increase was observed in dim = 100 where the DMN-A—DMN-V connection was statistically significantly greater in TDs compared to ASD participants after scrubbing, but just below the significance threshold without scrubbing.

DISCUSSION

The present ICA results with adolescent participants support the notion of antero-posterior DMN hypoconnectivity in ASD. The motion scrubbing only minimally altered the results over conventional methods. The result with high dimensional ICA showed a particularly interesting dissociation between anterior and ventral DMN nodes (**Figure 2**). Excluding limitations in physiological noise correction, our findings indicate that network level interplay is affected in adolescents with ASDs and indeed, interaction between distinct brain networks has been acknowledged as critical for understanding the cognitive and behavioral symptoms in ASD (Uddin and Menon, 2009). We did not detect any local DMN FC differences in ICA dual-regression analysis, which is in concordance with a recent whole brain analysis showing no changes in adult participants with ASDs (Tyszka et al., 2013). However, our FC analysis between DM-SN time-courses complements the study by Tyszka and colleagues by showing alterations in network-level interplay. A lack of local alterations in DMN suggests rather normal regional functionality in ASD. Age or symptom measures were not found to correlate with DMN hypoconnectivity.

Analysis results after motion scrubbing point out that the antero-posterior DMN hypoconnectivity in ASD does not emerge from motion artifact and thereby supports the hypoconnectivity theory in ASD. Motion scrubbing did not coherently alter the investigated DMN correlations across ICA dimensionality or across DM-SNs (**Table 1**). Overall, the additive effect of scrubbing was diminutive compared to ICA results with conventional methods of motion artefact suppression that included removal of considerably moving subjects and gross motion estimates as covariates in the statistical testing. Based on the present results, the ICA dual-regression carried out with conventional motion control measures is resilient against motion artefacts in static FC analysis. Motion scrubbing can presumably give slightly more accurate results but the changes are small in this context.

Local DMN FC alterations in ASD were not detected in our ICA dual-regression analysis, and even noteworthy supra-threshold differences could not be observed. The lack of differences slightly contradicts with earlier resting state studies reporting diverse findings (Kennedy and Courchesne, 2008; Monk et al., 2009; Weng et al., 2010), although the spatial extent of the findings was fairly small for instance in an ICA study of an adolescent ASD population (Assaf et al., 2010) that has the most comparable analysis to ours. The type of resting state scanning in these earlier studies was similar to ours, namely visual fixation, so the main dissimilarities remain in the analysis methods and in the heterogeneity of participants. In their recent study, (Tyszka et al., 2013) discuss reasons for possible overemphasis on group differences in earlier ASD studies. Such reasons may be targeting brain networks already thought to be abnormal (e.g., DMN), bias induced by prior task-fMRI on successive resting state scans, excess head motion in ASD and publication bias toward group differences. Additionally the sample characteristics will have an effect on the analysis outcome with probably more differences occurring with lower level of functioning and younger age in the sample. Although our study targeted the DMN and participants were relatively young, there were no local differences in ICA dual-regression. In the present study there were also aspects that made the groups more equal: resting state data were acquired before any task-fMRI scans eliminating cognitive carry-over effects, and the effect of motion was practically eliminated in the analysis.

During the preparation of the present study new results on default mode FC in ASD have been published with findings indicating that the "underconnectivity" theory of ASD is too simplistic and that ASD has to be considered more from a developmental viewpoint. Nevertheless, the findings of the present study did not correlate with age, nor was there any DMN hyper-connectivity observed in ASD. In other studies the findings also do not seem fully consistent, although comparison is difficult due to varying methodology. In young children (7–12 years) there was mainly increased FC found in the DMN (Lynch et al., 2013). On the other hand, in another study utilizing the rest periods from task-fMRI, the older half (10–17 years) of the population clearly presented decreased FC between DM-SNs (also between PCC and MPFC), while in the younger half (6–9 years) the decreases were more subtle (Washington et al., 2013). Finally, in adult participants with ASDs no marked FC differences at the whole brain level were found either with atlas-based inter-regional correlation or ICA dual-regression analyses (Tyszka et al., 2013). Overall, the FC results in the literature seem relatively variable still and it remains to be conclusively determined how DMN connectivity alters during the developmental stages in ASD.

DM-SN time-series' correlations (**Table 1**) demonstrated clearly lowered DMN connectivity in those with ASDs between DMN-A and DMN-P at dim = 20 and between DMN-A and DMN-D at dim = 30. However, at dim = 100 dysconnectivity was detected between DMN-A and DMN-V with more confined DMN parcellations. This finding does not conflict with those at lower model orders since the connectivity in the DMN-A—DMN-V—pair was already near-significant ($p = 0.08$) at dim = 30. Interestingly though, the DMN-A—DMN-D connectivity was very similar for the TD and ASD groups at dim = 100, which is a prominent difference compared to lower dimensionalities. This altering result pattern across dimensionalities is certainly related to the correspondingly changing spatial DMN characteristics. A major difference in DM-SN constellations is that the parietal lobule connectivity at dim = 100 is dedicated to DMN-L and DMN-R, and largely eliminated from DMN-D compared to dim = 30. Secondly, DMN-A is more ventrally weighted at dim = 100.

Our attempt to relate the findings to ASD symptoms as measured by SRS scores (obtained 4 years prior to MRI) did not give any indications about relevant symptoms. Also, interpreting the altered resting state antero-posterior DMN connectivity via psychological processes is challenging due to the various cognitive functions that have often simultaneously been attributed to both the anterior and posterior DMN nodes (e.g., Schilbach et al., 2008). However, our DM-SN constellation from dim = 100 decomposition is highly similar to a compelling study by Andrews-Hanna et al. (2010) wherein the DMN FC was mapped in the resting state and the relation of several tasks on the self-relevancy and present-future axis to the DMN were investigated. The DMN was split into anterior and posterior midline core nodes (vs. DMN-D and DMN-A) and into two distinct subsystems termed the medial temporal lobe (MTL) subsystem (vs. DMN-V) and the dorsal medial prefrontal cortex (dMPFC) subsystem (vs. combined DMN-R and DMN-L). Core midline nodes DMN-D and DMN-A are active during tasks related to present and future self whereas DMN-V is particularly related to future self, not present self. In more detail, the fMRI stimulus variables that disentangle DMN-V from core nodes include memory, imagination and spatial content. As a summary, the combination of anterior, dorsal, and ventral DM-SNs was most prominently activated when the subject was thinking about themself in the future (Andrews-Hanna et al., 2010). Intriguingly, the decreased coupling between DMN-V and DMN-A could be linked to delayed imaginative play, another symptom in autism (Levy et al., 2009), as imagination and self-referential processing are elementary for such activity. Also related to our main finding, autobiographical episodic memory and self-referential processing in the past temporal domain are particularly impaired in those with ASDs (Lind, 2010). Our findings indicate the need for brain imaging studies of autobiographical memory in people with ASDs as earlier noted by Uddin (2011).

The antero-posterior DMN dissociation has also been robustly shown in aging and wide domain decline in the cognitive performance of older adults is associated with this finding too (Andrews-Hanna et al., 2007). Interestingly, a psychedelic state induced by psilocybin manifests as a significant decoupling in antero-posterior DMN connectivity, implying that the DMN has an imperative role in cognitive integration (Carhart-Harris et al., 2012). The reverse finding of increased antero-posterior DMN connectivity with ICA has been reported in schizophrenia (Jafri et al., 2008). Altogether these studies and our findings again emphasize the central role of the DMN in sound function of the brain.

In task-fMRI the DMN brain regions are known to normally deactivate during the task and activate during rest periods. However, diminished DMN deactivation in diverse task-fMRI studies has been a characteristic finding for participants with ASDs (Kennedy et al., 2006; Murdaugh et al., 2012; Rahko et al., 2012; Spencer et al., 2012; Christakou et al., 2013). From task-fMRI studies it is not straightforward to conclude whether abnormal baseline activity or failure to deactivate is the ultimate driver for group differences, but our results support the view that DMN connectivity is already altered at baseline.

In our previous diffusion tensor imaging study (Bode et al., 2011), with almost the same participants with ASDs as the present study, a decreased diffusivity in the transverse direction was detected in the inferior fronto-occipital fasciculus. That fiber formation directly connects the IPL of DMN-V with the MPFC of DMN-A. Inferior fronto-occipital fasciculus is also in close connection with the RSC, a main node of DMN-V, which provides a potential structural explanation for our decreased FC findings in DMN.

The investigation of optimally determined ICA model order is a persistent topic in resting state connectivity research, but our aim was to study the DMN connectivity at very different dimensionalities without restricting the analysis on one data representation. The unitary DMN obtained from very low ICA dimensionality is highly similar to the conjunction analysis result of several DMN seed correlations (Fox et al., 2005). The diverse DMN manifestations demonstrated also in the present study suggests that if one aims to study the DMN FC with temporal-concatenation based group ICA, either very low dimensionality (<10) should be used or several DM-SNs should be incorporated into the analysis already at around typical 20–30 dimensionality. A high dimensional group ICA has a disadvantage that component estimates become more variable across ICA runs and less generalizable across subjects (Pendse et al., 2012), and also the risk of unwanted component splitting arises due to inter-individual spatial variability (Allen et al., 2012). However, high dimensionality has been found to be useful, for example, in a group ICA based fMRI data classification study comparing a wide range of dimensionalities (Duff et al., 2012), it was found that prediction accuracy was highest using 80 or more components. The prediction accuracy did not deteriorate when using even several 100 components. Based on our earlier investigations (e.g., Abou-Elseoud et al., 2010) regarding DMN core regions, DM-SNs seem to converge to a relatively stable decomposition at very high model orders, which supports the validity of analysis on such decomposition.

A limitation of the present study is the lack of specific subject-level control over physiological signal sources, although on the group level, the ICA dual regression procedure models physiological noise with a wide set of spatial components.. If there are systematic differences between ASD and TD groups in the physiological noise processes, they might account for the observed DMN hypoconnectivity in ASDs. Mixing of physiological nuisance sources with RSNs of interest has also been shown to occur on the DMN (Birn et al., 2008) but less on high ICA dimensionality (Beall and Lowe, 2010; Starck et al., 2010). Therefore, the fact that the differences are potentiated at high ICA dimensionality support our findings. Also, physiological noise signal strength is less in our 1.5 T data as compared to 3 T data (Krüger et al., 2001). Additionally, recently the ICA dual-regression procedure without explicit physiological correction was shown to produce robust DMNs that were not notably different for physiologically corrected (RETROICOR or RVHRCOR) data (Khalili-Mahani et al., 2013).

In conclusion, we have shown antero-posterior hypoconnectivity in ASD despite additional elimination of motion effects by means of motion scrubbing. Detailed views on the altered DMN connectivity in adolescents with ASDs were obtained by multi-dimensional ICA analysis and the results suggest that the aberrant FC manifests particularly in the network-level interplay rather than in local abnormalities. In particular, high ICA dimensionality analysis showed a significant decrease of aDMN—vDMN connectivity in ASD. Our findings of resting state DMN dissociation in adolescents with ASDs could be related to deficits in autobiographical memory and self-referential processing, which provides an interesting future prospect in autism research.

ACKNOWLEDGMENTS

We wish to thank the adolescents and their families for participating. This study received financial support from the Alma and K. A. Snellman Foundation, Oulu, Finland, the Child Psychiatric Research Foundation, Finland, the Emil Aaltonen Foundation, Finland, the Rinnekoti Research Foundation, Espoo, Finland, the Sigrid Jusélius Foundation, Finland and the Thule Institute, Oulu, Finland. This study was funded by Finnish Academy Grant #117111 and Finnish Medical Foundation grants. The Graduate School of Circumpolar Wellbeing Health and Adaptation is acknowledged for its support. We would also like to thank the National Alliance for Autism Research for financial support granted to Prof David Pauls.

REFERENCES

Abou Elseoud, A., Littow, H., Remes, J., Starck, T., Nikkinen, J., Nissilä, J., et al. (2011). Group-ICA model order highlights patterns of functional brain connectivity. Front. Syst. Neurosci. 5:37. doi: 10.3389/fnsys.2011.00037

Abou-Elseoud, A., Starck, T., Remes, J., Nikkinen, J., Tervonen, O., and Kiviniemi, V. J. (2010). The effect of model order selection in group PICA. Hum. Brain Mapp. 31, 1207–1216. doi: 10.1002/hbm.20929

Allen, E. A., Erhardt, E. B., Wei, Y., Eichele, T., and Calhoun, V. D. (2012). Capturing inter-subject variability with group independent component analysis of fMRI data: a simulation study. Neuroimage 59, 4141–4159. doi: 10.1016/j.neuroimage.2011.10.010

American Psychiatric Association (APA). (2000). Diagnostic and Statistical Manual of Mental Disorders: DSM-IV-TR, 4th Edn, text revision. Washington, DC: American Psychiatric Association. doi: 10.1176/appi.books.9780890423349

Anderson, J. S., Nielsen, J. A., Froehlich, A. L., DuBray, M. B., Druzgal, T. J., Cariello, A. N., et al. (2011). Functional connectivity magnetic resonance imaging classification of autism. Brain 134, 3742–3754. doi: 10.1093/brain/ awr263

Andreasen, N. C., O'Leary, D. S., Cizadlo, T., Arndt, S., Rezai, K., Watkins, G. L., et al. (1995). Remembering the past: two facets of episodic memory explored with positron emission tomography. Am. J. Psychiatry 152, 1576–1585.

Andrews-Hanna, J. R., Snyder, A. Z., Vincent, J. L., Lustig, C., Head, D., Raichle, M. E., et al. (2007). Disruption of large-scale brain systems in advanced aging. Neuron 56, 924–935. doi: 10.1016/j.neuron.2007.10.038

Andrews-Hanna, J. R., Reidler, J., Sepulcre, R., Poulin, C., and Buckner, R. L. (2010). Functional-anatomic Fractionation of the Brain's default network. Neuron 65, 550–562. doi: 10.1016/j.neuron.2010.02.005

Assaf, M., Jagannathan, K., Calhoun, V. D., Miller, L., Stevens, M. C., Sahl, R., et al. (2010). Abnormal functional connectivity of default mode sub-networks in autism spectrum disorder patients. Neuroimage 53, 247–256. doi: 10.1016/j.neuroimage.2010.05.067

Beall, E. B., and Lowe, M. J. (2010). The non-separability of physiologic noise in functional connectivity MRI with spatial ICA at 3T. J. Neurosci. Methods 191, 263–276. doi: 10.1016/j.jneumeth.2010.06.024

Beckmann, C. F., and Smith, S. M. (2004). Probabilistic independent component analysis for functional magnetic resonance imaging. IEEE Trans. Med. Imaging 23, 137–152. doi: 10.1109/TMI.2003.822821

Birn, R. M., Murphy, K., and Bandettini, P. A. (2008). The effect of respiration variations on independent component analysis results of resting state functional connectivity. Hum. Brain Mapp. 29, 740–750. doi: 10.1002/hbm.20577

Bode, M. K., Mattila, M.-L., Kiviniemi, V., Rahko, J., Moilanen, I., Ebeling, H., et al. (2011). White matter in autism spectrum disorders - evidence of impaired fiber formation. Acta Radiol. 52, 1169–1174. doi: 10.1258/ar.2011.110197

Buckner, R. L., Andrews-Hanna, J. R., and Schacter, D. L. (2008). The brain's default network: anatomy, function, and relevance to disease. Ann. N.Y. Acad. Sci. 1124, 1–38. doi: 10.1196/annals.1440.011

Calhoun, V. D., Adali, T., Pearlson, G. D., and Pekar, J. J. (2001). A method for making group inferences from functional MRI data using independent component analysis. Hum. Brain Mapp. 14, 140–151.

doi: 10.1002/hbm.1048

Calhoun, V. D., Kiehl, K. A., and Pearlson, G. D. (2008). Modulation of temporally coherent brain networks estimated using ICA at rest and during cognitive tasks. Hum. Brain Mapp. 29, 828–838. doi: 10.1002/hbm.20581

Carhart-Harris, R. L., Leech, R., Erritzoe, D., Williams, T. M., Stone, J. M., Evans, J., et al. (2012). Functional connectivity measures after psilocybin inform a novel hypothesis of early psychosis. Schizophr. Bull. 39, 1343–1351. doi: 10.1093/schbul/sbs117

Cherkassky, V. L., Kana, R. K., Keller, T. A., and Just, M. A. (2006). Functional connectivity in a baseline resting-state network in autism. Neuroreport 17, 1687–1690. doi: 10.1097/01.wnr.0000239956.45448.4c

Christakou, A., Murphy, C. M., Chantiluke, K., Cubillo, A. I., Smith, A. B., Giampietro, V., et al. (2013). Disorder-specific functional abnormalities during sustained attention in youth with Attention Deficit Hyperactivity Disorder (ADHD) and with autism. Mol. Psychiatry 18, 236–244. doi: 10.1038/mp. 2011.185

Constantino, J. N. (2002). The Social Responsiveness Scale. Los Angeles, CA: Western Psychological Services.

Damoiseaux, J. S., Beckmann, C. F., Arigita, E. J., Barkhof, F., Scheltens, P., Stam, C. J., et al. (2008). Reduced resting-state brain activity in the "default network" in normal aging. Cereb. Cortex 18, 1856–1864. doi: 10.1093/cercor/bhm207

Dastjerdi, M., Foster, B. L., Nasrullah, S., Rauschecker, A. M., Dougherty, R. F., Townsend, J. D., et al. (2011). Differential electrophysiological response during rest, self-referential, and non-self-referential tasks in human posteromedial cortex. Proc. Natl. Acad. Sci. U.S.A. 108, 3023–3028. doi: 10.1073/pnas.1017098108

Deen, B., and Pelphrey, K. (2012). Perspective: Brain scans need a rethink. Nature 491:S20. doi: 10.1038/491S20a

Duff, E. P., Trachtenberg, A. J., Mackay, C. E., Howard, M. A., Wilson, F., Smith, S. M., et al. (2012). Task-driven ICA feature generation for accurate and interpretable prediction using fMRI. Neuroimage 60, 189–203. doi: 10.1016/j.neuroimage.2011.12.053

Ehlers, S., Gillberg, C., and Wing, L. (1999). A screening guestionnaire for asperger syndrome and other high-functioning autism spectrum disorders in school age children. J. Autism Dev. Disord. 29, 129–141. doi: 10.1023/A:1023040610384

Esposito, F., and Goebel, R. (2011). Extracting functional networks with spatial independent component analysis: the role of dimensionality, reliability and aggregation scheme. Curr. Opin. Neurol. 24, 378–385. doi: 10.1097/WCO.0b013e32834897a5

Filippini, N., MacIntosh, B. J., Hough, M. G., Goodwin, G. M., Frisoni, G. B., Smith, S. M., et al. (2009). Distinct patterns of brain activity in young carriers of the APOE-epsilon4 allele. Proc. Natl. Acad. Sci. U.S.A. 106, 7209–7214. doi: 10.1073/pnas.0811879106

Fox, M. D., Snyder, A. Z., Vincent, J. L., Corbetta, M., Van Essen, D. C., and Raichle, M. E. (2005). The human brain is intrinsically organized into dynamic, anticor- related functional networks. Proc. Natl. Acad. Sci. U.S.A. 102, 9673–9678. doi: 10.1073/pnas.0504136102

Himberg, J., Hyvärinen, A., and Esposito, F. (2004). Validating the independent components of neuroimaging time series via clustering and visualization. Neuroimage 22, 1214–2122. doi: 10.1016/j.neuroimage.2004.03.027

Horwitz, B., Rumsey, J. M., Grady, C. L., and Rapoport, S. I. (1988). The cerebral metabolic landscape in autism. Intercorrelations of regional glucose utilization. Arch. Neurol. 45, 749–755. doi: 10.1001/archneur.1988.0052031 0055018

Jafri, M. J., Pearlson, G. D., Stevens, M., and Calhoun, V. D. (2008). A method for functional network connectivity among spatially independent resting-state components in schizophrenia. Neuroimage 39, 1666–1681. doi: 10.1016/j.neuroimage.2007.11.001

Jansson-Verkasalo, E., Kujala, T., Jussila, K., Mattila, M. L., Moilanen, I., Näätänen, R., et al. (2005). Similarities in the phenotype of the auditory neural substrate in children with Asperger syndrome and their parents. Eur. J. Neurosci. 22, 986–990. doi: 10.1111/j.1460-9568.2005.04216.x

Jenkinson, M., Bannister, P., Brady, M., and Smith, S. (2002). Improved optimization for the robust and accurate linear registration and motion correction of brain images. Neuroimage 17, 825–841. doi: 10.1006/nimg.2002.1132

Jenkinson, M., and Smith, S. (2001). A global optimisation method for robust affine registration of brain images. Med. Image Anal. 5, 143–156. doi: 10.1016/S1361-8415(01)00036-6

Just, M. A., Cherkassky, V. L., Keller, T. A., and Minshew, N. J. (2004). Cortical activation and synchronization during sentence comprehension in high- functioning autism: evidence of underconnectivity. Brain 127, 1811–1821. doi: 10.1093/brain/awh199

Just, M. A., Cherkassky, V. L., Keller, T. A., Kana, R. K., and Minshew, N. J. (2007). Functional and anatomical cortical underconnectivity in autism: evidence from an FMRI study of an executive function task and corpus callosum morphometry. Cereb. Cortex 17, 951–961. doi: 10.1093/cercor/bhl006

Kaufman, J., Birmaher, B., Brent, D., Rao, U., Flynn, C., Moreci, P., et al. (1997). Schedule for affective disorders and schizophrenia for school-age children- present and lifetime version (K-SADSPL): initial reliability and validity data. J. Am. Acad. Child Adolesc. Psychiatry 36, 980–988. doi: 10.1097/00004583- 199707000-00021

Kennedy, D. P., and Courchesne, E. (2008). The intrinsic functional organi- zation of the brain is altered in autism. Neuroimage 39, 1877–1885. doi: 10.1016/j.neuroimage.2007.10.052

Kennedy, D. P., Redcay, E., and Courchesne, E. (2006). Failing to deactivate: resting functional abnormalities in autism. Proc. Natl. Acad. Sci. U.S.A. 103, 8275–8280. doi: 10.1073/pnas.0600674103

Khalili-Mahani, N., Chang, C., van Osch, M. J., Veer, I. M., van Buchem, M. A., Dahan, A., et al. (2013). The impact of "physiological correction" on functional connectivity analysis of pharmacological resting state fMRI. Neuroimage 65, 499–510. doi: 10.1016/j.neuroimage.2012.09.044

Kim, D. I., Manoach, D. S., Mathalon, D. H., Turner, J. A., Mannell, M., Brown, G. G., et al. (2009). Dysregulation of working memory and default-mode networks in schizophrenia using independent component analysis, an fBIRN and MCIC study. Hum. Brain Mapp. 30, 3795–3811. doi: 10.1002/hbm.20807

Kiviniemi, V., Starck, T., Remes, J., Long, X., Nikkinen, J., Haapea, M., et al. (2009). Functional segmentation of the brain cortex using high model order group PICA. Hum. Brain Mapp. 30, 3865–3886. doi: 10.1002/hbm.20813

Krüger, G., Kastrup, A., and Glover, G. H. (2001). Neuroimaging at 1.5 T and 3.0 T: comparison of oxygenation-sensitive magnetic resonance imaging. Magn. Reson. Med. 45, 595–604. doi: 10.1002/mrm.1081

Kuusikko, S., Haapsamo, H., Jansson-Verkasalo, E., Hurtig, T., Mattila, M. L., Ebeling, H., et al. (2009). Emotion recognition in children and adolescents with autism spectrum disorders. J. Autism Dev. Disord. 39, 938–945. doi: 10.1007/s10803-009-0700-0

Kuusikko, S., Pollock-Wurman, R., Jussila, K., Carter, A. S., Mattila, M. L., Ebeling, H., et al. (2008). Social anxiety in high-functioning children and adolescents with autism and asperger syndrome. J. Autism Dev. Disord. 38, 1697–1709. doi: 10.1007/s10803-008-0555-9

Leech, R., Kamourieh, S., Beckmann, C. F., and Sharp, D. J. (2011). Fractionating the default mode network: distinct contributions of the ventral and dorsal posterior cingulate cortex to cognitive control. J. Neurosci. 31, 3217–3224. doi: 10.1523/JNEUROSCI.5626-10.2011

Levy, S. E., Mandell, D. S., and Schultz, R. T. (2009). Autism. Lancet 7, 1627–1638. doi: 10.1016/S0140-6736(09)61376-3

Lind, S. E. (2010). Memory and the self in autism: A review and theoretical framework. Autism 14, 430–456. doi: 10.1177/1362361309358700

Lord, C., Rutter, M., DiLavore, P. C., and Risi, S. (2000). Autism Diagnostic Observation Schedule (ADOS). Los Angeles, CA: Western Psychological Services. Lord, C., Rutter, M., and LeCouteur, A. (1995). Autism Diagnostic Interview–Revised, 3rd Edn. Los Angeles, CA: Western psychological services.

Lynch, C. J., Uddin, L. Q., Supekar, K., Khouzam, A., Phillips, J., and Menon, V. (2013). Default mode network in childhood autism: posteromedial cortex het rogeneity and relationship with social deficits. Biol. Psychiatry 74, 212–219. doi: 10.1016/j.biopsych.2012.12.013

Malinen, S., Hlushchuk, Y., and Hari, R. (2007). Towards natural stimulation in fMRI–issues of data analysis. Neuroimage 35, 131–139. doi: 10.1016/j.neuroimage.2006.11.015 •

Margulies, D. S., Vincent, J. L., Kelly, C., Lohmann, G., Uddin, L. Q., Biswal, B. B., et al. (2009). Precuneus shares intrinsic functional architecture in humans and monkeys. Proc. Natl. Acad. Sci. U.S.A. 106, 20069–20074. doi: 10.1073/pnas.0905314106

Marrelec, G., and Fransson, P. (2011). Assessing the influence of different ROI selection strategies on functional connectivity analyses of fMRI data acquired during steady-state conditions. PLoS

ONE 6:e14788. doi: 10.1371/journal.pone.0014788

Mattila, M.-L., Jussila, K., Kuusikko, S., Kielinen, M., Linna, S.-L., Ebeling, H., et al. (2009). When does the Autism Spectrum Screening Questionnaire (ASSQ) predict autism spectrum disorders in primary school-aged children? Eur. Child Adolesc. Psychiatry 18, 499–509. doi: 10.1007/s00787-009- 0044-5

Mattila, M.-L., Jussila, K., Linna, S. L., Kielinen, M., Ebeling, H., Joseph, R. M., et al. (2012). Validation of the Finnish Autism Spectrum Screening Questionnaire (ASSQ) for clinical settings and total population screening. J. Autism Dev. Disord. 42, 2162–2180. doi: 10.1007/s10803-012-1464-5

Mattila, M.-L., Kielinen, M., Jussila, K., Linna, S.-L., Bloigu, R., Ebeling, H., et al. (2007). An epidemiological and diagnostic study of Asperger syndrome according to four sets of diagnostic criteria. J. Am. Acad. Child Adolesc. Psychiatry 46, 636–646. doi: 10.1097/chi.0b013e318033ff42

Mattila, M.-L., Kielinen, M., Linna, S. L., Jussila, K., Ebeling, H., Bloigu, R., et al. (2011). Autism spectrum disorders according to DSM-IV-TR and comparison with DSM-5 draft criteria: an epidemiological study. J. Am. Acad. Child Adolesc. Psychiatry 50, 583–592. doi: 10.1016/j.jaac.2011.04.001

Monk, C. S., Peltier, S. J., Wiggins, J. L., Weng, S. J., Carrasco, M., Risi, S., et al. (2009). Abnormalities of intrinsic functional connectivity in autism spectrum disorders. Neuroimage 47, 764–772. doi: 10.1016/j.neuroimage.2009.04.069

Mowinckel, A. M., Espeseth, T., and Westlye, L. T. (2012). Network-specific effects of age and in-scanner subject motion: a resting-state fMRI study of 238 healthy adults. Neuroimage 63, 1364–1373. doi: 10.1016/j.neuroimage.2012.08.004

Murdaugh, D. L., Shinkareva, S. V., Deshpande, H. R., Wang, J., Pennick, M. R., and Kana, R. K. (2012). Differential deactivation during mentalizing and classification of autism based on default mode network connectivity. PLoS One 7:e50064. doi: 10.1371/journal.pone.0050064

Nichols, T. E., and Holmes, A. P. (2002). Nonparametric permutation tests for functional neuroimaging: a primer with examples. Hum. Brain Mapp. 15, 1–25. doi: 10.1002/hbm.1058

Pendse, G. V., Borsook, D., and Becerra, L. (2012). A simple and objective method for reproducible resting state network (RSN) detection in fMRI. PLoS ONE 6:e27594. doi: 10.1371/journal.pone.0027594

Power, J. D., Barnes, K. A., Snyder, A. Z., Schlaggar, B. L., and Petersen, S. E. (2012). Spurious but systematic correlations in functional connectivity MRI networks arise from subject motion. Neuroimage 59, 2142–2154. doi: 10.1016/j.neuroimage.2011.10.018

Rahko, J. S., Paakki, J. J., Starck, T. H., Nikkinen, J., Pauls, D. L., Kätsyri, J. V., et al. (2012). Valence scaling of dynamic facial expressions is altered in high-functioning subjects with autism spectrum disorders: an fMRI study. J. Autism Dev. Disord. 42, 1011–1024. doi: 10.1007/s10803-011-1332-8

Satterthwaite, T. D., Elliott, M. A., Gerraty, R. T., Ruparel, K., Loughead, J., Calkins, M. E., et al. (2013). An improved framework for confound regression and filtering for control of motion artifact in the preprocessing of resting-state functional connectivity data. Neuroimage 64, 240–256. doi: 10.1016/j.neuroimage.2012.08.052

Satterthwaite, T. D., Wolf, D. H., Loughead, J., Ruparel, K., Elliott, M. A., Hakonarson, H., et al. (2012). Impact of in-scanner head motion on multiple measures of functional connectivity: relevance for studies of neurodevelopment in youth. Neuroimage 60, 623–632. doi: 10.1016/j.neuroimage.2011. 12.063 Schilbach, L., Eickhoff, S. B., Rotarska-Jagiela, A., Fink, G. R., and Vogeley, K. (2008). Minds at rest? Social cognition as the default mode of cognizing and its putative relationship to the "default system" of the brain. Conscious. Cogn. 17, 457–467. doi: 10.1016/j.concog.2008.03.013

Schipul, S. E., Keller, T. A., and Just, M. A. (2011). Inter-regional brain communication and its disturbance in autism. Front. Syst. Neurosci. 5:10. doi: 10.3389/fnsys.2011.00010

Smith, S. M. (2002). Fast robust automated brain extraction. Hum. Brain Mapp. 17, 143–155. doi: 10.1002/hbm.10062

Smith, S. M., Fox, P. T., Miller, K. L., Glahn, D. C., Fox, P. M., Mackay, C. E., et al. (2009). Correspondence of the brain's functional architecture during activation and rest. Proc. Natl. Acad. Sci. U.S.A. 106, 13040–13045. doi: 10.1073/pnas.0905267106

Smith, S. M., and Nichols, T. (2009). Threshold-free cluster enhancement: addressing problems of smoothing, threshold dependence and localisation in cluster inference. Neuroimage 44, 83–98. doi: 10.1016/j.neuroimage.2008.03.061

Spencer, M. D., Chura, L. R., Holt, R. J., Suckling, J., Calder, A. J., Bullmore, E. T., et al. (2012). Failure to deactivate the default mode network indicates a possible endophenotype of autism. Mol. Autism 3:15. doi: 10.1186/2040-2392-3-15

Starck, T., Remes, J., Nikkinen, J., Tervonen, O., and Kiviniemi, V. (2010). Correction of low-frequency physiological noise from the resting state BOLD fMRI–Effect on ICA default mode analysis at 1.5 T. J. Neurosci. Methods 186, 179–185. doi: 10.1016/j.jneumeth.2009.11.015

Tyszka, J. M., Kennedy, D. P., Paul, L. K., and Adolphs, R. (2013). Largely typical patterns of resting-state functional connectivity in high-functioning adults with autism. Cereb. Cortex doi: 10.1093/cercor/bht040. [Epub ahead of print].

Uddin, L. Q. (2011). The self in autism: an emerging view from neuroimaging. Neurocase 17, 201–208. doi: 10.1080/13554794.2010.509320

Uddin, L. Q., Kelly, A. M., Biswal, B. B., Xavier Castellanos, F., and Milham, M. P. (2009). Functional connectivity of default mode network components: cor- relation, anticorrelation, and causality. Hum. Brain Mapp. 30, 625–637. doi: 10.1002/hbm.20531

Uddin, L. Q., and Menon, V. (2009). The anterior insula in autism: under-connected and under-examined. Neurosci. Biobehav. Rev. 33, 1198–1203. doi: 10.1016/j.neubiorev.2009.06.002

Van Dijk, K. R., Sabuncu, M. R., and Buckner, R. L. (2012). The influence of head motion on intrinsic functional connectivity MRI. Neuroimage 59, 431–438. doi: 10.1016/j.neuroimage.2011.07.044

Washington, S. D., Gordon, E. M., Brar, J., Warburton, S., Sawyer, A. T., Wolfe, A., et al. (2013). Dysmaturation of the default mode network in autism. Hum. Brain Mapp. doi: 10.1002/hbm.22252. [Epub ahead of print].

Wechsler, D. (1991). Wechsler Intelligence Scale for Children (WISCIII), 3rd Edn. New York, NY: The Psychological Corporation.

Weiss, L. A., Arking, D. E., Gene Discovery Project of Johns Hopkins, and the Autism Consortium, Daly, M. J., and Chakravarti, A. (2009). A genome-wide linkage and association scan reveals novel loci for autism. Nature 461, 802–808. doi: 10.1038/nature08490

Weng, S.-J., Lee Wiggins, J., Peltier, S. J., Carrasco, M., Risi, S., Lord, C., et al. (2010). Alterations of resting state functional connectivity in the default net- work in adolescents with autism spectrum disorders. Brain Res. 1313, 202–214. doi: 10.1016/j.brainres.2009.11.057

Wiggins, J. L., Bedoyan, J. K., Peltier, S. J., Ashinoff, S., Carrasco, M., Weng, S. J., et al. (2012). The impact of serotonin transporter (5-HTTLPR) geno-type on the development of resting-state functional connectivity in children and adolescents: a preliminary report. Neuroimage 59, 2760–2770. doi: 10.1016/j.neuroimage.2011.10.030

Ystad, M., Eichele, T., Lundervold, A. J., and Lundervold, A. (2010). Subcortical functional connectivity and verbal episodic memory in healthy elderly–a resting state fMRI study. Neuroimage 52, 379–388. doi: 10.1016/j.neuroimage.2010.03.062

15

Approaches to local connectivity in autism using resting state functional connectivity MRI

Jose O. Maximo[1], Christopher L. Keown[1,2], Aarti Nair[1,3] and Ralph-Axel Müller[1]*

[1] *Brain Development Imaging Laboratory, Department of Psychology, San Diego State University, San Diego, CA, USA*
[2] *Computational Science Research Center, San Diego State University, San Diego, CA, USA*
[3] *Joint Doctoral Program in Clinical Psychology, San Diego State University and University of California at San Diego, San Diego, CA, USA*

Edited by:
Lucina Q. Uddin, Stanford University, USA

Reviewed by:
Chandan J. Vaidya, Georgetown University, USA
Jeffrey D. Rudie, University of California at Los Angeles, USA

****Correspondence:***
Ralph-Axel Müller, Brain Development Imaging Laboratory, Department of Psychology, San Diego State University, 6363 Alvarado Court, Suite 200, San Diego, CA 92120, USA
e-mail: rmueller@mail.sdsu.edu

While the literature on aberrant long-distance connectivity in autism spectrum disorder (ASD) has grown fast over the past decade, little is known about local connectivity. We used regional homogeneity and local density approaches at different spatial scales to examine local connectivity in 29 children and adolescents with ASD and 29 matched typically developing participants, using resting state functional magnetic resonance imaging data. Across a total of 12 analysis pipelines, the gross pattern of between-group findings was overall stable, with local overconnectivity in the ASD group in occipital and posterior temporal regions and underconnectivity in middle/posterior cingulate, and medial prefrontal regions. This general pattern was confirmed in secondary analyses for low-motion subsamples ($n = 20$ per group), in which time series segments with >0.25 mm head motion were censored, as well as in an analysis including global signal regression. Local overconnectivity in visual regions appears consistent with preference for local over global visual processing previously reported in ASD, whereas cingulate and medial frontal underconnectivity may relate to aberrant function within the default mode network.

Keywords: autism, local connectivity, functional MRI, regional homogeneity, graph theory, BOLD signal, intrinsic connectivity

INTRODUCTION

Autism spectrum disorder (ASD) is a highly prevalent neurodevelopmental disorder (Kim et al., 2011; CDC, 2012). There is growing consensus that sensorimotor, cognitive, and sociocommunicative impairments in ASD are linked to abnormalities of functional and anatomical connectivity (Wass, 2011; Vissers et al., 2012). Evidence of aberrant white matter growth anomalies early in life (Courchesne et al., 2011), atypical white matter maturation in infants and toddlers (Weinstein et al., 2011; Wolff et al., 2012), and white matter compromise in children and adolescents with ASD (Shukla et al., 2011a) all support the relevance of connectivity as source for biomarkers of ASD. A growing body of functional connectivity magnetic resonance imaging (fcMRI) studies indeed indicates aberrant long-distance connectivity, with the predominant, though not universally replicated, finding of underconnectivity in ASD (Müller et al., 2011; Schipul et al., 2011; Vissers et al., 2012). In strange contrast, rather little is known about *short-distance* connectivity in ASD, despite evidence from postmortem studies suggesting that cytoarchitectonic abnormalities in cerebral cortex (Amaral et al., 2008), in particular the reported tight packing of cortical minicolumns with reduced lateral inhibition (Casanova and Trippe, 2009), could likely affect local connections in ASD. Theoretical arguments suggesting that local connectivity may be atypically increased in ASD (Belmonte et al., 2004; Courchesne and Pierce, 2005; Rippon et al., 2007) have been mostly speculative, although they appear consistent with some findings indicating increased cortical excitation/inhibition ratios (Rubenstein and Merzenich, 2003).

Few studies available to date have used magnetic resonance imaging (MRI) techniques to examine local connectivity, with rather divergent findings. Note, however, that the concept of "local connectivity" is not well defined and with its typically low spatial resolution, functional MRI (fMRI) detects "local" connectivity at a much coarser spatial scale than, for example, the postmortem studies of minicolumnar organization cited above (as discussed in detail in Sections "Overall Pattern of Findings and the Effect of Spatial Scale" and "Regional Patterns and Implications for the Study of Local Connectivity in ASD"). One fMRI approach uses the regional homogeneity (ReHo) approach, which implements Kendall's coefficient of concordance (KCC) to test the homogeneity of time courses of the blood oxygen level dependent (BOLD) signal in small clusters of neighboring voxels. While originally designed for cluster purification (Zang et al., 2004), the technique has been increasingly used to examine local connectivity in a variety of clinical disorders (Dai et al., 2012; Farb et al., 2012; Yin et al., 2012; Zalesky et al., 2012; Weaver et al., 2013) as well as in the typically developing (TD) brain (Zou et al., 2009; Lopez-Larson et al., 2011; Wang et al., 2011; Anderson et al., 2013; Dong et al., 2013). Two studies have implemented ReHo in ASD. In ReHo analyses of resting state fMRI (rs-fMRI) data for 27 nearest neighboring voxels, Paakki et al. (2010) detected mixed between-group effects, with decreased ReHo in adolescents with ASD (compared to matched TD participants) in right temporal, frontal, and insular sites, accompanied by increased ReHo in right thalamus and left occipital regions. Shukla et al. (2010) used fMRI data acquired during visual search, but regressed out the modeled task effects. Nonetheless, ReHo findings for seven nearest neighbors differed heavily from those reported by Paakki et al. (2010), with increased ReHo in children and adolescents with ASD in right temporal regions, and decreased ReHo in numerous bilateral fronto-parietal sites. Notably, both of these studies used standardized ReHo (in which the KCC in each voxel is normalized by dividing it by the mean KCC), which is in principle insensitive to any potential global group differences in local connectivity. The mixed pattern of over- and underconnectivity findings in these studies was thus mandated by the analysis. However, the inconsistencies in regional patterns require further explanation, being potentially related to the finer spatial scale in the study by Shukla et al. (2010). Furthermore neither study addressed head motion, which can severely confound local BOLD correlations, at a level that can be considered adequate based on recent relevant publications (Power et al., 2012; Van Dijk et al., 2012; Satterthwaite et al., 2013; Yan et al., 2013).

The present study used a sample of rs-fMRI data that was well controlled for motion for a systematic investigation of local connectivity in ASD and matched TD adolescents, examining effects of spatial scale of local connectivity, standardization in ReHo, and the impact of head motion. A comparison analysis using the local density approach from graph theory, which has been applied to the study of local connectivity in TD adults (Sepulcre et al., 2010), was also performed.

Table 1 | Demographic and diagnostic information.

	Groups		
	TD ($n = 29$)	**ASD ($n = 29$)**	***p***
Gender	7 female	4 female	0.31
Handedness	25 R, 4 L	26 R, 3 L	0.57
Age in years	13.5 (2.2)	13.8 (2.4)	0.74
Verbal IQ	106.2 (9.5)	105.4 (20.9)	0.84
Non-verbal IQ	108.1 (10.0)	106.3 (18.51)	0.65
Full-scale IQ	108 (8.9)	107.9 (19.0)	0.97
RMSD	0.15 (0.14)	0.14 (.11)	0.78
ADOS algorithm score			
Communication	–	3.4 (1.8)	–
Social reciprocity	–	8.2 (3.0)	–
Repetitive behavior	–	2.1 (1.4)	–
ADI-R algorithm score			
Social interaction	–	17.4 (6.2)	–
Communication	–	14.4 (6.0)	–
Repetitive behavior	–	6.3 (2.3)	–

Values for age, IQ, and Autism Diagnostic Observation Schedule (ADOS) scores are presented as mean, with standard deviation in brackets. The p-value reflects group differences from χ^2 tests (for gender and handedness) and independent t-tests (for all other variables). The IQ scores were missing for one individual with ASD. ADOS scores were not available for one individual, and ADI-R scores were not available for three ASD individuals. RMSD, root-mean-square of displacement; R, right; L, left.

MATERIALS AND METHODS

PARTICIPANTS

Magnetic resonance imaging data were collected from 37 high-functioning adolescents with ASD and 33 TD control participants. Six ASD participants with excessive head motion (as defined in Section "Motion") were excluded from the analysis. Two further ASD and four TD participants were excluded to restore group matching on age, handedness, non-verbal IQ, and motion (see below), resulting in a final sample of 29 ASD and 29 TD participants (**Table 1**). Diagnoses in the ASD group were established using the Autism Diagnostic Interview-Revised (ADI-R; Lord et al., 1994), and the Autism Diagnostic Observation Schedule (ADOS; Lord et al., 2000). Children with ASD-related medical conditions (e.g., Fragile-X syndrome, tuberous sclerosis) or other neurological conditions (e.g., epilepsy, Tourette's syndrome) were excluded. Participants in the TD group had no reported history of ASD or any other neurological or psychiatric condition. IQ was assessed using the Wechsler Abbreviated Scale of Intelligence–2nd edition (WASI-2; Wechsler, 1999). All participants scored above the cutoff for intellectual disability ($IQ > 70$). Hand preference was assessed through the Edinburgh Handedness Inventory (Oldfield, 1971). The Institutional Review Boards of San Diego State University and the University of California San Diego approved the experimental protocol. Parental informed consent was obtained for all participants, along with written assent from each participant.

MRI DATA ACQUISITION

Resting state imaging data were acquired on a GE 3T MR750 scanner with an eight-channel head coil at the University of California at San Diego Center for Functional MRI. High-resolution structural images were acquired with a standard FSPGR T1-weighted sequence (TR: 11.08 ms; TE: 4.3 ms; flip angle: 45°; FOV: 256 mm; matrix: 256 × 256; 180 slices; resolution: 1 mm^3). Functional T2-weighted images were obtained using a single-shot gradient-recalled, echo-planar pulse sequence. One 6:10-min scan was acquired consisting of 185 whole-brain volumes (TR: 2000 ms; TE: 30 ms; slice thickness: 3.4 mm; flip angle: 90°; field of view: 220 mm; matrix: 64 × 64; in-plane resolution: 3.4 mm^2). The first five time points were discarded to allow for T1 equilibration effects, leaving 180 time points (6 min) for analysis. Participants were instructed to keep their eyes directed on a cross-hair in the center of the projector, relax, and try not to fall asleep for the duration of the scan.

DATA PREPROCESSING

Functional images were processed using Analysis of Functional NeuroImages software (AFNI; Cox, 1996) and FMRI software library (FSL; Smith et al., 2004). Functional images were slice-time corrected, and correction for head motion was performed by registering each functional volume to the middle time point of the scan. Field map correction was applied on each participant using in-house software for correcting magnetic resonance image distortion due to field inhomogeneity. Functional images were registered to the anatomical images via FSL's FLIRT (Jenkinson and Smith, 2001; Jenkinson et al., 2002). Both images were resampled (3 mm isotropic) and standardized to the atlas space of the MNI152 template via FSL's nonlinear registration tool (FNIRT) for group comparisons. In order to isolate spontaneous low-frequency BOLD fluctuations (Cordes et al., 2001), fMRI time series were bandpass filtered ($0.008 < f < 0.08$ Hz), using a second-order Butterworth filter, which was also applied to all nuisance regressors described below.

Spatial smoothing preceding ReHo statistics is an obvious critical question, because smoothness directly impacts time series correlations between neighboring voxels (Zuo et al., 2013). Our primary preprocessing pipeline therefore did not include a smoothing step. However, spatial smoothness may differ across data sets due to varying interpolation associated with motion correction and spatial normalization. In order to minimize effects of varying smoothness, a secondary analysis setting the effective smoothness of all data sets to a Gaussian FWHM of 6 mm, using AFNI's 3dBlurToFWHM, was performed. Results are presented in **Figure 2D**. For density analyses, we followed the preprocessing pipeline by Sepulcre et al. (2010), which included smoothing with a Gaussian kernel (FWHM 6 mm). Linear effects attributable to scanner drift were removed during regression.

Six rigid-body motion parameters acquired from motion correction and their derivatives were regressed from the images. In order to remove signal from cerebral white matter and lateral ventricles, masks were created at the participant level, using FSL's FAST automated segmentation (Zhang et al., 2001). Masks were trimmed to avoid partial-volume effects, and an average time series for each region was extracted and removed via regression. Derivatives for white matter and ventricular time series were also computed and removed, for a total of 16 nuisance regressors. All main analyses were performed without global signal regression (GSR) to avoid the creation of spurious anti-correlations (Murphy et al., 2009), which may substantially distort group differences (Saad et al., 2012). Nonetheless, an additional ReHo analysis including GSR was performed using a cluster size of 27 voxels. Results are presented in **Figure 2E**.

MOTION

Motion was quantified as the Euclidean distance calculated from the six rigid-body motion parameters for two consecutive time points. For any instance >1.0 mm, considered excessive motion, the time point as well as the immediately preceding and subsequent time points were censored, or "scrubbed" (Power et al., 2012). If two censored time points occurred within 10 time points of each other, all time points between them were also censored. Participants with fewer than 80% of time points remaining after censoring were excluded from the analysis. The two groups did not significantly differ in the number of retained time points ($M = 177$ in each group, $p = 0.94$). Average head motion over each participant's session was defined as the root mean square of displacement (RMSD) and did not significantly differ between groups ($p = 0.78$). For more detailed analysis of head motion, a two-way analysis of variance (ANOVA) was conducted to test the effects of group and type of motion (three translational and three rotational). The interaction of group and motion type was not significant, $F(5,342) = 0.307$, $p = 0.91$. Additionally, we correlated KCC from ReHo27, averaged across all brain voxels, for cluster size 27 with RMSD values to determine the relationship between connectivity and motion. There was no significant correlation between these two measures, $r = -0.135$, $p = 0.54$.

For further protection against potential effects of head motion on local connectivity measures, a low-motion subsample was identified and a more conservative censoring threshold of >0.25 mm was applied. Participants who had less than 80% of their time points remaining after censoring were excluded from both analysis. Both groups were matched for gender, handedness, age, verbal IQ, non-verbal IQ, full-scale IQ, and motion (**Table 2**). The final low-motion subsample consisted of 42 participants (TD = 22; ASD = 20).

LOCAL FUNCTIONAL CONNECTIVITY MEASURES

Regional homogeneity

Regional homogeneity implements KCC, which relies on rank correlations of time series to assess the homogeneity of a given center voxel and its neighboring voxels. KCC within a given cluster of voxels is equal to the parameter W (ranging from 0 to 1)

$$W = \frac{\sum (R_i)^2 - n(\bar{R})^2}{\frac{1}{12}K^2(n^3 - n)},$$

where R_i is the sum rank of the ith time point; $\bar{R}$ is the mean of the R_is; K is the number of time series within a selected cluster (7, 19, or 27 voxels), and n is the number of ranks, as determined by the number of time points (Zang et al., 2004).

Table 2 | Demographic and diagnostic information for low-motion subsamples.

	Groups		
	TD ($n = 22$)	**ASD ($n = 20$)**	***p***
Gender	4 female	2 female	0.44
Handedness	18 R, 4 L	14 R, 3 L	0.97
Age in years	14.0 (1.82)	14.37 (2.07)	0.65
Verbal IQ	107.5 (9.76)	110.79 (20.37)	0.50
Non-verbal IQ	107.95 (10.39)	109.32 (18.74)	0.77
Full-Scale IQ	108.68 (9.46)	110.45 (19.93)	0.71
RMSD	0.05 (0.02)	0.05 (0.03)	0.84
ADOS algorithm score			
Communication	–	3.1 (1.9)	–
Social reciprocity	–	7.8 (2.8)	–
Repetitive behavior	–	1.8 (1.2)	–
ADI-R algorithm score			
Social interaction	–	16.8 (6.5)	–
Communication	–	13.8 (6.0)	–
Repetitive behavior	–	6.2 (2.4)	–

Values for age, IQ, and Autism Diagnostic Observation Schedule (ADOS) scores are presented as mean and standard deviation (SD). The p-value is from χ^2 tests and independent t-tests for differences between groups. Handedness scores were missing for three ASD participants, IQ scores were missing for one ASD participant, and ADI-R scores were not available for another ASD participant. RMSD, root-mean-square difference; R, right; L, left.

For this study, ReHo was computed for cluster sizes of 7, 19, and 27 voxels (abbreviated "ReHo7," "ReHo19," and "ReHo27," respectively), which correspond to the smallest cluster (a reference voxel and its six immediate neighbors) and small gradual symmetric expansions of this cluster. In order to further examine spatial scale effects, ReHo was also computed using a radius of 14 mm (407 voxels; "ReHo14mm"), corresponding to a radius used in the density analysis (described below). A gray-matter mask was used to avoid partial-volume effects. All individual ReHo maps were obtained using AFNI's 3dReHo command. Individual voxel-wise ReHo maps were standardized into KCC–ReHo z-values by subtracting the mean voxel-wise KCC–ReHo obtained for the entire whole-brain mask (i.e., global KCC–ReHo), and then dividing by the standard deviation. An additional analysis without standardization was performed (for ReHo27 only) to detect any potential global group differences in local connectivity. All ReHo maps were smoothed to a Gaussian FWHM of 6 mm for better anatomical comparability of ReHo values on the group level, using AFNI's 3dBlurToFWHM. Group differences were examined with two-sample t-tests (3dttest). To correct for multiple comparisons, Monte Carlo simulations via AFNI's 3dClustSim command were applied to obtain a corrected significance level of $p < 0.05$ (using a voxelwise threshold of $p < 0.05$, uncorrected, and a minimum cluster size of 55 voxels).

The relationship between local connectivity and symptom severity was further examined focusing on regions with significant group differences. Two separate combined clusters were created (all clusters of overconnectivity and all clusters of underconnectivity) based on group comparison for ReHo27 (yellow and blue clusters in **Figure 1E**, respectively) and Pearson's correlation analyses were performed between z-scores from KCC (averaged across all voxels within combined over- and underconnectivity clusters, respectively) and ADOS, and ADI scores (as listed in **Table 1**).

Density analysis

Local functional connectivity was further examined using connection density, as previously applied in neurotypical adults (Sepulcre et al., 2010). In graph theory, connection "density" is defined as the number of "edges" (connections) of a "node" (here: voxel) in proportion to the total number of possible edges (Bullmore and Sporns, 2009). We implemented this measure by calculating the "degree" of each voxel, i.e., the number of neighboring voxels with BOLD time series correlation at $r > 0.25$ ($p < 0.001$) within a 6 and 14 mm radius from the reference voxel, based on the Euclidean distance between the centers of voxel pairs. A 14 mm radius allowed comparison of results with those reported by Sepulcre et al. (2010) who used the same radius, whereas an additional 6 mm radius was chosen for comparison with ReHo27. To generate a connectivity map for each group, local degrees were converted to z-scores. Group comparisons were performed using two-sample t-tests. Multiple comparison correction was performed as described above.

RESULTS

ReHo

We first inspected ReHo within each group for the most commonly used cluster size of 27 voxels (**Figures 1A,B**). Patterns were highly similar for TD and ASD groups, with bilateral hotspots in posterior cingulate gyrus extending into precuneus. A hotspot in the ASD group in striate and extrastriate cortex appeared less pronounced in the TD group. Further regions of relatively high ReHo were seen in superior parietal, frontopolar, and medial frontal regions.

Despite the overall similar patterns on within-group maps, localized group differences were detected for ReHo at all four spatial scales (7, 19, 27 voxels, 14 mm radius; **Figures 1C–F**; **Table 3**). All of these analyses showed underconnectivity in the ASD group compared to the TD group in left superior frontal gyrus and bilateral cingulate cortex, accompanied by overconnectivity in right middle frontal gyrus. Generally, between-group effects were more modest at the finer spatial scales, and additional clusters of under- and overconnectivity were detected with increasingly coarse spatial scale. For example, underconnectivity in the ASD group was detected in right paracentral regions only for ReHo27 and ReHo14mm. Extensive overconnectivity effects were detected in bilateral striate and extrastriate cortices at 14 mm radius, which were smaller for ReHo27 and ReHo19, and absent for ReHo7. Overconnectivity effects in parahippocampal, temporal, and supramarginal regions were also only detected at the coarsest spatial scale (14 mm radius). Non-standardized ReHo27 (**Figure 1G**) yielded very similar group differences compared to standardized ReHo at the same spatial scale.

Local connectivity from ReHo27 was positively correlated with ADI-R communicative scores in clusters of underconnectivity in the ASD group (all blue clusters in **Figure 1E** combined), $r = 0.43$, $p = 0.04$, as well as in clusters of overconnectivity (all yellow clusters in **Figure 1E** combined), $r = 0.48$, $p = 0.02$. There were no significant correlations with ADOS scores. However, note that these analyses were performed for exploratory purposes and caution is required given that no correction for multiple comparisons was performed.

DENSITY ANALYSIS

The patterns of group differences for local degrees (density of connections) were overall similar to the ReHo findings (**Figures 1H,I**; **Table 4**). Comparing only two spatial scales (radii of 6 mm, corresponding to ReHo27, and 14 mm), we again found much more robust between-group effects for the coarser spatial scale. However, there was less regional consistency: only a single effect – local overconnectivity in right middle frontal gyrus in the ASD group – was found in both analyses. Overconnectivity in right medial paracentral cortex and underconnectivity in bilateral anterior cingulate cortex were detected only for a 6 mm radius. Conversely, extensive overconnectivity clusters in bilateral striate and extrastriate as well as right temporopolar cortices were only detected at a 14 mm radius, as was underconnectivity in middle/posterior cingulate gyri bilaterally.

SECONDARY ANALYSIS IN LOW-MOTION SUBSAMPLE

ReHo

Additional analyses using ReHo27 (**Figure 2A**) and ReHo14mm (**Figure 2B**) were performed for the low-motion subsample. For both scales, underconnectivity in the ASD group was found

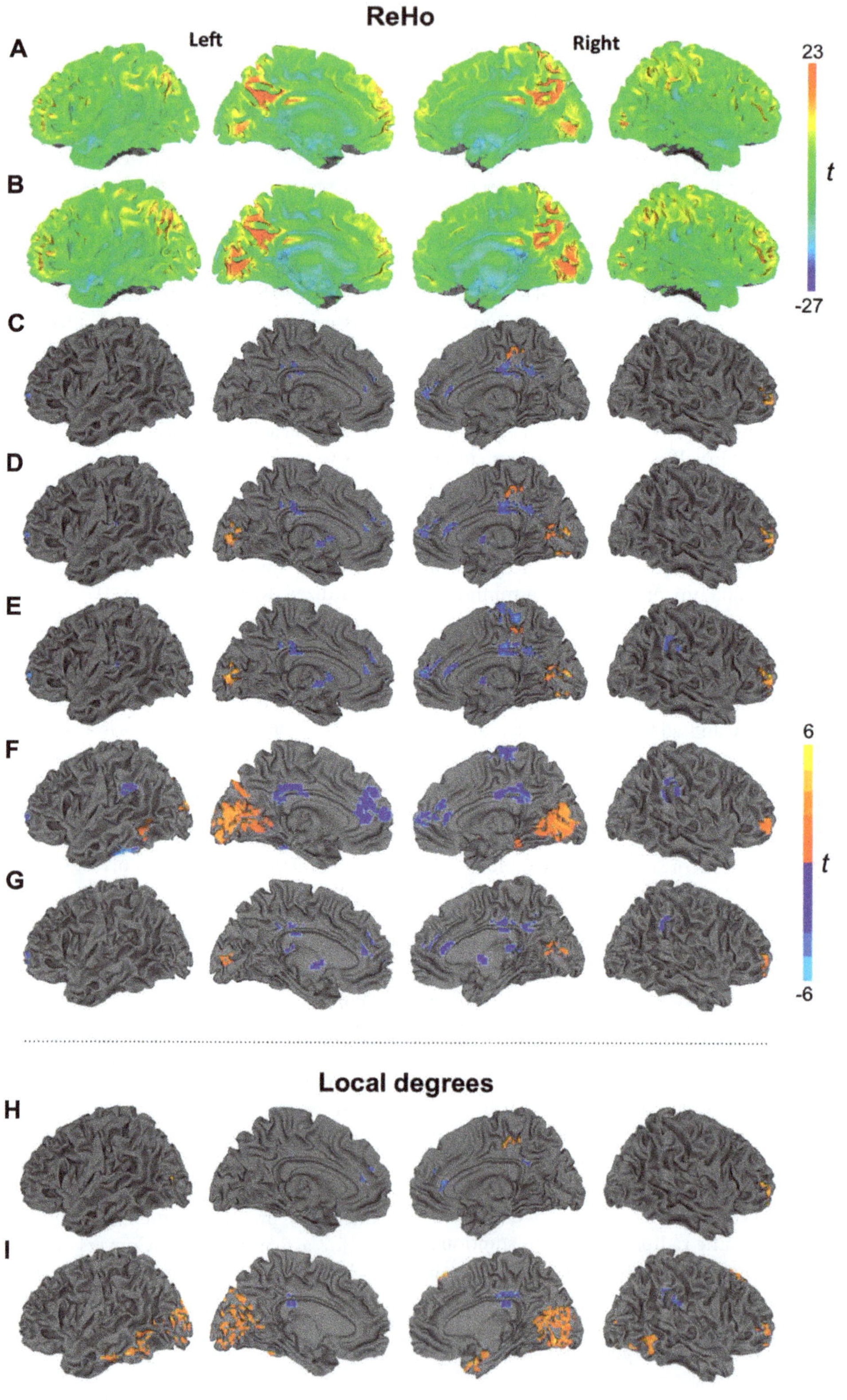

FIGURE 1 | Surface renderings of ReHo (27 voxels) for TD **(A)** and ASD groups **(B)**. Clusters of significant group differences between TD and ASD groups in ReHo using cluster sizes of 7 **(C)**, 19 **(D)**, 27 voxels **(E)**, 14 mm radius **(F)**, and non-standardized ReHo (27 voxels) **(G)**. Significant group differences between TD and ASD groups of density analysis using radii of 6 **(H)** and 14 mm **(I)**. All clusters $p < 0.05$, corr. warm colors: ASD > TD; cool colors: TD > ASD.

Table 3 | Clusters of significant group differences in ReHo.

ReHo cluster size (voxels)	Region	Cluster volume (μl)	Peak coordinates			Peak
			x	*Y*	*z*	*t*
7	TD > ASD					
	Right precuneus	3888	14.5	−50.5	33.5	−3.8
	Left superior frontal gyrus	1944	−18.5	60.5	3.5	−5.0
	Left anterior cingulate cortex	1917	−0.5	45.5	18.5	−3.9
	ASD > TD					
	Right middle cingulate cortex	2349	17.5	−20.5	48.5	4.5
	Right middle frontal gyrus	1809	41.5	54.5	6.5	5.0
19	TD > ASD					
	Left middle cingulate cortex	4941	−0.5	−29.5	33.5	−4.2
	Right anterior cingulate cortex	3456	2.5	39.5	9.5	−4.2
	Left putamen	2322	−27.5	−14.5	12.5	−3.8
	Left superior frontal gyrus	2025	−18.5	60.5	3.5	−4.6
	Left caudate	1917	−6.5	12.5	6.5	−4.7
	ASD > TD					
	Left calcarine gyrus	3753	−3.5	−86.5	3.5	3.2
	Right middle frontal gyrus	3267	41.5	54.5	6.5	4.9
	Right paracentral lobule	2403	17.5	−35.5	48.5	4.1
	Right fusiform gyrus	2295	32.5	−68.5	−8.5	3.6
27	TD > ASD					
	Left middle cingulate cortex	5400	−0.5	−29.5	33.5	−4.2
	Right superior medial gyrus	4077	8.5	57.5	9.5	−4.1
	Left putamen	2349	−27.5	−14.5	12.5	−3.3
	Right paracentral lobule	2106	2.5	−32.5	60.5	−3.1
	Left superior frontal gyrus	2079	−18.5	60.5	3.5	−4.7
	Left caudate	2052	−6.5	12.5	6.5	−4.8
	Right supramarginal gyrus	1809	65.5	−38.5	30.5	−3.3
	ASD > TD					
	Left calcarine gyrus	4239	−3.5	−86.5	3.5	3.2604
	Right middle frontal gyrus	3240	41.5	54.5	6.5	4.5738
	Right fusiform gyrus	2997	32.5	−68.5	−8.5	3.3385
	Right middle cingulate gyrus	1971	20.5	−32.5	51.5	3.8254
27 (Non−standardized)	TD > ASD					
	Right middle cingulate cortex	4536	2.5	−23.5	33.5	−3.8
	Right anterior cingulate cortex	2862	2.5	39.5	9.5	−3.5
	Left caudate	2484	−6.5	9.5	6.5	−4.5
	Left superior frontal gyrus	2052	−18.5	60.5	3.5	−4.3
	Right supramarginal gyrus	1809	65.5	−38.5	30.5	−2.9
	Left thalamus	1566	−3.5	−29.5	12.5	−3.0
	ASD > TD					
	Right calcarine gyrus	2268	5.5	−68.5	12.5	2.8
	Right middle frontal gyrus	2133	41.5	54.5	6.5	4.2

(Continued)

Table 3 | Continued

ReHo cluster size (voxels)	Region	Cluster volume (μl)	Peak coordinates			Peak
			x	*Y*	*z*	*t*
407 (14 mm)	TD > ASD					
	Left superior medial gyrus	5265	−3.5	42.5	27.5	−2.9
	Left cingulate gyrus	4131	−3.5	−26.5	27.5	−3.7
	Left inferior temporal gyrus	3348	−51.5	−35.5	−26.5	−3.4
	Right supramarginal gyrus	1836	65.5	−35.5	27.5	−3.7
	Right anterior cingulate cortex	1755	2.5	42.5	9.5	−2.9
	Left supramarginal gyrus	1701	−57.5	−38.5	27.5	−2.8
	Right superior medial gyrus	1215	2.5	54.5	9.5	−2.9
	ASD > TD					
	Left lingual gyrus	29808	−15.5	−68.5	3.5	4.3
	Right parahippocampal gyrus	3051	29.5	−29.5	−17.5	3.1
	Right middle frontal gyrus	2511	44.5	54.5	3.5	3.5
	Left middle temporal gyrus	1620	−66.5	−47.5	−8.5	2.8
	Right supp. motor area	1161	5.5	−14.5	75.5	−3.0

Table 4 | Clusters of significant group differences in density analysis.

Radius (mm)	Region	Cluster volume (μl)	Peak coordinates			Peak
			x	*y*	*z*	*t*
6	TD > ASD					
	Right posterior cingulate cortex	2133	2.5	−41.5	24.5	−4.1
	Left anterior cingulate cortex	1701	−3.5	42.5	21.5	−4.1
	ASD > TD					
	Right middle frontal gyrus	2376	41.5	51.5	6.5	4.3
	Right postcentral gyrus	2025	23.5	−26.5	48.5	4.0
	Left middle temporal gyrus	1485	−54.5	−65.5	12.5	3.5
14	TD > ASD					
	Right supramarginal gyrus	1809	−65.5	32.5	24.5	−3.7
	Right middle cingulate cortex	1512	−2.5	29.5	33.5	−3.6
	ASD > TD					
	Right cuneus	41013	5.5	−74.5	18.5	4.5
	Left inferior temporal gyrus	9126	−48.5	−47.5	−23.5	4.1
	Right inferior temporal gyrus	3915	53.5	−53.5	−8.5	4.1
	Left cuneus	2565	−9.5	−92.5	30.5	3.4
	Right superior medial gyrus	2349	5.5	33.5	57.5	4.0
	Right middle orbital gyrus	2187	35.5	54.5	−2.5	3.4
	Right middle temporal gyrus	1755	44.5	6.5	−26.5	3.0
	Right parahippocampal gyrus	1620	23.5	6.5	−29.5	3.9

in left perisylvian and frontopolar regions, as well as in bilateral middle/posterior cingulate gyrus and right paracentral cortex, accompanied by overconnectivity in right middle frontal and middle temporal gyri. Extensive overconnectivity in visual regions around the calcarine fissure was only seen at the 14 mm radius.

Density analysis

For a 14 mm radius (**Figure 2C**), results were mostly consistent with the corresponding ReHo analysis and the corresponding density analysis for the full sample. Widespread overconnectivity was detected in bilateral occipital and posterior temporal regions, as well as right middle frontal gyrus, while underconnectivity was

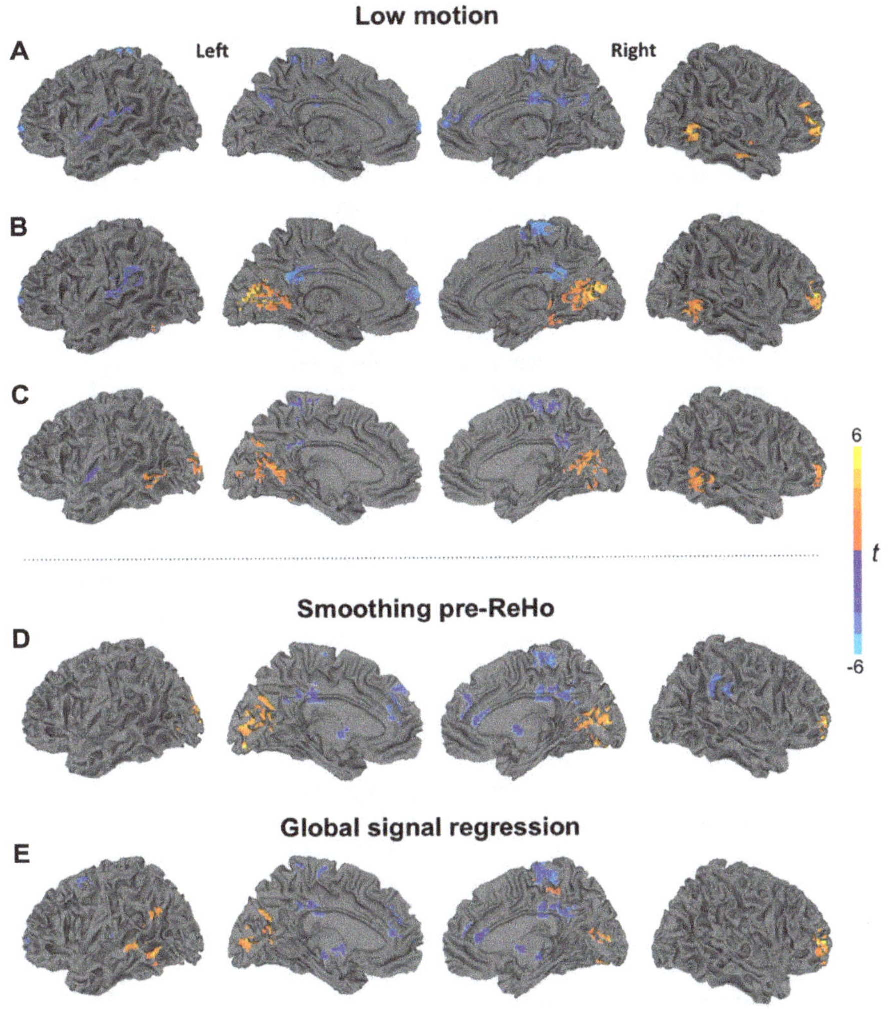

FIGURE 2 | Clusters of significant group differences between low-motion TD and ASD groups for ReHo using **(A)** a cluster size of 27 voxels, and **(B)** a radius of 14 mm, and **(C)** for 14 mm density analysis. Analyses of ReHo (27 voxels) showing clusters of significant group differences **(D)** for pipeline applying spatial smoothing before ReHo statistics and **(E)** for pipeline including global signal regression. All clusters $p < 0.05$, corr; warm colors: ASD > TD; cool colors: TD > ASD.

found in left insula, bilateral precuneus, and middle/posterior cingulate gyrus.

DISCUSSION

OVERALL PATTERN OF FINDINGS AND THE EFFECT OF SPATIAL SCALE

Across 12 different analysis pipelines (**Figures 1C–I** and **2A–E**), regional patterns of between-group differences were overall stable, with increased local connectivity in the ASD group detected in bilateral striate and extrastriate as well as right lateral prefrontal cortices, accompanied by reduced local connectivity in anterior and posterior cingulate and medial prefrontal regions. We generally observed a trend toward more robust between-group findings for coarser spatial scales, corresponding to radii of ≥6 mm. This may be primarily attributed to sampling from a larger number of voxels, which probably improved the signal-to-noise ratio. Effects that were seen at lower, but not at higher spatial scales, such as overconnectivity in ASD in right inferior paracentral regions (**Figures 1C–E** vs. **Figure 1F**) are therefore noteworthy, as they might reflect group differences occurring only at the more local levels. Some effects, such as underconnectivity in anterior and posterior cingulate gyrus as well as medial prefrontal cortex, were also remarkably stable across radii from c. 3 to 14 mm. On the other hand, effects in striate and extrastriate visual cortices were much more robust at higher spatial scales and in fact not at all detected in ReHo7 analysis (for interpretation of regional patterns, see Regional Patterns and Implications for the Study of "Local Connectivity" in ASD).

While these findings may suggest an overall superiority of analyses at coarser spatial scales (when assessed on the basis of robustness of between-group effects), any such conclusion very much depends on the exact goals of the investigation. The study of local connectivity by fMRI is generally hampered by this technique's typically modest spatial resolution, which limits its sensitivity to abnormalities of local cortical organization suspected in ASD. For example, smaller size and increased density of cortical minicolumns with reduced lateral inhibition has been reported in postmortem studies from one group (Casanova et al., 2006; Casanova and Trippe, 2009). As minicolumns measure c. 30–50 μm in width, the spatial resolution in our study was too low by at least a factor of 100 to capture individual minicolumns. Although it is possible that basic abnormalities of minicolumnar organization, such as the suspected reduced lateral inhibition, could affect the BOLD signal and its local correlations at the resolution common in fMRI, this remains speculative. Widening the spatial scale, beyond what is dictated by raw image resolution (3.4 mm in this study), may therefore yield cleaner or more robust results; however, these probably reflect abnormalities at a different level of complexity, compared to those described in the postmortem literature. Nonetheless, it is likely that anatomical parameters, such as cortical thickness, may have some impact on measures of local functional connectivity. Given the mentioned relatively low spatial resolution of fMRI data, some voxels in a ReHo cluster, for example, may show partial volume effects (part of the voxel falling onto the gray/white boundary), which would be expected to reduce BOLD correlations with a neighboring reference voxel in pure gray matter. Resulting reductions in ReHo will most likely occur to a lesser extent in cortex with greater thickness. However, investigation of such links was beyond the scope of the current study. The described issue here solely serves to illustrate the intimate links between local functional connectivity and local cortical anatomy.

Density analyses showed a similar pattern of between-group effects compared to ReHo analyses, although underconnectivity clusters were overall less robust and one overconnectivity cluster in right anterior mediotemporal cortex was seen only in the density analysis for a 14 mm radius (but not in ReHo14mm). This may relate to methodological differences: Whereas ReHo is based on rank ordering of time series to assess the homogeneity in voxels within a cluster of chosen size, density reflects degrees, i.e., the number of voxels exceeding a threshold Pearson's correlation (here, $r > 0.25$). ReHo is therefore more sensitive to the strength of correlations within a cluster of selected volume (e.g., 7 or 27 voxels), whereas in our density analysis, weak correlations were discarded and local connectivity was solely assessed with respect to the number (not the strength) of the connections exceeding the correlation threshold. Differences in sensitivity are therefore not unexpected.

MOTION, SMOOTHNESS, GLOBAL SIGNAL, AND ReHo STANDARDIZATION

Recent investigations have highlighted the significant impact of even small amounts of head motion on fcMRI measures (Power et al., 2012; Van Dijk et al., 2012; Satterthwaite et al., 2013; Yan et al., 2013). We therefore also ran analyses in a low-motion subsample, including only the 42 participants with >80% time points remaining after applying a more conservative censoring threshold of 0.25 mm. The pattern of findings for this subsample was overall similar to the one seen in the full sample, suggesting that our results were well protected against motion confounds.

Image smoothness is of particular importance in *local* connectivity analyses because smoothing by definition inflates the correlation between neighboring voxels. In order to avoid this issue, our primary analysis pipeline implemented smoothing only subsequent to ReHo statistics. However, even without an explicit smoothing step, preprocessing requires intermodal alignment (of functional to high-resolution structural volumes), motion correction (alignment across time points), and spatial normalization, which unavoidably increases image smoothness (even when intermodal alignment and spatial normalization are performed in a single interpolation, as in our study). Smoothness may therefore vary across individual datasets, and more importantly, across groups, potentially confounding comparisons of local connectivity. We therefore performed an additional ReHo27 analysis, setting the smoothness of all datasets to an effective Gaussian FWHM of 6 mm. This analysis (**Figure 2D**) yielded almost identical results to the primary analysis without pre-statistic smoothing (**Figure 1C**), indicating that differences in image smoothness did not confound our group comparisons.

We further considered the question of GSR, the pros and cons of which have been debated for several years in the fcMRI literature. Arguments against the procedure include findings that at least some components of global signal fluctuations likely reflect true neuronal activity (Schölvinck et al., 2010) and that GSR may induce spurious negative correlations of BOLD time series (Murphy et al., 2009). Nonetheless, GSR has been found highly effective in removing noise, especially reducing the effects of head motion on BOLD correlations (Yan et al., 2013). We therefore included GSR in one analysis (ReHo27) and found that removal of the global signal had some effect (e.g., highlighting overconnectivity effects in the ASD group in left lateral temporal cortex not seen in ReHo27 without GSR), but did not dramatically change the overall pattern of findings. Thus, while GSR may in principle bear the risk of distorting fcMRI group comparisons (Saad et al., 2012), this was not the case in our data set.

A final methodological issue concerned ReHo standardization. As initially advocated by Zang et al. (2004), conversion of KCC (W) into z-maps was performed in both previous ReHo studies of ASD (Paakki et al., 2010; Shukla et al., 2010). This standardization mandates a distribution of whole brain ReHo maps around zero. While advantageous for teasing out regionally specific differences in ReHo, this procedure bears the risk of type II error in group comparisons, if there are global differences in ReHo between groups (because the whole brain mean ReHo in each individual participant from both groups is equally set to zero). It is therefore possible in principle that the mixed pattern of effects seen on our ReHo analyses (with both clusters of overconnectivity and underconnectivity) could be due to the standardization step – a possibility not considered in previous ASD ReHo studies. However, non-standardized ReHo27 (i.e., without conversion of KCC to z) yielded highly similar results to standardized ReHo27 (**Figure 1G** vs. **Figure 1E**). Overall subtly more robust between-group effects for standardized ReHo can be attributed to lower variance due to z-conversion. It is therefore unlikely that the mixed pattern of over- and underconnectivity findings in our study was an artifact of ReHo standardization.

COMPARISON WITH PREVIOUS STUDIES

As noted, the two previous ReHo studies of ASD by Paakki et al. (2010) and Shukla et al. (2010) reported highly divergent findings. The convergence between either of them and the current study was equally modest, with only a few roughly consistent findings. These included local overconnectivity in ASD in occipital lobe (also detected by Paakki et al., 2010) and underconnectivity in ASD in left superior frontal gyrus, precuneus, and posterior cingulate gyrus, and overconnectivity in right fusiform gyrus (also observed by Shukla et al., 2010). While differences between our study and the study by Shukla et al. (2010) may be attributed to the use of resting vs. task-activated fMRI data, respectively, the even more pronounced inconsistencies with the study by Paakki et al. (2010) may appear less transparent at first, given that these authors also used resting state data. Participants were probably overall older in the study by Paakki et al. (2010), although no exact demographic data are provided and matching on important variables, such as age, sex, handedness, and non-verbal IQ, is either not mentioned or not available due to lack of data (e.g., IQ). It is therefore hard to determine whether demographic factors may have affected the pattern of results in the study by Paakki et al. (2010).

There were also differences in imaging methods. While acquisition at lower spatial resolution (70.4 vs. 39.3 μl voxels) and at lower field strength (1.5 vs. 3T) in the study by Paakki et al. (2010), compared to ours, may have had some effect, the differential treatment of head motion (and other noise components) is probably crucial in explaining differential findings. Paakki et al. (2010) performed solely conventional motion correction. Noise components removed through regression of six translational and rotational motion times series, time series from white matter and ventricles (and their derivatives) in our study were thus retained in this earlier study. In view of recent methods investigations (Power et al., 2012; Van Dijk et al., 2012; Satterthwaite et al., 2013; Yan et al., 2013), which were not available to Paakki et al. (2010) and which highlight the exquisite sensitivity of fcMRI (including local connectivity and ReHo) analyses to even small amounts of motion, the confidence in these earlier findings therefore has to be low. Furthermore, no group matching for head motion or censoring ("scrubbing") of motion-affected time points was reported by Paakki et al. (2010). Conversely, the study by Shukla et al. (2010) performed censoring (albeit at an all-too liberal threshold of 2 mm) and ascertained approximate group matching for motion ($p = 0.7$ for translations; $p = 0.3$ for rotations). In this context, the relatively greater (though still modest) consistency of findings between this study and the present one may be noted.

REGIONAL PATTERNS AND IMPLICATIONS FOR THE STUDY OF "LOCAL CONNECTIVITY" IN ASD

As already alluded to above, the term "local connectivity" is ill-defined, encompassing spatial scales from a few microns to millimeters and even centimeters. While there has been some indirectly supporting evidence (Rubenstein and Merzenich, 2003; Casanova and Trippe, 2009), the theoretical idea of atypically increased local connectivity in ASD (Belmonte et al., 2004; Courchesne and Pierce, 2005; Rippon et al., 2007) therefore requires specification of scale. The expectation that fMRI, using ReHo or local density techniques, or diffusion tensor imaging (Shukla et al., 2011b) may provide empirical tests of the local overconnectivity hypothesis applies at best to the coarsest spatial scales included under the vague umbrella term of "local connectivity." At these relative coarse scales, the mixed pattern of our findings (with regions of both atypically increased and decreased connectivity) does not support *general* local overconnectivity in ASD. This compares with a study by Anderson et al. (2011) who found no general overconnectivity for connections at a distance below 25 mm in adolescents and adults with ASD. As measures were collapsed across the whole brain in this latter study, such non-finding can be reconciled with regionally specific effects in both directions (increased and reduced), as detected in our study. Note that the conclusion in the study by Anderson et al. (2011) of short-distance connections not being strongly informative for machine learning classification (ASD vs. TD) may be due to the mentioned whole brain approach and does not rule out predictive power for region-specific local connectivity patterns.

The finding of robust and extensive overconnectivity in striate and extrastriate visual cortex, at scales above 6 mm, is intriguing in view of potential local biases in visual perception, supported thus far mainly by findings from behavioral studies (Dakin and Frith, 2005; Mottron et al., 2006). Unusual profiles of visual perception have been observed in many studies (as reviewed in Simmons et al., 2009). Remarkable are islets of superior abilities in visual search (O'Riordan, 2004), associated with increased functional connectivity during visual search performance (Keehn et al., 2012). In a meta-analysis, Samson et al. (2012) found overall greater activity in ASD groups compared to TD control groups in posterior brain regions for a variety of visual processing tasks (from studies using face, object, and word stimuli), including occipitotemporal regions, for which local overconnectivity was detected in the present study. Greater activation and increased local connectivity could be directly related, as increased spontaneous BOLD signal correlations in visual cortex (as detected in our ReHo and density analyses) may also enhance BOLD signal changes in response to a task (as in the studies reviewed by Samson et al., 2012). Indeed, effects of resting state signal fluctuations on amplitude of stimulus-induced response have been observed in a number of fMRI and electrophysiological studies (as reviewed in Northoff et al., 2010). Specifically with respect to visual cortex, Liu et al. (2011) reported that local BOLD correlations were positively associated with amplitude of response to simple visual stimuli.

Conversely, regions that consistently (across different analysis pipelines) showed local underconnectivity in ASD included posterior cingulate cortex and medial prefrontal lobe. Both of these belong to a system that has been found active during the resting state and is considered a "default mode network" (DMN; Raichle et al., 2001). Several fcMRI studies have examined the DMN in ASD, with the overall consistent finding of reduced connectivity between DMN nodes, such as posterior cingulate and medial prefrontal cortices (Monk et al., 2009; Assaf et al., 2010; von dem Hagen et al., 2012). The present findings suggest that such reduced long-distance connectivity between regions of the

DMN is accompanied by local underconnectivity *within* these regions. This is consistent with a recent finding by Lynch et al. (2013) who observed underconnectivity in children with ASD between posterior cingulate gyrus and neighboring regions (precuneus, retrosplenial cortex). Notably, this latter study as well as the one by Monk et al. (2009) found that underconnectivity within the DMN was accompanied by atypically increased functional connectivity of DMN regions with regions outside this network, such as medial and lateral temporal cortices. Our finding may also be consistent with atypically reduced connectivity in bilateral precuneus observed by Di Martino et al. (2013) in children with ASD. Note, however, that this latter finding compares only indirectly to ours, as Di Martino et al. (2013) tested degree centrality, which is a graph theory construct reflecting both short- and long-distance connectivity of each node.

A further finding that was overall stable across analysis pipelines was an asymmetry of reduced connectivity in left, but increased connectivity in right anterior prefrontal regions. The asymmetric effects in anterior prefrontal cortex may be related to a recent finding of right-hemisphere shifts of functional networks in ASD (Cardinale et al., 2013). Expanding on a few previous studies (e.g., Boddaert et al., 2003; Eyler et al., 2012) that had suggested greater right-hemisphere participation in language-related processing in ASD, the study by Cardinale et al. (2013) indicated that such right-hemisphere shifts may be a pervasive feature of functional brain organization in ASD, applying to many functional networks, including non-verbal ones and those with participation of anterior prefrontal cortices. Such rightward shifts may be associated by atypically increased local connectivity in right compared to left prefrontal cortex in ASD, as observed in the pattern of group differences detected in our study. However, such potential links need to be considered with caution, given that this asymmetric pattern of group differences was solely found in anterior prefrontal cortex, whereas the rightward shifts observed by Cardinale et al. (2013) occurred in widely distributed functional networks.

Local connectivity abnormalities, as detected in our study, may relate to recent evidence suggesting reduced functional differentiation of cerebral cortex. Shih et al. (2011) first reported such reduced functional differentiation in posterior superior temporal sulcus in children and adolescents with ASD. Neighboring subregions were found to be less differentiated, both in the temporal domain (with respect to BOLD time series) and in the spatial domain (with respect to whole brain connectivity patterns). Analogous findings for primary motor cortex have been reported by Nebel et al. (2012) who observed that functional differentiation between lower limb and trunk regions vs. upper limb and hand regions was reduced in children with ASD. Findings from these two studies may be consistent with a general model of reduced network segregation in ASD, as proposed in two studies by Rudie et al. (2012, 2013). Reduced network segregation, accompanied by impaired local functional differentiation, may relate to findings of regional local overconnectivity. For example, reduced differentiation in posterior superior temporal sulcus, as reported by Shih et al. (2011), is equivalent to atypically increased correlations in neighboring voxels, and thus corresponds to local overconnectivity in ASD in this region, as detected by us in analyses at coarser spatial scales (**Figures 1F,I**). On the other hand, local underconnectivity could reflect reduced integration within specialized functional networks, such as the DMN, as discussed above. However, these potential links across studies remain speculative, as long as direct comparisons of local connectivity and network segregation in the same cohort are unavailable.

Our results also compare in interesting ways to a recent magnetoencephalography (MEG) study by Khan et al. (2013), who reported reduced local functional connectivity within the fusiform face area in response to face and house stimuli in adolescents with ASD. This may at first glance appear at odds with our findings of overconnectivity in fusiform gyrus in some of the analyses. However, note that the cited MEG study operationalized "local connectivity" by testing the phase–amplitude coupling between alpha and gamma bands, which presumably reflects *inhibitory* connectivity. This differs fundamentally from physiological mechanisms boosting correlations of the BOLD signal, which likely rely primarily on excitatory connectivity. Ours and the findings from Khan et al. (2013) may thus well be compatible, indicating increased excitatory and reduced inhibitory local connectivity in inferior occipitotemporal regions, respectively.

CHALLENGES AND CONCLUSIONS

We found that local connectivity was atypical in adolescents with ASD, with overconnectivity – mostly in occipital and posterior temporal regions – accompanied by underconnectivity in cingulate and medial frontal sites. While the consistency of findings across different analysis pipelines and in low-motion subsamples was reassuring, many challenges remain for a full understanding of local connectivity, both at the methodological and conceptual levels. Methodologically, limits of spatial and temporal resolution may best be approached in future studies combining hemodynamic and electrophysiological techniques. However, a spatial resolution adequate for the *in vivo* study of cytoarchitectonic anomalies, which may affect local connectivity in ASD, is unlikely in the foreseeable future and there is a need for mechanistic models that will allow a prediction of effects that can be detected with fMRI, based on post mortem findings on cellular organization.

Although only a first step in this direction, our findings indicate that local connectivity at a relatively coarse spatial scale is aberrant in ASD. However, the patterns of these aberrations were inconsistent with previous simple hypotheses about "local overconnectivity contrasting with long-distance underconnectivity" (as described in the Introduction), suggesting instead regionally specific abnormalities of local connectivity, whose functional significance (e.g., in the visual system) is only beginning to emerge.

ACKNOWLEDGMENTS

This study was supported by the National Institutes of Health R01-MH081023, with additional funding from NIH/NIGMS IMSD 5R25GM058906-13 (Jose O. Maximo) and Autism Speaks (Dennis Weatherstone Predoctoral Fellowship #7850; to Aarti Nair). Special thanks to the participants and their families.

REFERENCES

Amaral, D. G., Schumann, C. M., and Nordahl, C. W. (2008). Neuroanatomy of autism. *Trends Neurosci.* 31, 137–145. doi: 10.1016/j.tins.2007.12.005

Anderson, J. S., Nielsen, J. A., Froehlich, A. L., Dubray, M. B., Druzgal, T. J., Cariello, A. N., et al. (2011). Functional connectivity magnetic resonance imaging classification of autism. *Brain* 134, 3742–3754. doi: 10.1093/brain/awr263

Anderson, J. S., Zielinski, B. A., Nielsen, J. A., and Ferguson, M. A. (2013). Complexity of low-frequency blood oxygen level-dependent fluctuations covaries with local connectivity. *Hum. Brain Mapp.* doi: 10.1002/hbm.22251 [Epub ahead of print].

Assaf, M., Jagannathan, K., Calhoun, V. D., Miller, L., Stevens, M. C., Sahl, R., et al. (2010). Abnormal functional connectivity of default mode sub-networks in autism spectrum disorder patients. *Neuroimage* 53, 247–256. doi: 10.1016/j.neuroimage.2010.05.067

Belmonte, M. K., Allen, G., Beckel-Mitchener, A., Boulanger, L. M., Carper, R. A., and Webb, S. J. (2004). Autism and abnormal development of brain connectivity. *J. Neurosci.* 24, 9228–9231. doi: 10.1523/JNEUROSCI.3340-04.2004

Boddaert, N., Belin, P., Chabane, N., Poline, J. B., Barthelemy, C., Mouren-Simeoni, M. C., et al. (2003). Perception of complex sounds: abnormal pattern of cortical activation in autism. *Am. J. Psychiatry* 160, 2057–2060. doi: 10.1176/appi.ajp.160.11.2057

Bullmore, E., and Sporns, O. (2009). Complex brain networks: graph theoretical analysis of structural and functional systems. *Nat. Rev. Neurosci.* 10, 186–198. doi: 10.1038/nrn2575

Cardinale, R. C., Shih, P., Fishman, I., Ford, L. M., and Müller, R.-A. (2013). Pervasive rightward asymmetry shifts of functional networks in autism spectrum disorder: an fMRI study using independent component analysis. *JAMA Psychiatry* 70, 975–982. doi: 10.1001/jamapsychiatry.2013.382

Casanova, M., and Trippe, J. (2009). Radial cytoarchitecture and patterns of cortical connectivity in autism. *Philos. Trans. R. Soc. Lond. B Biol. Sci.* 364, 1433–1436. doi: 10.1098/rstb.2008.0331

Casanova, M. F., Van Kooten, I. A., Switala, A. E., Van Engeland, H., Heinsen, H., Steinbusch, H. W., et al. (2006). Minicolumnar abnormalities in autism. *Acta Neuropathol. (Berl.)* 112, 287–303. doi: 10.1007/s00401-006-0085-5

CDC. (2012). Prevalence of autism spectrum disorders: autism and developmental disabilities monitoring network, 14 sites, United States. *MMWR Surveill. Summ.* 61, 12–19.

Cordes, D., Haughton, V. M., Arfanakis, K., Carew, J. D., Turski, P. A., Moritz, C. H., et al. (2001). Frequencies contributing to functional connectivity in the cerebral cortex in "resting-state" data. *Am. J. Neuroradiol.* 22, 1326–1333.

Courchesne, E., Campbell, K., and Solso, S. (2011). Brain growth across the life span in autism: age-specific changes in anatomical pathology. *Brain Res.* 1380, 138–145. doi: 10.1016/j.brainres.2010.09.101

Courchesne, E., and Pierce, K. (2005). Why the frontal cortex in autism might be talking only to itself: local over-connectivity but long-distance disconnection. *Curr. Opin. Neurobiol.* 15, 225–230. doi: 10.1016/j.conb.2005.03.001

Cox, R. W. (1996). AFNI: software for analysis and visualization of functional magnetic resonance neuroimages. *Comput. Biomed. Res.* 29, 162–173. doi: 10.1006/cbmr.1996.0014

Dai, Z., Yan, C., Wang, Z., Wang, J., Xia, M., Li, K., et al. (2012). Discriminative analysis of early Alzheimer's disease using multi-modal imaging and multi-level characterization with multi-classifier (M3). *Neuroimage* 59, 2187–2195. doi: 10.1016/j.neuroimage.2011.10.003

Dakin, S., and Frith, U. (2005). Vagaries of visual perception in autism. *Neuron* 48, 497–507. doi: 10.1016/j.neuron.2005.10.018

Di Martino, A., Zuo, X. N., Kelly, C., Grzadzinski, R., Mennes, M., Schvarcz, A., et al. (2013). Shared and distinct intrinsic functional network centrality in autism and attention-deficit/hyperactivity disorder. *Biol. Psychiatry* doi: 10.1016/j.biopsych.2013.02.01 [Epub ahead of print].

Dong, M., Qin, W., Zhao, L., Yang, X., Yuan, K., Zeng, F., et al. (2013). Expertise modulates local regional homogeneity of spontaneous brain activity in the resting brain: an fMRI study using the model of skilled acupuncturists. *Hum. Brain Mapp.* doi: 10.1002/hbm.22235 [Epub ahead of print].

Eyler, L. T., Pierce, K., and Courchesne, E. (2012). A failure of left temporal cortex to specialize for language is an early emerging and fundamental property of autism. *Brain* 135, 949–960. doi: 10.1093/brain/awr364

Farb, N. A., Grady, C. L., Strother, S., Tang-Wai, D. F., Masellis, M., Black, S., et al. (2012). Abnormal network connectivity in frontotemporal dementia: evidence for prefrontal isolation. *Cortex* 49, 1856–1873. doi: 10.1016/j.cortex.2012.09.008

Jenkinson, M., Bannister, P., Brady, M., and Smith, S. (2002). Improved optimization for the robust and accurate linear registration and motion correction of brain images. *Neuroimage* 17, 825–841. doi: 10.1006/nimg.2002.1132

Jenkinson, M., and Smith, S. (2001). A global optimisation method for robust affine registration of brain images. *Med. Image Anal.* 5, 143–156. doi: 10.1016/S1361-8415(01)00036-6

Keehn, B., Shih, P., Brenner, L., Townsend, J., and Müller, R.-A. (2012). Functional connectivity for an "island of sparing" in autism spectrum disorder: an fMRI study of visual search. *Hum. Brain Mapp.* doi: 10.1002/hbm.22084 [Epub ahead of print].

Khan, S., Gramfort, A., Shetty, N. R., Kitzbichler, M. G., Ganesan, S., Moran, J. M., et al. (2013). Local and long-range functional connectivity is reduced in concert in autism spectrum disorders. *Proc. Natl. Acad. Sci. U.S.A.* 110, 3107–3112. doi: 10.1073/pnas.1214533110

Kim, Y. S., Leventhal, B. L., Koh, Y. J., Fombonne, E., Laska, E., Lim, E. C., et al. (2011). Prevalence of autism spectrum disorders in a total population sample. *Am. J. Psychiatry* 168, 904–912. doi: 10.1176/appi.ajp.2011.10101532

Liu, X., Zhu, X. H., and Chen, W. (2011). Baseline BOLD correlation predicts individuals' stimulus-evoked BOLD responses. *Neuroimage* 54, 2278–2286. doi: 10.1016/j.neuroimage.2010.10.001

Lopez-Larson, M. P., Anderson, J. S., Ferguson, M. A., and Yurgelun-Todd, D. (2011). Local brain connectivity and associations with gender and age. *Dev. Cogn. Neurosci.* 1, 187–197. doi: 10.1016/j.dcn.2010.10.001

Lord, C., Risi, S., Lambrecht, L., Cook, E. H. Jr., Leventhal, B. L., Dilavore, P. C., et al. (2000). The autism diagnostic observation schedule-generic: a standard measure of social and communication deficits associated with the spectrum of autism. *J. Autism Dev. Disord.* 30, 205–223. doi: 10.1023/A:1005592401947

Lord, C., Rutter, M., and Le Couteur, A. (1994). Autism diagnostic interview-revised: a revised version of a diagnostic interview for caregivers of individuals with possible pervasive developmental disorders. *J. Autism Dev. Disord.* 24, 659–685. doi: 10.1007/BF02172145

Lynch, C. J., Uddin, L. Q., Supekar, K., Khouzam, A., Phillips, J., and Menon, V. (2013). Default mode network in childhood autism: posteromedial cortex heterogeneity and relationship with social deficits. *Biol. Psychiatry* 74, 212–219. doi: 10.1016/j.biopsych.2012.12.013

Monk, C. S., Peltier, S. J., Wiggins, J. L., Weng, S. J., Carrasco, M., Risi, S., et al. (2009). Abnormalities of intrinsic functional connectivity in autism spectrum disorders. *Neuroimage* 47, 764–772. doi: 10.1016/j.neuroimage.2009.04.069

Mottron, L., Dawson, M., Soulieres, I., Hubert, B., and Burack, J. (2006). Enhanced perceptual functioning in autism: an update, and eight principles of autistic perception. *J. Autism Dev. Disord.* 36, 27–43. doi: 10.1007/s10803-005-0040-7

Müller, R.-A., Shih, P., Keehn, B., Deyoe, J. R., Leyden, K. M., and Shukla, D. K. (2011). Underconnected, but how? A survey of functional connectivity MRI studies in autism spectrum disorders. *Cereb. Cortex* 21, 2233–2243. doi: 10.1093/cercor/bhq296

Murphy, K., Birn, R. M., Handwerker, D. A., Jones, T. B., and Bandettini, P. A. (2009). The impact of global signal regression on resting state correlations: are anti-correlated networks introduced? *Neuroimage* 44, 893–905. doi: 10.1016/j.neuroimage.2008.09.036

Nebel, M. B., Joel, S. E., Muschelli, J., Barber, A. D., Caffo, B. S., Pekar, J. J., et al. (2012). Disruption of functional organization within the primary motor cortex in children with autism. *Hum. Brain Mapp.* doi: 10.1002/hbm.22188 [Epub ahead of print].

Northoff, G., Qin, P., and Nakao, T. (2010). Rest-stimulus interaction in the brain: a review. *Trends Neurosci.* 33, 277–284. doi: 10.1016/j.tins.2010.02.006

Oldfield, R. C. (1971). The assessment and analysis of handedness: the Edinburgh inventory. *Neuropsychologia* 9, 97–113. doi: 10.1016/0028-3932(71)90067-4

O'Riordan, M. A. (2004). Superior visual search in adults with autism. *Autism* 8, 229–248. doi: 10.1177/1362361304045219

Paakki, J. J., Rahko, J., Long, X., Moilanen, I., Tervonen, O., Nikkinen, J., et al. (2010). Alterations in regional homogeneity of resting-state brain activity in autism spectrum disorders. *Brain Res.* 1321, 169–179. doi: 10.1016/j.brainres.2009.12.081

Power, J. D., Barnes, K. A., Snyder, A. Z., Schlaggar, B. L., and Petersen, S. E. (2012). Spurious but systematic correlations in functional connectivity MRI networks arise from subject motion. *Neuroimage* 59, 2142–2154. doi: 10.1016/j.neuroimage.2011.10.018

Raichle, M. E., Macleod, A. M., Snyder, A. Z., Powers, W. J., Gusnard, D. A., and Shulman, G. L. (2001). A default mode of brain function. *Proc. Natl. Acad. Sci. U.S.A.* 98, 676–682. doi: 10.1073/pnas.98.2.676

Rippon, G., Brock, J., Brown, C., and Boucher, J. (2007). Disordered connectivity in the autistic brain: challenges for the "new psychophysiology." *Int. J. Psychophysiol.* 63, 164–172. doi: 10.1016/j.ijpsycho.2006.03.012

Rubenstein, J. L., and Merzenich, M. M. (2003). Model of autism: increased ratio of excitation/inhibition in key neural systems. *Genes Brain Behav.* 2, 255–267. doi: 10.1034/j.1601-183X.2003.00037.x

Rudie, J. D., Brown, J. A., Beck-Pancer, D., Hernandez, L. M., Dennis, E. L., Thompson, P. M., et al. (2013). Altered functional and structural brain network organization in autism. *Neuroimage Clin.* 2, 79–94. doi: 10.1016/j.nicl.2012.11.006

Rudie, J. D., Shehzad, Z., Hernandez, L. M., Colich, N. L., Bookheimer, S. Y., Iacoboni, M., et al. (2012). Reduced functional integration and segregation of distributed neural systems underlying social and emotional information processing in autism spectrum disorders. *Cereb. Cortex* 22, 1025–1037. doi: 10.1093/cercor/bhr171

Saad, Z. S., Gotts, S. J., Murphy, K., Chen, G., Jo, H. J., Martin, A., et al. (2012). Trouble at rest: how correlation patterns and group differences become distorted after global signal regression. *Brain Connect.* 2, 25–32. doi: 10.1089/brain.2012.0080

Samson, F., Mottron, L., Soulieres, I., and Zeffiro, T. A. (2012). Enhanced visual functioning in autism: an ALE meta-analysis. *Hum. Brain Mapp.* 33, 1553–1581. doi: 10.1002/hbm.21307

Satterthwaite, T. D., Elliott, M. A., Gerraty, R. T., Ruparel, K., Loughead, J., Calkins, M. E., et al. (2013). An improved framework for confound regression and filtering for control of motion artifact in the preprocessing of resting-state functional connectivity data. *Neuroimage* 64, 240–256. doi: 10.1016/j.neuroimage.2012.08.052

Schipul, S. E., Keller, T. A., and Just, M. A. (2011). Inter-regional brain communication and its disturbance in autism. *Front. Syst. Neurosci.* 5:10. doi: 10.3389/fnsys.2011.00010

Schölvinck, M. L., Maier, A., Ye, F. Q., Duyn, J. H., and Leopold, D. A. (2010). Neural basis of global resting-state fMRI activity. *Proc. Natl. Acad. Sci. U.S.A.* 107, 10238–10243. doi: 10.1073/pnas.0913110107

Sepulcre, J., Liu, H., Talukdar, T., Martincorena, I., Yeo, B. T., and Buckner, R. L. (2010). The organization of local and distant functional connectivity in the human brain. *PLoS Comput. Biol.* 6:e1000808. doi: 10.1371/journal.pcbi.1000808

Shih, P., Keehn, B., Oram, J. K., Leyden, K. M., Keown, C. L., and Müller, R.-A. (2011). Functional differentiation of posterior superior temporal sulcus in autism: a functional connectivity magnetic resonance imaging study. *Biol. Psychiatry* 70, 270–277. doi: 10.1016/j.biopsych.2011.03.040

Shukla, D. K., Keehn, B., and Müller, R.-A. (2011a). Tract-specific analyses of diffusion tensor imaging show widespread white matter compromise in autism spectrum disorder. *J. Child Psychol. Psychiatry* 52, 286–295. doi: 10.1111/j.1469-7610.2010.02342.x

Shukla, D. K., Keehn, B., Smylie, D. M., and Müller, R.-A. (2011b). Microstructural abnormalities of short-distance white matter tracts in autism spectrum disorder. *Neuropsychologia* 49, 1378–1382. doi: 10.1016/j.neuropsychologia.2011.02.022

Shukla, D. K., Keehn, B. M., and Müller, R.-A. (2010). Regional homogeneity of fMRI time series in autism spectrum disorders. *Neurosci. Lett.* 476, 46–51. doi: 10.1016/j.neulet.2010.03.080

Simmons, D. R., Robertson, A. E., Mckay, L. S., Toal, E., Mcaleer, P., and Pollick, F. E. (2009). Vision in autism spectrum disorders. *Vis. Res.* 49, 2705–2739. doi: 10.1016/j.visres.2009.08.005

Smith, S. M., Jenkinson, M., Woolrich, M. W., Beckmann, C. F., Behrens, T. E., Johansen-Berg, H., et al. (2004). Advances in functional and structural MR image analysis and implementation as FSL. *Neuroimage* 23(Suppl. 1), S208–S219. doi: 10.1016/j.neuroimage.2004.07.051

Van Dijk, K. R., Sabuncu, M. R., and Buckner, R. L. (2012). The influence of head motion on intrinsic functional connectivity MRI. *Neuroimage* 59, 431–438. doi: 10.1016/j.neuroimage.2011.07.044

Vissers, M. E., Cohen, M. X., and Geurts, H. M. (2012). Brain connectivity and high functioning autism: a promising path of research that needs refined models, methodological convergence, and stronger behavioral links. *Neurosci. Biobehav. Rev.* 36, 604–625. doi: 10.1016/j.neubiorev.2011.09.003

von dem Hagen, E. A., Stoyanova, R. S., Baron-Cohen, S., and Calder, A. J. (2012). Reduced functional connectivity within and between 'social' resting state networks in autism spectrum conditions. *Soc. Cogn. Affect. Neurosci.* 8, 694–701. doi: 10.1093/scan/nss053

Wang, L., Song, M., Jiang, T., Zhang, Y., and Yu, C. (2011). Regional homogeneity of the resting-state brain activity correlates with individual intelligence. *Neurosci. Lett.* 488, 275–278. doi: 10.1016/j.neulet.2010.11.046

Wass, S. (2011). Distortions and disconnections: disrupted brain connectivity in autism. *Brain Cogn.* 75, 18–28. doi: 10.1016/j.bandc.2010.10.005

Weaver, K. E., Chaovalitwongse, W. A., Novotny, E. J., Poliakov, A., Grabowski, T. G., and Ojemann, J. G. (2013). Local functional connectivity as a pre-surgical tool for seizure focus identification in non-lesion, focal epilepsy. *Front. Neurol.* 4:43. doi: 10.3389/fneur.2013.00043

Wechsler, D. (1999). *Wechsler Abbreviated Scale of Intelligence.* San Antonio, TX: Harcourt Assessment.

Weinstein, M., Ben-Sira, L., Levy, Y., Zachor, D. A., Ben Itzhak, E., Artzi, M., et al. (2011). Abnormal white matter integrity in young children with autism. *Hum. Brain Mapp.* 32, 534–543. doi: 10.1002/hbm.21042

Wolff, J. J., Gu, H., Gerig, G., Elison, J. T., Styner, M., Gouttard, S., et al. (2012). Differences in white matter fiber tract development present from 6 to 24 months in infants with autism. *Am. J. Psychiatry* 169, 589–600. doi: 10.1176/appi.ajp.2011.11091447

Yan, C. G., Cheung, B., Kelly, C., Colcombe, S., Craddock, R. C., Di Martino, A., et al. (2013). A comprehensive assessment of regional variation in the impact of head micromovements on functional connectomics. *Neuroimage* 76C, 183–201. doi: 10.1016/j.neuroimage.2013.03.004

Yin, Y., Jin, C., Eyler, L. T., Jin, H., Hu, X., Duan, L., et al. (2012). Altered regional homogeneity in post-traumatic stress disorder: a resting-state functional magnetic resonance imaging study. *Neurosci. Bull.* 28, 541–549. doi: 10.1007/s12264-012-1261-3

Zalesky, A., Fornito, A., Egan, G. F., Pantelis, C., and Bullmore, E. T. (2012). The relationship between regional and inter-regional functional connectivity deficits in schizophrenia. *Hum. Brain Mapp.* 33, 2535–2549. doi: 10.1002/hbm.21379

Zang, Y., Jiang, T., Lu, Y., He, Y., and Tian, L. (2004). Regional homogeneity approach to fMRI data analysis. *Neuroimage* 22, 394–400. doi: 10.1016/j.neuroimage.2003.12.030

Zhang, Y., Brady, M., and Smith, S. (2001). Segmentation of brain MR images through a hidden Markov random field model and the expectation-maximization algorithm. *IEEE Trans. Med. Imaging* 20, 45–57. doi: 10.1109/42.906424

Zou, Q., Wu, C. W., Stein, E. A., Zang, Y., and Yang, Y. (2009). Static and dynamic characteristics of cerebral blood flow during the resting state. *Neuroimage* 48, 515–524. doi: 10.1016/j.neuroimage.2009.07.006

Zuo, X. N., Xu, T., Jiang, L., Yang, Z., Cao, X. Y., He, Y., et al. (2013). Toward reliable characterization of functional homogeneity in the human brain: preprocessing, scan duration, imaging resolution and computational space. *Neuroimage* 65, 374–386. doi: 10.1016/j.neuroimage.2012.10.017

Conflict of Interest Statement: The authors declare that the research was conducted in the absence of any commercial or financial relationships that could be construed as a potential conflict of interest.

Received: 14 June 2013; accepted: 05 September 2013; published online: 08 October 2013.

Citation: Maximo JO, Keown CL, Nair A and Müller R-A (2013) Approaches to local connectivity in autism using resting state functional connectivity MRI. Front. Hum. Neurosci. 7:605. doi: 10.3389/fnhum.2013.00605

This article was submitted to the journal Frontiers in Human Neuroscience.

16

Abnormal functional connectivity during visuospatial processing is associated with disrupted organisation of white matter in autism

Jane McGrath*[1]*, *Katherine Johnson*[1,2], *Erik O'Hanlon*[3], *Hugh Garavan*[1,4], *Alexander Leemans*[5] and *Louise Gallagher*[1]

[1] *Department of Psychiatry, Trinity College Dublin, Ireland*
[2] *Department of Psychology, University of Melbourne, Melbourne, Victoria, Australia*
[3] *Department of Psychiatry, Royal College of Surgeons in Ireland, Dublin, Ireland*
[4] *Department of Psychology, University of Vermont, Burlington, VT, USA*
[5] *Image Sciences Institute, University Medical Centre Utrecht, Utrecht, Netherlands*

Edited by:
Rajesh K. Kana, University of Alabama at Birmingham, USA

Reviewed by:
Brittany Travers, University of Wisconsin-Madison, USA
Franco Pestilli, Stanford University, USA

****Correspondence:***
Jane McGrath, Department of Psychiatry, Trinity Centre for Health Sciences, St. James's Hospital, Dublin 8, Ireland
e-mail: jane.mcgrath@tcd.ie

Disruption of structural and functional neural connectivity has been widely reported in Autism Spectrum Disorder (ASD) but there is a striking lack of research attempting to integrate analysis of functional and structural connectivity in the same study population, an approach that may provide key insights into the specific neurobiological underpinnings of altered functional connectivity in autism. The aims of this study were (1) to determine whether functional connectivity abnormalities were associated with structural abnormalities of white matter (WM) in ASD and (2) to examine the relationships between aberrant neural connectivity and behavior in ASD. Twenty-two individuals with ASD and 22 age, IQ-matched controls completed a high-angular-resolution diffusion MRI scan. Structural connectivity was analysed using constrained spherical deconvolution (CSD) based tractography. Regions for tractography were generated from the results of a previous study, in which 10 pairs of brain regions showed abnormal functional connectivity during visuospatial processing in ASD. WM tracts directly connected 5 of the 10 region pairs that showed abnormal functional connectivity; linking a region in the left occipital lobe (left BA19) and five paired regions: left caudate head, left caudate body, left uncus, left thalamus, and left cuneus. Measures of WM microstructural organization were extracted from these tracts. Fractional anisotropy (FA) reductions in the ASD group relative to controls were significant for WM connecting left BA19 to left caudate head and left BA19 to left thalamus. Using a multimodal imaging approach, this study has revealed aberrant WM microstructure in tracts that directly connect brain regions that are abnormally functionally connected in ASD. These results provide novel evidence to suggest that structural brain pathology may contribute (1) to abnormal functional connectivity and (2) to atypical visuospatial processing in ASD.

Keywords: neuroimaging, autism spectrum disorders, functional connectivity, diffusion tractography, constrained spherical deconvolution, visuospatial processing, structural connectivity, mental rotation

INTRODUCTION

There is extensive evidence to suggest that autism is a disorder characterized by disrupted functional and structural neural connectivity. Abnormal inter- and intra-regional functional connectivity has been described whilst participants have performed various neuropsychological paradigms and whilst in the resting state. In parallel with functional connectivity research, a number of diffusion imaging studies in autism have demonstrated aberrant "structural connectivity"—a term referring to the integrity of white matter (WM) micro- and macrostructure. Abnormal functional connectivity between brain regions in autism may arise from disrupted organization of WM, but its pathophysiology is unknown. Despite the numerous studies that have consistently reported abnormal functional connectivity in autism, there is a surprising lack of research attempting to integrate analysis of functional and structural connectivity in the same study population, an approach that may provide key insights into the specific neurobiological underpinnings of altered functional connectivity in autism.

BEHAVIORAL EFFECTS OF DISRUPTED NEURAL CONNECTIVITY IN ASD

There appear to be significant behavioral effects of disrupted structural and functional connectivity in autism. In relation to structural connectivity, several studies have explored the correlation between WM organization and autism symptom severity. Fractional anisotropy (FA) is a widely used measure that provides information about the degree of WM organization. Increased severity of restricted and repetitive behaviors was correlated with increased FA in left precentral gyrus and posterior brain regions (Cheung et al., 2009), with reduced FA in the right anterior cingulate cortex (Thakkar et al., 2008) and with the number of tracts in the forceps minor (Thomas et al., 2011). More severe social-communicative deficits have been correlated with reduced FA in WM of fronto-striatal regions, temporal regions, the posterior part of the corpus callosum (Cheung et al., 2009), left and right uncinate fasciculus, left superior longitudinal fasciculus, left and right fornix (Poustka et al., 2011), the dorsolateral prefrontal cortex (Noriuchi et al., 2010), right anterior thalamic radiation and right uncinate fasciculus (Cheon et al., 2011) and left cerebellar peduncle (Catani et al., 2008) and with increased fiber length and density in the corpus callosum (Kumar et al., 2010). Alexander et al. found a relationship between Autism Spectrum Disorder (ASD) symptom severity (Social Responsiveness Scale) and WM measures (although it was only seen across both groups combined and not just within the ASD group; Alexander et al., 2007). Some studies however have found no correlation between ASD symptomatology and WM measures (Sundaram et al., 2008; Barnea-Goraly et al., 2010; Shukla et al., 2010; Hong et al., 2011; Jou et al., 2011). Reduced microstructural organization of WM in autism has also been correlated with lower performance IQ scores (Alexander et al., 2007) and with increased response times in a pictorial problem-solving task (Sahyoun et al., 2010).

A number of studies have also investigated the behavioral effects of functional connectivity abnormalities in ASD and have reported correlations between altered functional connectivity and core symptoms of autism. Reduced fronto-posterior functional connectivity was found to correlate with increased severity of autism (Just et al., 2007). Poorer social functioning in individuals with ASD has been associated with reduced functional connectivity between the superior frontal gyrus and posterior cingulate (Monk et al., 2009; Weng et al., 2010) and communication deficits have been associated with increased functional connectivity between regions of the default mode network during the resting state (Weng et al., 2010). Increased severity of repetitive behaviors in autism has been associated with reduced functional connectivity between frontal structures and the posterior cingulate (Weng et al., 2010), and also with increased functional connectivity between the posterior cingulate and parahippocampal gyrus (Monk et al., 2009) and between the anterior cingulate and frontal eye fields (Agam et al., 2010). In summary, results from both anatomical and functional studies suggest that disrupted neural connectivity in autism may impact negatively on core features of the condition.

EVIDENCE FOR A RELATIONSHIP BETWEEN DISRUPTED BRAIN WHITE MATTER STRUCTURE AND FUNCTIONAL CONNECTIVITY ABNORMALITIES IN ASD

The direct impact of WM abnormalities on functional connectivity in ASD has been less well-studied. This is surprising given the extensive literature that has documented abnormal functional connectivity in the disorder, and the lack of knowledge about the pathophysiology of this abnormal functional connectivity. A small number of studies have used a measure of the size of the corpus callosum as an index of "anatomical connectivity" and demonstrated a relationship between reduced size of the corpus callosum and reduced functional connectivity during a number of neuropsychological paradigms, including the Tower of London task (Just et al., 2007), a sentence comprehension and visual imagery task (Kana et al., 2006), the Embedded Figures task (Damarla et al., 2010), a narrative comprehension task (Mason et al., 2008), and whilst participants were at rest (Cherkassky et al., 2006). No previous studies in autism have attempted to identify whether there are abnormal WM connections that directly link brain regions showing abnormal functional connectivity, nor have any studies examined the relationship between alterations in structural connectivity and functional connectivity.

EVIDENCE FOR A RELATIONSHIP BETWEEN BRAIN WHITE MATTER STRUCTURE AND FUNCTIONAL CONNECTIVITY IN NEUROTYPICAL POPULATIONS

In neurotypical populations, a number of multimodal (functional MRI and diffusion MRI) imaging studies have integrated structural and functional connectivity analyses in the same study population and have shown that there is evidence of substantial correspondence between structural and functional connectivity.

Studies that have combined analyses of structural and functional connectivity during the resting state have revealed a structural basis for resting state functional connectivity. Regions of the default mode network are linked by WM tracts (Greicius et al., 2009), the level of WM organization in the cingulum is correlated with resting state functional connectivity between midline brain regions (van den Heuvel et al., 2008) and maps of resting state functional connectivity in adult macaque monkeys were shown to be markedly similar to maps of structural connectivity obtained from tracer studies (Vincent et al., 2007; Margulies et al., 2009).

These combined structural/resting state studies have also provided evidence for a relationship (albeit complex) between anatomical and functional connectivity. Studies that have generated whole brain maps of functional and anatomical connectivity on the same cohort of participants have demonstrated that structural connection patterns and functional interactions between regions of the cortex are significantly correlated (Hagmann et al., 2008; Skudlarski et al., 2008; Honey et al., 2009; Hermundstad et al., 2013). This relationship between structural and functional connectivity is not a simple one however; strong functional connections often exist between regions with no direct anatomical connection (Honey et al., 2009). Such functional connections may arise from indirect WM connections, or from the two regions receiving common input from a third region (Behrens and Sporns, 2012).

There is also some evidence supporting a direct relationship between anatomical and functional connectivity at the level of individual pathways. The strength of functional connectivity within the default mode network was positively correlated with the level of WM organization in the cingulum, as estimated by FA (van den Heuvel et al., 2008). Consistent with the hypothesis that functional connectivity is directly related to anatomical connectivity, a study of three patients with callosal agenesis revealed reduced interhemispheric functional connectivity in the motor and auditory cortices (Quigley et al., 2003). Complete section of the corpus callosum in a young boy with intractable epilepsy resulted in a striking loss of interhemispheric resting state functional connectivity, with preservation of intrahemispheric functional connectivity (Johnston et al., 2008). In patients with multiple sclerosis, disease-related reduction of functional connectivity between left and right primary sensorimotor cortices was associated with increased radial diffusivity in the WM tracts connecting these regions, again indicating a relationship between reduced anatomical connectivity and reduced functional connectivity (Lowe et al., 2008).

To date, studies investigating a link between structural and functional connectivity in neurotypical populations have indicated that functional connectivity has a structural basis, and that there is evidence of substantial correspondence between the strength of structural and functional connectivity.

FUNCTIONAL CONNECTIVITY DURING VISUOSPATIAL PROCESSING IN ASD

Atypical visuospatial processing is common in autism spectrum disorders. In brief, enhanced visuospatial processing in ASD has been described in behavioral studies during a variety of cognitive tasks (see McGrath et al., 2012, for review). A number of neuroimaging studies have revealed that brain activity and connectivity differs markedly between ASD and control groups during visuospatial processing (Lee et al., 2007; Manjaly et al., 2007; Damarla et al., 2010). Recent work from our group used functional connectivity MRI (fcMRI) to investigate the neural correlates of visuospatial processing during a mental rotation task, whereby two rotated stimuli were judged to be the same ("Same" trials) or mirror-imaged ("Mirror" trials; McGrath et al., 2012). Results of this study indicated that there was a relative advantage of mental rotation in the ASD group. The ASD group performed Same and Mirror trials at similar speeds, but the control group slowed significantly on Mirror trials relative to Same trials. Functional connectivity analysis revealed marked abnormalities in the ASD group that were characterized by long-range fronto-posterior underconnectivity and short-range intra-occipital overconnectivity. This study concluded that atypical visuospatial processing in ASD appears to be associated with both quantitative and qualitative differences in functional connectivity, which may result in a combination of enhanced low-level visual perceptual processing and a reduction of higher-level cortical control. A further study from our group investigated the structural properties of major WM tracts that are thought to play an important role in visuospatial processing (McGrath et al., 2013) This research demonstrated that there were significant alterations in the microstructural organization of WM in the right inferior fronto-occipital fasciculus (IFOF) in ASD. This alteration was associated with poorer visuospatial processing performance in the ASD group. This study provided an insight into structural brain abnormalities that may influence atypical visuospatial processing in autism, however it did not provide any information on how WM abnormalities may impact on functional connectivity in the disorder.

AIMS AND HYPOTHESES

In ASD, there is strong evidence for disrupted functional and anatomical connectivity but no previous studies have attempted to integrate these types of connectivity analyses. The integration of functional and structural connectivity analysis in the same study population allows for the investigation of inter-participant variability in structural connectivity and provides an opportunity to relate this variability to differences in individual functional connectivity and behavior (Hagmann et al., 2008). As discussed above, such multimodal connectivity studies in neurotypical populations have revealed strong relationships between WM organization, functional connectivity and behavior. Thus, the aims of this study were two-fold; first to investigate the structural integrity of WM that directly connected brain regions showing abnormal functional connectivity in ASD, and second to investigate relationships between brain WM structure, functional connectivity and behavior. To do this, brain regions from a previously reported functional connectivity analysis (McGrath et al., 2012) were used as regions of interest (ROIs) for diffusion tractography in order to isolate WM tracts that directly linked the two regions. Microstructural organization of these WM tracts was assessed and correlated with both functional connectivity and behavioral measures to provide a comprehensive examination of the relationships between brain structural connectivity, functional connectivity and behavior in ASD. It was hypothesized that there would be WM tracts linking some, but not all, pairs of brain regions that showed abnormal functional connectivity. This hypothesis was based on the knowledge that functional connectivity between regions does not always require a direct WM connection, but can be mediated by indirect connections or input from unrelated regions (Behrens and Sporns, 2012). It was also hypothesized that WM structure would be abnormal in tracts directly connecting the functionally defined ROIs and that there would be correlation between microstructural organization of WM, functional connectivity and behavior. It is difficult to make specific predictions about the correlations in this study because there is such a limited literature that has investigated relationships between structural connectivity, functional connectivity and behavior. Nevertheless, it was theorized that if ASD and control groups do use qualitatively and quantitatively neural networks for successful visuospatial processing as hypothesized in McGrath et al. (2012), there should be differential relationships between WM organization, functional connectivity and response time data in the ASD and control groups.

MATERIALS AND METHODS

PARTICIPANTS

Twenty-two right-handed male individuals with ASD and 22 right-handed age- and IQ-matched male neurotypical controls were included in the analysis (see **Table 1**). Participants with ASD were recruited from an existing autism genetics sample at the Department of Psychiatry, Trinity College Dublin, and through additional recruitment from local schools and child and adolescent mental health services. The diagnosis of autism was established using two structured research diagnostic tools; the Autism Diagnostic Interview-Revised [ADI-R, (Lord et al., 1994)] and the Autism Diagnostic Observation Schedule-Generic [ADOS-G, (Lord et al., 2000)]. Administrators of the ADI-R and ADOS-G were trained to reliability and maintained reliability. Community-recruited control participants were selected to match participants with autism on age, handedness, gender, race and IQ (full-scale IQ was estimated based on four sub-scales of the WISC/WAIS [Wechsler Intelligence Scale for Children

Table 1 | Demographics of study participants *Full scale IQ was estimated based on four sub-scales of the WISC/WAIS [Wechsler Intelligence Scale for Children (WISC-III or IV UK), (Wechsler, 2004) and Wechsler Adult Intelligence Scale (WAIS-III), (Wechsler, 1997)].

	Control	ASD	*p*-value
Number	22	22	
Gender	Male (22)	Male (22)	
Age mean (SD, Range)	17.51 (2.76, 13.6–21.3)	17.56 (2.91, 13.0–21.8)	0.76
Full scale IQ* Mean (SD, Range)	110.50 (16.97, 84–147)	105.95 (13.46, 84–127)	0.25
Verbal IQ^ Mean (SD, Range)	117.60 (12.69, 93–134)	105.60 (18.48, 79–134)	0.11
Performance IQ~ Mean (SD, Range)	120.80 (26.39, 91–155)	124.35 (17.46, 99–155)	0.73
Handedness	Right (22)	Right (22)	
Medication	None	None	
Ethnicity	Irish (22)	Irish (22)	

^Verbal IQ was estimated using the Information and Vocabulary subtests of the WISC III for n = 10 participants with ASD and n = 10 matched controls, using Sattler's method (Sattler, 1992). It was not possible to produce a Verbal IQ for n = 12 participants with ASD and n = 12 controls, as the WISC IV was used to estimate full scale IQ for these participants. ~Performance IQ was estimated using the Picture Completion and Block Design subtests of the WISC III for n = 10 participants with ASD and n = 10 for controls, using Sattler's method (Sattler, 1992). It was not possible to produce a Performance IQ for n = 12 participants with ASD and n = 12 controls, as the WISC-IV was used to estimate full scale IQ for these participants. Subtests of the WISC-IV that were used to calculate full scale IQ included Similarities, Block Design, Digit Span, and Coding. Subtests of the WAIS that were used to calculate full scale IQ included Similarities, Block Design, Digit Span and Matrix Reasoning.

(WISC-III and IV UK)], (Wechsler, 2004) and Wechsler Adult Intelligence Scale (WAIS-III), (Wechsler, 1997)]. Verbal IQ and performance IQ were estimated from the verbal and performance subtests of the WISC-III and WAIS-III data. Exclusion criteria included known causes for autism, e.g., tuberous sclerosis/fragile-X syndrome, current/past neurological or psychiatric conditions, serious head injuries, MR contraindications, below-average intelligence (full-scale IQ <80) and current use of psychoactive medication. Additional exclusion criteria for controls included history of developmental delay or first-degree relatives with ASD. The study was approved by the Irish Health Services Executive Linn Dara-Beechpark Research Ethics committee and by the School of Psychology Ethics Committee, Trinity College Dublin. Written informed consent was obtained from parents (where appropriate) and participants prior to scanning. Demographics of participants are detailed in **Table 1**.

OVERVIEW OF METHODS

To investigate the links between brain structural connectivity and functional connectivity, diffusion MRI data, and previously analysed functional connectivity data (see McGrath et al., 2012) from the same participants were combined. Three questions were posed:

1. Were there WM tracts directly linking pairs of brain regions that showed abnormal functional connectivity in the ASD group?
2. If there were WM tracts that directly linked pairs of brain regions showing abnormal functional connectivity, were there structural abnormalities of this WM in the ASD group?
3. Was there evidence for relationships between structural connectivity, functional connectivity and behavior?

To answer question 1, ROIs were defined from the results of a previously reported functional connectivity analysis, in which significant abnormalities of functional connectivity were reported in the ASD group (McGrath et al., 2012). These functionally defined ROIs were then used in diffusion tractography analysis to determine whether WM tracts linked brain regions that were abnormally functionally connected in the ASD group. In the methods sections below, there is a brief overview of the previously reported functional connectivity analysis (section Review of Functional Connectivity Analysis), a description of the diffusion MRI acquisition and pre-processing (section Diffusion MRI Acquisition/Preprocessing), a description of how functionally defined ROIs for tractography were selected (section Selection of Functionally Defined Seed Regions for Diffusion Tractography) and prepared for diffusion tractography (section Preparation of Functionally Defined ROIs for Tractography), and a description of the diffusion tractography protocol (section Diffusion Tractography Protocol).

To answer question 2, diffusion measures were extracted from the isolated tracts and compared between groups. Methods for this analysis are outlined in sections Dependent Measures and Between-Group Differences in White Matter Structure.

To answer question 3, a series of exploratory correlation analyses were performed to investigate the relationships between structural connectivity, functional connectivity and behavior (visuospatial processing speed). Methods for the correlation analyses are outlined in sections Correlation Analyses and Measures of White Matter Structure, Functional Connectivity and Behavior Included in the Correlation Analyses.

REVIEW OF FUNCTIONAL CONNECTIVITY ANALYSIS

fcMRI data was available on all participants who completed the diffusion MRI scan. In a previous study (McGrath et al., 2012), *psychophysiological interaction (PPI) functional connectivity analysis* (Friston et al., 1997) was used to examine functional connectivity between six seed ROIs and the rest of the brain during performance of a mental rotation task. Please see

McGrath et al. (2012) for full details of the mental rotation task, functional MRI acquisition, and PPI functional connectivity analysis. A brief summary of the functional connectivity analysis performed in McGrath et al. (2012) follows. PPI analyses were performed separately for each ROI for the Same and Mirror trials for ASD and control groups. For each PPI analysis, a multiple regression analysis was carried out for each subject. This analysis comprised seven task-related regressors (one for each experimental condition in the mental rotation task) and the motion-corrected time-series regressors to accommodate nuisance variance (for fMRI analysis). In addition, there were two other regressors. The first regressor, the physiological variable, was the detrended subject-specific time course of activity in the ROI (averaged across all voxels in the 8 mm sphere). The second regressor—the PPI term—was created by calculating the product of the detrended activation time-course from the seed region and the task regressor. The parameter estimate for the interaction term was converted to a Z-score through Fisher transformation for each subject. To investigate between-group differences in functional connectivity, Z-scores from each PPI analysis were entered into a Two-Way repeated-measures ANOVA [Group (ASD/Control) × Trial-type (Same/Mirror)]. The dependent variables that result from this PPI analysis are negative and positive connectivity. Negative connectivity indicates that the influence the task has on activity in the seed region produces a correlated opposite effect on the correlated region, which is consistent with (but not proof of) one region suppressing the other. In contrast positive connectivity between a pair of brain regions indicates that as activity in one brain region increases, there is a correlated increase in activity in the other region.

This previous study identified between-group differences in functional connectivity between all seed ROIs and numerous brain regions. These findings are summarized in **Table 2**, which is a modified version of Table 3 from McGrath et al. (2012).

DIFFUSION MRI ACQUISITION/PREPROCESSING

Whole-brain high angular resolution diffusion imaging (HARDI) data were acquired on a Philips Intera Achieva 3.0 Tesla MR system (Best, Netherlands) equipped with an eight-channel head coil. A parallel Sensitivity Encoding (SENSE) approach (Pruessmann et al., 1999) with a reduction factor of 2 was utilized for all diffusion weighted image (DWI) acquisitions. Single shot spin echo-planar imaging was used to acquire diffusion weighted data using the following parameters (Jones and Leemans, 2011): echo time (TE) 79 ms, repetition time (TR) 20,122 ms, field of view 248 × 248 mm^2, matrix 128 × 128, isotropic voxel resolution 2 × 2 × 2 mm^3, 65 slices with 2 mm thickness with no gap between slices. Diffusion gradients were applied in 61 isotropically distributed orientations with $b = 1500$ s/mm^2 and also four images with $b = 0$ s/mm^2 were acquired. Total DWI scan time was 24.3 min.

Pre-processing and tractography analyses were performed with the diffusion MR toolbox ExploreDTI (http://www.ExploreDTI.com; Leemans et al., 2009). Each DW-MRI dataset was corrected for eddy current induced geometric distortions and subject motion by realigning all DWIs to the $b = 0$ images using Elastix (Klein et al., 2010), with an affine co-registration technique (with 12 degrees of freedom) and mutual information as the cost function (Pluim et al., 2003). In this procedure, the required reorientation of the B-matrix was performed (Leemans and Jones, 2009) and the tensor model was fitted to the data using the RESTORE approach (Chang et al., 2005), which uses a process of iteratively reweighted least-square regression for outlier identification and subsequent removal, thus minimizing estimation errors originating from gross signal artifacts (e.g., cardiac pulsation and subject motion).

SELECTION OF FUNCTIONALLY DEFINED SEED REGIONS FOR DIFFUSION TRACTOGRAPHY

Results of the functional connectivity analysis, discussed in detail in McGrath et al. (2012), revealed that there were significant group differences in functional connectivity between a large number of brain regions (see **Table 2**). In the current study, pairs of brain regions showing abnormal functional connectivity in ASD were used as ROIs for diffusion tractography analysis. To minimize the number of tractography analyses, only ipsilateral pairs of brain regions that showed abnormal functional connectivity were selected for analysis (i.e., the pair of brain regions had to be either in right or left hemisphere). The analysis was limited to ipsilateral pairs as it was thought less likely that there would be direct long-range WM connections between left and right hemispheres. For example, unless the two regions showing abnormal connectivity both were in the region of the corpus callosum, it was unlikely that there would be one direct WM tract linking them. In total there were 16 ipsilateral pairs of brain regions that showed abnormal functional connectivity in ASD in this previous study. These are shown shaded in **Table 2**, which is a modified version of Table 3 in McGrath et al. (2012), in which the results of between-group differences in functional connectivity are summarized.

PREPARATION OF FUNCTIONALLY DEFINED ROIs FOR TRACTOGRAPHY

To prepare the 16 pairs of ROIs for tractography, each cluster of interest was isolated from the fcMRI analysis and was projected back from standard MNI space into the space of the original subjects' diffusion data (native space) using the FSL TBSS Deproject tool (http://www.fmrib.ox.ac.uk/fsl/tbss/index.html). These ROIs were subsequently used to select the fiber trajectories that were computed with the constrained spherical deconvolution (CSD) based tractography approach (discussed in section Diffusion Tractography Protocol below).

Three of these ROIs (namely, the right superior frontal gyrus, right superior temporal gyrus, and left inferior semilunar lobule) failed to deproject successfully into native space. This failure to deproject occurred because the fcMRI clusters fell solely within the external extremity of the gray matter cortex and did not extend into subcortical WM regions. These subcortical regions are used by (and required by) the TBSS analysis during construction of the FA skeleton that is needed for transformation between native and standard space. Therefore, after deprojection, there were 10 pairs of brain regions in native diffusion space that were used as ROIs for CSD-based tractography. The location of these 10 pairs of brain regions are reported in **Table 3**.

Table 2 | A modified version of Table 3 in McGrath et al. (2012), in which the results of between-group differences in functional connectivity are summarized.

Seed ROI	Region		Cluster location	BA	Voxels	*X*	*Y*	*Z*	Effect
Right BA8	Frontal	L	Medial frontal gyrus	6	2024	1.6	−4.5	52.3	C − ASD +
		L	Inferior frontal gyrus	47	1154	22	−30.4	2.2	C − ASD +
		L	Superior frontal gyrus	11	253	23.6	−44	−18.2	C − > ASD −
		L	Inferior frontal gyrus	47	187	50.2	−25.8	−7	C + > ASD+
		R	Superior frontal gyrus	11	162	−27	−42.6	−16.6	C − ASD +
	Parietal	L	Precuneus	7	673	27.4	55.7	51.5	C − ASD +
	Cingulate	L	Posterior cingulate	23	331	1.1	32	23.1	C − ASD +
	Temporal	L	Superior temporal gyrus	38	461	34.9	−15.9	−21.9	C − ASD +
		L	Fusiform gyrus		277	28.9	58.1	−9.5	C − ASD +
	Occipital	L	Cuneus	19	1330	18.7	85.3	30.1	C − ASD +
			Cuneus	17	222	1.4	91.8	2.8	C − ASD +
	Cerebellum	L	Culmen		244	10.1	48.2	−0.1	C − ASD +
	Subcortical	L	Thalamus		1106	1.4	19.8	9.6	C − ASD +
Right fusiform	Frontal	R	Precentral gyrus	4	170	−32	21.5	60.6	C − > ASD −
	Parietal	L	Postcentral gyrus	1	346	33.8	33.9	66.4	C − ASD +
	Temporal	L	Parahippocampal gyrus	20	162	43.2	14.7	−15.7	C − > ASD −
	Subcortical	L	Pons		264	8.9	16.7	−35.2	C − ASD +
Right cuneus	Parietal	L	Inferior parietal lobule	40	404	55.5	53.9	39	C + > ASD +
		R	Inferior parietal lobule	40	222	−58.1	32.2	28.2	C + ASD −
		R	Supramarginal gyrus	39	180	−53.8	58	30.1	C + > ASD +
	Temporal	L	Superior temporal gyrus	39	1439	51.2	61.2	20.5	C + ASD −
		R	Middle temporal gyrus	22	720	−52	39.1	5.4	C + ASD −
Left BA19	Frontal	R	Middle frontal gyrus	6	977	−18.3	10	59.1	C − > ASD −
		R	Medial frontal gyrus	6	935	−1.8	−3.6	51.5	C − > ASD −
	Parietal	L	Postcentral gyrus	3	541	46.2	15.4	52.2	C − > ASD −
	Temporal	L	Uncus	20	165	28.3	−0.1	−33.1	C − ASD +
	Occipital	L	Cuneus	18	657	19.2	84.4	26.1	C − > ASD −
		R	Cuneus	17	459	−4.9	91.5	4.7	C − ASD +
		R	Cuneus	18	177	−16.1	86.8	19.2	C − ASD +
	Subcortical	L	Caudate head		1198	10.2	−7	4.7	C − > ASD −
		L	Thalamus		1026	4.6	23.1	8.9	C − > ASD −
		L	Caudate body		337	24.5	18.3	28.9	C − ASD +
		R	Caudate		598	−13.4	−13.6	12.1	C − > ASD −
		R	Lentiform		233	−17.6	−4.2	−4.6	C − > ASD −
Left inferior semilunar lobule	Frontal	L	Precentral gyrus	6	347	48.4	−2.3	34.4	C − > ASD −
		R	Middle frontal gyrus	6	653	−27.5	7.4	48.5	C − > ASD −
	Parietal	L	Precuneus	7	255	17.2	77.1	45.7	C − > ASD −
		L	Superior parietal lobule	7	173	25.3	59.9	55.7	C − > ASD −
		R	Superior parietal lobule	7	325	−22.9	65.1	46.4	C − > ASD −
	Occipital	L	Cuneus	19	566	21.3	88.2	25.4	C − > ASD −
Right caudate	Temporal	R	Superior temporal gyrus	22	317	−62.2	44.4	6.2	C + ASD −
	Cerebellar	L	Cerebellar tonsil		380	34.9	35.6	−44.1	C + > ASD +
		L	Cerebellum (XIII)		347	41.8	50.6	−51.9	C + > ASD +
	Subcortical	L	Thalamus		218	6.1	18.7	8	C − > ASD −

Gray shading indicates ipsilateral brain region pairs that were used as regions of interest for CSD based tractography in the current study. [Direction of between-group difference denoted with arrows (−, Negative functional connectivity, +, Positive functional connectivity), >, greater than (note that when both groups show negative connectivity the > means a larger negative value), C, Control group, ASD, Autism Spectrum Disorder group].

Table 3 | Summary of results from functional connectivity and tractography analysis.

ROI 1	*X*	*Y*	*Z*	ROI 2	*X*	*Y*	*Z*	Mean functional connectivity	Tractography result
Right Fusiform	−55	51	−19	Right precentral gyrus	−32	22	61	C −0.046 ASD −0.013	No direct tracts
Right Cuneus	−11	75	6	Right inferior parietal lobule	−58	32	28	C +0.029 ASD −0.013	No direct tracts
				Right supramarginal gyrus	−54	58	30	C +0.046 ASD +0.004	No direct tracts
				Right middle temporal gyrus	−52	39	5	C +0.017 ASD −0.018	No direct tracts
Left BA19	42	73	−2	Left postcentral gyrus	46	15	52	C −0.059 ASD −0.010	No direct tracts
				Left caudate head	10	−7	5	C −0.050 ASD −0.011	Tracts in 9 controls, 11 ASD
				Left thalamus	5	23	9	C −0.051 ASD −0.003	Tracts in 12 controls, 13 ASD
				Left caudate body	25	18	29	C −0.004 ASD +0.027	Tracts in 22 controls, 22 ASD
				Left cuneus	19	84	26	C − 0.066 ASD −0.010	Tracts in 22 controls, 22 ASD
				Left Uncus	28	0	−33	C −0.020 ASD +0.005	Tracts in 5 controls, 6 ASD

ROI_1 and ROI_2 refer to the regions used in tractography analysis. [Direction of between-group difference for functional connectivity is denoted with arrows (−, Negative functional connectivity, +, Positive functional connectivity), C, Control group, ASD, Autism Spectrum Disorder group].

DIFFUSION TRACTOGRAPHY PROTOCOL

CSD based tractography was used in this study. Typically a model of diffusion tensor tractography has been used in ASD research, however in recent years it has become evident that there are significant limitations associated with this method, in particular in voxels containing more than one coherently oriented fiber population (e.g., in "crossing fibers" configurations; Wedeen et al., 2000; Alexander et al., 2002; Frank, 2002; Wedeen et al., 2008; Tournier et al., 2011; Jeurissen et al., 2012). The CSD method allows reliable estimation of one or more fiber orientations in the presence of intra-voxel orientational heterogeneity (Tournier et al., 2004, 2007, 2008), it overcomes partial volume effects associated with diffusion tensor imaging (Vos et al., 2011, 2012), permits fiber-tracking through regions of crossing fibers (Tournier et al., 2008), and has recently shown promising results in other clinical applications (Metzler-Baddeley et al., 2012; Reijmer et al., 2012, 2013).

The WM tracts between each pair of ROIs were reconstructed using CSD based tractography (Jeurissen et al., 2011). This tractography procedure consisted of the following steps: (i) CSD, using a spherical harmonics model with maximum harmonic degree $L = 8$ was used to extract the fiber orientation distribution (FOD) from the diffusion weighted signal in each voxel (Tournier et al., 2007), (ii) Seed points were defined on a uniform $2 \times 2 \times 2\,\text{mm}^3$ grid to cover the entire brain; (iii) For each step during tract propagation, the FOD peak direction that was closest to the previous stepping direction was extracted; (iv) The trajectory was advanced with a fixed step size (1 mm) along the peak direction obtained with step (iii). Tracking ended when the FOD peak magnitude was beneath a fixed threshold (i.e., 0.1), or when a maximum angle (30°) was exceeded. Subsequently, from this whole-brain tractography result, WM tracts that ran directly between each pair of ROIs were identified by coding the two regions as "AND" regions (i.e., only WM tracts that passed through ROI 1 and ROI 2 were isolated).

Preliminary tractography analysis was carried out using the exact clusters from functional connectivity analysis as outlined in **Table 2**, however this analysis indicated that there were no (or very few) WM tracts between the pairs of brain regions. One possible reason for this is that these are functionally defined ROIs, which are essentially generated by BOLD signal fluctuation in gray matter, and therefore they may not have projected far enough into the adjacent WM. A pragmatic approach was thus adopted using larger ROIs in the analysis to increase projection into WM. These larger ROIs were created in standard space by generating a sphere 8×8 mm for each cluster with its center-point the center of mass of the original fcMRI derived cluster. This size of sphere was chosen as it corresponded with the size of the seed spheres used in the corresponding functional connectivity analysis (McGrath et al., 2012). These spheres were then back projected from standard MNI space to each participants' native diffusion space and used as the ROIs for CSD based tractography as outlined above. All tractography analyses were performed in native diffusion space.

DEPENDENT MEASURES

For each tract in each participant, microstructural measures of FA and the Westin measures of linear diffusion coefficient (CL) and planar diffusion coefficient (CP; Westin et al., 2002) were computed from the tracts. The mean values for FA, CL, and CP were extracted from all tracts using Explore DTI software (Leemans et al., 2009). FA was the primary measure of interest as it is the most widely used measure in the literature, and shows high sensitivity. In regions of complex fiber architecture however, tensor derived measures such as FA are unreliable (Jones and Cercignani, 2010) and the interpretation of these measures can be ambiguous (Jeurissen et al., 2012) and see McGrath et al. (2013) for discussion. In order to reduce the ambiguity about the biological interpretation of FA changes, alternative measures of diffusion anisotropy are often measured in conjunction with FA. One example of such alternative tensor-based metrics are the Westin measures of CL and CP. Although these measures are indeed still based on the eigenvalues, they can describe the geometrical shape of the diffusion tensor and, therefore, can provide a more meaningful interpretation of microstructural changes that are occurring in the ASD group compared to the FA (Westin et al., 2002; Reijmer et al., 2013). A high value of CL implies that there is only one dominant fiber orientation within a voxel (Vos et al., 2012) and a high value of CP indicates the presence of crossing fiber configurations (Vos et al., 2012).

STATISTICAL ANALYSIS

Between-group differences in white matter structure

Statistical comparisons of the data were performed using PASW (SPSS) software version 18 (SPSS Inc., Chicago, IL). For all analyses the level of statistical significance was defined as $p < 0.05$ (two-tailed) and Bonferroni corrections were used for within-test comparisons. To investigate whether there were between-group differences in the WM of tracts that directly connected a pair of brain regions, univariate ANOVA with Group (ASD/Control) as the between-subjects factor was performed for the dependent measures FA, CL, and CP in each separate set of these WM tracts.

Correlation analyses

To explore how brain WM structure, functional connectivity and behavior are related, a number of exploratory correlation analyses (using bivariate Pearson correlation analysis) were performed to investigate the relationships between (1) WM structure and functional connectivity, (2) WM structure and behavior, (3) functional connectivity and behavior. Given the extremely limited data in current literature, in both autism and healthy populations, on relationships between brain structural connectivity, functional connectivity, and behavior, it was felt important that all these measures were included to comprehensively explore the possible associations. Pearson correlation analysis was used as behavioral response times, fcMRI and DTI data in this study are normally distributed, as indicated by p-values of >0.05 following Kolmgorov–Smirnov and Shapiro–Wilk tests of normality. The correlation analyses were exploratory in nature, and correction for multiple comparisons was not performed.

Measures of white matter structure, functional connectivity and behavior included in the correlation analyses. For WM structure, FA was included in the correlation analysis. This measure of WM structure is the most widely used measure in the literature, and shows high sensitivity.

Four measures of functional connectivity were included in the correlation analyses; negative functional connectivity on Same trials, negative functional connectivity on Mirror trials, positive functional connectivity on Same trials and positive functional connectivity on Mirror trials. The distinction between Same and Mirror trials was included in the correlations as behavioral and functional connectivity analyses both demonstrated an interesting dissociation between ASD and control groups on Same vs. Mirror trials (McGrath et al., 2012). These findings may indicate that visuospatial processing in ASD is achieved using qualitatively (and quantitatively) different neural networks. A primary aim of the current study was to increase our understanding of the structural correlates of atypical visuospatial processing in ASD. We hypothesized that correlation analyses would demonstrate differential relationships between ASD and control groups on Same and Mirror trials. A distinction was also made between negative and positive functional connectivity. Unfortunately, there is very limited literature investigating the relationships between structural and functional connectivity in neurotypical populations, therefore it is not possible to make specific predictions about how structural connectivity may relate differentially to these types of functional connectivity. Nevertheless, there is an important difference between these measures in terms of functional interactions between brain regions (see McGrath et al., 2012, for discussion). While it seems plausible that the level of WM organization should be correlated with the overall strength of functional connectivity, it was felt that it would not be appropriate to combine negative and positive functional connectivity into a composite measure as doing so might obscure important relationships between WM organization and functional connectivity. Functional connectivity values were individual z-scores extracted from the PPI Main effect of Group results. These were extracted for each participant for each pair of brain regions in which there were WM connections.

The behavioral data used in the correlation analyses provided a measure of visuospatial processing speed. This was calculated using mean response times (MRTs) for the Same and Mirror trials during a mental rotation task (McGrath et al., 2012).

A set of correlation analyses was performed for every set of brain regions that had direct WM connections. The groups (ASD and controls) were analysed separately for the correlation analyses.

RESULTS

OVERVIEW OF RESULTS

Section 3.1

Results relate to Question 1 outlined in Methods section Overview of Methods—are there WM tracts between all pairs of ROIs that are functionally connected? This section includes a summary of the between-group differences in functional connectivity, which are reported in McGrath et al. (2012).

Section 3.2

Results relate to Question 2 outlined in the Methods section Overview of Methods—if there were WM tracts that directly linked pairs of brain regions showing abnormal functional connectivity, were there structural abnormalities of this WM in the ASD group? This section outlines the between-group comparisons of diffusion measures extracted from the isolated WM tracts.

Section 3.3

Results relate to Question 3 outlined in the Methods section Overview of Methods—was there evidence for relationships between structural connectivity, functional connectivity and behavior? This section outlines the results of the correlation analyses.

ARE THERE WHITE MATTER TRACTS BETWEEN ALL PAIRS OF ROIs THAT ARE FUNCTIONALLY CONNECTED?

Table 3 summarizes the results of the tractography analyses between the 10 pairs of ROIs that showed abnormal functional connectivity. In summary, there were WM tracts directly connecting the left BA19 ROI to five other ROIs including the left uncus, left cuneus, left caudate head, left caudate body, and left thalamus (see **Figures 1–5**). There were no WM tracts in any participants between the other five pairs of seed regions. Consequently, the subsequent analyses of diffusion measures and the correlation analyses are restricted to the five pairs of ROIs with direct WM tracts.

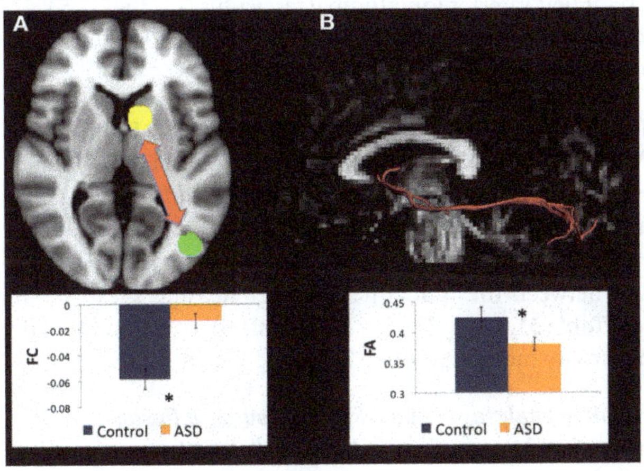

FIGURE 1 | (A) Regions for tractography in left BA19 (green sphere) and left caudate head (yellow sphere). The ASD group showed weaker functional connectivity relative to controls between these regions during a mental rotation task. The bar graph shows the strength of functional connectivity (FC) in the Control group (blue) and ASD group (orange) between these seed regions. **(B)** Example of white matter tracts that directly connect the left BA19 and left caudate head regions in one participant. The bar graph shows Fractional Anisotropy (FA) in the Control group (blue) and ASD group (orange) in these white matter tracts. *indicates statistical significance with $p < 0.05$.

IF THERE WERE WHITE MATTER TRACTS THAT DIRECTLY LINKED PAIRS OF BRAIN REGIONS SHOWING ABNORMAL FUNCTIONAL CONNECTIVITY, WERE THERE STRUCTURAL ABNORMALITIES OF THIS WHITE MATTER IN THE ASD GROUP?

Changes in white matter between left BA19 and left caudate head

There were WM tracts directly connecting the regions in left BA19 and left caudate head in 9 controls and 11 participants

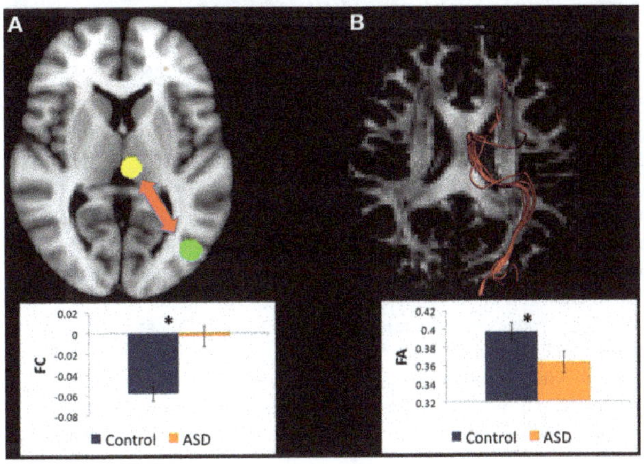

FIGURE 2 | (A) Regions for tractography in left BA19 (green sphere) and left thalamus (yellow sphere). The ASD group showed much weaker functional connectivity relative to controls between these regions during a mental rotation task. The bar graph shows the strength of functional connectivity (FC) in the Control group (blue) and ASD group (orange) between these regions. **(B)** Example of white matter tracts that directly connect the left BA19 and left thalamus regions in one participant. The bar graph shows Fractional Anisotropy (FA) in the Control group (blue) and ASD group (orange) in these white matter tracts. *indicates statistical significance with $p < 0.05$.

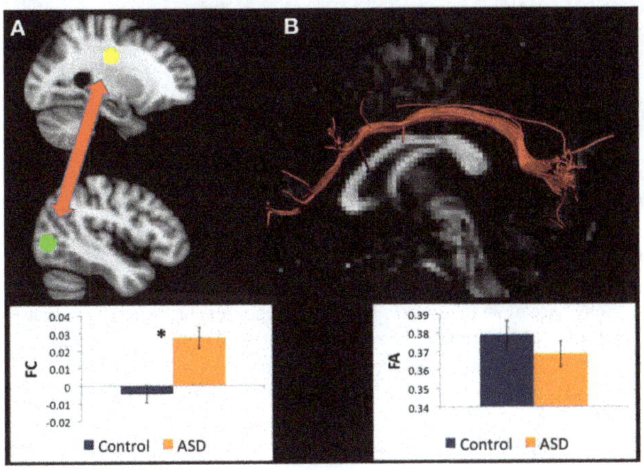

FIGURE 3 | (A) Regions for tractography in left BA19 (green sphere) and left caudate body (yellow sphere). The ASD group showed increased functional connectivity relative to controls between these regions during a mental rotation task. The bar graph shows the strength of functional connectivity (FC) in the Control group (blue) and ASD group (orange) between these regions. **(B)** Example of white matter tracts that directly connect the left BA19 and left caudate body regions in one participant. The bar graph shows Fractional Anisotropy (FA) in the Control group (blue) and ASD group (orange) in these white matter tracts. *indicates statistical significance with $p < 0.05$.

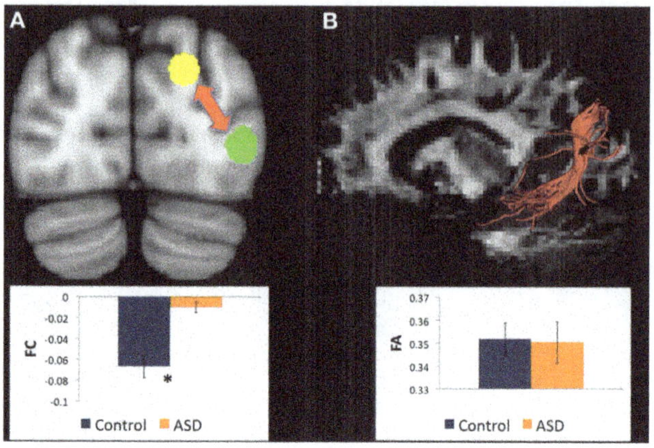

FIGURE 4 | (A) Regions for tractography in left BA19 (green sphere) and left cuneus (yellow sphere). The ASD group showed weaker functional connectivity relative to controls between these regions during a mental rotation task. The bar graph shows the strength of functional connectivity (FC) in the Control group (blue) and ASD group (orange) between these regions. **(B)** Example of white matter tracts that directly connect the left BA19 and left cuneus regions in one participant. The bar graph shows Fractional Anisotropy (FA) in the Control group (blue) and ASD group (orange) in these white matter tracts. *indicates statistical significance with $p < 0.05$.

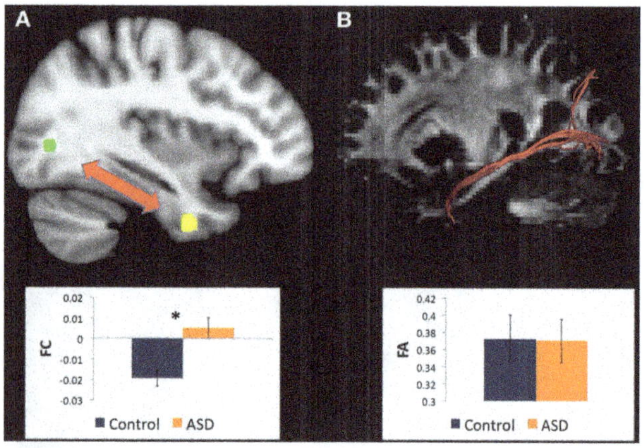

FIGURE 5 | (A) Regions for tractography in left BA19 (green sphere) and left uncus (yellow sphere). The ASD group showed weaker functional connectivity relative to controls between these regions during a mental rotation task. The bar graph shows the strength of functional connectivity (FC) in the Control group (blue) and ASD group (orange) between these regions. **(B)** Example of white matter tracts that run through the left BA19 and left uncus regions in one participant. The bar graph shows Fractional Anisotropy (FA) in the Control group (blue) and ASD group (orange) in these white matter tracts. *indicates statistical significance with $p < 0.05$.

with ASD, and the WM tracts linking these regions formed part of the left IFOF (see **Figure 1**). Univariate ANOVA of the dependent measures from diffusion analysis revealed that there was significantly reduced FA (mean FA ASD 0.38, *SD* 0.04, controls 0.42, *SD* 0.05, $F = 5.972$, $p = 0.027$, $\eta_p^2 = 0.272$) and CL (mean CL ASD 0.35, *SD* 0.04, controls 0.40, *SD* 0.06, $F = 5.074$, $p = 0.039$, $\eta_p^2 = 0.199$) in the ASD group relative to controls (**Table 4**), indicating that WM microstructural organization was reduced in these tracts in the ASD group.

Changes in white matter between left BA19 and left thalamus

There were WM tracts directly connecting left BA19 and left thalamus in 12 controls and 13 participants with ASD, and this WM appeared to comprise part of the left IFOF (see **Figure 2**). Univariate ANOVA revealed significantly reduced FA (mean FA ASD 0.36, *SD* 0.04, controls 0.40, *SD* 0.04, $F = 4.306$, $p < 0.050$, $\eta_p^2 = 0.170$) and CL (mean CL ASD 0.34, *SD* 0.04 controls 0.38, *SD* 0.03, $F = 8.085$, $p < 0.010$, $\eta_p^2 = 0.278$) in the ASD group relative to controls in the WM directly connecting left BA19 and left thalamus regions.

Changes in white matter between left BA19 and left caudate body

There were WM tracts directly connecting left BA19 and left caudate body in 22 controls and 22 participants with ASD, and this WM appeared to be part of the superior longitudinal fasciculus (see **Figure 3**). There were no between-group differences in microstructural measures of the WM linking left BA19 and left caudate body.

Changes in white matter between left BA19 and left cuneus

There were WM tracts directly connecting the regions in left BA19 and left cuneus in 22 controls and 22 participants with ASD (see **Table 3**). This WM tract ran intra-occipitally in the left hemisphere (see **Figure 4**). There were no between-group differences in microstructural organization of this tract (see **Table 4**).

Changes in white matter between left BA19 and left uncus

There were WM tracts directly connecting the regions in left BA19 and the left uncus in only 5 controls and 6 participants with ASD (see **Table 3**). This WM appeared to be part of the left IFOF/left inferior longitudinal fasciculus (see **Figure 5**). There were no between-group differences in WM microstructure in this tract (see **Table 4**).

IS THERE EVIDENCE FOR RELATIONSHIPS BETWEEN STRUCTURAL CONNECTIVITY, FUNCTIONAL CONNECTIVITY AND BEHAVIOR?

Correlation analyses of behavioral measures, diffusion measure, and functional connectivity in left BA19/left caudate head region

For both control and ASD groups, no significant correlations were found between the functional connectivity and mean RT measures (**Table 5**), FA and mean RTs (**Table 6**), or FA and functional connectivity measures (**Table 7** and see **Figure 6**).

Correlation analyses of behavioral measures, diffusion measures, and functional connectivity in left BA19/left thalamus region

Controls. In controls, there was a significant correlation between negative functional connectivity during Same trials, and MRT during these trials ($r = 0.80$, $p < 0.006$), indicating that a reduction in MRT (i.e., faster task performance) was associated with stronger negative connectivity (see **Table 5** and see **Figure 6**).

There was no significant correlation between the diffusion measure of FA and MRT.

There were correlations between structural organization of the WM connecting the regions in left BA19 and left thalamus and

Table 4 | The mean, standard deviation and *p*-values for the three micro-structural dependent measures (FA, CP, CL) for white matter tracts connecting functionally defined regions in the ASD and control groups.

Tract		Left BA19 – Left uncus		Left BA19 – Left cuneus		Left BA19 – Left caudate head		Left BA19 – Left thalamus		Left BA19 – Left caudate body	
		ASD $n = 6$ Con $n = 5$		ASD $n = 22$ Con $n = 22$		ASD $n = 9$ Con $n = 11$		ASD $n = 12$ Con $n = 13$		ASD $n = 22$ Con $n = 22$	
Measure	**Group**	**Mean (*SD*)**	***p***	**Mean (*SD*)**	***p***	**Mean (*SD*)**	***p***	**Mean (*SD*)**	***p***	**Mean (*SD*)**	***p***
FA	ASD	0.37 (0.06)	0.69	0.35 (0.04)	0.98	**0.38* (0.04)**	**0.02***	**0.36* (0.04)**	**0.05***	0.37 (0.03)	0.23
	Con	0.37 (0.07)		0.35 (0.03)		**0.42* (0.05)**		**0.39* (0.04)**		0.38 (0.03)	
CP	ASD	0.16 (0.03)	0.65	0.17 (0.03)	0.81	0.16 (0.02)	0.93	0.16 (0.04)	0.48	0.19 (0.03)	0.85
	Con	0.17 (0.04)		0.17 (0.02)		0.16 (0.01)		0.15 (0.02)		0.19 (0.02)	
CL	ASD	0.35 (0.05)	0.78	0.32 (0.05)	0.96	**0.35* (0.04)**	**0.04***	**0.34** (0.04)**	**0.01****	0.33 (0.03)	0.26
	Con	0.34 (0.08)		0.32 (0.04)		**0.40* (0.06)**		**0.38** (0.03)**		0.34 (0.03)	

**Indicates statistical significance $p < 0.05$; **indicates statistical significance $p < 0.01$.*

Table 5 | Results of correlation analysis between functional connectivity and mean response times during Same and Mirror trials of a mental rotation task (*p*: *p*-value, r: Pearson correlation co-efficient, FC_S – Negative functional connectivity on Same trials, FC_S + Positive functional connectivity on Same trials, FC_M – Negative functional connectivity on Mirror trials, FC_M + Positive functional connectivity on Mirror trials, MRT: mean response time, ^1 Insufficient data for correlation as all functional connectivity values were negative between seed regions in left BA19 and left caudate head).

			MRT_S *r* (*p*)			**MRT_M *r* (*p*)**
Left BA19 – Left cuneus	FC_S –	ASD	0.18 (0.53	FC_M –	ASD	0.16 (0.55)
		Control	−0.17 (0.51)		Control	0.02 (0.93)
	FC_S +	ASD	−0.52 (0.29)	FC_M +	ASD	0.03 (0.97)
		Control	−0.08 (0.92)		Control	^1
Left BA19 – Left caudate head	FC_S –	ASD	−0.22 (0.58)	FC_M –	ASD	0.03 (0.95)
		Control	0.63 (0.07)		Control	0.15 (0.69)
	FC_S +	ASD	^1	FC_M +	ASD	^1
		Control	^1		Control	^1
Left BA19 – Left thalamus	FC_S –	ASD	−0.63 (0.37)	FC_M –	ASD	0.17 (0.57)
		Control	0.80 (0.006)**		Control	0.18 (0.42)
	FC_S +	ASD	−0.35 (0.33)	FC_M +	ASD	−0.16 (0.77)
		Control	^1		Control	^1
Left BA19 – Left caudate body	FC_S –	ASD	−0.50 (0.31)	FC_M –	ASD	^1
		Control	−0.03 (0.93)		Control	−0.18 (0.53)
	FC_S +	ASD	0.23 (0.36)	FC_M +	ASD	0.53 (0.02)*
		Control	0.53 (0.14)		Control	0.34 (0.41)

**Indicates statistical significance $p < 0.05$; **indicates statistical significance $p < 0.01$.*

functional connectivity between these regions. FA was significantly correlated ($r = 0.69$, $p < 0.03$) with negative functional connectivity on Same trials in controls (see **Table 7** and see **Figure 6**). This correlation indicates that as WM organization increases (with increasing FA), there is a correlated reduction in the strength of negative functional connectivity.

ASD. In the ASD group, there were no correlations between mental rotation performance (MRT) and functional connectivity or WM integrity of tracts between left BA19 and left thalamus (see **Tables 5**, **6** and see **Figure 6**). WM organization was significantly correlated with functional connectivity. FA was associated with positive functional connectivity in Same trials (FA $r = -0.92$, $p < 0.01$; see **Table 7** and see **Figure 6**). These results indicate that a greater level of microstructural organization in the WM between left BA19 and left thalamus (increased FA) is associated with a reduction in positive functional connectivity.

Table 6 | Results of correlation analysis between mean response times during a mental rotation task and the micro-structural diffusion measure of FA extracted from the white matter tracts linking functionally defined regions.

		Left BA19 – Left cuneus		Left BA19 – Left caudate head		Left BA19 – Left thalamus		Left BA19 – Left caudate body	
		MRT_S *r (p)*	MRT_M *r (p)*	MRT_S *r (p)*	MRT_M *r (p)*	MRT_S *r (p)*	MRT_M *r (p)*	MRT_S *r (p)*	MRT_M *r (p)*
FA	ASD	−0.04 (0.85)	0.17 (0.44)	−0.31 (0.39)	−0.09 (0.80)	−0.01 (0.98)	−0.05 (0.89)	−0.48 (0.03)*	−0.57 (0.01)**
	Con	−0.14 (0.53)	−0.33 (0.13)	0.12 (0.77)	−0.32 (0.39)	0.25 (0.43)	0.09 (0.79)	−0.01 (0.98)	0.02 (0.94)

*(p, p value; r, Pearson correlation co-efficient; MRT_S, mean response time on Same trials; MRT_M, mean response time on Mirror trials). *Indicates statistical significance $p < 0.05$; **indicates statistical significance $p < 0.01$.*

Table 7 | Results of correlation analysis between diffusion measures in white matter tracts and functional connectivity during Same and Mirror trials of a mental rotation task (*p*, *p*-value; *r*, Pearson correlation co-efficient; FC_S – Negative functional connectivity on Same trials; FC_S + Positive functional connectivity on Same trials, FC_M – Negative functional connectivity on Mirror trials, FC_M + Positive functional connectivity on Mirror trials, Con: Control, ^1 Insufficient data for correlation as all functional connectivity values were negative between seed regions in left BA19 and left caudate head).

		FC_S – *r (p)*	FC_S + *r (p)*	FC_M – *r (p)*	FC_M + *r (p)*
LEFT BA19 – LEFT CUNEUS					
FA	ASD	0.09 (0.75)	−0.13 (0.81)	−0.10 (0.70)	0.01 (0.99)
	Con	−0.49 (0.06)	0.89 (0.11)	−0.01 (0.96)	^1
		FC_S –	**FC_S +**	**FC_M –**	**FC_M +**
LEFT BA19 – LEFT CAUDATE HEAD					
FA	ASD	0.09 (0.82)	^1	−0.08 (0.84)	^1
	Con	0.31 (0.42)	^1	0.31 (0.42)	^1
LEFT BA19 – LEFT THALAMUS					
FA	ASD	0.23 (0.72)	−0.92 (0.01)**	0.40 (0.60)	0.53 (0.28)
	Con	0.69 (0.03)*	^1	0.21 (0.55)	^1
LEFT BA19 – LEFT CAUDATE BODY					
FA	ASD	0.30 (0.57)	0.16 (0.56)	0.09 (0.84)	−0.48 (0.04)*
	Con	0.36 (0.28)	−0.23 (0.54)	0.31 (0.33)	−0.53 (0.18)

**Indicates statistical significance $p < 0.05$; **indicates statistical significance $p < 0.01$.*

Correlation analyses of behavioral measures, diffusion measures, and functional connectivity in left BA19/left caudate body region

Controls. In controls, there were no correlations between the diffusion measure, functional connectivity, and MRT during mental rotation (see **Tables 5–7** and see **Figure 6**).

ASD. In the ASD group there was a significant correlation between the behavioral measure of MRT during Mirror trials and positive functional connectivity ($r = 0.53$, $p < 0.02$; see **Table 5** and see **Figure 6**). This indicates that faster MRT on Mirror trials is associated with reduced strength of positive functional connectivity.

There was a significant correlation between FA and MRT on Same ($r = -0.48$, $p < 0.03$) and Mirror ($r = -0.57$, $p < 0.01$) trials indicating that as microstructural organization of the WM linking left BA19 and left caudate body increases (characterized by an increase in FA), there is an associated reduction in MRT (i.e., faster MRT) in the ASD group (see **Table 6** and see **Figure 6**).

There was also correlation between FA and functional connectivity in the ASD group. FA was significantly correlated with positive functional connectivity on Mirror trials ($r = -0.48$, $p < 0.04$; see **Table 7** and see **Figure 6**) indicating that increased structural organization of WM (increased FA) is associated with reduced strength of positive functional connectivity.

Correlation analyses of behavioral measures, diffusion measure, and functional connectivity in left BA19/left cuneus region

For both control and ASD groups, no significant correlations were found between the functional connectivity and MRT data (**Table 5**), the diffusion data and mean RTs (**Table 6**), or the diffusion data and functional connectivity data (**Table 7**).

Correlation analyses of behavioral measures, diffusion measure, and functional connectivity in left BA19/left uncus region

There were no significant correlations between the diffusion measure and behavior (see **Table 6**). Power was limited however, by the small sample size. There was insufficient data to perform correlation analyses of functional connectivity and diffusion measures or functional connectivity and behavioral measures.

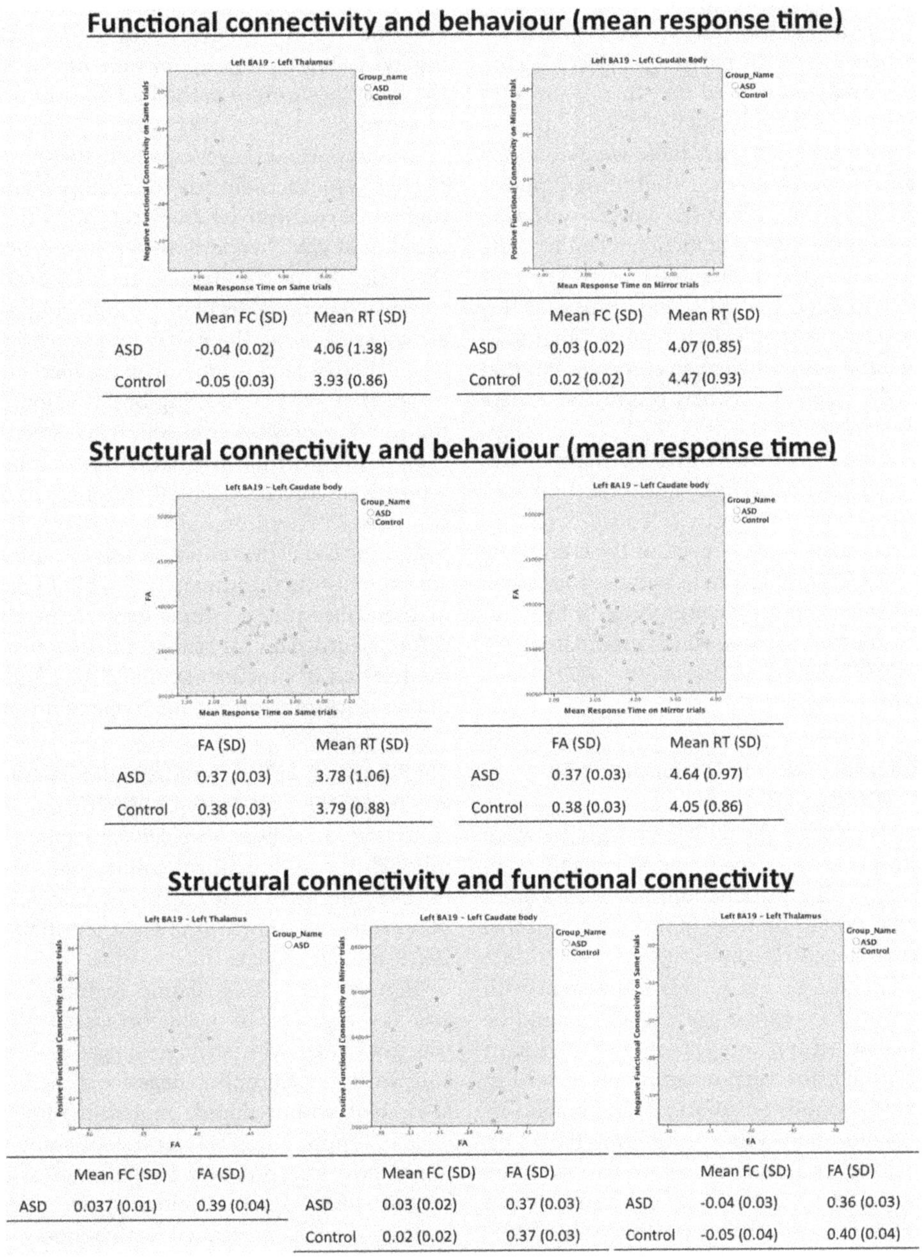

	Mean FC (SD)	Mean RT (SD)
ASD	-0.04 (0.02)	4.06 (1.38)
Control	-0.05 (0.03)	3.93 (0.86)

	Mean FC (SD)	Mean RT (SD)
ASD	0.03 (0.02)	4.07 (0.85)
Control	0.02 (0.02)	4.47 (0.93)

	FA (SD)	Mean RT (SD)
ASD	0.37 (0.03)	3.78 (1.06)
Control	0.38 (0.03)	3.79 (0.88)

	FA (SD)	Mean RT (SD)
ASD	0.37 (0.03)	4.64 (0.97)
Control	0.38 (0.03)	4.05 (0.86)

	Mean FC (SD)	FA (SD)
ASD	0.037 (0.01)	0.39 (0.04)

	Mean FC (SD)	FA (SD)
ASD	0.03 (0.02)	0.37 (0.03)
Control	0.02 (0.02)	0.37 (0.03)

	Mean FC (SD)	FA (SD)
ASD	-0.04 (0.03)	0.36 (0.03)
Control	-0.05 (0.04)	0.40 (0.04)

FIGURE 6 | Scatterplots of correlation analyses showing significant relationships between functional connectivity, structural connectivity and behavior.

DISCUSSION

The main finding of this study is that there are microstructural abnormalities in WM tracts that directly connect brain regions showing abnormal functional connectivity in participants with ASD. In addition, there are significant correlations between measures of WM microstructure, functional connectivity and behavior, which provide insight into the relationships between brain structure, brain function, and information processing in both neurotypical controls and individuals with ASD.

This discussion focuses on the implications these results have for the original hypotheses of this study, which predicted firstly that there would be WM tracts linking some, but not all pairs of brain regions showing abnormal functional connectivity, secondly that WM structure would be abnormal in tracts directly connecting the functionally defined regions and finally that there would be relationships between microstructural organization of WM, functional connectivity and behavior.

FUNCTIONAL CONNECTIVITY IS NOT ALWAYS ASSOCIATED WITH DIRECT WHITE MATTER CONNECTIONS

In this study, 10 pairs of brain regions were used as regions for selecting fiber pathways, reconstructed with CSD-based tractography. These regions were generated from functional connectivity maps during a mental rotation task, and indicated brain regions between which there was abnormal functional connectivity in ASD. Tractography analysis revealed that there were WM tracts directly connecting five of these 10 pairs of regions in most participants. For the other five region pairs there were no direct structural connections in any participants. This finding supports the first hypothesis. This finding of a direct structural connection between only half of the regions showing functional connectivity is consistent with results of imaging studies that have used a similar multimodal approach to integrate fcMRI and diffusion MRI. One of the first studies to use this approach reported that high functional and low structural connectivity can co-occur, but that low functional connectivity rarely occurs between regions where there is high structural connectivity (Koch et al., 2002). In keeping with this finding, a more recent study investigating the links between resting state functional connectivity and structural connectivity revealed that functional connectivity between regions is not indicative of a direct structural connection between those regions (Honey et al., 2009). This is likely to be because functional connectivity can be mediated by indirect connections or by input from a third region into the two regions, which modulates connectivity in the two primary regions (Koch et al., 2002; Honey et al., 2009; Behrens and Sporns, 2012).

ABNORMAL FUNCTIONAL CONNECTIVITY IS ASSOCIATED WITH ABNORMAL STRUCTURAL CONNECTIVITY

As discussed in section Evidence for a Relationship Between Brain White Matter Structure and Functional Connectivity in Neurotypical Populations of the introduction, previous studies have demonstrated a relationship between abnormal functional connectivity and abnormal structural connectivity (Quigley et al., 2003; Johnston et al., 2008; Lowe et al., 2008). Consistent with the prediction that abnormal functional connectivity would be associated with abnormal structural connectivity in the current study, there was reduced microstructural organization of WM in two of the five tracts linking regions of abnormal functional connectivity. In the ASD group, there was a significant reduction in the strength of functional connectivity between an occipital region (left BA19) and the left caudate head and also between this occipital seed region and the left thalamus. Analysis of diffusion measures in the WM directly linking these occipito-striatal and occipito-thalamic regions revealed significant microstructural abnormalities in the ASD group, which were characterized by reduced FA and CL, two measures that provide an indication of the level of organization of WM fibers. This finding of altered structural connectivity between brain regions that also show reduced functional connectivity is particularly interesting as it provides novel evidence to suggest that structural brain pathology may contribute to the abnormal functional connectivity that has been widely reported in the autism literature.

It is also noteworthy that the WM in both these tracts formed part of the left IFOF, a major WM association tract in the human brain. Interestingly, this study revealed structural abnormalities in this sub-region of the left IFOF, whereas a previous analysis of the whole left IFOF using the same data from the same study population found no abnormalities of WM (McGrath et al., 2013). This is of relevance as it supports a concern that current whole brain or even tract-specific analyses of WM may lack sensitivity in detecting WM abnormalities, and may not be specific enough about the exact locations of pathology in cases where abnormalities are reported.

It is important however to note that for the remaining three of the five WM tracts directly connecting regions showing abnormal functional connectivity, there was no evidence of disrupted organization of WM. In addition, in only one of these three tracts were there significant correlations between DTI and fcMRI measures (discussed in more detail in the following section). These findings are consistent with the theory that functional connectivity can be modulated by factors other than the level of microstructural organization of WM connecting brain regions. Such factors include the number of WM connections between regions; Hermudstat et al. recently demonstrated that the number of WM connections is positively correlated with the strength of resting state functional connectivity (Hermundstad et al., 2013). There are numerous diffusion measures that could be used to infer a level of "structural connectivity" in the human brain, but to date, the impact of most of these measures on functional connectivity is poorly understood. Neurochemical factors may also play an important role in modulation of functional connectivity, but a detailed discussion of these factors is outside the scope of this manuscript.

CORRELATIONS BETWEEN MICROSTRUCTURAL ORGANIZATION OF WHITE MATTER, FUNCTIONAL CONNECTIVITY AND BEHAVIOR

Correlation analysis revealed intriguing links between WM microstructure, functional connectivity and behavior in two of the five pairings in which there were direct WM tract connections; between regions in left BA19 and left thalamus, and between left BA19 and left caudate.

Between occipito-thalamic regions, functional connectivity was associated with behavior (faster visuospatial processing was associated with stronger negative functional connectivity) and with FA (stronger negative functional connectivity was associated with reduced microstructural organization) in the control group only. These correlation analyses suggest that during visuospatial processing, neurotypical controls benefit from increased functional inhibition between left BA19 and left thalamus, which is associated with reduced organization in WM between these regions. In the ASD group, structural and functional connectivity between occipito-thalamic regions were correlated (reduced microstructural organization was associated with reduced strength of positive functional connectivity). There were no statistically significant correlations between visuospatial processing speed and structural or functional connectivity, therefore the effect of altered connectivity in this tract on visuospatial processing is not known. It is interesting that both groups show a similar (statistically significant) relationship between structural and functional connectivity whereby less well-organized WM (reduced FA) is associated with increased functional suppression between regions. This may indicate that both ASD and control groups use this occipito-thalamic tract in a qualitatively similar way during visuospatial processing. This study has shown a reduction in FA in this tract in the ASD group. Given the correlation in the control group that shows a relationship between reduced FA and faster response times, it is possible that the reduced FA in the ASD group may contribute to their relative behavioral advantage in visuospatial processing.

Functional connectivity between left BA 19 and left caudate body was significantly increased in the ASD group relative to controls, but WM organization in the tracts directly connecting these regions was normal. The correlation analyses however implied that there were significant between-group differences in the functional use of this tract during visuospatial processing. Controls showed no association between structural, functional, and behavioral measures, whereas structural connectivity, functional connectivity, and visuospatial processing speed appeared to be strongly related in the ASD group. The lack of correlations in controls is in sharp contrast to the strong relationships found in the ASD group and might indicate that the ASD group relies on connectivity between these regions during visuospatial processing, whereas the controls do not. In relation to correlations observed in the ASD group, firstly greater organization of WM (higher FA) was associated with reduced functional connectivity between left BA19 and left caudate. Secondly, reduced functional connectivity between these regions was associated with faster MRT. Finally, faster MRT was correlated with greater microstructural organization of the WM between left BA19 and left caudate body. When considered together, these correlations suggest that a higher level of structural organization of this tract confers a benefit to visuospatial processing speed in ASD that may be mediated by increased functional suppression between left BA19 and left caudate. This finding is perplexing, as higher levels of WM organization have previously been associated with stronger rather than weaker functional connectivity; van de Heuvel reported a positive correlation between strength of functional connectivity in the default mode network and the level of FA in the cingulum (van den Heuvel et al., 2008) and another study demonstrated that increased radial diffusivity in WM connecting right and left primary sensorimotor cortices was associated with reduction of functional connectivity between these regions (Lowe et al., 2008). A recent paper specifically investigating the relationships between structural connectivity and resting state/task-based functional connectivity in the human brain' (Hermundstad et al., 2013), did not investigate the degree of organization of WM, but revealed that it is a high number of connections that facilitate strong resting state functional connectivity. In the current study, FA rather than number of connections was chosen as the measure of structural connectivity. In future studies investigating relationships between structural and functional connectivity, the measure(s) used to infer structural connectivity should be carefully considered.

Correlation analyses of connectivity and behavior between left BA19 and left caudate head and between left BA19 and left cuneus regions did not yield such strong evidence for an interrelationship of structure, function, and behavior. There were no relationships between brain structure, functional connectivity or behavior. It is difficult to speculate on the reasons for this relative lack of structure/function/behavior correlations between these regions because, as discussed already, there is very little literature documenting relationships between brain WM structure and functional connectivity. There is however increasing recognition of the urgent need for research investigating links between anatomical connectivity, functional connectivity and behavior; this knowledge is crucial to understand the "capabilities of and constraints on human cognitive function" (Hermundstad et al., 2013).

DIRECT IMPLICATIONS OF THIS STUDY

Together, these findings offer a fascinating insight into the relationships between brain structure, brain function, and information processing in both neurotypical controls and individuals with ASD. This multimodal imaging study has used a novel approach to integrate functional and structural neuroimaging data. It has demonstrated, for the first time in ASD research that there is reduced microstructural organization of WM in tracts that directly connect brain regions that show abnormal functional connectivity. It also reveals that in some brain regions, individual differences in WM organisation are related to the level of functional connectivity during a visuospatial processing task, and further that this relationship has consequences on behavior.

There are many studies investigating functional or structural connectivity in ASD; however to date none have attempted to relate the two types of connectivity, an approach that is vital to increase understanding of the underlying neurobiology. The approach that is described in this study is rational and clinically feasible. It is hoped that future neuroimaging research in ASD will follow this type of methodology to integrate investigation of functional and structural connectivity. It will be interesting to see the impact of abnormal structural connectivity on functional connectivity during other neuropsychological paradigms and at rest.

POTENTIAL IMPLICATIONS OF FINDINGS FROM CURRENT STUDY ON THERAPEUTIC INTERVENTIONS FOR AUTISM

A greater understanding of the specific deficits in functional and anatomical connectivity in autism is particularly salient as there is some evidence to suggest that connectivity abnormalities are amenable to training interventions. Neuroplasticity in humans is well-documented (Doidge, 2007) and two fascinating studies have demonstrated training-related changes in brain WM structure (Keller and Just, 2009; Scholz et al., 2009). One study demonstrated that healthy adults who were trained on a complex visuo-spatial skill (juggling) developed an increase in FA in WM underlying the intraparietal sulcus (Scholz et al., 2009), while the other reported that after 100 h of intensive remedial instruction, children with impaired reading ability showed an increase in FA in a brain region that, prior to instruction, had showed significantly lower FA relative to good readers (Keller and Just, 2009). In addition, a recent study in patients with schizophrenia reported that improvement in brain functioning following cognitive remediation therapy might be based on an increase of the interhemispheric information transfer between the bilateral prefrontal cortexes via the corpus callosum (Penades et al., 2013).

That WM structure can be influenced by experience is highly relevant for autism research. WM integrity is abnormal in numerous regions in autism; but it may be possible to introduce therapeutic training to stimulate improvement in WM organization. Although this study focuses on visuospatial processing, a cognitive function that is enhanced in ASD, it has revealed abnormal WM in a number of discrete brain regions. It is crucial to characterize the WM deficits in ASD to develop targets for future treatments, which could conceivably focus on interventions that improve WM organization and inter-regional brain connectivity. Improved brain connectivity in ASD may lead to improvements in the behaviors that are often impaired in this condition.

LIMITATIONS

There were a number of limitations to this study. Participants with ASD were limited to male, right-handed individuals with average or above-average IQ. Results are therefore very specific to this group and are not representative for all individuals on the spectrum. In this study, we adopted a novel approach whereby we specifically isolated WM tracts that directly connected brain regions showing abnormal functional connectivity. This approach was chosen as a primary aim of this research was to try to increase understanding of the neural correlates of atypical visuospatial processing in ASD and it was felt that a rational approach would be to use functionally defined ROIs from the connectivity analysis for diffusion tractography. This method allowed specific examination of the microstructural organization of WM in tracts that directly connected brain regions showing abnormal connectivity. It is important to point out however that there were a number of difficulties inherent in this approach. For example, it was not possible to back-project all functionally generated regions into native diffusion space and it is likely that valuable information about frontal and cerebellar WM abnormalities was not analysed in this study as a result. In addition, tracts between most of the fcMRI-defined ROIs are traceable in only a subset of participants. Also, we did not analyse any pairs of interhemispheric brain regions. It is also important to note that there are alternative approaches to investigating brain structural-functional connectivity relationships that were not adopted in the current study. For example one approach might be to define ROIs for tractography based on the location of between-group differences in diffusion measures, and move forward toward looking at the functional connectivity of the connected regions. In this study the diffusion measures used to infer structural connectivity were FA, CL, and CP. Recent research however has shown significant correlations between the number of tracts and functional connectivity, and researchers investigating relationships between functional and structural connectivity should carefully consider the measure(s) of "structural connectivity" selected.

In an attempt to increase understanding of the relationships between brain structural connectivity, functional connectivity and behavior, a large number of correlation analyses were carried out. Given the extremely limited data in both autism and healthy populations on the relationships between WM structure, functional connectivity and behavior, it was felt that it was reasonable to perform this number of exploratory correlation analyses; however, it is important to point out that correction for multiple comparisons was not carried out, thus some of the significant correlations reported may have been due to chance. In addition it is important to note that sample sizes for some of these correlation analyses were very small, which limited power. Nonetheless, it is illuminating to note the significant inter-relatedness of structure, function, and visuospatial processing speed in two of the WM tracts investigated (between the left occipital lobe and left caudate, and left occipital lobe and left thalamus). The correlations between these three measures lend strength to the hypothesis that there are indeed relationships, albeit complex, between structure, function, and behavior.

CONCLUSION

This novel multimodal imaging study has identified aberrant WM microstructure in tracts that directly connect brain regions that are abnormally functionally connected during visuospatial processing in ASD. Exploratory correlation analyses have revealed associations between structural connectivity, functional connectivity and visuospatial processing speed in both ASD and control groups, however the dearth of literature on normal relationships between DTI, fcMRI, and behavior makes it difficult to speculate on the true meaning of these associations. There is an urgent need for further research investigating links between structural connectivity, functional connectivity and behavior in both neurotypical and ASD populations. It is critical to understand the complex neural pathophysiology of autism in order to develop rational, targeted therapeutic interventions to improve WM organization and inter-regional neural connectivity.

ACKNOWLEDGMENTS

We wish to thank all the families who participated in this study, Mr. Sean Brennan and Dr. Miriam Law-Smith for help with recruitment, and Dr. Flavio Dell'Acqua, Dr. Marco Catani, Dr. Dara Cannon, and Dr. Stephen Meredith for expert advice on setting up the study. We gratefully acknowledge the support of Molecular Medicine Ireland who funded this work (grant number 4AA-G04005-0-S06), IITAC, the HEA, the National Development Plan and the Trinity Centre for High Performance Computing and thank Mr. Brendan Behan, Mr. Sojo Joseph, and many others for their invaluable assistance during the study.

REFERENCES

Agam, Y., Joseph, R. M., Barton, J. J., and Manoach, D. S. (2010). Reduced cognitive control of response inhibition by the anterior cingulate cortex in autism spectrum disorders. *Neuroimage* 52, 336–347. doi: 10.1016/j.neuroimage.2010.04.010

Alexander, A. L., Lee, J. E., Lazar, M., Boudos, R., Dubray, M. B., Oakes, T. R., et al. (2007). Diffusion tensor imaging of the corpus callosum in Autism. *Neuroimage* 34, 61–73. doi: 10.1016/j.neuroimage.2006.08.032

Alexander, D. C., Barker, G. J., and Arridge, S. R. (2002). Detection and modeling of non-Gaussian apparent diffusion coefficient profiles in human brain data. *Magn. Reson. Med.* 48, 331–340. doi: 10.1002/mrm.10209

Barnea-Goraly, N., Lotspeich, L. J., and Reiss, A. L. (2010). Similar white matter aberrations in children with autism and their unaffected siblings: a diffusion tensor imaging study using tract-based spatial statistics. *Arch. Gen. Psychiatry* 67, 1052–1060. doi: 10.1001/archgenpsychiatry.2010.123

Behrens, T. E., and Sporns, O. (2012). Human connectomics. *Curr. Opin. Neurobiol.* 22, 144–153. doi: 10.1016/j.conb.2011.08.005

Catani, M., Jones, D. K., Daly, E., Embiricos, N., Deeley, Q., Pugliese, L., et al. (2008). Altered cerebellar feedback projections in Asperger syndrome. *Neuroimage* 41, 1184–1191. doi: 10.1016/j.neuroimage.2008.03.041

Chang, L. C., Jones, D. K., and Pierpaoli, C. (2005). RESTORE:

robust estimation of tensors by outlier rejection. *Magn. Reson. Med.* 53, 1088–1095. doi: 10.1002/mrm.20426

Cheon, K. A., Kim, Y. S., Oh, S. H., Park, S. Y., Yoon, H. W., Herrington, J., et al. (2011). Involvement of the anterior thalamic radiation in boys with high functioning autism spectrum disorders: a diffusion tensor imaging study. *Brain Res.* 1417, 77–86. doi: 10.1016/j.brainres.2011.08.020

Cherkassky, V. L., Kana, R. K., Keller, T. A., and Just, M. A. (2006). Functional connectivity in a baseline resting-state network in autism. *Neuroreport* 17, 1687–1690. doi: 10.1097/01.wnr.0000239956.45448.4c

Cheung, C., Chua, S. E., Cheung, V., Khong, P. L., Tai, K. S., Wong, T. K., et al. (2009). White matter fractional anisotrophy differences and correlates of diagnostic symptoms in autism. *J. Child Psychol. Psychiatry* 50, 1102–1112. doi: 10.1111/j.1469-7610.2009.02086.x

Damarla, S. R., Keller, T. A., Kana, R. K., Cherkassky, V. L., Williams, D. L., Minshew, N. J., et al. (2010). Cortical underconnectivity coupled with preserved visuospatial cognition in autism: evidence from an fMRI study of an embedded figures task. *Autism Res.* 3, 273–279. doi: 10.1002/aur.153

Doidge, N. (2007). *The Brain That Changes Itself: Stories of Personal Triumph from the Frontiers of Brain Science.* James H. Silberman.

Frank, L. R. (2002). Characterization of anisotropy in high angular resolution diffusion-weighted MRI. *Magn. Reson. Med.* 47, 1083–1099. doi: 10.1002/mrm.10156

Friston, K. J., Buechel, C., Fink, G. R., Morris, J., Rolls, E., and Dolan, R. J. (1997). Psychophysiological and modulatory interactions in neuroimaging. *Neuroimage* 6, 218–229. doi: 10.1006/nimg.1997.0291

Greicius, M. D., Supekar, K., Menon, V., and Dougherty, R. F. (2009). Resting-state functional connectivity reflects structural connectivity in the default mode network. *Cereb. Cortex* 19, 72–78.

Hagmann, P., Cammoun, L., Gigandet, X., Meuli, R., Honey, C. J., Wedeen, V. J., et al. (2008). Mapping the structural core of human cerebral cortex. *PLoS Biol.* 6:e159. doi: 10.1371/journal.pbio.0060159

Hermundstad, A. M., Bassett, D. S., Brown, K. S., Aminoff, E. M., Clewett, D., Freeman, S., et al. (2013). Structural foundations of resting-state and task-based functional connectivity in the human brain. *Proc. Natl. Acad. Sci. U.S.A.* 110, 6169–6174. doi: 10.1073/pnas.1219562110

Honey, C. J., Sporns, O., Cammoun, L., Gigandet, X., Thiran, J. P., Meuli, R., et al. (2009). Predicting human resting-state functional connectivity from structural connectivity. *Proc. Natl. Acad. Sci. U.S.A.* 106, 2035–2040. doi: 10.1073/pnas.0811168106

Hong, S., Ke, X., Tang, T., Hang, Y., Chu, K., Huang, H., et al. (2011). Detecting abnormalities of corpus callosum connectivity in autism using magnetic resonance imaging and diffusion tensor tractography. *Psychiatry Res.* 194, 333–339. doi: 10.1016/j.pscychresns.2011.03.009

Jeurissen, B., Leemans, A., Jones, D. K., Tournier, J. D., and Sijbers, J. (2011). Probabilistic fiber tracking using the residual bootstrap with constrained spherical deconvolution. *Hum. Brain Mapp.* 32, 461–479. doi: 10.1002/hbm.21032

Jeurissen, B., Leemans, A., Tournier, J. D., Jones, D. K., and Sijbers, J. (2012). Investigating the prevalence of complex fiber configurations in white matter tissue with diffusion MRI. *Hum. Brain Mapp.* doi: 10.1002/hbm.22099. [Epub ahead of print].

Johnston, J. M., Vaishnavi, S. N., Smyth, M. D., Zhang, D., He, B. J., Zempel, J. M., et al. (2008). Loss of resting interhemispheric functional connectivity after complete section of the corpus callosum. *J. Neurosci.* 28, 6453–6458. doi: 10.1523/JNEUROSCI.0573-08.2008

Jones, D. K., and Cercignani, M. (2010). Twenty-five pitfalls in the analysis of diffusion MRI data. *NMR Biomed.* 23, 803–820. doi: 10.1002/nbm.1543

Jones, D. K., and Leemans, A. (2011). Diffusion tensor imaging. *Methods Mol. Biol.* 711, 127–144. doi: 10.1007/978-1-61737-992-5_6

Jou, R. J., Jackowski, A. P., Papademetris, X., Rajeevan, N., Staib, L. H., and Volkmar, F. R. (2011). Diffusion tensor imaging in autism spectrum disorders: preliminary evidence of abnormal neural connectivity. *Aust. N.Z. J. Psychiatry* 45, 153–162. doi: 10.3109/00048674.2010.534069

Just, M. A., Cherkassky, V. L., Keller, T. A., Kana, R. K., and Minshew, N. J. (2007). Functional and anatomical cortical underconnectivity in autism: evidence from an FMRI study of an executive function task and corpus callosum morphometry. *Cereb. Cortex* 17, 951–961.

Kana, R. K., Keller, T. A., Cherkassky, V. L., Minshew, N. J., and Just, M. A. (2006). Sentence comprehension in autism: thinking in pictures with decreased functional connectivity. *Brain* 129, 2484–2493. doi: 10.1093/brain/awl164

Keller, T. A., and Just, M. A. (2009). Altering cortical connectivity: remediation-induced changes in the white matter of poor readers. *Neuron* 64, 624–631. doi: 10.1016/j.neuron.2009.10.018

Klein, S., Staring, M., Murphy, K., Viergever, M. A., and Pluim, J. P. (2010). elastix: a toolbox for intensity-based medical image registration. *IEEE Trans. Med. Imaging* 29, 196–205. doi: 10.1109/TMI.2009.2035616

Koch, M. A., Norris, D. G., and Hund-Georgiadis, M. (2002). An investigation of functional and anatomical connectivity using magnetic resonance imaging. *Neuroimage* 16, 241–250. doi: 10.1006/nimg.2001.1052

Kumar, A., Sundaram, S. K., Sivaswamy, L., Behen, M. E., Makki, M. I., Ager, J., et al. (2010). Alterations in frontal lobe tracts and corpus callosum in young children with autism spectrum disorder. *Cereb. Cortex* 20, 2103–2113. doi: 10.1093/cercor/bhp278

Lee, P., Foss-Feig, J., Henderson, J., Kenworthy, L., Gilotty, L., Gaillard, W., et al. (2007). Atypical neural substrates of embedded figures task performance in children with autism spectrum disorder. *Neuroimage* 38, 184–193. doi: 10.1016/j.neuroimage.2007.07.013

Leemans, A., Jeurissen, B., Sijbers, J., and Jones, D. K. (2009). "ExploreDTI: a graphical toolbox for processing, analyzing, and visualizing diffusion MR data," in *Proceedings of the 17th Annual Meeting of International Society for Magnetic Resonance in Medicine* (Hawaii), 3536.

Leemans, A., and Jones, D. K. (2009). The B-matrix must be rotated when correcting for subject motion in DTI data. *Magn. Reson. Med.* 61, 1336–1349. doi: 10.1002/mrm.21890

Lord, C., Risi, S., Lambrecht, L., Cook, E. H. Jr., Leventhal, B. L., Dilavore, P. C., et al. (2000). The autism diagnostic observation schedule-generic: a standard measure of social and communication deficits associated with the spectrum of autism. *J. Autism Dev. Disord.* 30, 205–223. doi: 10.1023/A:1005592401947

Lord, C., Rutter, M., and Le Couteur, A. (1994). Autism diagnostic interview-revised: a revised version of a diagnostic interview for caregivers of individuals with possible pervasive developmental disorders. *J. Autism Dev. Disord.* 24, 659–685. doi: 10.1007/BF02172145

Lowe, M. J., Beall, E. B., Sakaie, K. E., Koenig, K. A., Stone, L., Marrie, R. A., et al. (2008). Resting state sensorimotor functional connectivity in multiple sclerosis inversely correlates with transcallosal motor pathway transverse diffusivity. *Hum. Brain Mapp.* 29, 818–827. doi: 10.1002/hbm.20576

Manjaly, Z. M., Bruning, N., Neufang, S., Stephan, K. E., Brieber, S., Marshall, J. C., et al. (2007). Neurophysiological correlates of relatively enhanced local visual search in autistic adolescents. *Neuroimage* 35, 283–291. doi: 10.1016/j.neuroimage.2006.11.036

Margulies, D. S., Vincent, J. L., Kelly, C., Lohmann, G., Uddin, L. Q., Biswal, B. B., et al. (2009). Precuneus shares intrinsic functional architecture in humans and monkeys. *Proc. Natl. Acad. Sci. U.S.A.* 106, 20069–20074.

Mason, R. A., Williams, D. L., Kana, R. K., Minshew, N., and Just, M. A. (2008). Theory of mind disruption and recruitment of the right hemisphere during narrative comprehension in autism. *Neuropsychologia* 46, 269–280. doi: 10.1016/j.neuropsychologia.2007.07.018

McGrath, J., Johnson, K., Ecker, C., O'Hanlon, E., Gill, M., Gallagher, L., et al. (2012). Atypical visuospatial processing in autism: insights from functional connectivity analysis. *Autism Res.* 5, 314–330. doi: 10.1002/aur.1245

McGrath, J., Johnson, K., O'Hanlon, E., Garavan, H., Gallagher, L., and Leemans, A. (2013). White matter and visuospatial processing in autism: a constrained spherical deconvolution tractography study. *Autism Res.* doi: 10.1002/aur.1290. [Epub ahead of print].

Metzler-Baddeley, C. M., Hunt, S., Jones, D. K., Leemans, A., Aggleton, J. P., and O'Sullivan, M. J. (2012). Temporal association tracts and the breakdown of episodic memory in mild cognitive impairment. *Neurology* 79, 2233–2240. doi: 10.1212/WNL.0b013e31827689e8

Monk, C. S., Peltier, S. J., Wiggins, J. L., Weng, S.-J., Carrasco, M., Risi, S., et al. (2009). Abnormalities of intrinsic functional connectivity in autism spectrum disorders. *Neuroimage* 47, 764–772.

Noriuchi, M., Kikuchi, Y., Yoshiura, T., Kira, R., Shigeto, H., Hara, T., et al. (2010). Altered white matter fractional anisotropy and social impairment in children with autism spectrum disorder. *Brain Res.* 1362, 141–149. doi: 10.1016/j.brainres.2010.09.051

Penades, R., Pujol, N., Catalan, R., Massana, G., Rametti, G., Garcia-Rizo, C., et al. (2013). Brain effects of cognitive remediation therapy in schizophrenia: a structural and functional neuroimaging study. *Biol. Psychiatry* 73, 1015–1023. doi: 10.1016/j.biopsych.2013.01.017

Pluim, J. P., Maintz, J. B., and Viergever, M. A. (2003). Mutual-information-based registration of medical images: a survey. *IEEE Trans. Med. Imaging* 22, 986–1004. doi: 10.1109/TMI.2003.815867

Poustka, L., Jennen-Steinmetz, C., Henze, R., Vomstein, K., Haffner, J., and Sieltjes, B. (2011). Fronto-temporal disconnectivity and symptom severity in children with autism spectrum disorder. *World J. Biol. Psychiatry* 13, 269–280.

Pruessmann, K. P., Weiger, M., Scheidegger, M. B., and Boesiger, P. (1999). SENSE: sensitivity encoding for fast MRI. *Magn. Reson. Med.* 42, 952–962.

Quigley, M., Cordes, D., Turski, P., Moritz, C., Haughton, V., Seth, R., et al. (2003). Role of the corpus callosum in functional connectivity. *AJNR Am. J. Neuroradiol.* 24, 208–212.

Reijmer, Y. D., Brundel, M., de Bresser, J., Kappelle, L. J., Leemans, A., and Biessels, G. J. (2013). Microstructural white matter abnormalities and cognitive functioning in type 2 diabetes: a diffusion tensor imaging study. *Diabetes Care* 36, 137–144. doi: 10.2337/dc12-0493

Reijmer, Y. D., Leemans, A., Heringa, S. M., Wielaard, I., Jeurissen, B., Koek, H. L., et al. (2012). Improved sensitivity to cerebral white matter abnormalities in alzheimer's disease with spherical deconvolution based tractography. *PLoS ONE* 7:e44074. doi: 10.1371/journal.pone.0044074

Sahyoun, C. P., Belliveau, J. W., and Mody, M. (2010). White matter integrity and pictorial reasoning in high-functioning children with autism. *Brain Cogn.* 73, 180–188. doi: 10.1016/j.bandc.2010.05.002

Sattler, J. M. (1992). *Assessement of Children. Revised and Updated 3rd Edn (Table L-12).* San Diego, CA: Sattler, Jerome M.

Scholz, J., Klein, M. C., Behrens, T. E., and Johansen-Berg, H. (2009). Training induces changes in white-matter architecture. *Nat. Neurosci.* 12, 1370–1371. doi: 10.1038/nn.2412

Shukla, D. K., Keehn, B., Lincoln, A. J., and Muller, R. A. (2010). White matter compromise of callosal and subcortical fiber tracts in children with autism spectrum disorder: a diffusion tensor imaging study.*J. Am. Acad. Child Adolesc. Psychiatry* 49, 1269–1278, 1278 e1–e2.

Skudlarski, P., Jagannathan, K., Calhoun, V. D., Hampson, M., Skudlarska, B. A., and Pearlson, G. (2008). Measuring brain connectivity: diffusion tensor imaging validates resting state temporal correlations. *Neuroimage* 43, 554–561. doi: 10.1016/j.neuroimage.2008.07.063

Sundaram, S. K., Kumar, A., Makki, M. I., Behen, M. E., Chugani, H. T., and Chugani, D. C. (2008). Diffusion tensor imaging of frontal lobe in autism spectrum disorder. *Cereb. Cortex* 18, 2659–2665. doi: 10.1093/cercor/bhn031

Thakkar, K., Polli, F., Joseph, R., Tuch, D., Hadjikhani, N., Barton, J., et al. (2008). Response monitoring, repetitive behaviour and anterior cingulate abnormalities in autism spectrum disorders (ASD). *Brain* 131, 2464–2478. doi: 10.1093/brain/awn099

Thomas, C., Humphreys, K., Jung, K. J., Minshew, N., and Behrmann, M. (2011). The anatomy of the callosal and visual-association pathways in high-functioning autism: a DTI tractography study. *Cortex* 47, 863–873. doi: 10.1016/j.cortex.2010.07.006

Tournier, J. D., Calamante, F., and Connelly, A. (2007). Robust determination of the fibre orientation distribution in diffusion MRI: non-negativity constrained super-resolved spherical deconvolution. *Neuroimage* 35, 1459–1472. doi: 10.1016/j.neuroimage.2007.02.016

Tournier, J. D., Calamante, F., Gadian, D. G., and Connelly, A. (2004). Direct estimation of the fiber orientation density function from diffusion-weighted MRI data using spherical deconvolution. *Neuroimage* 23, 1176–1185. doi: 10.1016/j.neuroimage.2004.07.037

Tournier, J. D., Mori, S., and Leemans, A. (2011). Diffusion tensor imaging and beyond. *Magn. Reson. Med.* 65, 1532–1556. doi: 10.1002/mrm.22924

Tournier, J. D., Yeh, C. H., Calamante, F., Cho, K. H., Connelly, A., and Lin, C. P. (2008). Resolving crossing fibres using constrained spherical deconvolution: validation using diffusion-weighted imaging phantom data. *Neuroimage* 42, 617–625. doi: 10.1016/j.neuroimage.2008.05.002

van den Heuvel, M., Mandl, R., Luigjes, J., and Hulshoff Pol, H. (2008). Microstructural organization of the cingulum tract and the level of default mode functional connectivity. *J. Neurosci.* 28, 10844–10851. doi: 10.1523/JNEUROSCI.2964-08.2008

Vincent, J. L., Patel, G. H., Fox, M. D., Snyder, A. Z., Baker, J. T., Van Essen, D. C., et al. (2007). Intrinsic functional architecture in the anaesthetized monkey brain. *Nature* 447, 83–86. doi: 10.1038/nature05758

Vos, S. B., Jones, D. K., Jeurissen, B., Viergever, M. A., and Leemans, A. (2012). The influence of complex white matter architecture on the mean diffusivity in diffusion tensor MRI of the human brain. *Neuroimage* 59, 2208–2216. doi: 10.1016/j.neuroimage.2011.09.086

Vos, S. B., Jones, D. K., Viergever, M. A., and Leemans, A. (2011). Partial volume effect as a hidden covariate in DTI analyses. *Neuroimage* 55, 1566–1576. doi: 10.1016/j.neuroimage.2011.01.048

Wechsler, D. (1997). *WAIS–III Administration and Scoring Manual.* San Antonio, TX: Psychological Corporation.

Wechsler, D. (2004). *The Wechsler Intelligence Scale for Children, 4th Edn.* London: Pearson Assessment.

Wedeen, V. J., Reese, T. G., Tuch, D. S., Weigel, M. R., Dou, R. M., Weiskoff, R. M., et al. (2000). "Mapping fibre orientation spectra in cerebral white matter with Fourier-transform diffusion MRI," in *International Society of Magnetic Resonance in Medicine,* (Denver, CO), 82.

Wedeen, V. J., Wang, R. P., Schmahmann, J. D., Benner, T., Tseng, W. Y., Dai, G., et al. (2008). Diffusion spectrum magnetic resonance imaging (DSI) tractography of crossing fibers. *Neuroimage* 41, 1267–1277. doi: 10.1016/j.neuroimage.2008.03.036

Weng, S. J., Wiggins, J. L., Peltier, S. J., Carrasco, M., Risi, S., Lord, C., et al. (2010). Alterations of resting state functional connectivity in the default network in adolescents with autism spectrum disorders. *Brain Res.* 1313, 202–214. doi: 10.1016/j.brainres.2009.11.057

Westin, C. F., Maier, S. E., Mamata, H., Nabavi, A., Jolesz, F. A., and Kikinis, R. (2002). Processing and visualization for diffusion tensor MRI. *Med. Image Anal.* 6, 93–108. doi: 10.1016/S1361-8415(02)00053-1

17

Evidence for dysregulation of axonal growth and guidance in the etiology of ASD

Kathryn McFadden[1] and Nancy J. Minshew[2]*

[1] *Department of Neurobiology, University of Pittsburgh, Pittsburgh, PA, USA*
[2] *Department of Psychiatry and Neurology, University of Pittsburgh Medical School, Pittsburgh, PA, USA*

Edited by:
Rajesh Kumar Kana, University of Alabama at Birmingham, USA

Reviewed by:
Andrew L. Alexander, University of Arizona, USA
Lucina Q. Uddin, Stanford University, USA
Tianming Liu, University of Georgia, USA

****Correspondence:***
Nancy J. Minshew, Western Psychiatric Institute and Clinic of University of Pittsburgh Medical Center, Webster Hall, Suite 300, 3811 O'Hara Street, Pittsburgh, PA 15213, USA
e-mail: minshewnj@upmc.edu

Current theories concerning the cause of autism spectrum disorders (ASDs) have converged on the concept of abnormal development of brain connectivity. This concept is supported by accumulating evidence from functional imaging, diffusion tensor imaging, and high definition fiber tracking studies which suggest altered microstructure in the axonal tracts connecting cortical areas may underly many of the cognitive manifestations of ASD. Additionally, large-scale genomic studies implicate numerous gene candidates known or suspected to mediate neuritic outgrowth and axonal guidance in fetal and perinatal life. Neuropathological observations in postmortem ASD brain samples further support this model and include subtle disturbances of cortical lamination and subcortical axonal morphology. Of note is the relatively common finding of poor differentiation of the gray–white junction associated with an excess superficial white matter or "interstitial" neurons (INs). INs are thought to be remnants of the fetal subplate, a transient structure which plays a key role in the guidance and morphogenesis of thalamocortical and cortico-cortical connections and the organization of cortical columnar architecture. While not discounting the importance of synaptic dysfunction in the etiology of ASD, this paper will briefly review the cortical abnormalities and genetic evidence supporting a model of dysregulated axonal growth and guidance as key developmental processes underlying the clinical manifestations of ASD.

Keywords: autism spectrum disorders, connectivity, neuritic outgrowth, axonal guidance, subplate

INTRODUCTION

Autism spectrum disorders (ASDs) are characterized by deficits across apparently disparate domains; language, social reciprocity, sensory integration, and repetitive/restricted behavior patterns among others. Within each domain, however, functioning is often markedly uneven, and the coexistence of significant impairments with areas of normal or even enhanced performance is a long recognized paradox. Cognitive-neurologic testing (Minshew et al., 1997, Minshew et al., 2002; Williams et al., 2006) has indicated the common denominator across domains is a normal or enhanced ability to perform perceptual and simple information processing tasks coupled with significant deficits in the ability to perform tasks requiring complex information processing, even in high-functioning, high-IQ subjects with ASD. Rather than implicating dysfunction in a particular brain area/structure, this cognitive profile is most consistent with altered functioning of the distributed cortical neural network, i.e., how and how well cortical functional areas, particularly association areas, communicate with each other and their subcortical targets (Minshew and Payton, 1988). This model of aberrant connectivity in ASD is now widely accepted, although the details vary (e.g., Belmonte et al., 2004; Geschwind and Levitt, 2007).

Functional magnetic resonance imaging (fMRI), which allows for examination at the neural systems level, has been key to demonstrating the above impairments and modeling altered connectivity in ASD. Numerous fMRI studies have reported decreased synchronization of critical cortical areas during the performance of complex tasks (or at rest) in subjects with ASD relative to age and IQ-matched controls. This appears to be particularly marked in tasks requiring high functional connectivity between frontal association (e.g., anterior cingulate and prefrontal cortices), and more posterior cortical regions (reviewed in Schipul et al., 2011) such as complex sentence comprehension (Just et al., 2004), social inference (Just et al., 2007), or inhibition (Kana et al., 2007).

Altered anatomic connectivity is the most likely substrate for reduced functional connectivity (**Figure 1**), although the exact basis of the relationship is not established and much debated. At the physical level, neural circuitry is comprised of neurons, their processes (axons and dendrites), and their synapses on neighboring or distant neurons. Wiring the brain, therefore, requires the coordinated interactions of numerous molecular cascades and environmental exposures during development so that neurons proliferate, migrate to the appropriate locations, extend axons with a high degree of spatial and temporal fidelity, and establish synaptic connections with appropriate target neurons. Clearly, one or more of these developmental processes does not unfold in the typical fashion in ASD. In recent years, much attention has been paid to altered synaptic function as the central event explaining altered brain connectivity in ASD. However, the view of ASD as predominately an intrinsic synaptopathy is unsatisfying in view of the cerebral white matter alterations documented in many subjects and outlined below.

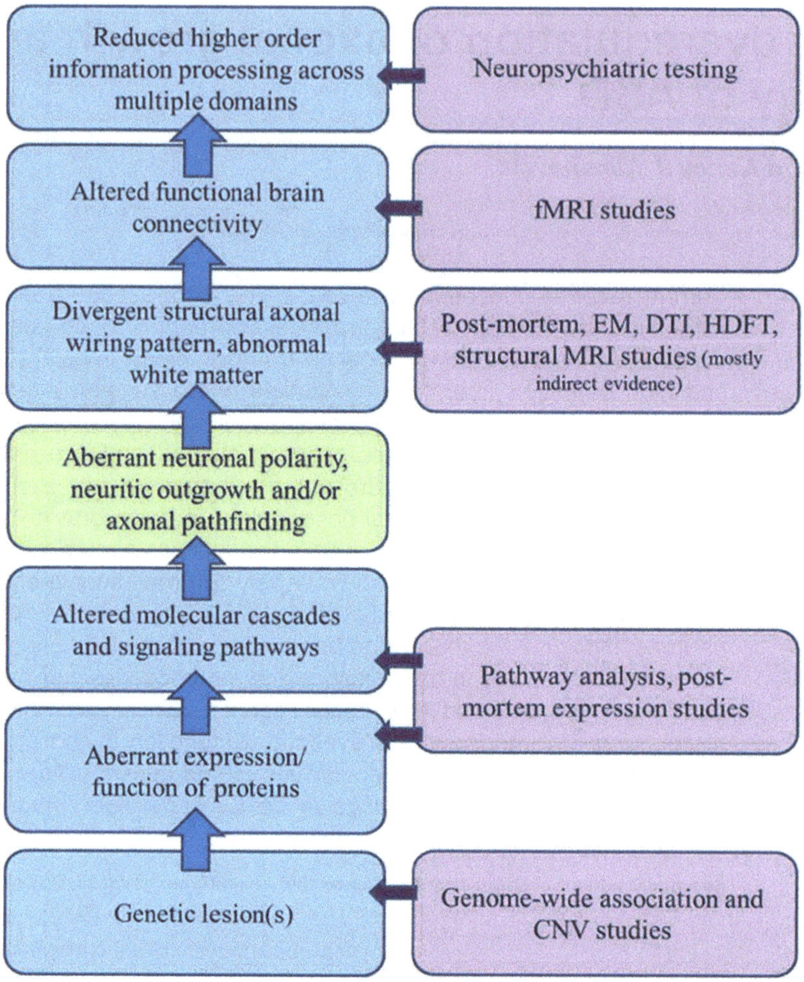

FIGURE 1 | Sources of evidence for a model of dysregulated axonal development in ASD. A broad gap exists between the clinical manifestations of ASD and growing list of genetic candidates; a gap only incompletely bridged by a general model of altered connectivity. A significant component of dysregulated axonal development (polarity, outgrowth, and guidance/targeting should be considered in constructing a model of ASD etiology that encompasses all of the clinical, functional, structural, and genetic observations.

ALTERED BRAIN GROWTH TRAJECTORIES: EVIDENCE FROM STRUCTURAL MRI STUDIES

Structural MRI, morphometric, and neuropathologic studies provide ample evidence of altered neocortical growth and organization in ASD. Studies examining head circumference and brain volume in individuals with ASD have demonstrated altered brain growth trajectories across the lifespan. While not significantly different from controls at birth, up to 70% of infants later diagnosed with ASD exhibit abnormally accelerated brain growth in the first year of life (Courchesne et al., 2003). Approximately 20–25% of infants in this subset meet formal criteria for macrocephaly in the first year. Brain volume ascertained by MRI is significantly larger in 90% of infants with ASD by 2–4 years of life as well (Courchesne et al., 2003). Many studies note a marked rostral–caudal gradient in these altered growth trajectories (reviewed in Lainhart, 2006). At the time of maximal brain growth in very early childhood, cerebral gray matter and white matter are both increased (by approximately 20 and 40%, respectively). The frontal cortical gray and white matter show the most enlargement followed by the temporal and parietal lobes. The occipital gray and white matter and parietal gray matter tend not to vary significantly from normal (Carper et al., 2002). Within the frontal lobes, the gray matter areas most affected are the dorsolateral and mesial prefrontal cortex. Similarly, the white matter most involved appears to be the radiate compartment and U-fibers immediately underlying these cortical areas which represent intrahemispheric, cortico-cortical connections originating from cortical layers II and III (Herbert et al., 2003). The corpus callosum, conversely, is often reduced in autism (e.g., Hardan et al., 2000; Keary et al., 2009). Therefore, increased brain size in toddlers with ASD appears to be largely driven by enlargement of the white matter compartment underlying the frontal and temporal cortices (Carper et al., 2002; Herbert et al., 2004; Carper and Courchesne, 2005).

Following this initial acceleration, growth rates decline significantly causing an apparent normalization of brain volume by adolescence and early adulthood (Courchesne et al., 2001,

Courchesne et al., 2004; Waiter et al., 2005). This relative decrease is most marked in the white matter in that children with autism experience only a 10% increase in cerebral white matter between the ages of 3 and 12 years (Courchesne et al., 2001). Gray matter volumes remain elevated into adulthood as does mean head circumference. Rates of macrocephaly, although lower, remain increased overall. This pattern stands in stark contrast to the age related cerebral white matter increase (60%) and gray matter decrease observed in typically developing individuals between the ages of 4 and 22 years (Tau and Peterson, 2010) which are generally thought to be a function of the concurrent processes of synaptic/collateral pruning and myelination. It must be noted that the above pattern does not hold true for all individuals with ASD. Many show typical rates of head and brain growth and a small subset even meet criteria for microencephaly, although this is more common in the setting of syndromic ASD (see Activating Mutations in the mTOR Pathway are Associated with Syndromic ASD for discussion of this concept).

ALTERED CORTICAL MICROSTRUCTURE: EVIDENCE FROM POSTMORTEM STUDIES

A number of studies have reported gross and microscopic changes that may relate to increased gray matter and alterations in relative compartmental volumes. One recent report of seven autistic children with increased brain size (Courchesne et al., 2011) involved a 67% increase in the numbers of neurons in the prefrontal cortex relative to age-matched controls. Neurogenesis, the birth and early proliferation of neurons, is largely a prenatal process. At birth, cortical neurons are typically small, so that an appreciable excess might not translate into a significant change in head size. However, in the first years of life, the typical dramatic increase in cytoplasmic volumes (both of the cell body and axons/dendrites) occurring in more than the usual complement of frontal neurons, could account for abnormally accelerated brain growth in the first years of life. It would also explain why maturational synaptic/neuritic pruning may not register as an appreciable loss of cerebral gray matter in these individuals.

Related to this is the finding of subtle microstructural abnormalities in cortical architecture, even in the absence of more obvious dysgenic lesions. Although most of these analyzes are not rigorously stereologic, the impression is of increased numbers of narrow minicolumns containing increased densities of neurons (Casanova et al., 2002, 2006; Buxhoeveden et al., 2006) in the frontal cortex of ASD brains. This trend appears to be most pronounced in the frontal lobe, particularly the dorsolateral prefrontal cortex, and is not seen in more posterior regions such as the visual cortex. Minicolumns are the vertical cell columns created by sequential waves of migrating neurons traveling along radial glial fibers during early corticogenesis. Increased numbers of such arrays may reflect excess early divisions of radial glial cells immediately prior to the onset of neurogenesis and migration. Furthermore, the distribution of minicolumn abnormalities correlates with patterns of accelerated growth and excess neurons in the early postnatal period.

More than half of all postmortem investigations have uncovered additional features of cortical dysgenesis, presumably caused by abnormal neurogenesis, neuronal migration or maturation, in ASD brains. Bailey et al. (1998) observed significant and widespread cortical dysgenic lesions in four of six subjects with ASD. Similarly, in a recent large-scale study, Wegiel et al. (2010) reported a wide variety of dysgenic lesions and heterotopias in multiple cortical regions in 12 of 13 subjects with ASD. These included excess subependymal neurons, subcortical and periventricular heterotopias, and additional minor disruptions of cytoarchitecture. In the seminal postmortem studies by Kemper and Bauman (Bauman and Kemper, 1985, 1998; Kemper and Bauman, 1993, 2002), the only consistent abnormality in the cerebral cortex was relatively small neuronal cell size and increased cell packing in the anterior cingulate cortex. Simms et al. (2009) also found decreased cell size and decreased cell packing in different sub-regions of the anterior cingulate. Van Kooten et al. (2008) conducted a stereologic study on the fusiform gyrus, involved in face processing, and found significantly lower neuronal densities within layer III and lower total neuron numbers in layers III, V, and VI, as well as smaller average cell volumes of neurons in layers V and VI. Hutsler and Zhang (2010) found increased dendritic spine densities in the temporal lobes of individuals with ASD and intellectual disability relative to age-matched controls. Most of the reported cortical microstructural finding in ASD are very subtle. It must be noted that even the non-subtle dysgenic lesions reported in the literature are not specific to ASD and are more often found in non-ASD individuals both with and without seizures or other neurologic symptoms. Conversely, the vast majority of ASD brains show relatively normal cortical cytoarchitecture.

ALTERED CORTICAL WHITE MATTER: EVIDENCE FROM DTI AND POSTMORTEM STUDIES

It is very possible that an increase in absolute numbers and densities of neurons in the frontal cortex could have an adverse effect on anterior–posterior connectivity. The mismatch created by relatively too few afferent and/or too many efferent axonal terminals attempting to form circuits could potentially be disruptive. But converging lines of evidence also point to microstructural differences in white matter. Much of this evidence is indirect and relatively non-specific, but white matter is notoriously hard to study. While MRI-based studies allow the direct examination of the general course and volume of major white matter tracts, they have lacked the necessary resolution to directly examine even large axon fascicles or to trace these entering the cortex. Histologic techniques, conversely, have permitted the direct examination of axons and their myelin coverings, but are too laborious and time consuming to feasibly trace connections over large distances in the brain. Fortunately, recent advances in high definition fiber tracking (HDFT) promise to soon permit the best (or the best compromise) of both worlds. HDFT is a novel tractography method using high-angular-resolution diffusion imaging and diffusion spectrum imaging (DSI) techniques in order to track white matter fibers from cortical origins, through complex fiber crossings, to cortical and subcortical targets with at least millimeter resolution (a few hundred axons; Verstynen et al., 2011; Fernandez-Miranda et al., 2012). Initial reports (only in the popular media for now) have demonstrated significant alterations in the morphology (i.e., wiring plan) of a number of major white matter tracts in a few individuals with ASD (e.g., Schneider, 2011, 2012). These highly preliminary findings indicate the physical alterations of ASD in the brain may prove to be quite unsubtle, but until now, almost completely invisible.

Much of the current evidence for altered white matter comes from studies employing diffusion tensor imaging (DTI). DTI measures apparent diffusibility of water molecules as a function of direction over time and is a method to characterize the organization and microstructural properties of white matter. The most common DTI measure is fractional anisotropy (FA) which characterizes the directional variation in the apparent diffusions. White matter, which is arranged in parallel arrays of axonal bundles (fascicles) tends to have a higher FA than gray matter as diffusion of water in neuropil has less directionality (i.e., is more isotropic). A complementary measure, radial diffusivity (RD), describes the tendency of perpendicular water movement and is, therefore, lower in white matter compared to gray matter (reviewed in Travers et al., 2012). Numerous studies have found widespread decreases in FA (and concurrent increases in RD or similar measures) in children (>4 years of age) and adults with ASD (reviewed in Travers et al., 2012). This tendency is most pronounced in the corpus callosum (e.g., Shukla et al., 2010; Jeong et al., 2011), cingulum bundle, and various white matter tracts involving the temporal and frontal lobes (e.g., Jou et al., 2011; Shukla et al., 2011) thereby correlating, generally, with both the fMRI and structural MRI growth trajectory data. These white matter alterations are attributed to reduced tract coherence and/or loss of microstructural integrity, but are not specific to a particular etiology as similar effects could potentially be produced by reduced myelination, increased axonal diameter, alterations of axonal density, or more complex white matter (i.e., turning or crossing fibers, or excess branching) or reduced axonal fasciculation (Travers et al., 2012).

Microscopic tissue studies, although limited by the time necessary to perform, allow a greater degree of resolution and may potentially being able to resolve these differences. In a rare and recent study, Zikopoulos and Barbas (2010) stereologically investigated the fine structure (by light and electron microscopy) of myelinated axons in the white matter below the anterior cingulate cortex, orbitofrontal cortex, and lateral prefrontal cortex in individuals with ASD relative to age-matched controls. They found similar overall axonal density between groups below all prefrontal areas. However, the ASD group had significantly fewer large axons (likely representing the more long-range cortico-cortical connections) in the deep white matter below the anterior cingulate cortex. This was associated with the presence of a significantly greater density of smaller axons (thought to connect more adjacent cortical areas) in the corresponding superficial white matter. There were no discernible differences in neuronal densities or distributions in the overlying gray matter. The white matter below the anterior cingulate cortex also exhibited a significantly higher proportion of branched axons of medium caliber. Axons in the superficial white matter below the orbitofrontal exhibited significantly thinner myelin sheaths when controlled for axon diameter despite similar numbers of oligodendrocytes (Zikopoulos and Barbas, 2010). Azmitia et al. (2010, 2011) also found a significant excess of morphologically abnormal serotonin axons in principle ascending fiber bundles of the medialand lateral forebrain bundles as well as target areas in the temporal cortex, amygdala, and globus pallidus.

THE POTENTIAL ROLE OF THE FETAL SUBPLATE IN WIRING ALTERATIONS IN ASD

Probably the most pervasive cortical finding in ASD, documented in both neuropathologic and structural MRI studies, is the relatively poor differentiation of the gray–white junction associated with excess superficial white matter or interstitial neurons (INs; Bailey et al., 1998; Casanova et al., 2002; Hutsler et al., 2007; Simms et al., 2009; Wegiel et al., 2010; Avino and Hutsler, 2011). This is noted particularly in the white matter just below the frontal association cortices and superior temporal gyrus (e.g., Avino and Hutsler, 2010). The presence of excess INs in ASD has been long attributed to abnormalities of cortical migration despite the very limited findings of gross laminar alterations within the cortex proper. An alternative theory, however, is that these INs represent excess remnants of the fetal subplate instead of arrested neurons destined for the upper layers of the cortical plate (Avino and Hutsler, 2010). This is an attractive hypothesis as this structure performs numerous developmental functions related to formation of neocortical circuits. Interestingly, this finding is also not specific to autism. Increased numbers of INs, particularly in the dorsolateral prefrontal and temporal cortices of schizophrenic patients, have been reported in five of six studies to date, making it one of the most replicated postmortem finding in this disorder as well (Eastwood and Harrison, 2003; Fung et al., 2011; Yang et al., 2011).

The subplate is a transient cortical compartment which becomes fully established during the second trimester and mostly resolves by the sixth postnatal month in humans. Many subplate neurons are actually born before the appearance of the cortical plate proper, and are the first cortical neurons to mature functionally, differentiating into diverse subpopulations in terms of morphology, molecular markers, and neurotransmitter identity (Kostovic and Rakic, 1990). Throughout fetal development, the subplate serves as the major, albeit transient, postsynaptic target for all classes of cortical afferents, both in terms of location of origin and neurotransmitter system (Kanold and Luhmann, 2010). This function is reflected by subplate-enriched or specific expression of numerous extracellular matrix (Chun and Shatz, 1988) and axon guidance molecules, e.g., cadherins, ephrins, semaphorins, and Rho-GTPases (Oeschger et al., 2012).

The earliest afferents, which enter the subplate and synapse on subplate neurons between 8 and 12 gestational weeks, derive from the brainstem nuclei and basal forebrain (Kostovic et al., 2012). Thalamocortical afferents then arrive in huge numbers beginning approximately 13 gestational weeks. All of the above afferents accumulate and remain within the subplate until approximately 22–24 gestational weeks when they begin to penetrate the cortical plate roughly in the order in which they arrived in the subplate (Kostovic and Judas, 2010). At the same time, significant numbers of cortico-cortical and callosal afferents begin arriving in the subplate where they will wait as well. In the case of thalamocortical connections, the most studied in this context, it is thought that the role of the subplate neurons during the "waiting" period is to act as an intermediary between the thalamic neuron and the cortical target thereby relaying thalamic input to layer IV. The subplate neuron then serves as a pioneer axon to guide the afferent to the target cell. The early thalamocortical synapse is weak, but by co-activating the target neuron, the subplate neuron assists in maturing and strengthening the connection (Kanold and Luhmann, 2010). Subplate neurons likely play the same role for other classes of cortical afferents, but this has not been established.

When an adequately strong final synaptic connections are finally established, it is thought that subplate neurons receive an unknown signal to undergo developmental apoptosis. During the perinatal period of subplate dissolution, afferents representing long associative cortico-cortical pathways are still present in the diminishing subplate (Vasung et al., 2010; Kostovic et al., 2012). Subplate dissolution can be seen to begin earlier in primary motor and sensory cortices and later in association areas (e.g., prefrontal cortex and operculum) and coincides somewhat with the development gyral complexity. The postnatal persistence of the subplate in frontal association areas has been related to the ongoing growth of short-range cortico-cortical connections Finally, the subplate is still present in the early postnatal frontal cortex and contains developing short cortico-cortical pathways (Kostović and Judas, 2007; Kostovic et al., 2012).

Neurons surviving dissolution of the subplate persist into adulthood as INs, dispersed among the cortico-cortical "U-fibers" of the superficial white matter. In humans and other primates they remain quite numerous in frontal and prefrontal areas relative to more caudal regions, e.g., visual cortex and are represented by both excitatory, glutamatergic and inhibitory, GABAergic cells (reviewed in Suárez-Solá et al., 2009). What role they may play in adult brain function is unknown, although it is hypothesized that abnormal axonal connectivity during fetal life may cause, or be reflected by, abnormalities in the numbers and/or distribution of INs that persist into adulthood. The presence of excess INs in ASD could potentially be explained by either abnormal proliferation early in embryonic life or reduced developmental apoptosis in the later fetal/perinatal period (Chun and Shatz, 1989; Avino and Hutsler, 2010). Because the subplate is an early structure, the same frontal overgrowth causing excess radial glia/minicolumns and cortical neurons may also be responsible for (or related to) the production of excess subplate neurons. This could potentially be tested. Conversely, subplate neurons not capable of "hooking up" their dependent cortical afferents to the proper targets, for one reason or another, might not receive or properly process the signal for programed cell death. This would be much more difficult to test.

GENETIC MODELS OF ASD

A predominately genetic etiology for ASD is well established and supported by twin and family studies. An estimated 10–15% of children evaluated for ASD have a known genetic syndrome (e.g., Fragile X or tuberous sclerosis), and an additional 25% or so are found to have an identifiable chromosomal deletion or duplication (i.e., copy number variation, CNV; Sebat et al., 2007). However, despite the recent use of microarray technology to perform CNV analysis and whole genome expression profiling and association studies on large samples, the genetic structure underlying most idiopathic autism is still poorly known. There is considerable debate concerning this architecture, and arguments may be made for either effects of single, rare risk alleles, or interactions of numerous common low-risk alleles. Although these models are not mutually exclusive, only a few identified genetic lesions are recurrent to any appreciable extent. Therefore, the majority of the dozens of candidate loci (and hundreds of associated genes) currently under investigation are derived from rare Mendelian mutations, CNVs, and genes/chromosomal regions associated with syndromic forms of ASD (Marshall and Scherer, 2012). A number of schemes have been generated to organize this growing list in order to both identify a common, underlying pathophysiology as well as point to new potential candidate genes. Most of these models group candidates according to (1) participation in a common signaling pathway, (2) shared molecular or cellular function, or (3) participation in a common developmental pathway.

ACTIVATING MUTATIONS IN THE mTOR PATHWAY ARE ASSOCIATED WITH SYNDROMIC ASD

Approximately 10–15% of children being evaluated for ASD are found to have a syndromic form, i.e., an ASD or ASD-like behavioral phenotype occurring in the context of a recognized single gene or chromosomal syndrome and/or associated with one or more dysmorphic features (e.g., fragile X or tuberous sclerosis). Many common syndromic disorders with a significant ASD component are caused by alterations in genes that directly or indirectly participate in the mammalian target of rapamycin (mTOR) signaling pathway, i.e., tuberous sclerosis (TSC1/2), fragile X mental retardation 1 (FMR1), neurofibromatosis type 1 (NF1), PTEN mutation syndrome, and Rett's syndrome (MECP2; reviewed in Levitt and Campbell, 2009). The mTOR signaling pathway serves to integrate extracellular signals (e.g., growth factors) with downstream intracellular activities. In response to upstream tyrosine kinase signaling, ERK and PI3K activate mTOR which, via further kinase signaling, activates multiple downstream genes responsible for cellular proliferation, growth, survival, fate decision, and motility. PTEN, NF1, and TSC1/2 are all inhibitors of mTOR so that their pathogenic mutations all have the downstream effect of increasing mTOR signaling. MECP2 encodes a protein that regulates the transcription of multiple downstream genes involved either directly in the ERK/PI3K pathway or the upstream MET RTK pathway. Again, the net effect of MECP2 mutation is to increase mTOR signaling.

While the consequences of increased ERK/PI3K/mTOR signaling are consistent with many of the anatomic and neuropathologic findings in ASD (e.g., excess brain growth and neuronal proliferation), it must be noted that this pathway is a central cellular regulator in most organ systems and pathogenic mutations in key members produce more diverse, severe, and widespread clinical manifestations than is generally seen in non-syndromic or idiopathic ASD. However, this convergence on a single molecular pathway is considered a significant clue to the pathogenesis of idiopathic ASD. It is likely that many ASD mutations occur in genes further upstream, thereby imparting a more subtle and brain region specific orientation to the downstream effect of mTOR activation. Probably the most studied and well known of such upstream activators is a receptor tyrosine kinase coded by the MET gene, located in the 7q31 ASD candidate region. MET is known to be important in forebrain development and exhibits altered expression in ASD cortical tissue (Campbell et al., 2007). A common promoter variant which affects MET function *in vitro* (Campbell et al., 2006), as well as a number of MET mutations, has been found to be associated with a subset of ASD cases (Campbell et al., 2009).

ALTERATIONS IN SYNAPSE-RELATED GENES ARE ASSOCIATED WITH ASD

A second model for the pathogenesis of ASD focuses on abnormal formation or function of synaptic connections. This was first suggested by findings of abnormal dendritic spine morphology in the above syndromic forms of ASD as well as the high prevalence of seizures in both syndromic and idiopathic ASD. This model was supported by the identification of NLGN3, NLGN4X, NRXN1, and SHANK3 in ASD candidate loci. These are all synaptic cell adhesion molecules (CAMs) which are crucial for the dendrite development, initial contact between pre- and postsynaptic neurons, and/or assembly and anchoring of synaptic scaffolding proteins (reviewed by Betancur et al., 2009; Bourgeron, 2009). Overall, alterations in most candidate CAM genes do not appear to account for an appreciable proportion of ASD individually and are as likely to be found in association with other conditions or non-affected individuals alike. Additionally, single gene mouse models of these synaptic candidates usually have no discernable behavioral phenotype, although this alone does not exclude any candidate gene as potentially contributing to risk for ASD in humans.

Numerous other CAMs and synaptic scaffolding proteins are also under investigation as ASD susceptibility genes. These include various cadherins and protocadherins, members of the Ig CAM superfamily (e.g., L1CAM), and the contactins. One functional grouping (SHANK2/3, SYNGAP1, DLGAP2) converge on the postsynaptic density. Additionally, recent large-scale molecular and functional pathway analyses of CNV and association candidates (e.g., Pinto et al., 2010; Gilman et al., 2011; Hussman et al., 2011) have identified large functional groups converging on regulation of actin filament network dynamics. One group specifically, the Rho family of small GTPases, is particularly central to this process and therefore essential to dendrite morphogenesis and spine remodeling.

ALTERATIONS IN GENES REGULATING NEURONAL POLARITY, NEURITIC OUTGROWTH, AND AXONAL

Guidance are associated with ASD

A third model for the pathogenesis of ASD, more recently advanced, reinterprets many of the above functional groupings in terms of axon outgrowth, guidance, and targeting. Many of these proteins can be thought of more generally as providing positional information and mediating motility and are, therefore, re-cycled for various developmental processes mechanistically requiring specific recognition and/or movement (**Figure 2**). An axonal model is therefore also supported by the identification of many of the aforementioned synaptic CAMs (e.g., L1CAM, SHANKs, and NRXN1), which are often involved in neuritic outgrowth and axon guidance and targeting (Sheng and Kim, 2000; Gjorlund et al., 2012; Tagliavacca et al., 2013). The Rho-GTPases

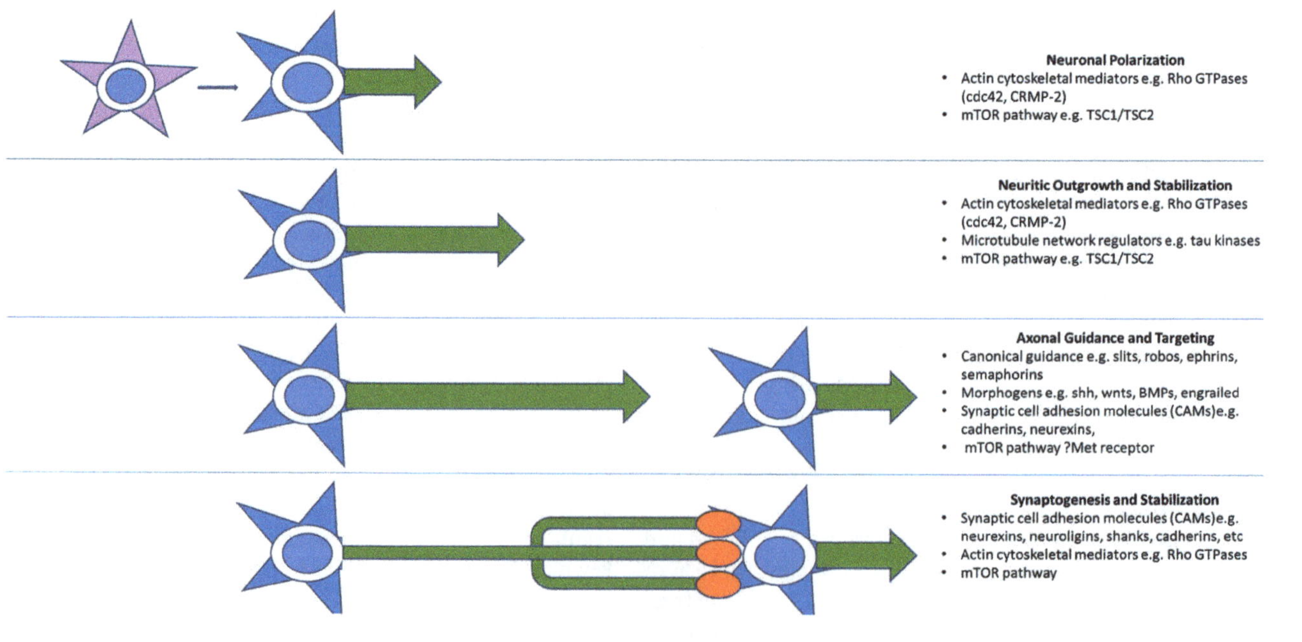

FIGURE 2 | Key molecular pathways of axonal development implicated by genetic studies. Genome-wide association and CNV studies have implicated numerous molecules and molecular pathways involved in neuritic outgrowth, neuronal polarity, axonal-dendritic targeting, and synaptogenesis. Many of these are common to multiple related developmental processes as they serve the more general functions of providing positional information. This recycling phenomenon may explain the link between arealization/proliferation abnormalities, axonal and dendritic abnormalities, and synaptic dysfunction in ASD.

and their regulators also act long before synaptogenesis to induce neurite formation and differentiation, mediate axonal extension and branching, and cause growth cone collapse in response to repulsive axonal guidance cues (Gilman et al., 2011). They do this by coordinating the interactions between the actin cytoskeleton of the axonal growth cone which interprets CAM-based guidance cues, and the microtubule network which stabilizes the growing neurite (Govek et al., 2011). Two recent ASD candidates, cdc42 and CRMP-2 (Gilman et al., 2011) are particularly important in early neuronal polarization, i.e., the differentiation of early neuritic processes into a single axon and multiple dendrites. This process forms the basis of directional information flow in neuronal circuits (Govek et al., 2011). Alterations in expression of these candidates in developing neurons causes either inhibition of axon formation or the production of supernumerary axons (Govek et al., 2011). No doubt as more "synaptic" molecules are investigated more closely in terms of developmental expression, axonal functions will continue to come to light.

The mTOR pathway, while important for synaptic function, it is also critical for neuritic growth and neuronal polarity. TSC1 and TSC2, mutated in tuberous sclerosis, form a complex which permits the functioning of a TSC2 GTPase activating protein for Rheb GTPase which inhibits the mTOR pathway. TSC pathway components are expressed in a polarized manner in developing neurons so that TSC2 is inactivated (and mTOR activity is increased) in the developing axon (Choi et al., 2008). Choi et al. (2008) found that overexpression of Tsc1/2 significantly inhibited axon formation in cultured mouse hippocampal neurons. Knockdown of Tsc2 and knockout of Tsc1 in hippocampal cultures, conversely, caused developing neurons to have multiple axons. This was born out *in vivo* by examinations of cortical sections derived from $Tsc1^{-/-}$ mice, which have relatively a normal cortical and hippocampal architecture, but develop seizures at postnatal day 5 and die in a few weeks. Neurofilament stained sections demonstrated numerous ectopic axons throughout the cortex of these mice, even in the usually dendrite-rich upper layers (Choi et al., 2008).

The Met receptor, long known to be present (at low levels) and active in synapses of the mature brain (Tyndall and Walikonis, 2006) has now been found to be more highly expressed, before most synaptogenesis occurs, in extending forebrain axons of the developing mouse brain. Judson et al. (2009) demonstrated peak Met expression by Western blot at birth in the developing mouse brain; the period at which neurons are finished migrating and are actively extending axons and dendrites. These levels declined during synaptogenesis to low, adult baseline levels (Judson et al., 2009). Strong mRNA expression of Met was visualized in cortical neurons of layers II/III and V/VI and exhibited a strong caudal (high) to rostral (low) gradient in the cortical plate but uniform expression in the subplate. Protein expression by immunohistochemistry was visualized in the callosal, cingulated, anterior commissure, and internal and external capsule white matter tracts as well as in axons extending from the hippocampus, septum, and amygdala (Judson et al., 2009). No appreciable dendritic or synaptic staining was detected with this method.

Recently published association and CNV studies have also identified numerous candidate genes coding for canonical axonal guidance molecules including multiple members of the Slit (Duvall et al., 2006; Hu et al., 2009), Robo (Anitha et al., 2008), Ephrin (Sbacchi et al., 2010), and Semaphorin (Melin et al., 2006; Sbacchi et al., 2010) families. Sbacchi et al. (2010) used gene ontogeny and pathway analyses to determine common functions of duplicated or deleted genes lying within CNVs derived from four large ASD microarray data sets. They identified a substantial number of canonical axonal guidance genes as well as certain BMP, Wnt, Engrailed morphogens which are also known to participate in axon guidance (Charron and Tessier-Lavigne, 2005) and linked to ASD by previous studies (Kalkman, 2012). Hussman et al. (2011), similarly identified a substantial group of ASD candidate genes involved in neurite outgrowth by genome-wide association. Specific functions included axonal guidance, Rho-GTPase signaling, cytoskeletal regulation, and cadherin–catenin function. Interestingly, while different canonical axonal guidance genes are implicated in different studies, SEM5A appears to be listed in practically all of them. Sema5a has also been recently found to be enriched in the mouse subplate during development along with other ASD candidates such as Nrxn1, and cadherins 10, 18, and 9 (Hoerder-Suabedissen et al., 2013).

CONCLUSION

Structural studies of brain development indicate a large subset of individuals with ASD experience dramatic overgrowth of frontal white matter in the first years of life. Excess fetal neuronal proliferation is likely responsible for much of the added volume, but may not explain abnormalities of white matter integrity and microstructure seen by DTI and microscopy. Abnormalities that persist into adult life, even as volumes "normalize." Frontal and temporal cortical areas overlying this white matter are not as functionally integrated with more posterior cortical regions. Subtle (for the most part) abnormalities of cortical neuronal migration and lamination are variably seen, but there is little consistency in the findings. An exception to this is a relatively frequent excess of INs, presumed remnants of the fetal subplate. This excess may be a function of a general overproliferation of cortical neurons or a reflection of aberrant axonal and/or synaptic connectivity during fetal life causing a subsequent failure of appropriate developmental apoptosis. Certainly, morphologic abnormalities reported in superficial subcortical white matter axons indicate a possible role for disordered organization of cortical afferent and/or efferent wiring through the subplate region.

Recently published association and CNV studies have identified, not only multiple axonal guidance molecules, but also numerous ASD candidate genes involved in neuritic outgrowth, neuronal polarity, and axonal–dendritic targeting. These include various participants in the mTOR signaling cascade, neuronal CAMs, Rho-GTPases, and traditional morphogens known to mediate axonal guidance. Many of these, particularly the CAMs and morphogens, can be thought of more generally as providing positional information, cues that may be variously interpreted by responding cells as division, fate specification, migration, neuritic sprouting/pathfinding, or synaptogenesis signals. In other words, they are re-cycled for various developmental processes mechanistically requiring positional information. Other candidates, such as those involved in mTOR and Rho-GTPase signaling, mediate neuronal interpretation of positional information and direct the response in a context-dependent manner. This recycling phenomenon may explain the link between arealization/proliferation abnormalities (frontal overgrowth), axonal and dendritic abnormalities, and synaptic dysfunction in ASD. Current interpretations of the genetic and neuropathologic data are more a matter of emphasis than mutual exclusion, however, the concept of a significant axonal component to the pathogenesis of ASD should be considered in constructing a model that encompasses all of the clinical, structural, and functional observations.

ACKNOWLEDGMENTS

The authors gratefully acknowledge support by the Pennsylvania Department of Health, grant 4100047862 (Kathryn McFadden and Nancy J. Minshew), and Eunice Kennedy Shriver National Institute of Child Health and Human Development (NICHD), grant HD055748 (Nancy J. Minshew).

REFERENCES

Anitha, A., Nakamura, K., Yamada, K., Suda, S., Thanseem, I., Tsujii, M., et al. (2008). Genetic analyses of roundabout (ROBO) axon guidance receptors in autism. *Am. J. Med. Genet. B Neuropsychiatr. Genet.* 147B, 1019–1027. doi: 10.1002/ajmg.b.30697

Avino, T. A., and Hutsler, J. J. (2010). Abnormal cell patterning at the cortical gray-white matter boundary in autism spectrum disorders. *Brain Res.* 1360, 138–146. doi: 10.1016/j.brainres.2010.08.091

Avino, T., and Hutsler, J. (2011). Abnormal cell pattering at the cortical gray–white boundary in autism spectrum disorders. *Brain Res.* 1360, 138–146. doi: 10.1016/j.brainres.2010.08.091

Azmitia, E. C., Singh, J. S., Hou, X. P., and Wegiel, J. (2011). Dystrophic serotonin axons in postmortem brains from young autism patients. *Anat. Rec.* 294, 1653–1662. doi: 10.1002/ar.21243

Azmitia, E. C., Singh, J. S., and Whi taker-Azmitia, P. M. (2010). Increased serotonin axons (immu noreactive to 5-HT transporter) in postmortem brains from young autism donors. *Neuropharmacology* 60, 1347–1354. doi: 10.1016/j.neuropharm.2011.02.002

Bailey, A., Luthert, A., Dean, A., Harding, B., Janota, I., Montgomery, M., et al. (1998). A clinicopathological study of autism. *Brain* 121, 889–905. doi: 10.1093/brain/121.5.889

Bauman, M., and Kemper, T. (1985). Histoanatomic observations of the brain in early infantile autism. *Neurology* 35, 66–867. doi: 10.1212/WNL.35.6.866

Bauman, M., and Kemper, T. (1998). Neuropathology of early infantile autism. *J. Neuropathol. Exp. Neurol.* 57, 645–652. doi: 10.1097/00005072-199807000-00001

Belmonte, M. K., Allen, G., Beckel-Mitchener, A., Boulanger, L. M., Carper, R. A., and Webb, S. J. (2004). Autism and abnormal development of brain connectivity. *J. Neurosci.* 24, 9228–9231. doi: 10.1523/JNEUROSCI.3340-04.2004

Betancur, C., Sakurai, T., and Buxbaum, J. D. (2009). The emerging role of synaptic cell-adhesion pathways in the pathogenesis of autism spectrum disorders. *Trends Neurosci.* 32, 402–412. doi: 10.1016/j.tins.2009.04.003

Bourgeron, T. (2009). A synaptic trek to autism. *Curr. Opin. Neurobiol.* 19, 231–234. doi: 10.1016/j.conb.2009.06.003

Buxhoeveden, D. P., Semendeferi, K., Buckwalter, J., Schenker, N., Switzer, R., and Courchesne, E. (2006). Reduced minicolumns in the frontal cortex of patients with autism. *Neuropathol. Appl. Neurobiol.* 32, 483–491. doi: 10.1111/j.1365-2990.2006.00745.x

Campbell, D. B., D'Oronzio, R., Garbett, K., Ebert, P. J., Mirnics, K., Levitt, P., et al. (2007). Disruption of cerebral cortex MET signaling in autism spectrum disorder. *Ann. Neurol.* 62, 243–250. doi: 10.1002/ana.21180

Campbell, D. B., Sutcliffe, J. S., Ebert, P. J., Militerni, R., Bravaccio, C., Trillo, S., et al. (2006). A genetic variant that disrupts MET transcription is associated with autism. *Proc. Natl. Acad. Sci. U.S.A.* 103, 16834–16839. doi: 10.1073/pnas.0605296103

Campbell, D. B., Warren, D., Sutcliffe, J. S., Lee, E. B., and Levitt, P. (2009). Association of MET with social and communication phenotypes in individuals with autism spectrum disorder. *Am. J. Med. Genet. B Neuropsychiatr. Genet.* 153B, 438–446.

Carper, R. A., and Courchesne, E. (2005). Localized enlargement of the frontal cortex in early autism. *Biol. Psychiatry* 57, 126–133. doi: 10.1016/j.biopsych.2004.11.005

Carper, R. A., Moses, P., Tigue, Z. D., and Courchesne, E. (2002). Cerebral lobes in autism: early hyperplasia and abnormal age effects. *Neuroimage* 16, 1038–1051. doi: 10.1006/nimg.2002.1099

Casanova, M., Buxhoeveden, D. P., Switala, A. E., and Roy, E. (2002). Minicolumnar pathology in autism. *Neurology* 58, 428–432. doi: 10.1212/WNL.58.3.428

Casanova, M., van Kooten, I. A., Switala, A. E., van Engeland, H., Heinsen, H., Steinbusch, H. W., et al. (2006). Minicolumnar abnormalities in autism. *Acta Neuropathol.* 112, 287–303. doi: 10.1007/s00401-006-0085-5

Charron, F., and Tessier-Lavigne, M. (2005). Novel brain wiring functions for classical morphogens: a role as graded positional cues in axon guidance. *Development* 132, 2251–2262. doi: 10.1242/dev.01830

Choi, Y. J., Di Nardo, A., Kramvis, I., Meikle, L., Kwiatkowski, D. J., Sahin, M., et al. (2008). Tuberous sclerosis complex proteins control axon formation. *Genes Dev.* 22, 2485–2495. doi: 10.1101/gad.1685008

Chun, J., and Shatz, C. (1988). A fibronectin-like molecule is present in the developing cat cerebral cortex and is correlated with subplate neurons. *J. Cell Biol.* 106, 857–872. doi: 10.1083/jcb.106.3.857

Chun, J. J., and Shatz, C. J. (1989). Interstitial cells of the adult neocortical white matter are the remnant of the early generated subplate neuron population. *J. Comp. Neurol.* 282, 555–569.

Courchesne, E., Carper, R., and Akshoomoff, N. (2003). Evidence of brain overgrowth in the first year of life in autism. *JAMA* 290, 337–344. doi: 10.1001/jama.290.3.337

Courchesne, E., Karns, C. M., Davis, H. R., Ziccardi, R., Carper, R. A., Tigue, Z. D., et al. (2001). Unusual brain growth patterns in early life in patients with autistic disorder: an MRI study. *Neurology* 57, 245–254. doi: 10.1212/WNL.57.2.245

Courchesne, E., Mouton, P. R., Calhoun, M. E., Semendeferi, K., Ahrens-Barbeau, C., Hallet, M. J., et al. (2011). Neuron number and size in prefrontal cortex of children with autism. *JAMA* 9, 2001–2010. doi: 10.1001/jama.2011.1638

Courchesne, E., Redcay, E., and Kennedy, D. P. (2004). The autistic brain: birth through adulthood. *Curr. Opin. Neurol.* 17, 489–496. doi: 10.1097/01.wco.0000137542.14610.b4

Duvall, J. A., Stone, J. L., Cantor, R. M., Nelson, S. F., and Geschwind, D. H. (2006). "Independent replication of autism association in several neuronal connectivity genes," in *Proceedings of the Annual Meeting of the American Society of Human Genetics*, New Orleans, LA. Available at: http://www.ashg.org/genetics/ashg06s/

Eastwood, S. L., and Harrison, P. J. (2003). Interstitial white matter neurons express less reelin and are abnormally distributed in schizophrenia: towards an integration of molecular and morphologic aspects of the neurodevelopmental hypothesis. *Mol. Psychiatry* 8, 821–831. doi: 10.1038/sj.mp.4001371

Fernandez-Miranda, J. C., Pathak, S., Engh, J., Jarbo, K., Verstynen, T., Yeh, F. C., et al. (2012). High-definition fiber tractography of the human brain: neuroanatomical validation and neurosurgical applications. *Neurosurgery* 71, 430–453. doi: 10.1227/NEU.0b013e3182592faa

Fung, S. J., Joshi, D., Allen, K. M., Sivagnanasundaram, S., Rothmond, D. A., Saunders, R., et al. (2011). Developmental patterns of doublecortin expression and white matter neuron density in the postnatal primate prefrontal cortex and schizophrenia. *PLoS ONE* 6:e25194. doi: 10.1371/journal.pone.0025194

Geschwind, D. H., and Levitt, P. (2007). Autism spectrum disorders: developmental disconnection syndromes. *Curr. Opin. Neurobiol.* 17, 103–111. doi: 10.1016/j.conb.2007.01.009

Gilman, S. R., Iossifov, I., Levy, D., Ronemus, M., Wigler, M., and Vitkup, D. (2011). Rare de novo variants associated with autism implicate a large functional network of genes involved in formation and function of synapses. *Neuron* 70, 898–907. doi: 10.1016/j.neuron.2011.05.021

Gjorlund, M., Nielsen, J., Pankratova, S., Li, S., Korshunova, I., Bock, E., et al. (2012). Neuroligin-1 induces neurite outgrowth through interaction with neurexin-1β and activation of fibroblast growth factor receptor-1. *FASEB J.* 26, 4174–4186. doi: 10.1096/fj.11-202242

Govek, E. E., Newey, S. E., and Van Aelst, L. (2011). The role of Rho GTPases in neuronal development. *Genes Dev.* 19, 1–49. doi: 10.1101/gad.1256405

Hardan, A. Y., Minshew, N. J., and Keshavan, M. S. (2000). Corpus callosum size in autism. *Neurology* 55, 1033–1036. doi: 10.1212/WNL.55.7.1033

Herbert, M. R., Ziegler, D. A., Deutsch, C. K., O'Brien, L. M., Lange, N., Bakardjiev, A., et al. (2003). Dissociations of cerebral cortex, subcortical and cerebral white matter volumes in autistic boys. *Brain* 126, 1182–1192. doi: 10.1093/brain/awg110

Herbert, M. R., Ziegler, D. A., Makris, N., Filipek, P. A., Kemper, T. L., Normandin, J. J., et al. (2004). Localization of white matter volume increase in autism and developmental language disorder. *Ann. Neurol.* 55, 530–540. doi: 10.1002/ana.20032

Hoerder-Suabedissen, A., Oeschger, F. M., Krishnan, M. L., Belgard, T. G., Wang, W. Z., Lee, S., et al. (2013). Expression profiling of mouse subplate reveals a dynamic gene network and disease association with autism and schizophrenia. *Proc. Natl. Acad. Sci. U.S.A.* 110, 3555–3560. doi: 10.1073/pnas.1218510110

Hu, V. W., Nguyen, A., Kim, K. S., Steinberg, M. E., Sarachana, T., Scully, M. A., et al. (2009). Gene expression profiling of lymphoblasts from autistic and nonaffected sib pairs, altered pathways in neuronal development and steroid biosynthesis. *PLoS ONE* 4:e5775. doi: 10.1371/journal.pone.0005775

Hussman, J. P., Chung, R. H., Griswold, A. J., Jaworski, J. M., Salyakina, D., Ma, D., et al. (2011). A noise-reduction GWAS analysis implicates altered regulation of neurite outgrowth and guidance in autism. *Mol. Autism* 2, 1–16. doi: 10.1186/2040-2392-2-1

Hutsler, J. J., and Zhang, H. (2010). Increased dendritic spine densities on cortical projection neurons in autism spectrum disorders. *Brain Res.* 1309, 83–94. doi: 10.1016/j.brainres.2009.09.120

Hutsler, J. J., Love, T., and Zhang, H. (2007). Histological and magnetic resonance imaging assessment of cortical layering and thickness in autism spectrum disorders. *Biol. Psychiatry* 61, 449–457. doi:10.1016/j.biopsych.2006.01.015

Jeong, J. W., Kumar, A. K., Sundaram, S. K., Chugani, H. T., and Chugani, D. C. (2011). Sharp curvature of frontal lobe white matter pathways in children with autism spectrum disorders: tract-based morphometry analysis. *AJNR Am. J. Neuroradiol.* 32, 1600–1606. doi: 10.3174/ajnr.A2557

Jou, R. J., Mateljevic, N., Kaiser, M. D., Sugrue, D. R., Volkmar, F. R., and Pelphrey, K. A. (2011). Structural neural phenotype of autism: preliminary evidence from a diffusion tensor imaging study using tract-based spatial statistics. *AJNR Am. J. Neuroradiol.* 32, 1607–1613. doi: 10.3174/ajnr.A2558

Judson, M., Bergman, M. Y., Campbell, D. B., Eagleson, K. L., and Levitt, P. (2009). Dynamic gene and protein expression patterns of the autism-associated Met receptor tyrosine kinase in the developing mouse forebrain. *J. Comp. Neurol.* 513, 511–531. doi: 10.1002/cne.21969

Just, M. A., Cherkassky, V. L., Keller, T. A., Kana, R. K., and Minshew, N. J. (2007). Functional and anatomical cortical underconnectivity in autism: evidence from an fMRI study of an executive function task and corpus callosum morphometry. *Cereb. Cortex* 17, 951–961. doi: 10.1093/cercor/bhl006

Just, M. A., Cherkassky, V. L., Keller, T. A., and Minshew, N. J. (2004). Cortical activation and synchronization during sentence comprehension in high-functioning autism: evidence of underconnectivity. *Brain* 127, 1811–1821. doi: 10.1093/brain/awh199

Kalkman, H. O. (2012). A review of the evidence for the canonical Wnt pathway in autism spectrum disorders. *Mol. Autism* 3, 10. doi: 10.1186/2040-2392-3-10

Kana, R. K., Keller, T. A., Minshew, N. J., and Just, M. A. (2007). Inhibitory control in high-functioning autism: decreased activation and underconnectivity in inhibition networks. *Biol. Psychiatry* 62, 198–206. doi: 10.1016/j.biopsych.2006.08.004

Kanold, P. O., and Luhmann, H. J. (2010). The subplate and early cortical circuits. *Annu. Rev. Neurosci.* 33, 23–48. doi: 10.1146/annurev-neuro-060909-153244

Keary, C. J., Minshew, N. J., Bansal, R., Goradia, D., Fedorov, S., Keshavan, M. S., et al. (2009). Corpus callosum volume and neurocognition in autism. *J. Autism Dev. Dis.* 39, 834–841. doi: 10.1007/s10803-009-0689-4

Kemper, T. L., and Bauman, M. L. (1993). The contribution of neuropathologic studies to the understanding of autism. *Neurol. Clin.* 11, 175–187.

Kostović, I., and Judas, M. (2007). Transient patterns of cortical lamination during prenatal life: do they have implications for treatment? *Neurosci. Biobehav. Rev.* 31, 1157–1168. doi: 10.1016/j.neubiorev.2007.04.01868

Kemper, T. L., and Bauman, M. L. (2002). Neuropathology of infantile autism. *Mol. Psychiatry* 7, S12–S13. doi: 10.1038/sj.mp.4001165

Kostovic, I., Jovanov-Milošević, N., Radoš, M., Sedmak, G., Benjak, V., Kostović-Srzentić, M., et al. (2012). Perinatal and early postnatal reorganization of the subplate and related cellular compartments in the human cerebral wall as revealed by histological and MRI approaches. *Brain Struct. Funct.* doi 10.1007/s00429-012-0496-0 [Epub ahead of print].

Kostovic, I., and Judas, M. (2010). The development of the subplate and thalamocortical connections in the human foetal brain. *Acta Paediatr.* 99, 1119–1127. doi: 10.1111/j.1651-2227.2010.01811.x

Kostovic, I., and Rakic, P. (1990). Developmental history of the transient subplate zone in the visual and somatosensory cortex of the macaque monkey and human brain. *J. Comp. Neurol.* 297, 441–470. doi: 10.1002/cne.902970309

Lainhart, J. (2006). Advances in autism neuroimaging research for the clinician and geneticist. *Am. J. Med. Genet. C Semin. Med. Genet.* 142C, 33–39. doi: 10.1002/ajmg.c.30080

Levitt, P., and Campbell, D. (2009). The genetic and neurobiologic compass points toward common signaling dysfunctions in autism spectrum disorders. *J. Clin. Invest* 119, 747–754. doi: 10.1172/JCI37934

Marshall, C. R., and Scherer, S. W. (2012). "Detection and characterization of copy number variation in autism spectrum disorder," in *Genomic Structural Variants: Methods and Protocols, Methods in Molecular Biology*, Vol. 838, ed. L. Feuk (Totowa, NJ: Humana Press), 115–135.

Melin, M., Carlsson, B., Anckarsater, H., Rastam, M., Betancur, C., Isaksson, A., et al. (2006). Constitutional downregulation of SEMA5A expression in autism. *Neuropsychobiology* 54, 64–69. doi: 10.1159/000096040

Minshew, N. J., Goldstein, G., and Siegel, D. J. (1997). Neuropsychologic functioning in autism: profile of a complex information processing disorder. *J. Int. Neuropsychol. Soc.* 3, 303–316.

Minshew, N. J., and Payton, J. B. (1988). New perspectives in autism, Part II: the differential diagnosis and neurobiology of autism. *Curr. Probl. Pediatr.* 18, 613–694.

Minshew, N. J., Sweeney, J., and Luna, B. (2002). Autism as a selective disorder of complex information processing and underdevelopment of neocortical systems. *Mol. Psychiatry* 7(Suppl. 2), S14–S15. doi: 10.1038/sj.mp.4001166

Oeschger, F. M., Wang, W. Z., Lee, S., García-Moreno, F., Goffinet, A. M., Arbonés, M. L., et al. (2012). Gene expression analysis of the embryonic subplate. *Cereb. Cortex* 22, 1343–1359. doi: 10.1093/cercor/bhr197

Pinto, D., Pagnamenta, A. T., Klei, L., Anney, R., Merico, D., Regan, R., et al. (2010). Functional impact of global rare copy number variation in autism spectrum disorder. *Nature* 466, 368–372. doi: 10.1038/nature09146

Sbacchi, S., Acquadro, F., Calò, I., Calì, F., and Romano, V. (2010). Functional annotation of genes overlapping copy number variants in autistic patients: focus on axon pathfinding. *Curr. Genomics* 11, 136–145. doi: 10.2174/138920210790886880

Schipul, S., Keller, T. A., and Just, M. A. (2011). Inter-regional brain communication and its disturbances in autism. *Front. Syst. Neurosci.* 5:10. doi: 10.3389/fnsys.2011.00010

Schneider, W. (2011, 2012). *High Definition Fiber Tracking (HDFT) was Featured in this "60 Minutes" Feature: Apps for Autism.* Available at: http://schneiderlab.lrdc.pitt.edu/content/60-minutes-20120716 (accessed August 23, 2013).

Sebat, J., Lakshmi, B., Malhotra, D., Troge, J., Lese-Martin, C., Walsh, T., et al. (2007). Strong association of de novo copy number mutation with autism. *Science* 316, 445–449. doi: 10.1126/science.1138659

Sheng, M., and Kim, E. (2000). The Shank family of scaffold proteins. *J. Cell Sci.* 113, 1851–1856.

Shukla, D. K., Keehn, B., Lincoln, A. J., and Müller, R. A. (2010). White matter compromise of callosal and subcortical fiber tracts in children with autism spectrum disorder: a diffusion tensor imaging study. *J. Am. Acad. Child Adolesc. Psychiatry* 49, 1269–1278.

Shukla, D. K., Keehn, B., and Müller, R. A. (2011). Tract-specific analyses of diffusion tensor imaging show widespread white matter compromise in autism spectrum disorder. *J. Child Psychol. Psychiatry* 52, 286–295. doi: 10.1111/j.1469-7610.2010.02342.x

Simms, M., Kemper, T. L., Timbie, C. M., Bauman, M. L., and Blatt, G. J. (2009). The anterior cingulate cortex in autism: heterogeneity of qualitative and quantitative cytoarchitectonic features suggests possible subgroups. *Acta Neuropathol.* 118,

673–684. doi: 10.1007/s00401-009-0568-2

Suárez-Solá, M. L., González-Delgado, F. J., Pueyo-Morlans, M., Medina-Bolívar, O. C., Hernández-Acosta, N. C., González-Gómez, M., et al. (2009). Neurons in the white matter of the adult human neocortex. *Front. Neuroanat.* 3:7. doi: 10.3389/neuro.05.007.2009

Tagliavacca, L., Colombo, F., Racchetti, G., and Meldolesi, J. (2013). L1CAM and its cell-surface mutants: new mechanisms and effects relevant to the physiology and pathology of neural cells. *J. Neurochem.* 124, 397–409. doi: 10.1111/jnc.12015

Tau, G. Z., and Peterson, B. S. (2010). Normal development of brain circuits. *Neuropsychopharmacology* 35, 147–168. doi: 10.1038/npp.2009.115

Travers, B., Adluru, N., Ennis, C., Tromp do, P. M., Destiche, D., Doran, S., et al. (2012). Diffusion tensor imaging in autism spectrum disorder: a review. *Autism Res.* 5, 289–313. doi: 10.1002/aur.1243

Tyndall, S., and Walikonis, R. (2006). The receptor tyrosine kinase Met and its ligand hepatocyte growth factor are clustered at excitatory synapses and can enhance clustering of synaptic proteins. *Cell Cycle* 5, 1560–1568. doi: 10.4161/cc.5.14.2918

Van Kooten, I. A., Palmen, S. J., von Cappeln, P., Steinbusch, H. W., Korr, H., Heinsen, H., et al. (2008). Neurons in the fusiform gyrus are fewer and smaller in autism. *Brain* 131, 987–999. doi: 10.1093/brain/awn033

Vasung, L., Huang, H., Jovanov-Milošević, N., Pletikos, M., Mori, S., and Kostović, I. (2010). Development of axonal pathways in the human fetal fronto-limbic brain: histochemical characterization and diffusion tensor imaging. *J. Anat.* 217, 400–417. doi: 10.1111/j.1469-7580.2010.01260.x

Verstynen, T., Jarbo, K., Pathak, S., and Schneider, W. (2011). In vivo mapping of microstructural somatotopies in the human corticospinal pathways. *J. Neurophysiol.* 105, 336–346. doi: 10.1152/jn.00698.2010

Waiter, G. D., Williams, J. H., Murray, A. D., Gilchrist, A., Perrett, D. I., and Whiten, A. (2005). Structural white matter deficits in high-functioning individuals with autistic spectrum disorder: a voxel-based investigation. *Neuroimage* 24, 455–461. doi: 10.1016/j.neuroimage.2004.08.049

Wegiel, J., Kuchna, I., Nowicki, K., Imaki, H., Wegiel, J., Marchi, E., et al. (2010). The neuropathology of autism: defects of neurogenesis and neuronal migration, and dysplastic changes. *Acta Neuropathol.* 119, 755–770. doi: 10.1007/s00401-010-0655-4

Williams, D. L., Goldstein, G., and Minshew, N. J. (2006). Neuropsychologic functioning in children with autism: further evidence for disordered complex information-processing. *Child Neuropsychol.* 12, 279–298. doi: 10.1080/09297040600681190

Yang, Y., Fung, S. J., Rothwell, A., Tianmei, S., and Weickert, C. S. (2011). Increased interstitial white matter neuron density in the DLPFC of people with schizophrenia. *Biol. Psychiatry* 69, 63–70. doi: 10.1016/j.biopsych.2010.08.020

Zikopoulos, B., and Barbas, H. (2010). Changes in prefrontal axons may disrupt the network in autism. *J. Neurosci.* 30, 14595–14609. doi: 10.1523/JNEUROSCI.2257-10.2010

18

Brain connectivity in autism

Rajesh K. Kana[1]*, Lucina Q. Uddin[2], Tal Kenet[3], Diane Chugani[4] and Ralph-Axel Müller[5]

[1] *Psychology, University of Alabama at Birmingham, Birmingham, AL, USA*
[2] *Psychology, University of Miami, Coral Gables, FL, USA*
[3] *Department of Neurology, Massachusetts General Hospital, Boston, MA, USA*
[4] *Departments of Pediatrics and Neurology, Wayne State University, Detroit, MI, USA*
[5] *Department of Psychology, San Diego State University, San Diego, CA, USA*
**Correspondence: rkana@uab.edu*

Edited and reviewed by:
John J. Foxe, Albert Einstein College of Medicine, USA

Keywords: brain connectivity, multimodal imaging methods, diffusion tensor imaging, functional connectivity, autism spectrum disorders, white matter

With the increasing prevalence of autism spectrum disorders (ASD), the pace of research aimed at understanding the neurobiology of this complex neurodevelopmental disorder has accelerated. Neuroimaging and postmortem studies have provided evidence for disruptions in functional and structural connectivity in the brains of individuals with ASD (Vissers et al., 2012). This burgeoning literature continues to struggle with methodological and conceptual issues inherent to discovering relationships between brain and behavior. While there has been considerable progress, many open questions remain. In this special topic, a collection of empirical contributions and reviews from leaders in the field attempt to synthesize and extend prior work investigating brain connectivity in autism. Multiple theoretical perspectives and neuroimaging methods are brought together with the aim of addressing outstanding questions about the nature and extent of brain connectivity aberrations in autism.

Functional connectivity magnetic resonance imaging (fcMRI), which detect correlations of the blood oxygen level dependent (BOLD) signal, provided first findings (Just et al., 2004) suggesting that the brains of individuals with ASD may exhibit reduced long-distance connectivity (Just et al., 2012). However, many more recent studies have suggested that patterns of both hypo- and hyper-connectivity can be observed in the autistic brain (Müller et al., 2011). Redcay and colleagues (2013) present one of the few currently available studies examining whole brain functional connectivity in ASD using graph theory and resting state fcMRI. They find that in adolescents with ASD (aged 14–20 years), a right lateral parietal region show both increased betweenness centrality and increased functional connectivity with prefrontal regions, compared with typically developing (TD) participants. Another fcMRI study by You et al. (2013) suggests that atypically increased functional connectivity in ASD may be state-dependent. The authors find that in TD children, BOLD signal correlations become reduced and more localized during sustained attention (compared to rest), whereas this is not seen in children with ASD. The study raises the important question to what extent functional overconnectivity maybe maladaptive. Delmonte and colleagues (2013) examine fronto-striatal circuitry in adolescents and young adults with ASD, again finding atypically increased functional connectivity—consistent with and expanding upon an earlier study (Di Martino et al., 2011). Using independent component analysis in order to identify subnetworks within the default mode network, Starck and colleagues (2013) report decreased connectivity between anterior and posterior default mode subnetworks in adolescents with ASD.

Whereas the studies mentioned above focus on long-range connectivity, relatively little is known from fcMRI about local connectivity. The article by Maximo and colleagues (2013) uses a regional homogeneity approach to reveal local overconnectivity in posterior occipital and temporal cortices alongside local underconnectivity in posterior cingulate and medial prefrontal regions in adolescents with ASD.

The fcMRI studies described above suggest that differential findings are not only region- or network-specific (Redcay et al., 2013 and Delmonte et al., 2013 vs. Starck et al., 2013), but also state-specific (You et al., 2013). An important additional aspect is discussed in a review by Uddin et al. (2013), who suggest that research on brain connectivity in autism should be placed in a developmental framework in order to more precisely pinpoint the sources of age-related group differences in functional connectivity. In their review, the authors summarize recent evidence suggesting that at younger ages closer to disorder onset, the brains of children with ASD are hyper-connected in comparison with TD controls. Keehn and colleagues provide further empirical evidence in support of this claim. They used functional near-infrared spectroscopy to examine brain connectivity in infants in the first year of life who are at high risk for developing autism. They report that at 3 months, high-risk infants showed increased connectivity compared to low-risk infants, and that between 6 and 9 months these group differences disappear and even reverse in direction (Keehn et al., 2013). Another study by Padmanabhan and colleagues examine striatal functional connectivity in a relatively large ASD and TD samples (ages 8–36 years), using resting state functional MRI. Aside from a main group effect (increased connectivity with parietal and decreased connectivity with frontal areas in ASD), they identify numerous regions in cerebellum and temporal lobe showing age-related increases of functional connectivity with striatal seeds in TD children and adults, contrasted by decreases in ASD. These findings highlight the importance of studying autism across the lifespan using multimodal neuroimaging approaches.

In addition to age-related factors that may contribute to the conflicting hypo- vs. hyper-connectivity results in the literature, several methodological factors are beginning to be identified. It is now understood that group differences in functional connectivity studies can be dramatically affected by methodological details

(Jones et al., 2010; Nair et al., 2014), as for example the thorough treatment of head motion even in the sub-millimeter range (Power et al., 2012, 2014). Gotts and colleagues show how a related issue, i.e., fluctuations of the whole brain (global) signal across time, and its treatment in data preprocessing can influence the pattern of group differences observed. They find that the common practice of global signal regression can alter the location and direction of connectivity differences, obscuring neural findings. The empirical contributions by Starck et al. in this special issue carefully address these methodological concerns by explicitly characterizing and censoring motion artifacts to validate the robustness of their connectivity findings.

In contrast to the high spatial but low temporal resolution of functional connectivity MRI, MEG (magnetoencephalography) and EEG (electroencephalography) enable the measurement of functional connectivity with high temporal resolution and medium level spatial resolution. An additional advantage of these techniques is that they are not susceptible to motion artifacts that would confound connectivity results in the same way as fcMRI. Using EEG, Coben and colleagues (2014) propose a theory of mixed under- and over-connectivity in ASD, based on EEG data supporting both types of effects in ASD. The authors emphasize the use of more advanced statistical approaches to EEG coherence analysis, and discuss three different forms of multivariate connectivity analysis. In parallel, using MEG, Buard and colleagues (2013) investigate the differences in low frequency and high frequency oscillatory power in participants with ASD and their first degree relatives. They also find mixed results, with differing patterns of abnormalities in ASD across different frequency bands, opening the door to interesting potential mechanistic interpretations.

While functional connectivity studies of autism continue to reveal nuanced patterns of hypo- and hyper-connectivity associated with the disorder, studies of white matter connectivity using diffusion tensor imaging (DTI) and tractography provide complementary metrics. However, only few studies to date have combined functional and anatomical connectivity findings (Mueller et al., 2013; Nair et al., 2013). Delmonte and colleagues, despite detecting functional overconnectivity between striatum and frontal cortex during resting state, find no group differences in structural connectivity in corresponding fronto-striatal tracts, using DTI. The authors suggest that hyperconnectivity within certain circuits may be a reflection of complex functional reorganization in autism. Another study by Lewis and colleagues (2013) examines the potential impact of brain overgrowth in autism on conduction delays and long-distance connectivity, using DTI. They find network efficiency in adults with autism to be inversely correlated with intracranial volume, and suggest that the reduction in efficient connectivity in autism may be due to early brain overgrowth. Schaer and colleagues (2013) address the issue of connectivity by examining changes in cortical folding, comparing a local gyrification index with connectivity indices from DTI. This approach is based upon Van Essen's theory that mechanical tension exerted on long connections shapes cortical folds (Van Essen, 1997). While they do not observe a relationship between long-range connectivity and gyral patterns, they observe a higher gyrification index in ASD participants with higher short-range connectivity. McGrath and colleagues use a multimodal neuroimaging approach (functional MRI and High Angular Diffusion MRI) to examine the relationship between abnormal functional connectivity in a visuospatial task in autism and the integrity of corresponding white matter tracts. They find altered white matter microstructure to be related to disruptions in functional connectivity during visuospatial processing, especially in connections between left occipital lobe and five paired regions in the left hemisphere (caudate head, caudate body, uncus, thalamus, and cuneus). While findings from fcMRI and DTI do not always correspond in obvious ways (see Delmonte et al., 2013) the studies described above highlight the importance of multimodal neuroimaging approaches for a more comprehensive understanding of brain network abnormalities in ASD.

An important aspect of understanding the neurobiology of autism is to test the utility of the findings in aiding the diagnostic process, which may establish such findings as neural signatures or biomarkers. In a machine learning approach, Nielson and colleagues use a large fMRI autism database, the Autism Brain Imaging Data Exchange (ABIDE) (Di Martino et al., 2013), to classify participants with ASD from TD participants based on functional connectivity features. This study uses resting state functional connectivity data obtained from 964 participants across 16 international sites. Diagnostic classification accuracy in this study is 60% overall, disappointingly hovering just above chance. The authors suggest that additional sources of variability with use of multisite data are likely to blame, indicating a need for standardized data acquisition protocols. Their results may also indicate advantages of longer fMRI acquisition times. While this multisite study shows relatively low classification accuracy, Deshpande and colleagues (2013) use different connectivity measures, obtained from an fMRI study of theory-of-mind, in a classification analysis. They report that effective connectivity differences across 19 paths in the brain classify participants with autism from typical controls with 95% accuracy. A couple of interesting aspects of this study are: (1) While functional connectivity studies of autism are abundant, there are only a handful of studies examining effective connectivity (the causal influence of one brain area on another). This study presents differences in effective connectivity between autism and control participants. (2) The authors use different indices of connectivity (functional, effective, and white matter integrity) in their classification analysis and find effective connectivity results classifying the two groups with the highest level of accuracy. Connectivity-based pattern classification studies, with larger sample size and multiple indices, can provide valuable insight in identifying reliable neural markers of autism.

In a comprehensive review, McFadden and Minshew (2013) examine the findings of brain connectivity in autism and their underlying structural and genetic bases. Their review points to widespread abnormalities during different stages of brain development to be critical in altered brain connectivity in autism. They suggest that a relatively consistent finding involving excess of interstitial neurons may be a function of a general overproliferation of cortical neurons or a reflection of aberrant axonal and/or synaptic connectivity during fetal life causing a subsequent failure of appropriate developmental apoptosis. This review emphasizes that axonal abnormalities and their underlying genetic bases may be critical for characterizing the neurobiology of ASD. Similarly, Zikopoulos and Barbas focus their review of postmortem microscopic changes on axonal pathology in ASD. Their findings show a complex pattern of fewer large myelinated axons and increased numbers of thin myelinated axons in superficial white matter in anterior cingulate cortex, no change in lateral prefrontal cortex, and decreased thin myelinated axons in orbital frontal cortex. These results are consistent with the notion of regionally varying patterns of hypo- and hyper-connectivity associated with ASD, as discussed above. However, knowledge of brain anomalies at the cellular level in ASD is hampered by a lack of *in vivo* imaging techniques that can detect cytoarchitectonic changes. The study by Jeong and colleagues uses a sophisticated analysis of diffusion weighted MRI data in order to detect connectivity changes in the cerebellum related to Purkinje cell loss, as known from postmortem studies. They find evidence that tracts between cerebellar cortex and dentate nuclei (i.e., axonal efferents from Purkinje cells) are compromised in children with ASD, suggesting that *in vivo* diffusion weighted MRI can generate complementary evidence in support of cellular findings from the postmortem literature.

Returning to the basic questions regarding brain network connectivity in ASD raised in the initial announcement, the contributions to this Research Topic underline the need for differentiated interpretations of functional connectivity findings that consider the specificity of networks and cognitive states under investigation and the exact preprocessing pipelines and analysis tools implemented. The need for electrophysiological studies that provide a window onto the dynamic aspects of network connectivity is further emphasized by several contributions, as is the need for multimodal investigations that combine assays of functional and anatomical connectivity. The developmental trajectory of brain connectivity and the classification potential of different connectivity measures are important topics that are investigated by different studies. Finally, several articles contribute to a better understanding of the links between cellular abnormalities in autistic cortex (both cerebral and cerebellar) and disturbances in network connectivity.

REFERENCES

Buard, I., Rogers, S. J., Hepburn, S., Kronberg, E., and Rojas, D. C. (2013). Altered oscillation patterns and connectivity during picture naming in autism. *Front. Hum. Neurosci.* 7:742. doi: 10.3389/fnhum.2013.00742

Coben, R., Mohammad-Rezazadeh, I., and Cannon, R. L. (2014). Using quantitative and analytic EEG methods in the understanding of connectivity in autism spectrum disorders: a theory of mixed over- and under-connectivity. *Front. Hum. Neurosci.* 8:45. doi: 10.3389/fnhum.2014.00045

Delmonte, S., Gallagher, L., O'Hanlon, E., McGrath, J., and Balsters, J. H. (2013). Functional and structural connectivity of frontostriatal circuitry in Autism Spectrum Disorder. *Front. Hum. Neurosci.* 7:430. doi: 10.3389/fnhum.2013.00430

Deshpande, G., Libero, L. E., Sreenivasan, K. R., Deshpande, H. D., and Kana, R. K. (2013). Identification of neural connectivity signatures of autism using machine learning. *Front. Hum. Neurosci.* 7:670. doi: 10.3389/fnhum.2013.00670

Di Martino, A., Kelly, C., Grzadzinski, R., Zuo, X. N., Mennes, M., Mairena, M. A., et al. (2011). Aberrant striatal functional connectivity in children with autism. *Biol. Psychiatry* 69, 847–856. doi: 10.1016/j.biopsych.2010.10.029

Di Martino, A., Yan, C. G., Li, Q., Denio, E., Castellanos, F. X., Alaerts, K., et al. (2013). The autism brain imaging data exchange: towards a large-scale evaluation of the intrinsic brain architecture in autism. *Mol. Psychiatry*. doi: 10.1038/mp.2013.78. [Epub ahead of print].

Jones, T. B., Bandettini, P. A., Kenworthy, L., Case, L. K., Milleville, S. C., Martin, A., et al. (2010). Sources of group differences in functional connectivity: an investigation applied to autism spectrum disorder. Neuroimage 49, 401–414. doi: 10.1016/j.neuroimage.2009.07.051

Just, M., Cherkassky, V., Keller, T., and Minshew, N. (2004). Cortical activation and synchronization during sentence comprehension in high-functioning autism: evidence of underconnectivity. Brain 127, 1811–1821. doi: 10.1093/brain/awh199

Just, M. A., Keller, T. A., Malave, V. L., Kana, R. K., and Varma, S. (2012). Autism as a neural systems disorder: a theory of frontal-posterior underconnectivity. Neurosci. Biobehav. Rev. 36, 1292–1313. doi: 10.1016/j.neubiorev.2012.02.007

Keehn, B., Wagner, J. B., Tager-Flusberg, H., and Nelson, C. A. (2013). Functional connectivity in the first year of life in infants at-risk for autism: a preliminary near-infrared spectroscopy study. Front. Hum. Neurosci. 7:444. doi: 10.3389/fnhum.2013.00444

Lewis, J. D., Theilmann, R. J., Townsend, J., and Evans, A. C. (2013). Network efficiency in autism spectrum disorder and its relation to brain overgrowth. Front. Hum. Neurosci. 7:845. doi: 10.3389/fnhum.2013.00845

Maximo, J. O., Keown, C. L., Nair, A., and Müller, R.-A. (2013). Approaches to local connectivity in autism using resting state functional connectivity MRI. Front. Hum. Neurosci. 7:605. doi: 10.3389/fnhum.2013.00605

McFadden, K., and Minshew, N. J. (2013). Evidence for dysregulation of axonal growth and guidance in the etiology of ASD. *Front. Hum. Neurosci.* 7:671. doi: 10.3389/fnhum.2013.00671

Mueller, S., Keeser, D., Samson, A. C., Kirsch, V., Blautzik, J., Grothe, M., et al. (2013). Convergent findings of altered functional and structural brain connectivity in individuals with high functioning autism: a multimodal MRI study. PLoS ONE 8:e67329. doi: 10.1371/journal.pone.0067329

Müller, R.-A., Shih, P., Keehn, B., Deyoe, J. R., Leyden, K. M., and Shukla, D. K. (2011). Underconnected, but how? A survey of functional connectivity MRI studies in autism spectrum disorders. Cereb. Cortex 21, 2233–2243. doi: 10.1093/cercor/bhq296

Nair, A., Keown, C. L., Datko, M. C., Shih, P., Keehn, B. M., and Müller, R.-A. (2014). Impact of methodological variables on functional connectivity findings in Autism Spectrum Disorders. Hum. Brain Mapp. doi: 10.1002/hbm. 22456. [Epub ahead of print].

Nair, A., Treiber, J. M., Shukla, D. K., Shih, P., and Müller, R.-A. (2013). Thalamocortical connectivity in autism spectrum disorder: a study of functional and anatomical connectivity. Brain 136, 1942–1955. doi: 10.1093/brain/ awt079

Padmanabhan, A., Lynn, A., Foran, W., Luna, B., and O'Hearn, K. (2013). Age related changes in striatal resting state functional connectivity in autism. Front. Hum. Neurosci. 7:814. doi: 10.3389/fnhum.2013.00814

Power, J. D., Barnes, K. A., Snyder, A. Z., Schlaggar, B. L., and Petersen, S. E. (2012). Spurious but systematic correlations in functional connectivity MRI networks arise from subject motion. Neuroimage 59, 2142–2154. doi: 10.1016/j.neuroimage.2011.10.018

Power, J. D., Mitra, A., Laumann, T. O., Snyder, A. Z., Schlaggar, B. L., and Petersen, S. E. (2014). Methods to detect, characterize, and remove motion artifact in resting state fMRI. Neuroimage 84, 320–341. doi: 10.1016/j.neuroimage.2013. 08.048

Redcay, E., Moran, J. M., Mavros, P. L., Tager-Flusberg, H., Gabrieli, J. D. E., and Whitfield-Gabrieli, S. (2013). Intrinsic functional network organization in high- functioning adolescents with autism spectrum disorder. Front. Hum. Neurosci. 7:573. doi: 10.3389/fnhum.2013.00573

Schaer, M., Ottet, M.-C., Scariati, E., Dukes, D., Franchini, M., Eliez, S., et al. (2013). Decreased frontal gyrification correlates with altered connectivity in children with autism. Front. Hum. Neurosci. 7:750. doi: 10.3389/fnhum.2013.00750

Starck, T., Nikkinen, J., Rahko, J., Remes, J., Hurtig, T., Haapsamo, H., et al. (2013).

Resting state fMRI reveals a default mode dissociation between retrosplenial and medial prefrontal subnetworks in ASD despite motion scrubbing. Front. Hum. Neurosci. 7:802. doi: 10.3389/fnhum.2013.00802

Uddin, L. Q., Supekar, K., and Menon, V. (2013). Reconceptualizing functional brain connectivity in autism from a developmental perspective. Front. Hum. Neurosci. 7:458. doi: 10.3389/fnhum.2013.00458

Van Essen, D. C. (1997). A tension-based theory of morphogenesis and compact wiring in the central nervous system. Nature 385, 313–318. doi: 10.1038/385313a0

Vissers, M. E., Cohen, M. X., and Geurts, H. M. (2012). Brain connectivity and high functioning autism: a promising path of research that needs refined models, methodological convergence, and stronger behavioral links. Neurosci. Biobehav. Rev. 36, 604–625. doi: 10.1016/j.neubiorev.2011.09.003

You, X., Norr, M., Murphy, E., Kuschner, E. S., Bal, E., Gaillard, W. D., et al. (2013). Atypical modulation of distant functional connectivity by cognitive state in children with Autism Spectrum Disorders. Front. Hum. Neurosci. 7:482. doi: 10.3389/fnhum.2013.00482

Zikopoulos, B., and Barbas, H. (2013). Altered neural connectivity in excitatory and inhibitory cortical circuits in autism. Front. Hum. Neurosci. 7:609. doi: 10.3389/fnhum.2013.00609

Permissions

All chapters in this book were first published in BCA, by Frontiers Media SA; hereby published with permission under the Creative Commons Attribution License or equivalent. Every chapter published in this book has been scrutinized by our experts. Their significance has been extensively debated. The topics covered herein carry significant findings which will fuel the growth of the discipline. They may even be implemented as practical applications or may be referred to as a beginning point for another development.

The contributors of this book come from diverse backgrounds, making this book a truly international effort. This book will bring forth new frontiers with its revolutionizing research information and detailed analysis of the nascent developments around the world.

We would like to thank all the contributing authors for lending their expertise to make the book truly unique. They have played a crucial role in the development of this book. Without their invaluable contributions this book wouldn't have been possible. They have made vital efforts to compile up to date information on the varied aspects of this subject to make this book a valuable addition to the collection of many professionals and students.

This book was conceptualized with the vision of imparting up-to-date information and advanced data in this field. To ensure the same, a matchless editorial board was set up. Every individual on the board went through rigorous rounds of assessment to prove their worth. After which they invested a large part of their time researching and compiling the most relevant data for our readers.

The editorial board has been involved in producing this book since its inception. They have spent rigorous hours researching and exploring the diverse topics which have resulted in the successful publishing of this book. They have passed on their knowledge of decades through this book. To expedite this challenging task, the publisher supported the team at every step. A small team of assistant editors was also appointed to further simplify the editing procedure and attain best results for the readers.

Apart from the editorial board, the designing team has also invested a significant amount of their time in understanding the subject and creating the most relevant covers. They scrutinized every image to scout for the most suitable representation of the subject and create an appropriate cover for the book.

The publishing team has been an ardent support to the editorial, designing and production team. Their endless efforts to recruit the best for this project, has resulted in the accomplishment of this book. They are a veteran in the field of academics and their pool of knowledge is as vast as their experience in printing. Their expertise and guidance has proved useful at every step. Their uncompromising quality standards have made this book an exceptional effort. Their encouragement from time to time has been an inspiration for everyone.

The publisher and the editorial board hope that this book will prove to be a valuable piece of knowledge for researchers, students, practitioners and scholars across the globe.

List of Contributors

Jared A. Nielsen
Interdepartmental Program in Neuroscience, University of Utah, Salt Lake City, UT, USA
Department of Psychiatry, University of Utah, Salt Lake City, UT, USA

Brandon A. Zielinski
Departments of Pediatrics and Neurology, University of Utah and Primary Children's Medical Center, Salt Lake City, UT, USA

P. Thomas Fletcher
School of Computing and Scientific Computing and Imaging Institute, University of Utah, Salt Lake City, UT, USA

Andrew L. Alexander
Waisman Laboratory for Brain Imaging and Behavior, Department of Psychiatry, University of Wisconsin, Madison, WI, USA
Department of Medical Physics, University of Wisconsin, Madison, WI, USA

Nicholas Lange
Departments of Psychiatry and Biostatistics, Harvard University, Boston, MA, USA
Neurostatistics Laboratory, McLean Hospital, Belmont, MA, USA

Erin D. Bigler
Department of Psychology and Neuroscience Center, Brigham Young University, Provo, UT, USA
The Brain Institute of Utah, University of Utah, Salt Lake City, UT, USA

Janet E. Lainhart
Waisman Laboratory for Brain Imaging and Behavior, Department of Psychiatry, University of Wisconsin, Madison, WI, USA

Jeffrey S. Anderson
Interdepartmental Program in Neuroscience, University of Utah, Salt Lake City, UT, USA
The Brain Institute of Utah, University of Utah, Salt Lake City, UT, USA
Department of Bioengineering, University of Utah, Salt Lake City, UT, USA
Division of Neuroradiology, University of Utah, Salt Lake City, UT, USA

Elizabeth Redcay
Department of Psychology, University of Maryland, College Park, MD, USA

Joseph M. Moran
Center for Brain Science, Harvard University, Cambridge, MA, USA
United States Army Natick Soldier Research Development and Engineering Center, Natick, MA, USA

Penelope L. Mavros
Simons Center for the Social Brain at Massachusetts Institute of Technology, Cambridge, MA, USA

Helen Tager-Flusberg
Department of Psychology, Boston University, Boston, MA, USA

John D. E. Gabrieli and Susan Whitfield-Gabrieli
McGovern Institute for Brain Research at Massachusetts Institute of Technology, Cambridge, MA, USA
Department of Brain and Cognitive Sciences, Massachusetts Institute of Technology, Cambridge, MA, USA

Jeong-Won Jeong, Vijay N. Tiwari, Michael E. Behen, Harry T. Chugani and Diane C. Chugani
Department of Pediatrics and Neurology, Wayne State University, Detroit, MI, USA
Translational Imaging Laboratory, PET center, Children's Hospital of Michigan, Detroit, MI, USA

Gopikrishna Deshpande
AU MRI Research Center, Department of Electrical and Computer Engineering, Auburn University, Auburn, AL, USA
Department of Psychology, Auburn University, Auburn, AL, USA

Lauren E. Libero, Hrishikesh D. Deshpande and Rajesh K. Kana
Department of Psychology, University of Alabama at Birmingham, Birmingham, AL, USA

Karthik R. Sreenivasan
AU MRI Research Center, Department of Electrical and Computer Engineering, Auburn University, Auburn, AL, USA

Lucina Q.Uddin and Kaustubh Supekar
Department of Psychiatry and Behavioral Sciences, Stanford University School of Medicine, Stanford, CA, USA

Vinod Menon
Department of Psychiatry and Behavioral Sciences, Stanford University School of Medicine, Stanford, CA, USA
Program in Neuroscience, Stanford University School of Medicine, Stanford, CA, USA
Department of Neurology and Neurological Sciences, Stanford University School of Medicine, Stanford, CA, USA

Marie Schaer
Stanford Cognitive and Systems Neuroscience Laboratory, Stanford University School of Medicine, Palo Alto, CA, USA
Office Médico-Pédagogique, Department of Psychiatry, University of Geneva School of Medicine, Geneva, Switzerland

Marie-Christine Ottet, Elisa Scariati, Martina Franchini and Bronwyn Glaser
Office Médico-Pédagogique, Department of Psychiatry, University of Geneva School of Medicine, Geneva, Switzerland

Daniel Dukes
Cognitive Science Centre, University of Neuchâtel, Neuchâtel, Switzerland
Swiss Center for Affective Sciences, University of Geneva, Geneva, Switzerland

Stephan Eliez
Office Médico-Pédagogique, Department of Psychiatry, University of Geneva School of Medicine, Geneva, Switzerland
Department of Genetic Medicine and Development, University of Geneva School of Medicine, Geneva, Switzerland

John D. Lewis and Alan C. Evans
McConnell Brain Imaging Center, Montreal Neurological Institute, McGill University, Montreal, QC, Canada

Rebecca J. Theilmann
Department of Radiology, University of California, San Diego, La Jolla, CA, USA

Jeanne Townsend
Department of Neuroscience, University of California, San Diego, La Jolla, CA, USA
Research on Aging and Development Laboratory, University of California, San Diego, La Jolla, CA, USA

Isabelle Buard, Eugene Kronberg and Donald C. Rojas
UCD Magnetoencephalography Lab, Department of Psychiatry, University of Colorado at Denver - Anschutz Medical Campus, Aurora, CO, USA

Sally J. Rogers
Psychiatry and Behavioral Sciences, UC Davis MIND Institute, Sacramento, CA, USA

Susan Hepburn
University of Colorado/JFK Partners, Aurora, CO, USA

Sonja Delmonte and Jane Mc Grath
Department of Psychiatry, Trinity College Dublin, Dublin, Ireland
Trinity College Institute of Neuroscience, Trinity College Dublin, Dublin, Ireland

Louise Gallagher
Department of Psychiatry, Trinity College Dublin, Dublin, Ireland

Erik O'Hanlon
Department of Psychiatry, Royal College of Surgeons, Dublin, Ireland

Joshua H. Balsters
Trinity College Institute of Neuroscience, Trinity College Dublin, Dublin, Ireland
Neural Control of Movement Lab, Department of Health Sciences and Technology, ETH Zurich, Zurich, Switzerland

Stephen J. Gotts, Gregory L. Wallace and Alex Martin
Section on Cognitive Neuropsychology, Laboratory of Brain and Cognition, National Institute of Mental Health, National Institutes of Health, Bethesda, MD, USA

Ziad S. Saad, Hang Joon Jo, Robert W. Cox
Scientific and Statistical Computing Core, National Institute of Mental Health, National Institutes of Health, Bethesda, MD, USA

Basilis Zikopoulos and Helen Barbas
Neural Systems Laboratory, Department of Health Sciences, Boston University, Boston, MA, USA

Brandon Keehn and Charles A. Nelson
Laboratories of Cognitive Neuroscience, Division of Developmental Medicine, Boston Children's Hospital, Boston, MA, USA

Harvard Medical School, Boston, MA, USA
Jennifer B. Wagner
Department of Psychology, The College of Staten Island, The City University of New York, Staten Island, NY, USA
Department of Psychology, Boston University, Boston, MA, USA

Helen Tager-Flusberg
Department of Psychology, Boston University, Boston, MA, USA

Xiaozhen You, Megan Norr and Eric Murphy
Department of Psychology, Georgetown University, Washington, DC, USA

Emily S. Kuschner, Elgiz Bal, William D. Gaillard and Lauren Kenworthy
Children's Research Institute, Children's National Medical Center, Washington DC, USA

Chandan J. Vaidya
Department of Psychology, Georgetown University, Washington, DC, USA
Children's Research Institute, Children's National Medical Center, Washington DC, USA

Tuomo Starck, Osmo Tervonen and Vesa J. Kiviniemi
Department of Diagnostic Radiology, Oulu University Hospital, Oulu, Finland
Department of Diagnostic Radiology, Oulu University, Oulu, Finland

Juha Nikkinen
Department of Diagnostic Radiology, Oulu University Hospital, Oulu, Finland

Jukka Rahko, Tuula Hurtig, Helena Haapsamo, Katja Jussila, Sanna Kuusikko-Gauffin, Marja-Leena Mattila, Hanna Ebeling and Irma Moilanen
Department of Child Psychiatry, Institute of Clinical Medicine, Oulu University Hospital and Oulu University, Oulu, Finland

Jukka Remes
Department of Diagnostic Radiology, Oulu University Hospital, Oulu, Finland
Department of Electrical and Information Engineering, Oulu University, Oulu, Finland

Eira Jansson-Verkasalo
Department of Behavioral Sciences and Philosophy, Logopedics, University of Turku, Turku, Finland

David L. Pauls
Psychiatric and Neurodevelopmental Genetics Unit, Harvard Medical School, Boston, MA, USA

Jose O. Maximo and Ralph-Axel Müller
Brain Development Imaging Laboratory, Department of Psychology, San Diego State University, San Diego, CA, USA

Christopher L. Keown
Brain Development Imaging Laboratory, Department of Psychology, San Diego State University, San Diego, CA, USA
Computational Science Research Center, San Diego State University, San Diego, CA, USA

Aarti Nair
Brain Development Imaging Laboratory, Department of Psychology, San Diego State University, San Diego, CA, USA
Joint Doctoral Program in Clinical Psychology, San Diego State University and University of California at San Diego, San Diego, CA, USA

Jane McGrath
Department of Psychiatry, Trinity College Dublin, Ireland

Katherine Johnson
Department of Psychiatry, Trinity College Dublin, Ireland
Department of Psychology, University of Melbourne, Melbourne, Victoria, Australia

Hugh Garavan
Department of Psychiatry, Trinity College Dublin, Ireland
Department of Psychology, University of Vermont, Burlington, VT, USA

Alexander Leemans
Image Sciences Institute, University Medical Centre Utrecht, Utrecht, Netherlands

Kathryn McFadden
Department of Neurobiology, University of Pittsburgh, Pittsburgh, PA, USA

Nancy J. Minshew
Department of Psychiatry and Neurology, University of Pittsburgh Medical School, Pittsburgh, PA, USA

Rajesh K. Kana
Psychology, University of Alabama at Birmingham, Birmingham, AL, USA

Lucina Q. Uddin
Psychology, University of Miami, Coral Gables, FL, USA

Tal Kenet
Department of Neurology, Massachusetts General Hospital, Boston, MA, USA

Diane Chugani
Departments of Pediatrics and Neurology, Wayne State University, Detroit, MI, USA

Index

www.ingramcontent.com/pod-product-compliance
Lightning Source LLC
Chambersburg PA
CBHW081216180926
51613CB00003B/255
9781639272846